Ob/Gyn Sonography
An Illustrated Review

Ob/Gyn Sonography
An Illustrated Review

2nd Edition

Jim Baun, BS, RDMS, RVT, FSDMS
Professional Ultrasound Services
San Francisco, California

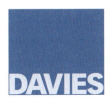

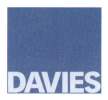

Copyright © 2016, 2004 by Davies Publishing, Inc.

All rights reserved. No part of this work may be reproduced, stored in a retrieval system, or transmitted in any form or by any means, electronic or mechanical, including photocopying, scanning, and recording, without prior written permission from the publisher.

Mike Davies

Davies Publishing, Inc.
Specialists in Ultrasound Education, Test Preparation, and Continuing Medical Education
32 South Raymond Avenue
Pasadena, California 91105-1961
Phone 626-792-3046
Facsimile 626-792-5308
Email info@daviespublishing.com
www.daviespublishing.com

Michael Davies, Publisher
Christina J. Moose, Editorial Director
Charlene Locke, Production Manager
Janet Heard, Operations Manager
Jim Baun, Illustration
Stephen Beebe, Illustration
Satori Design Group, Inc., Design

Notice to Users of This Publication:
In the field of ultrasonography, knowledge, technique, and best practices are continually evolving. With new research and developing technologies, changes in methodologies, professional practices, and medical treatment may become necessary. Sonography practitioners and other medical professionals and researchers must rely on their experience and knowledge when evaluating and using information, methods, technologies, experiments, and medications described herein, always remaining mindful of their own, their patients', their coworkers', and others' safety and well-being. Regarding any treatments, procedures, technologies, and/or pharmaceutical products identified, users of this publication are advised to check the most current information provided by product manufacturers and professional societies to verify their latest recommendations regarding methodologies, dosages, timing of administration, practice guidelines, standards of care, and contraindications. It is the responsibility of practitioners, relying on their own experience and knowledge of their patients, to report, make recommendations, and work within these standards, in consultation with other clinicians such as referring and supervisory physicians, to determine to take all appropriate safety procedures and to determine the best treatment of each individual patient. To the fullest extent of the law, neither Davies Publishing, Inc., nor the authors, contributors, reviewers, or editors assume any liability for any injury and/or damage to persons or property as a matter of products liability, negligence, or otherwise, or from any use or operation of any methods, products, instructions, or ideas contained in the material herein.

Library of Congress Cataloging-in-Publication Data

Names: Baun, Jim, author. | De Lange, Marie. Ob/Gyn sonography. Preceded by (work):
Title: Ob/Gyn sonography : an illustrated review / Jim Baun.
Description: 2nd edition. | Pasadena, California : Davies Publishing, Inc., [2016] | Preceded by Ob/Gyn sonography : an illustrated review / Marie De Lange, Glenn A. Rouse. 2004. | Includes bibliographical references and index.
Identifiers: LCCN 2015042279 | ISBN 9780941022873 (alk. paper)
Subjects: | MESH: Obstetrics--Atlases. | Obstetrics—Examination Questions. | Genital Diseases, Female—ultrasonography—Atlases. | Genital Diseases, Female--ultrasonography--Examination Questions. | Pregnancy Complications—ultrasonography—Atlases. | Pregnancy Complications—ultrasonography—Examination Questions.
Classification: LCC RG107.5.U4 | NLM WQ 18.2 | DDC 618.107/543--dc23
LC record available at http://lccn.loc.gov/2015042279

Printed and bound in China

ISBN 978-0-941022-87-3

*In loving memory of Mom and Dad,
who got this whole thing started.
And to my grandchildren Joey Carr
and Colin and Adalyn Showman,
who keep that love alive.*

Reviewers

Marveen Craig
Vice President, International Foundation for
 Sonography Education and Research (Retired)
Founder, International Ultrasound Institute
Tucson, Arizona

Nirvikar Dahiya, MD
Assistant Professor of Radiology
Department of Radiology
Mayo Clinic College of Medicine
Phoenix, Arizona

Marianna Desmond, EdM, RDMS, RT(R)
Clinical Coordinator, Diagnostic Medical Sonography
Triton College
River Grove, Illinois

Julia A. Drose, BA, RDMS, RDCS, RVT
Manager, Divisions of Ultrasound and Prenatal
 Diagnosis and Genetics
Associate Professor of Radiology
University of Colorado School of Medicine
Department of Radiology
Aurora, Colorado

Terry J. DuBose, MS, RDMS, FSDMS, FAIUM
Associate Professor Emeritus, Diagnostic Medical
 Sonography
College of Health Professions
University of Arkansas for Medical Sciences
Little Rock, Arkansas

Traci B. Fox, EdD, RT(R), RDMS, RVT
Assistant Professor, Department of Radiologic Sciences
Jefferson College of Health Professions
Assistant Research Professor, Department of Radiology
Sidney Kimmel Medical College at
 Thomas Jefferson University
Philadelphia, Pennsylvania

Diane Kawamura, PhD, RT(R), RDMS, FAIUM, FSDMS
Brady Presidential Distinguished Professor
Department of Radiologic Sciences
Weber State University
Ogden, Utah

Frederick W. Kremkau, PhD, FACR, FAIMBE, FAIUM, FASA
Professor of Radiologic Sciences
Director, Program for Medical Ultrasound
Center for Applied Learning
Wake Forest University School of Medicine
Winston-Salem, North Carolina

Annmarie Lobdell, MHS, RDMS, RDCS, RVT
Clinical Technology Consultant
ZONARE Medical Systems, Inc.
Mountain View, California

Darla J. Matthew, BAS, RT(R)(S), RDMS
Program Director
Diagnostic Medical Sonography
Doña Ana Community College
Las Cruces, New Mexico

Cynthia Reber-Bonhall, RDMS, RVT
Professor and Program Director
Diagnostic Medical Sonography
Orange Coast College
School of Allied Health Professions
Costa Mesa, California

Janice Hickey Scharf, BSc, RDMS, CRGS, FSC
Clinical Applications Specialist
Ultrasound, Philips Healthcare Canada
Markham, Ontario, Canada

Susan Raatz Stephenson, MS, MA.Ed., BSRT-U, RDMS, RVT, RT(R)(C), CIIP
Global Training and Education Radiology Project Manager
Siemens Medical Solutions USA, Inc.
Sandy, Utah

Regina K. Swearengin, BS, RDMS
Department Chair, Sonography
Austin Community College, Eastview Campus
Austin, Texas

Mark G. Torchia, MSc, PhD
Director, Centre for the Advancement of Teaching and Learning
Associate Professor of Surgery
University of Manitoba
Winnipeg, Manitoba, Canada

Jill D. Trotter, BS, RT(R), RDMS, RVT
Director, Diagnostic Medical Sonography Program
Vanderbilt University Medical Center
Nashville, Tennessee

Ellen T. Tuchinsky, BA, RDMS, RDCS
Director of Clinical Education (Retired)
Diagnostic Medical Sonography
School of Health Professions
Long Island University
Brooklyn, New York

Claudia von Zamory, BA, RDMS(A)(OB/GYN)(B), RVT
Ultrasound Program Director
Gurnick Academy of Medical Arts
San Mateo, California

Kerry E. Weinberg, PhD, RT(R), RDMS, RDCS, FSDMS
Associate Professor and Director
Diagnostic Medical Sonography Program
Long Island University
Brooklyn, New York

Preface to the 2nd Edition

When I undertook this project, my brief was to write a concise "silver bullet" review for RDMS candidates in obstetrics and gynecology. With this goal in mind, I found myself covering exam topics and key concepts and principles in somewhat greater depth than I had first imagined—and with an abundance of original illustrations and images—to satisfy the needs of registry candidates looking for a single-source review as well as the needs of students, veteran sonographers cross training in Ob/Gyn, and those seeking a convenient and inexpensive means of earning continuing medical education credit. It is therefore my hope and belief that you will find in this second edition the following:

- A one-volume, topic-by-topic, silver bullet review to help you study for the ARDMS Ob/Gyn specialty exam.
- A balanced and richly illustrated text for sonography students.
- A clinical reference for veteran and cross-training sonographers.
- A resource for interpreting physicians.
- A convenient and inexpensive means of earning 15 continuing medical education (CME) credits in Ob/Gyn sonography.

In approaching the content, I have referred to the last best ARDMS content outline as a guideline. You will find this exam outline in Appendix B, "Chapters Cross-Referenced to the ARDMS Exam Content Outline," wherein each exam topic is cross-referenced to the chapter or chapters that cover it. At the same time, I have organized the content using a comprehensive, subject-driven approach to ensure that all important topics are fully addressed. Current ARDMS exam outlines provide a generalized categorical overview together with very specific clinical tasks, but they can miss key intermediate topics you must know to pass your exam. Hence this hybrid approach, which gives you the best of both worlds. Mastery of the material in this book will help you not only pass the registry exam but also develop the habits of mind that form the foundation of success in your career as an ultrasound professional.

A complete CME application and exam at the end of the book also make it possible to earn 15 SDMS-approved continuing medical education credits toward satisfaction of ARDMS and other requirements for maintaining the active status of your professional credentials and facility accreditation.

A personal note: My strongly held faith-based values preclude me from providing information about or teaching individuals how to participate in elective abortions. For this reason, the topic of elective termination procedures has been intentionally excluded from this book; other authorities do address this issue and can easily be consulted if necessary.

For their tireless efforts to bring this book to print and ensure its completeness and accuracy I am indebted to the many reviewers listed in the front matter, as well as the editorial and production staff of Davies Publishing, Inc.

It is my hope that *Ob/Gyn Sonography: An Illustrated Review* will provide a strong educational foundation upon which those with less experience can build and those with more experience can expand—and remain a valuable reference for you in the years ahead. You have my best wishes for success!

Jim Baun, BS, RDMS, RVT, FSDMS
San Francisco, California

Contents

Reviewers **vii**

Preface to the 2nd Edition **ix**

PART I   OBSTETRICS   1

Chapter 1   The First Trimester   3

Chapter 2   The Placenta   31

Chapter 3   The Umbilical Cord   53

Chapter 4   Fetal Biometry   67

Chapter 5   The Fetal Face and Neck   87

Chapter 6   The Fetal Central Nervous System   111

Chapter 7   The Fetal Chest, Lungs, and Heart   151

Chapter 8   The Fetal Skeleton   197

Chapter 9   The Fetal Abdomen and Pelvis   219

Chapter 10   The Fetal Genitourinary Tract   247

Chapter 11   The Prenatal Genetic Workup   271

Chapter 12   At-Risk and Multiple-Gestation Pregnancies   301

PART II GYNECOLOGY 343

Chapter 13 Pelvic Anatomy and Physiology **345**

Chapter 14 Pelvic Pathology **371**

Chapter 15 Infertility **409**

Chapter 16 Pediatric and Postmenopausal Gynecologic Sonography **421**

PART III PHYSICAL PRINCIPLES, PROTOCOLS, AND PATIENT CARE 437

Chapter 17 Physical Principles and Instrumentation **439**

Chapter 18 Protocols and Patient Care **461**

Appendix A Answers to Chapter Review Questions **477**

Appendix B Chapters Cross-Referenced to the ARDMS Exam Content Outline **485**

Appendix C AIUM Practice Guidelines **491**

Appendix D Application for CME Credit **521**

Subject Index 539

PART I

Obstetrics

Chapter 1 | The First Trimester

Chapter 2 | The Placenta

Chapter 3 | The Umbilical Cord

Chapter 4 | Fetal Biometry

Chapter 5 | The Fetal Face and Neck

Chapter 6 | The Fetal Central Nervous System

Chapter 7 | The Fetal Chest, Lungs, and Heart

Chapter 8 | The Fetal Skeleton

Chapter 9 | The Fetal Abdomen and Pelvis

Chapter 10 | The Fetal Genitourinary Tract

Chapter 11 | The Prenatal Genetic Workup

Chapter 12 | At-Risk and Multiple-Gestation Pregnancies

CHAPTER 1

The First Trimester

Sonographic Protocols

Normal First Trimester

Abnormal First Trimester—Failed Pregnancy

SONOGRAPHIC PROTOCOLS

During the first trimester of pregnancy, the standard sonographic exam is performed to assess the following:

- Presence of gestational sac
- Size of sac
- Location of sac
- Number of sacs
- Presence of a yolk sac
- Presence of an embryo/fetus
- Cardiac activity (using a two-dimensional video clip or M-mode imaging)

Spectral and color Doppler imaging is avoided whenever possible during the first trimester as it is associated with a higher exposure to acoustic energy. In addition, the examination should assess the following structures:

- Uterus
- Cervix
- Adnexa
- Cul-de-sac

The rest of this chapter rehearses the development of a pregnancy during the first trimester, including both normal and abnormal sonographic findings, targeted protocols, and diagnostic criteria.

NORMAL FIRST TRIMESTER

The first trimester of a pregnancy begins with the first day of the woman's last menstrual period (LMP) and ends 10 weeks later. The end of the first trimester marks the point when all organ systems have been differentiated and are in place and the embryo has become a fetus. It is important to note that, although ovulation typically occurs 14 days after the first day of the menstrual period, the first day of the last menstrual period—not the date of conception—determines the beginning of a pregnancy in clinical obstetrics. The term for the gestational age based on this date is *menstrual age*, and it is this age on which ultrasound charts and biometric measurements are based. Embryologic tests, by contrast, are based on *conceptual age*, the age from conception, which lags behind menstrual age by 2 weeks. Gestational age is covered in more detail later in this chapter.

PREGNANCY DIAGNOSIS

Three main diagnostic tools are used in the diagnosis of pregnancy: patient history and physical examination (H&P), laboratory evaluation, and sonography.

Patient History and Physical Examination

Assessing the patient's history—particularly the date of the onset of the last menstrual period, along with information about historical frequency of menstrual periods, flow, and duration—is the initial approach. A missed menstrual period accompanied by nausea, vomiting, generalized malaise, and breast tenderness is often considered diagnostic of early pregnancy. However, normal implantation bleeding, which occurs at about the same time as an expected menstrual period, may confuse the clinical presentation.

A physical examination will reveal a *gravid uterus* (the uterus during pregnancy), which will be enlarged on bimanual examination, and *Chadwick's sign* (a bluish discoloration of the cervix), which will be observed by 8–10 weeks. *Goodell's sign* (softening of the vaginal portion of the cervix), *Hegar's sign* (softening of the uterine isthmus), and hyperpigmentation of the *linea alba* (the fibrous structure that runs down the abdominal midline) are other physical signs associated with early pregnancy.

Laboratory Evaluation

Laboratory evaluation typically centers on assays for the beta subunit of human chorionic gonadotropin (beta-hCG) in maternal serum, but other hormones that have been used in the early diagnosis of pregnancy include progesterone and early pregnancy factor.

Progesterone

In a normal first trimester pregnancy, progesterone levels rise to multiples of those observed during the nonpregnant state and are an indicator of the integrity of an intrauterine gestation. Typical serum levels range from 10 to 44 nanograms per milliliter (ng/ml); laboratory values less than expected raise suspicion for ectopic pregnancy and are also associated with an increased risk of failed intrauterine pregnancy.

Early Pregnancy Factor

Early pregnancy factor (EPF) is a protein produced by the conceptus within hours after fertilization and is the earliest laboratory evidence of pregnancy. Because EPF is produced prior to implantation, abnormal values may indicate embryo loss prior to implantation, earlier than can be discerned using hCG and/or progesterone assays. EPF is measured using the rosette inhibition test (RIT), which yields either positive or negative results.[1]

Human Chorionic Gonadotropin

Human chorionic gonadotropin is a glycoprotein similar in structure to follicle-stimulating hormone (FSH), luteinizing hormone (LH), and thyrotropin. It is composed of alpha and beta subunits and can be detected in the maternal serum as early as 6–8 days post conception. *Qualitative* serum beta-hCG testing, which yields a simple positive or negative result, has a threshold of about 25 million International Units per milliliter (mIU/ml). *Quantitative* serum evaluation is more sensitive, with a threshold as low as 1 mIU/ml, and provides a numeric value that can be followed serially and correlated with a normally progressing gestation to rule out a failed pregnancy.

Human chorionic gonadotropin is secreted by physiologically active trophoblastic tissue. Because every intact conceptus, intrauterine or ectopic, contains trophoblastic tissue, the presence of the beta subunit of this glycoprotein hormone in maternal blood is strong evidence of pregnancy. A "negative" beta-hCG blood test (that is, one resulting in undetectable levels by radioimmunoassay) essentially excludes the

Table 1-1.	Discriminatory levels of serum beta-hCG.	
US Method	1st IRP or 3IS (mIU/ml)	2IS (mIU/ml)
Endovaginal	1000–2000	500–1000
Transabdominal	3600	1800

Table 1-2.	Early pregnancy time line: menstrual vs. conceptual age.	
Event	Gestational Age (Days)	
	Menstrual (Clinical)	Conceptual (Embryologic)
LMP begins	1	n/a
Ovulation	14	n/a
Fertilization	15–16	1–2
Conceptus enters uterine cavity	18–19	4–5
Implantation	21–22	7–8
Gastrulation	29–30	15–16
Neurulation starts	35	21
Neurulation ends	42	28
Heart septation starts	43	29

diagnosis of a live pregnancy anywhere in the body. "Positive" results, which are evident at approximately 23 menstrual days (9 days post conception), confirm the presence of viable trophoblastic tissue somewhere.

Three different reference standards have been used to measure beta-hCG. The system known as the First International Reference Preparation (1st IRP, sometimes referred to as FIRP) was developed first, and later the Second International Standard (2IS) came into use.[2] In samples that have equivalent beta-hCG levels, the numeric result using the 2IS system is approximately double the result using the 1st IRP system. The Third International Standard (3IS) yields levels similar to those of the 1st IRP, and therefore many labs have reverted to using the 1st IRP in reporting results. While exact values can vary slightly from one laboratory to the next, typical values for the three measuring systems have been established (Table 1-1).

A correlation can be made between sonographic identification of the gestational sac in early pregnancy and maternal serum beta-hCG levels. *Discriminatory serum levels* are defined as those at which an intrauterine pregnancy (IUP) will always be seen if, indeed, it is present within the endometrial cavity. If an intrauterine pregnancy is not identified at these levels, a failed pregnancy, as discussed below, is highly suspected.

Sonographic Diagnosis of Pregnancy

Sonographic diagnosis of early pregnancy is the final piece of the diagnostic triad, providing visual information about the uterine contents and adnexa. The role of sonography in diagnosing the presence of early pregnancy is well established and is based on the identification of normal intrauterine gestational structures in a patient with correlative clinical and/or laboratory findings. The specific roles and diagnostic criteria used in evaluation of early pregnancy are discussed throughout the rest of this chapter.

GESTATIONAL AGE

As mentioned previously, the term *gestational age* can refer to either of two methods for dating a pregnancy. An embryologic approach calculates gestational age based on when fertilization occurs and is called *conceptual age*. In a theoretically perfect 28-day menstrual cycle, fertilization occurs 24–36 hours after ovulation. If ovulation transpires on day 14, as is assumed in this perfect menstrual cycle, then fertilization of the ovum happens 15–16 days after the beginning of the last menstrual period.

In clinical obstetrics, however, the exact date of ovulation is usually unknown, so gestational age is calculated based on the last menstrual period, a clinically observable event, and is called *menstrual age*. When calculated from the first day of the last menstrual period (LMP), gestational age is expressed as *menstrual weeks*; when calculated from the moment of conception, *conceptual weeks*. Conceptual age is roughly 2 weeks (14 days) less than menstrual age.

In this book, unless otherwise specified, all presentations of gestational age are calculated based on the beginning date of the last menstrual period. While the distinction is important in understanding first trimester events, it becomes less so as the gestation passes from the embryonic to the fetal period at about week 10. (Examples of the two systems for key events in early pregnancy appear in Table 1-2.)

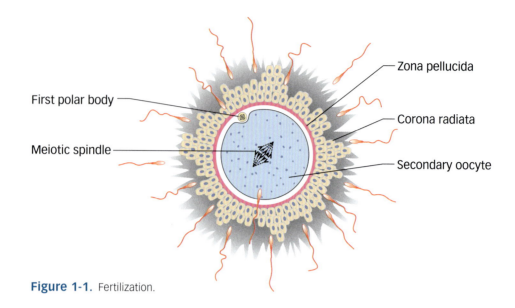

Figure 1-1. Fertilization.

FERTILIZATION AND EMBRYOLOGY

The early development of the conceptus/embryo can be summarized as follows, using menstrual ages.

Conceptus Period: Weeks 3–5

Menstrual weeks 3–5 (conceptual weeks 1–3) constitute the *conceptus period*.

Menstrual Week 3/Days 15–21: Early Development of the Conceptus

- Days 15–16: Fertilization of the *oocyte* or (when mature) *ovum* (the female gamete) by the *spermatozoon* or *sperm cell* (the male gamete) occurs within 24–36 hours of ovulation on day 14 (Figure 1-1).
- Days 16–18: The *zygote* (fertilized egg) traverses the fallopian tube (Figure 1-2).
- Day 17: 8-cell stage.
- Day 18: 12- to 16-cell stage, known as the *morula*.
- Day 18 or 19: The morula enters the uterus and begins transformation into the *blastocyst*, a hollow ball of cells with a single germ layer.
- Days 18–21: The blastocyst cavity and inner cell mass form; the blastocyst cavity becomes the *primary yolk sac*; amniotic cavity formation begins.

Menstrual Week 4/Days 22–28: Implantation, Bilaminar Embryonic Disc, Amnion, and Chorion

A normal intrauterine pregnancy begins with the implantation of the conceptus in the secretory endometrium in the central portion of the uterine cavity.

- Days 21–22: *Implantation* of the blastocyst in the uterine wall and formation of the *syncytiotrophoblast*,

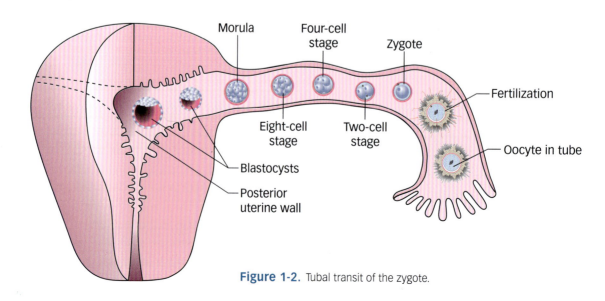

Figure 1-2. Tubal transit of the zygote.

the placental precursor (Figure 1-3). Vaginal bleeding may occur at this time.

- Days 23–26: Transformation of the inner cell mass into the *bilaminar embryonic disc* (Figure 1-4), which has two germ layers, the epiblast and the hypoblast.
- Days 27–28: Regression of the primary yolk sac and formation of a *secondary yolk sac* and the surrounding *chorionic cavity*. The *amniotic sac* enlarges on the side of the embryo opposite the yolk sac. The adjacent amnion and secondary yolk sac (Figure 1-5) are sometimes visible sonographically within the chorionic cavity. This finding is called the *double bleb sign*. At the beginning of the fourth week, the gestational sac is about 1 mm in diameter.

Menstrual Week 5/Days 29–30: Gastrulation

- *Trilaminar disc*: Formation of the trilaminar disc, comprising the three primary germ layers: ectoderm, endoderm, and mesoderm.
- *Notochord*: Formation of the primitive node and streak and the rod-shaped group of cells that defines the body's primary supporting axis (the notochord). The notochord forms within the embryonic plate between the endoderm and ectoderm.
- *Early embryo*: The notochord induces development of the structure of the early embryo and later develops into the nucleus pulposus of the discs of the spinal column.

Menstrual Weeks 5–6/Days 31–42: Neurulation and Vasculogenesis

- Days 31–42: *Neural tube* and *neural plate*: Formation of the neural plate, neural tube, and *somites* (blocks of mesoderm located on either side of the neural tube), which develop into the central nervous system.
  - Day 35: Neural tube formation (neurulation) begins (Figure 1-6A) and the first somites appear.
  - Day 40: The *rostral* (head) end of the neural tube closes.
  - Day 42: The *caudal* (sacral) end of the neural tube closes and neurulation ends (Figure 1-6B).
- Days 35–42: Formation of primitive blood cells (*hematogenesis*), blood vessels (*angiogenesis*), fetal heart, and placental vasculogenesis.

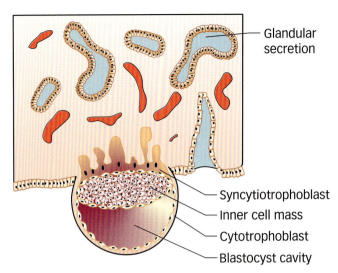

Figure 1-3. Implantation.

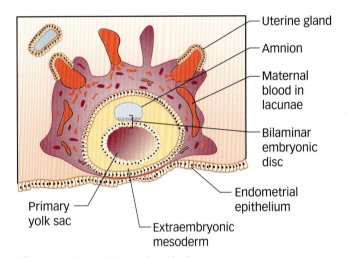

Figure 1-4. Bilaminar embryonic disc.

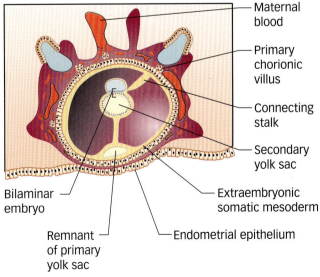

Figure 1-5. Secondary yolk sac.

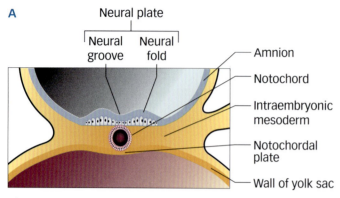
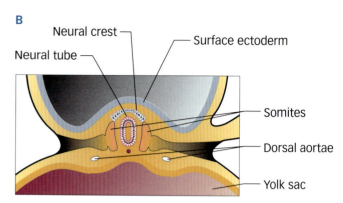

Figure 1-6. A Neurulation begins. **B** Neurulation ends.

Embryonic Period: Weeks 6–10

During menstrual weeks 6–10 (conceptual weeks 4–8)—the *embryonic period*—nearly all permanent internal and external structures are formed (a few of the morphologic developments listed below occur after 10 weeks).

Cardiovascular System
- Week 6: Unidirectional blood flow begins.
- Week 8: Formation of the heart is complete.
- Week 10: Formation of the peripheral vascular system is complete.
- For more on the fetal cardiovascular system, see Chapter 7.

Gastrointestinal System
- Week 6: Formation of the primitive gut is complete.
- Week 8: The rectum separates from the urogenital sinus.
- Weeks 8–12: The midgut herniates into the umbilical cord and then returns to the abdomen.
- Week 10: The anal membrane perforates.
- For more on the fetal gastrointestinal system, see Chapter 9.

Urogenital System
- Week 8: The primitive kidneys (metanephroi) begin to form and descend into the abdomen.
- Week 11: Kidneys are in the adult position; external genitalia are visually similar in males and females.
- Week 14: Differentiation of external male and female genitalia is complete.
- For more on the fetal urogenital system, see Chapter 10.

Musculoskeletal System
- Weeks 5.5–6: Formation of limb buds is complete.
- Weeks 7.5–8: Digital rays develop; arms are bent at the elbow.
- Week 8: The clavicle begins to ossify.
- Week 9: The mandible, palate, vertebral bodies, and neural arches begin to ossify.
- Week 11: The long bones begin to ossify.
- For more on the fetal musculoskeletal system, see Chapter 8.

Sonographic Signs—Early Intrauterine Pregnancy

The identification of a gestational sac (GS) within the endometrial cavity is the first sonographic evidence that a normal intrauterine pregnancy is present. A gestational sac is always seen in a normal intrauterine pregnancy when the following discriminatory levels[3] are achieved:

- Serum beta-hCG ≥ 800–1000 mIU/ml (endovaginal) using 2IS.
- Serum beta-hCG ≥ 1800 mIU/ml (transabdominal) using 2IS.
- Certain last menstrual period ≥ 5 weeks.
- Decidual thickening: The earliest sonographic sign of pregnancy is focal thickening of the echogenic decidua at the site of implantation.[4] This finding is quite subtle, and the predictive value of the finding has not been established.

GESTATIONAL SAC

The fluid-filled gestational sac is first visible at about 4.5–5 menstrual weeks, and it is the first definitive sonographic sign of pregnancy (Figure 1-7A).

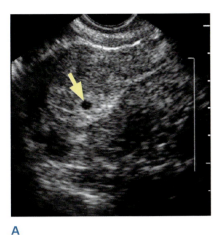 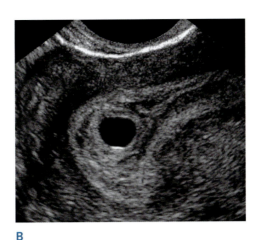

Figure 1-7. A Early intrauterine pregnancy: longitudinal view of a pregnant uterus containing a small echolucency (arrow) most likely representing an early intrauterine pregnancy. **B** Normal intrauterine gestational sac, 6 weeks. A well-circumscribed, anechoic sac positioned in the central portion of the uterine cavity. There are intact, echogenic borders representing developing chorionic trophoblastic tissue and decidual layers.

Endovaginal scanning can reliably visualize a gestational sac in the uterus by 5 weeks, when the mean sac diameter (MSD) is 2–3 mm, and transabdominal scanning can visualize the gestational sac by 6 weeks, when the mean sac diameter reaches 5 mm. A normal gestational sac appears as a small fluid collection surrounded by an echogenic rim. The central lucency represents fluid in the chorionic cavity, while the surrounding echogenic rim represents developing chorionic trophoblastic tissue and adjacent decidual layers. When the sac is measured, the largest diameter is selected.

Sonographic Signs—Gestational Sac

The following are the characteristic sonographic signs of a normal intrauterine gestational sac (Figure 1-7B):

- Round, oval, well defined.
- Echogenic, intact borders.
- Positioned in the fundus or mid uterus.
- Growth ≈ 1 mm/day.

- Yolk sac present when mean sac diameter is ≥ 13 mm.
- *Intradecidual sign*: The sonographic presence of a small gestational sac within the decidua at approximately 4–4.5 weeks, with a mean sac diameter of approximately 2.5 mm, is known as the *intradecidual sign*. To distinguish a true intradecidual sign from a decidual (endometrial) cyst, the sonographer must be sure that the gestational sac is directly adjacent to the endometrial canal. Because the intradecidual sign can sometimes mimic a pseudogestational sac of ectopic pregnancy, its value appears somewhat limited.
- *Double bleb sign*: At 5.5 menstrual weeks, the developing amniotic sac measures about 2 mm in diameter and becomes visible adjacent to the yolk sac (Figures 1-8A and B). This double sac appearance is called the *double bleb sign*. At this time the bilaminar embryonic disc lies between the yolk sac and the amnion. The double bleb sign is no longer visible by 7 menstrual weeks.

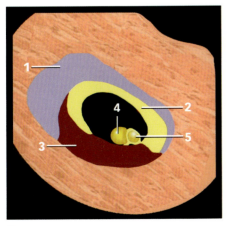 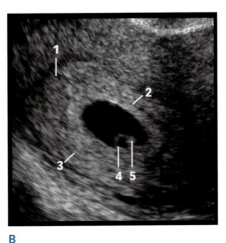

Figure 1-8. A Schematic and **B** correlative sonogram demonstrating the double bleb sign. An early amniotic sac is visible adjacent to the yolk sac. 1 = decidua vera, 2 = decidua capsularis, 3 = decidua basalis, 4 = yolk sac, 5 = amniotic sac.

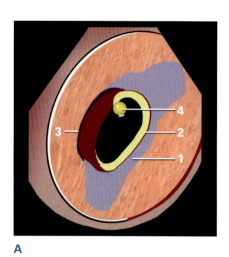 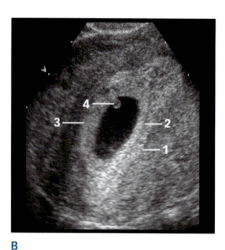

Figure 1-9. **A** Schematic and **B** correlative sonogram demonstrating the double decidual sac sign. Echogenic ring formed by two decidual layers surrounding the gestational sac. 1 = decidua vera, 2 = decidua capsularis, 3 = decidua basalis, 4 = yolk sac.

- *Double decidual sac sign*: The echogenic ring formed by the decidua vera (parietalis) and decidua capsularis is called the *double decidual sac sign* (or *double sac sign*). The decidua basalis (future placenta) may be visualized as an area of echogenic thickening on one portion of the sac. This sign can typically be visualized by 5.5–6 menstrual weeks (Figures 1-9A and B), when the mean sac diameter is ≥8 mm.[5] As the use of high-resolution transvaginal sonography has become more extensive, the double sac sign has come to play a less significant role in the diagnosis of pregnancy.

YOLK SAC

The secondary yolk sac is the earliest embryonic structure identified sonographically and is reliably demonstrated by 5 weeks in a normal gestation. The yolk sac initially produces red blood cells needed by the primitive circulatory system.

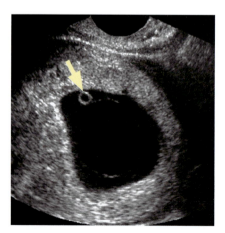

Figure 1-10. Sonogram of a gestational sac with a yolk sac (arrow) situated normally between the amnion and chorion.

High-frequency (7–10 MHz) transvaginal sonography is required to consistently visualize yolk sacs in 8 mm gestational sacs. The inability to demonstrate a yolk sac when the mean sac diameter is ≥ 8 mm or when serum beta-hCG levels have reached discriminatory levels is consistent with a failed pregnancy.

Sonographic Signs—Yolk Sac

The following are the characteristic sonographic signs of a normal yolk sac:

- Spherical in shape, with a sonolucent center and a clearly defined echogenic wall (Figure 1-10)
- May be visualized when the mean sac diameter is ≥ 5 mm (at 5 menstrual weeks)
- Always visualized when the mean sac diameter is ≥ 8 mm (at 5.5 menstrual weeks)

EMBRYO

In a very early intrauterine pregnancy (<6 weeks), endovaginal sonography may reveal a small "embryonic bud," measuring 1–2 mm and lying adjacent to the yolk sac, with or without cardiovascular activity (Figure 1-11). Absence of these findings at such an early embryonic moment does not portend pregnancy failure. By 6 weeks, however, an embryo with cardiovascular activity can be reliably demonstrated with endovaginal sonography.

Sonographic Signs—Cardiac Activity

Embryonic cardiac activity may be visualized when the crown-rump length (CRL) is approximately 2–4 mm and will be observed in normal embryos 5 mm or more in length. In normal pregnancies the embryo will be visualized when mean sac diameter is 5–12 mm, and

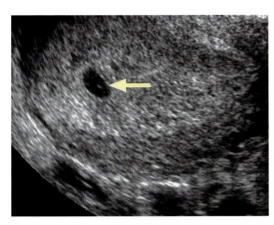

Figure 1-11. Embryonic bud (arrow) at 5.5 weeks, measuring 1–2 mm: echogenic focus within the gestational sac. The bud may or may not demonstrate cardiovascular activity.

cardiac activity when mean sac diameter is 13–18 mm. High-frequency (7–10 MHz) endovaginal sonography probes, appropriate focusing, and low-persistence settings are needed to image the embryo and heartbeat adequately (Figures 1-12A and B). Some investigators have correlated reduced cardiovascular activity in an embryo with unfavorable pregnancy outcomes. At 5–6 weeks, 100–115 beats per minute (bpm) is a normal range for embryonic cardiovascular activity. By about 9 weeks, mean heart rate increases to ≥140 bpm, where it remains for the duration of pregnancy. There is evidence to suggest a correlation between reduced embryonic cardiovascular activity and poor pregnancy outcomes. Table 1-3 summarizes the association between a reduced cardiac rate and pregnancy loss.

Documentation of embryonic cardiac activity during the first trimester ultrasound examination is best accomplished using M-mode rather than either color Doppler imaging or pulsed Doppler spectral display. Both Doppler modalities are associated with higher levels of acoustic output and, in compliance with ALARA[6] exposure standards, should not be used

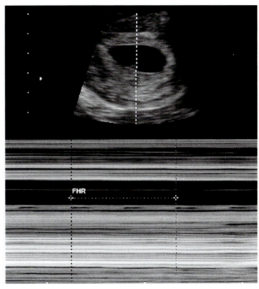

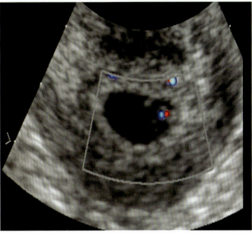

Figure 1-12. **A** M-mode and **B** color Doppler imaging demonstrating embryonic cardiac activity at 6 weeks.

routinely in obstetric imaging when M-mode capabilities are available. M-mode interrogation through the embryonic heart yields a two-axis tracing that permits calculation of heart rate by placing measurement cursors at similar points in two separate cardiac cycles. On-board software algorithms calculate heart rate.

Sonographic Signs—Gestational Viability

The primary value of endovaginal sonography in the first trimester of pregnancy is its great sensitivity and reliability in detecting early signs of gestational viability (Table 1-4). The close correlation between the appearance of specific sonographic signs and the normal progression of pregnancy allows early detection of abnormalities that portend a poor outcome.

Table 1-3. Embryonic bradycardia and pregnancy loss.

Heart Rate (bpm)	Pregnancy Loss Rate
<80	100%
80–90	64%
90–99	32%
>100	11%

Table 1-4. Measures of pregnancy viability using endovaginal sonography.

Viability Measure	Age (Menstrual Weeks)	Mean Sac Diameter (mm)
Gestational sac may be identified	4.5	2
Gestational sac always identified	5	5
Yolk sac identified	5	10
Embryo detection	5–6	5–12
Cardiac activity identified	6–6.5	13–18

Underpinning the reliability of the sonographic findings is the reliability of the dating of the pregnancy. As significant embryonic events are unfolding on a daily basis, uncertainty about the date of the last menstrual period introduces uncertainty into the sonographic findings. Normal variations in the first 14 days of the menstrual cycle that delay fertilization will render even firm dates for the last menstrual period somewhat unreliable. As always in clinical practice, correlation with physical findings and laboratory values, particularly quantitative serum beta-hCG titers, is essential for a proper diagnosis (see Table 1-1).

Sonographic Signs—Embryonic Anatomy

Embryonic development is rapid in the first trimester of pregnancy. By 10 weeks, all major organ systems have appeared and are in place; by 12 weeks, the embryo has transitioned into a fully formed fetus.

Identifying anatomic structural anomalies is not usually possible in the first trimester. However, there are three normal embryonic anatomic findings that, if detected in later trimesters, raise the specter of a major fetal anomaly: midgut herniation, a prominent rhombencephalon, and abnormal nuchal translucency.

Midgut Herniation

In an embryo, the primitive gastrointestinal tract resides in the base of the umbilical cord, as much of the abdominal cavity is filled with liver (Figure 1-13). This normal physiologic herniation of the bowel occurs at about 8 menstrual weeks (6 conceptual weeks) and is reduced into the abdominal cavity by menstrual week 12 (conceptual week 10). The sonographic appearance of midgut herniation when observed later than menstrual week 14 is consistent with an *omphalocele*, a pathologic protrusion of part of the large intestine—and, in many instances, other intra-abdominal structures—through the anterior abdominal wall. (See Chapter 9 for more on abdominal anatomy and pathology.)

Prominent Rhombencephalon

The embryonic brain is a collection of cystic cavities surrounded by thin mantles of neural tissue. The *rhombencephalon*, which in the fetus comprises the hindbrain structures, can appear prominent, a normal finding during the first and second trimesters. However, if seen after the second trimester, this sonographic finding suggests a *Dandy-Walker malformation*—cystic dilatation of the fourth ventricle, hypoplasia or complete absence of the vermis, an enlarged posterior fossa, and hydrocephalus (Figure 1-14).

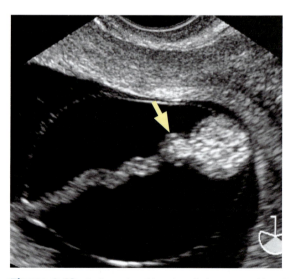

Figure 1-13. Embryonic midgut herniation: normal herniation of intra-abdominal contents into the base of the umbilical cord (arrow) at 10 weeks' gestation.

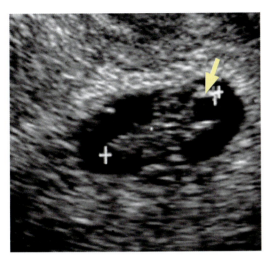

Figure 1-14. Prominent rhombencephalon (arrow). Normal cystic intracranial anatomy in an 8-week gestation.

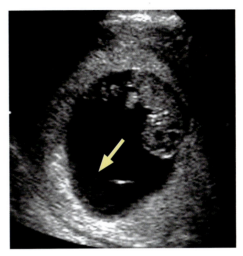

Figure 1-16. Curvilinear echogenic band representing the amnion (arrow). Low-level echoes are seen within the chorionic cavity.

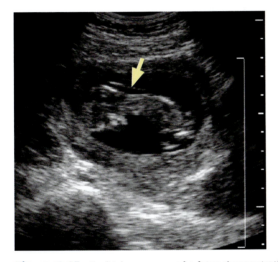

Figure 1-15. Sagittal sonogram of a fetus demonstrating abnormal nuchal translucency (arrow).

Nuchal Translucency

The *nuchal translucency*, sometimes called the *nuchal lucency* (Figure 1-15), is a collection of lymphatic fluid found in the posterior neck region of the embryo that is normal during the first trimester. Its diameter, when exceeding normal values and measured between 11 and 14 weeks, is a useful indicator of possible genetic abnormalities, notably trisomy 21. (See Chapter 11.)

AMNION

Gradually—by approximately 12–16 weeks—the amniotic sac grows to fill the chorionic cavity. In some pregnancies, it may be seen as a curvilinear, echogenic band separating amniotic fluid from the periphery of the gestational sac. Occasionally, with high-resolution equipment, diffuse low-level echoes may be observed filling the chorionic cavity (Figure 1-16). The cause of the low-level echoes is unknown but most likely represents the thick proteinaceous material contained within the cavity.

ABNORMAL FIRST TRIMESTER— FAILED PREGNANCY

Failed pregnancy is a common occurrence but one whose incidence is hard to measure. Some researchers have found a 30% loss of early pregnancy after implantation in normal, healthy volunteers.[7,8] Most failed pregnancies pass without any clinical signs or awareness on the part of the patient. Those that have implanted in the endometrial cavity and have begun growing trophoblastic connections to the uterus produce the signs and symptoms of failed pregnancy.

Typically the patient presents with a positive pregnancy test and a history of recent vaginal bleeding, spotting, and cramping. Vaginal bleeding, as an isolated symptom, is not uncommon and occurs in approximately 25% of patients during the first few weeks of pregnancy. *Implantation bleeding* is the temporary, normal passage of blood *per vaginam* (through the vagina) that occurs as the conceptus implants into the endometrium. However, heavy bleeding and cramping, especially if accompanied by the passage of clots and/or tissue, raise the legitimate concern that the pregnancy is failing.

The primary role of endovaginal sonography in the assessment of suspected failed pregnancy is to identify a viable intrauterine gestation. If a healthy-appearing, intact gestational sac is found in the central portion of the endometrial cavity, a failed or failing pregnancy can be excluded and the patient can be reassured. (One caveat with regard to taking this approach is the possibility of an uncommon and potentially overlooked *heterotopic pregnancy*—concomitant intra- and extra-uterine implantations—which can confuse the clinical scenario.)

If sonography fails to demonstrate an intrauterine pregnancy in the milieu of a positive pregnancy test, ectopic pregnancy becomes a primary consideration. If, on the other hand, sonographic examination of the uterine cavity provides evidence of an abortive process, appropriate therapeutic intervention can be instituted.

SONOGRAPHIC SIGNS AND DIAGNOSTIC CRITERIA

Reasonably reliable indicators of abnormal early pregnancy include:

- Mean sac diameter (MSD) ≥ 8 mm with absent yolk sac (Figure 1-17A)
- Crown-rump length (CRL) > 16 mm with absent embryo or heartbeat
- Amniotic sac noted within the gestational sac and embryo absent
- Embryo > 5 mm with cardiovascular activity absent
- MSD − CRL ≥ 5 mm between 5.5 and 9 weeks
- Gestational sac much larger than the embryo (Figure 1-17B)

Less reliable or not as well established indicators include:

- Irregular shape of the gestational sac (Figure 1-17C)
- Absent double sac sign
- Weak decidual echoes at the edge of the gestational sac
- Low position of the sac in the uterus (Figure 1-17D)
- Yolk sac < 2 mm or > 5.6 mm with irregular shape or calcifications
- Yolk sac disproportionately large for sac size (> 30% of total sac volume) (Figure 1-17E)
- Mean sac diameter growth < 0.6 mm per day (normal growth = 1.13 mm per day)
- Embryonic bradycardia—a reduction in embryonic cardiac rate has been associated with failed pregnancy (see Table 1-3)

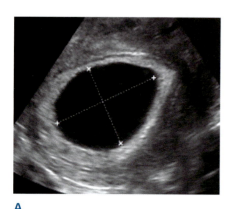

A

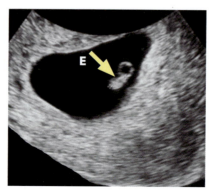

B

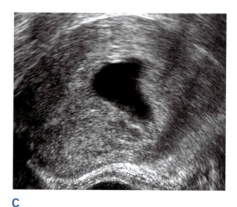

C

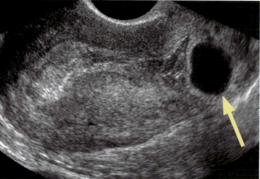

D

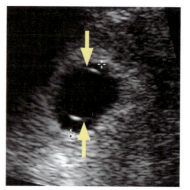

E

Figure 1-17. A Intrauterine gestational sac ≥8 mm without evidence of embryo. **B** Small demised embryo (E) relative to gestational sac size. **C** Poorly marginated and indistinct borders surround an irregularly shaped gestational sac. **D** Sagittal endovaginal image demonstrating a large, well-circumscribed gestational sac (arrow) implanted in the lower uterine segment. **E** Yolk sac (arrows) occupying more than 30% of total gestational sac volume.

SPONTANEOUS ABORTION

Spontaneous abortion (SAB), or *miscarriage*, is the physiologic termination of pregnancy prior to 20 weeks' gestation. Approximately 12% of all pregnancies end in spontaneous abortion, with 75% occurring before the 16th week.

Etiologies and Risk Factors

While its cause frequently cannot be determined in an individual patient, common etiologies include:

- Endocrine factors
- Failure of the corpus luteum
- Maternal müllerian defects
- Interruption of embryonic development
- Chromosomal causes
- Diabetes mellitus
- Polycystic ovary syndrome
- Cigarette smoking

Pathologically, spontaneous abortion begins with hemorrhage into the decidua basalis. Inflammation and necrosis occur around the region of implantation, with subsequent detachment of the conceptus. Uterine contractions and expulsion of intrauterine contents occur through a dilated cervix. An incomplete abortion occurs when some of the products of conception remain, and there may be organization of a blood clot surrounding the conceptus.

The primary role of sonography in patients presenting with the clinical signs of spontaneous abortion is to assess the presence and amount of retained products of conception in the uterine cavity.

Clinical Types

Complete Abortion

As its name implies, a *complete abortion* is a spontaneous abortion in which all gestational tissue, including the embryo, has been expelled from the uterus. Brisk vaginal bleeding with tissue and clots and a subsequent rapid decline in serum beta-hCG levels are clinical characteristics associated with a complete abortive event. As the uterine cavity has been emptied of its contents, the sonographic appearance is that of a normal uterus, although it may remain generously sized for several days. Color Doppler imaging may normally demonstrate high-amplitude trophoblastic blood flow patterns encircling the endometrium. Persistence of this hyperemic flow pattern after three days, however, is evidence of retained products of conception.

Sonographic Signs

The following are the characteristic sonographic signs of complete abortion:

- Empty uterus with a "clean" endometrial stripe
- Moderate to bright endometrial echoes
- Uterine enlargement

Incomplete Abortion

If gestational tissue remains within the uterus and bleeding persists, the appropriate term is *incomplete abortion* or *abortion in process*. The term *missed abortion* is vague and has fallen out of use. Sonographic appearances associated with incomplete abortion vary with the type and amount of products remaining in the uterine cavity following the initial abortive event. Doppler ultrasound is a useful adjunct in identifying hemodynamically active trophoblastic tissue still attached to the myometrium.

Sonographic Signs

The following are the characteristic sonographic signs of incomplete abortion:

- Presence of a complex collection of echoes within the endometrium (Figure 1-18A)
- Thin, irregular borders with hematoma (Figure 1-18B)
- Acoustic shadowing secondary to air bubbles or retained bony fragments

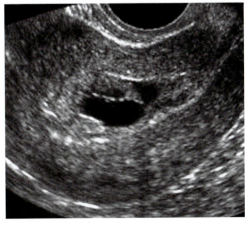

A

Figure 1-18. Sonographic appearance of incomplete abortion. **A** Sagittal endovaginal image demonstrating an irregularly shaped gestational sac containing complex, echogenic material consistent with products of conception and clot. (Figure continues . . .)

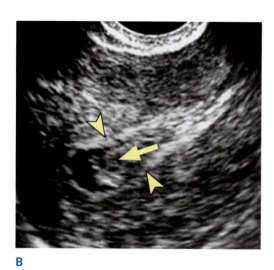 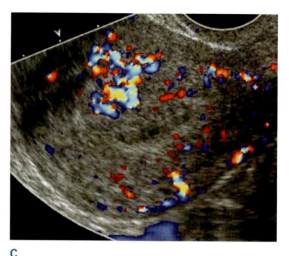

B   C

Figure 1-18, continued. B Sagittal endovaginal image from a different patient demonstrating thin, irregular borders (arrowheads) with a hematoma (arrow) present in the gestational sac. **C** Sagittal endovaginal image with color Doppler demonstrating high-amplitude, low-resistance blood flow consistent with persistent trophoblastic material retained within the uterine cavity.

- Persistence of trophoblastic waveforms near the endometrial cavity 5 or more days post abortion (Figure 1-18C)

Anembryonic Pregnancy (Blighted Ovum)

Anembryonic pregnancy or *blighted ovum* occurs when a gestational sac is present in the uterus but no embryo is identified in a sac large enough to expect one. In *embryonic demise*, an embryo > 5 mm is observed without a heartbeat. Anembryonic pregnancy is associated with variable serum levels, as beta-hCG–producing trophoblastic tissue may be present, intact, and functionally normal. The patient may or may not present with a history of vaginal bleeding or spotting.

Sonographic Signs

The following are the characteristic sonographic signs of anembryonic pregnancy:

- No identifiable embryo in a gestational sac ≥ 25 mm (Figure 1-19)
- Absence of the double sac sign

Threatened Abortion

Threatened abortion is defined as bleeding, spotting, or cramping during the first trimester, with a closed cervical os. About half of patients with these symptoms will have a normal outcome, while the other half will spontaneously abort. Loss rates are influenced by maternal age, smoking, and alcohol or caffeine consumption, as well as other causes, such as failure of the corpus luteum to support the implanted conceptus

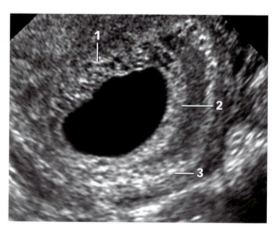

Figure 1-19. Anembryonic pregnancy: Endovaginal image demonstrating a large, smoothly marginated gestational sac without evidence of embryo or yolk sac. All three decidual layers are intact. 1 = decidua vera, 2 = decidua capsularis, 3 = decidua parietalis.

sufficiently. The corpus luteum secretes progesterone to support pregnancy until the placenta takes over the hormonal function. It forms during the secretory phase of the menstrual cycle and during pregnancy is usually less than 5 cm in diameter with a variety of appearances. The corpus luteum usually regresses or decreases in size by approximately 16–18 weeks. When the corpus luteum persists beyond 18 weeks, it is called a corpus luteum cyst and it should be followed sonographically.

Sonographic Signs

There are no sonographic findings associated with a threatened abortion that are predictive of outcome in a

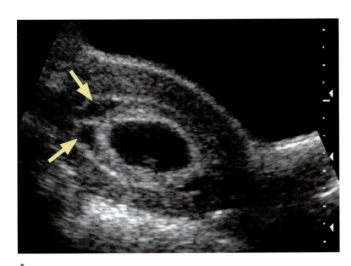
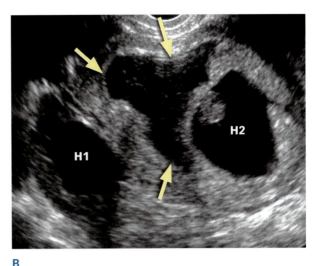

Figure 1-20. A Longitudinal view through the uterus demonstrating the gestational sac with hypoechoic area superiorly (arrows) representing subchorionic hemorrhage. **B** Transverse transabdominal image through a didelphic uterus demonstrating a subchorionic hemorrhage (arrows) associated with a normal, intact gestational sac in the left uterine horn (H2). The nongravid right uterine horn (H1) contains a small amount of free fluid.

particular pregnancy. The use of sonography is limited to the identification of an intact intrauterine pregnancy.

Subchorionic Hemorrhage

Subchorionic hemorrhage—blood within the uterine cavity and outside the gestational sac—is a marker for an increased risk of miscarriage. The blood collection may be identified adjacent to or opposite the placenta (Figures 1-20A and B), or it may be partly or completely retroplacental. During early pregnancy the blood visualized may be due to implantation of the *chorion frondosum* (the fetal contribution to the placenta) as it penetrates into the *decidua basalis* (the maternal contribution to the placenta). The risk of miscarriage increases with the size of a subchorionic hemorrhage. Abruption is more likely to result in miscarriage than is subchorionic hemorrhage.

Sonographic Signs

The following are the characteristic sonographic signs of subchorionic hemorrhage:

- Fluid collection identified beneath the chorionic plate
- Elevation of the membrane from the chorion frondosum (primitive placenta)

ECTOPIC PREGNANCY

Ectopic pregnancy is the implantation of a conceptus anywhere outside the endometrial cavity. It is also known as *extrauterine pregnancy*. While a full 90% of ectopic implantations occur in the fallopian tube, a conceptus that is expelled from the tube and into the peritoneal cavity can attach to the ovary, broad ligament, cervix, abdominal wall, or intestine and burrow in to establish a hemodynamic connection. The risk of significant morbidity and mortality to both mother and fetus that accompanies ectopic pregnancy results from the sudden rupture of the highly vascularized conceptus and, in some cases, of the organ upon which it is implanted.

Etiologies and Risk Factors

The causes and risk factors for ectopic pregnancy are many. Tubal scarring from prior infections, prior ectopic pregnancies, trauma from diagnostic or therapeutic instrumentation, or surgery can mechanically impede normal transport, causing the rapidly growing conceptus to become "stuck" in the tube, where it then dutifully implants.

Medical or genetic factors can cause a reduction in the normal ciliary action that massages a conceptus forward into the endometrial cavity. Retrograde menstruation can flush a conceptus out of the tube and into the peritoneal cavity. Other risk factors for ectopic pregnancy include the use of intrauterine contraceptive devices (IUDs), cigarette smoking, and advanced maternal age (i.e., ≥35 years). Women who are taking fertility drugs or who are participating in assisted reproductive technology protocols are also at a higher risk that one or more fertilized ova will find their way into an ectopic location.

Table 1-5.	Incidence of ectopic pregnancy by implantation site.
Site	Percentage of Ectopic Pregnancies
Fallopian tube, ampullary	80.0
Fallopian tube, isthmic	12.0
Fimbrial	5.0
Cornual/interstitial	2.0
Abdominal	1.4
Ovarian	0.2
Cervical	0.2

Note: Rounding errors account for percentages totaling more than 100.

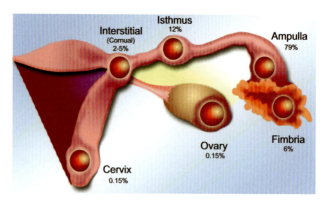

Figure 1-21. Common ectopic implantation sites.

Sites of Ectopic Pregnancy

The vast majority (>90%) of ectopic pregnancies occur in the fallopian tube; however, as Table 1-5 indicates, the conceptus can implant anywhere in the abdominal or pelvic cavity. Figure 1-21 shows the more common ectopic implantation sites.

Clinical Presentation

The clinical presentation associated with ectopic pregnancy sometimes includes the "classic triad": pain, bleeding, and a palpable adnexal mass. However, this combination of symptoms is present in only 45% of patients who have ectopic pregnancy. More valuable than vague clinical symptoms, by far, is the information provided by correlating serum beta-hCG levels with endovaginal sonography findings.

There are no specific clinical findings that are diagnostic for ectopic pregnancy. Common signs that should cause suspicion include:

- Positive pregnancy test
- Serum beta-hCG levels that may be appropriate for dates or may be decreased for dates
- Palpation of an adnexal mass (which in the presence of a positive serum beta-hCG is highly suspicious)
- Pelvic pain or bleeding within 1–8 weeks following the first missed menstrual period
- Leukocytosis
- Slight fever
- Pain referred to the shoulder caused by intraperitoneal hemorrhage

Sonographic Signs and Diagnostic Criteria

Sonography is one of the most important tools in diagnosing ectopic pregnancy. Most commonly it is used to confirm the presence of an intrauterine pregnancy in a patient with discriminatory levels of serum beta-hCG. Visualization of an intrauterine sac, particularly with identification of embryonic cardiac activity, often is adequate to exclude ectopic pregnancy. The exception to this is in the case of the heterotopic pregnancy, which occurs in 1:4000 to 1:30,000 naturally occurring, unassisted pregnancies.

In patients undergoing ovarian stimulation and assisted reproduction, examining the adnexa with sonography is mandatory despite visualization of an intrauterine pregnancy, because they have a tenfold increased risk of heterotopic pregnancy. The adnexa should also be examined carefully if an intrauterine pregnancy is not identified. When an adnexal mass is visualized, it should be examined for yolk sac, embryo, and cardiac activity. The cul-de-sac must also be evaluated for free fluid. A small amount of fluid is seen in both normal and abnormal pregnancies; however, a large amount of fluid, particularly complex fluid, is more highly suggestive of ectopic pregnancy. Complex fluid is suggestive of blood and possibly ectopic pregnancy.

The following are the characteristic sonographic signs of ectopic pregnancy. It is important to note, however, that approximately 25% of patients who have an ectopic pregnancy have a normal sonogram:

- *Extrauterine gestational sac*: Identification of an extrauterine gestational sac with yolk sac is pathognomonic for ectopic pregnancy (Figure 1-22A).
- *Empty uterus*: An intrauterine gestational sac should be identified with endovaginal sonography when the serum beta-hCG levels reach 800–1000 mIU/ml (2IS).

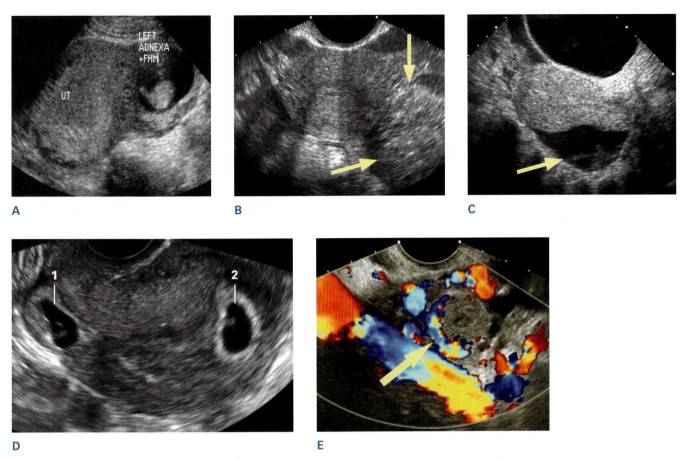

Figure 1-22. A Endovaginal coronal section demonstrating an empty uterus (UT) and an intact 8-week gestational sac in the left adnexa. Real-time imaging demonstrated embryonic cardiovascular activity. **B** Coronal endovaginal section demonstrating an empty uterus and a complex cystic and solid mass in the left adnexa (arrows). **C** Free fluid in the cul-de-sac: Sagittal transabdominal image demonstrating an empty uterus with a complex fluid collection in the posterior cul-de-sac (arrow). **D** Heterotopic pregnancy: Coronal endovaginal section demonstrating an ectopic pregnancy in the right adnexa (1) with a concomitant intrauterine gestational sac (2). **E** "Ring of fire" sign (arrow): Hemodynamically active trophoblastic tissue surrounding an ectopically implanted conceptus is demonstrated by high-amplitude, high-volume flow patterns when imaged with color Doppler.

- *Adnexal mass*: Visualization of extrauterine adnexal ring, yolk sac, and heartbeat is consistent with ectopic pregnancy. Also, a complex adnexal mass (Figure 1-22B) separate from the ovary is quite suspicious for ectopic pregnancy in a patient with a positive pregnancy test.
- *Free fluid* in the cul-de-sac (Figure 1-22C), adnexa, or paracolic gutters (spaces between the abdominal wall and the colon) is suspicious for ectopic pregnancy. Fluid is a nonspecific finding for ectopic pregnancy, though a large amount of fluid is suggestive of ectopic pregnancy. Complex fluid is consistent with hemoperitoneum (blood in the peritoneal cavity) and is associated with ectopic pregnancy but not necessarily rupture of the fallopian tube. Statistically, a viable conceptus implanted normally within the endometrial cavity excludes ectopic pregnancy.
- *Heterotopic pregnancy*: The risk of concomitant intra- and extrauterine implantations, *heterotopic pregnancy*, ranges from 1:4000 to 1:30,000 in a normal population and 1:2600 in patients participating in assisted reproductive technology protocols (Figure 1-22D).
- *Ring of fire sign*: Trophoblastic tissue surrounding an ectopically implanted conceptus is hemodynamically active and frequently demonstrates high-amplitude, high-volume flow patterns when imaged with color Doppler (Figure 1-22E).
- *Pseudogestational sac of ectopic pregnancy*: Visualization of an intrauterine fluid collection with a double sac sign is a more reliable indicator of normal

early intrauterine pregnancy than the intradecidual sac. However, the double sac sign does not absolutely rule out a *pseudogestational sac*: an anechoic, well-circumscribed intrauterine fluid collection that can mimic a normal early intrauterine gestation. The presence of the yolk sac and embryo further confirm the diagnosis of a normal intrauterine pregnancy. In any case, it is important to evaluate the adnexa, particularly in those patients who have undergone in vitro fertilization.

- *Decidual cyst*: The presence of simple cysts in the deciduas can also mimic an early intrauterine pregnancy. Cysts can be differentiated from normal gestational sacs in that they lack the normal decidual ring found around a normally implanted intrauterine pregnancy.

GESTATIONAL TROPHOBLASTIC DISEASE

Gestational trophoblastic disease (GTD) is a spectrum of pathologic entities resulting from the excessive proliferation of trophoblastic tissue. While gestational trophoblastic disease most commonly occurs during or shortly after intrauterine implantation of a fertilized ovum, it can occur months to years after any type of pregnancy. Maternal genomes control the growth of the embryo; paternal genomes control the proliferation of trophoblastic tissue that ultimately becomes the placenta. Excessive paternal genetic material resulting from duplicated chromosomes in the sperm, lack of chromosomes in the ovum, and fertilization of a single ovum by two spermatozoa is the generally accepted etiologic mechanism for primary gestational trophoblastic disease.

Clinical findings associated with gestational trophoblastic disease are often pathognomonic. Rapid enlargement of the uterus with the expulsion of cystic vesicles *per vaginam* is the classic presentation of hydatidiform mole. Correlation of less predictive clinical signs with laboratory evaluation—particularly serial serum beta-hCG levels, which rise rapidly in the presence of excessive trophoblastic proliferation—is the usual method of diagnosis. The spectrum of clinical findings associated with gestational trophoblastic disease includes:

- Grossly elevated beta-hCG levels
- Hyperemesis gravidarum
- Rapid enlargement of the uterus
- Expulsion of vesicles

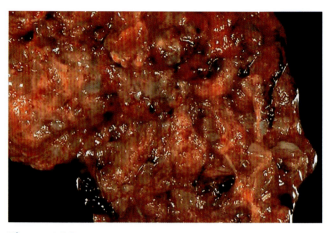

Figure 1-23. Gross pathologic specimen of a complete hydatidiform mole.

- Uterine bleeding in the first trimester
- Absence of fetal heart tones
- Theca-lutein cysts (also caused by multiple pregnancies)
- Onset of pre-eclampsia
- Hyperthyroidism

Complete Hydatidiform Mole

A complete hydatidiform mole is the most common form of gestational trophoblastic disease and occurs in 1 in 1200 pregnancies in the United States.[7] The chorionic villi in complete moles are diffusely hydropic and are enveloped by hyperplastic and atypical trophoblasts (Figure 1-23). No identifiable embryonic or fetal tissue is present. There is a 5% risk of recurrence, and up to 20% of complete moles develop persistent disease requiring additional therapy. Maternal risk factors include being very young (i.e., in the early teens), being over 40 years of age, and having a diet deficient in protein and folic acid.

Sonographic Signs

The following are the characteristic sonographic signs of complete hydatidiform mole:

- Filling of the endometrial cavity with heterogeneous echogenic material (Figure 1-24A)
- A vesicular appearance (Figure 1-24B)
- Increased uterine size
- Fluid collections surrounding a molar mass (not always but sometimes)
- Appearance that mimics a degenerating myoma
- Adnexal theca-lutein cysts (Figures 1-24C–E)

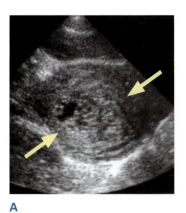 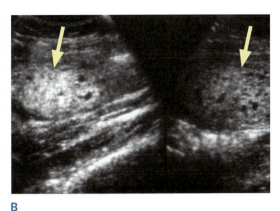 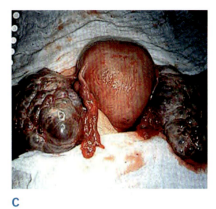

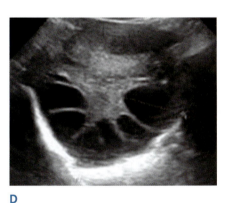 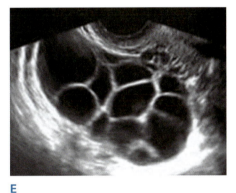

Figure 1-24. **A** Sagittal transabdominal image of a complete hydatidiform mole filling the uterine cavity with heterogeneous echogenic material (arrows). **B** Sagittal and transverse images demonstrating a vesicular pattern in a complete hydatidiform mole (arrows). **C** Gross pathologic specimen of bilateral theca-lutein cysts and an enlarged uterus containing a complete hydatidiform mole. **D** Endovaginal coronal sonographic appearance of a large theca-lutein cyst. **E** Endovaginal sagittal sonographic appearance of a different large theca-lutein cyst.

Partial Mole

A partial mole is the incomplete degeneration of a conceptus into trophoblastic tissue. Two types of chorionic villi are found in partial moles. While some villi appear relatively normal, others have hydropic swelling (trophoblastic hyperplasia). Fetal and/or embryonic tissue is frequently identified. These fetuses, however, typically exhibit the malformations of triploidy, including syndactyly, hydrocephalus, and intrauterine growth restriction (IUGR).

Sonographic Signs

The following are the characteristic sonographic signs of a partial mole:

- Grossly enlarged placenta with variously sized cystic places within (molar placenta) (Figure 1-25)
- Focal or diffuse areas of increased echogenicity in or about the placenta
- Presence of coexisting fetal tissue (in which case the diagnosis is virtually certain)
- Grossly abnormal fetus (triploidy malformations)

Mole with Coexisting Fetus

A *hydatidiform mole with a coexisting fetus* actually falls outside the realm of true gestational trophoblastic disease. Technically, two conceptions occur: One develops normally while one develops into a molar pregnancy, and both occupy the uterine cavity simultaneously. The fetus usually has a normal karyotype. This condition is rare, occurring in 1:10,000 to 1:100,000 of gestations.[8]

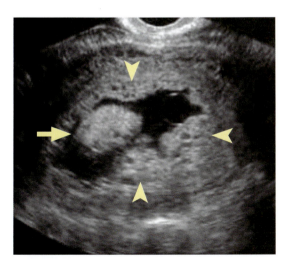

Figure 1-25. Coronal endovaginal image demonstrating an abnormal fetus (arrow) and molar-appearing placental tissue (arrowheads).

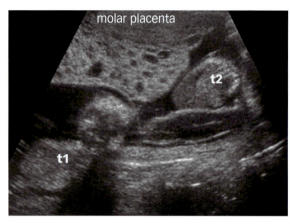 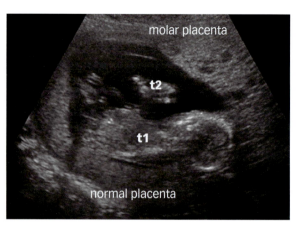

Figure 1-26. Hydatidiform mole with coexisting fetus in a twin pregnancy. **A** Transverse transabdominal image demonstrating a molar placenta belonging to twin 2 (t2) and a normal-appearing co-twin in a separate amniotic sac (t1). **B** Sagittal image in the same pregnancy demonstrating molar placental tissue on the anterior uterine wall associated with twin 2 (t2) and normal placenta on the posterior uterine wall associated with the normal twin 1 (t1).

Sonographic Signs
The sonographic signs of a hydatidiform mole with a coexisting fetus are similar to those for partial mole (Figures 1-26A and B).

Hydropic Degeneration of the Placenta
Hydropic degeneration of the placenta is a pathologic phenomenon characterized by the presence of numerous cystic areas within a generally enlarged placenta. It is not considered a part of the gestational trophoblastic disease spectrum; however, it may be associated with partial mole and paternal triploidy syndromes. When it occurs as simple hydropic degeneration in the first trimester, it is associated with an increased risk of fetal demise.[9]

Sonographic Signs
The following are the characteristic sonographic signs of hydropic degeneration of the placenta:
- May be similar to hydatidiform mole
- Focal cystic and echogenic areas within the placenta
- Placental enlargement

Persistent Trophoblastic Neoplasia
Persistent trophoblastic neoplasia (PTN) is a complication of pregnancy that most commonly follows gestational trophoblastic disease but can also (uncommonly) occur after normal term delivery, spontaneous abortion, or even ectopic pregnancy. Following evacuation and treatment of the initial type of gestational trophoblastic disease, some cells remain in situ and again begin to proliferate. If left untreated, persistent trophoblastic neoplasia can progress into one of the malignant types of recurrent gestational trophoblastic disease discussed in the next section. Patients with severe histologic types of initial trophoblastic proliferation are at highest risk for persistent trophoblastic neoplasia; the lowest risk is associated with partial molar pregnancy.[10]

Sonographic Signs
Characteristic sonographic signs of persistent trophoblastic neoplasia include the following:
- Heterogeneous uterine mass
- Multiple lacunae around the periphery of the mass with high-amplitude, low-resistance blood flow demonstrated with Doppler ultrasound

GESTATIONAL TROPHOBLASTIC NEOPLASIA
Gestational trophoblastic neoplasia (GTN) refers to the spectrum of pathologic entities that may follow treatment of either a complete or a partial hydatidiform mole. The typical clinical scenario has the patient returning for regular quantitative serum beta-hCG titers following molar evacuation—initially every week and then monthly for six months. An elevation of beta-hCG levels during this surveillance period raises the specter of the recurrent proliferation of trophoblastic tissue and warrants additional clinical, laboratory, and sonographic testing. Recurrent gestational trophoblastic disease has significant malignant potential and may

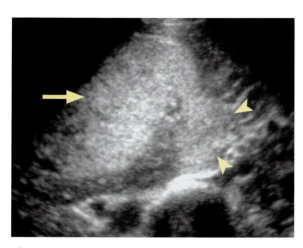

Figure 1-27. Transverse image through the lateral uterine wall demonstrating an echogenic, molar-appearing placenta (arrow) invading the uterine wall (arrowheads).

metastasize distantly to the patient's lungs, lower genital tract, brain, liver, kidney, and gastrointestinal tract. Pathologic classification of gestational trophoblastic neoplasia includes:

- Invasive mole
- Uterine choriocarcinoma
- Placental site trophoblastic tumors (PSTTs)
- Epithelioid trophoblastic neoplasia

Invasive Mole

An *invasive mole*, also called *chorioadenoma destruens*, is a rare form of gestational trophoblastic disease in which molar tissue invades the myometrium or adjacent anatomic structures. Complications of uterine invasion may include penetration of the uterine wall, causing uterine rupture and hemoperitoneum. Microscopic findings are the same as those seen in the hydatidiform mole.

Invasive mole is considered the malignant, nonmetastatic form of gestational trophoblastic disease and occurs in 2%–5% of all cases of gestational trophoblastic neoplasia. It is believed to follow hydatidiform mole in approximately 50% of cases; 25% follow term pregnancy, and 25% follow therapeutic abortion.

Sonographic Signs

The following are the characteristic sonographic signs of invasive mole:

- Presence of focal or diffuse echogenic material within the endometrial cavity
- Possible extension into the myometrium (Figure 1-27)
- Irregular, sonolucent areas that may be seen surrounding trophoblastic tissue
- Adnexal theca-lutein cysts

Uterine Choriocarcinoma

Uterine choriocarcinoma, also called *gestational choriocarcinoma*, is a pure epithelial tumor composed of syncytiotrophoblastic and cytotrophoblastic cells. Microscopic examination reveals the absence of the hydropic villi that are pathologically characteristic of other, primary forms of gestational trophoblastic disease. Instead, sheets or foci of trophoblasts are identified on a background of hemorrhage and necrosis. Choriocarcinoma is considered the malignant, metastatic form of gestational trophoblastic disease.

Choriocarcinoma accounts for approximately 5% of all gestational trophoblastic neoplasia and arises in about 1 in 40 patients with a previously existing molar pregnancy.[11] It may also arise following ectopic pregnancy.

Sonographic Signs

The following are the characteristic sonographic signs of uterine choriocarcinoma:

- Enlarged uterus
- Eccentrically situated irregular, complex mass within the uterus (Figure 1-28A)
- Low-resistance hemodynamic patterns in and around the mass (Figure 1-28B)

Placental Site Trophoblastic Tumor

Placental site trophoblastic tumor (PSTT) is a rare form of gestational trophoblastic disease that may occur after delivery of a normal pregnancy, following evacuation and treatment of a hydatidiform mole, or even after a terminated pregnancy. Time to presentation can vary widely—between 1 week and 14 years—and up to 30% of patients may present with metastatic lesions at the time of diagnosis.[12]

Sonographic Signs

The following are the characteristic sonographic signs of placental site trophoblastic tumor:

- Enlarged uterus
- Heterogeneous lesion within the uterus
- Anechoic lacunae surrounding the lesion with low-resistance blood flow demonstrated with Doppler ultrasound

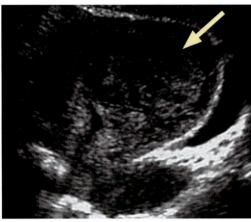
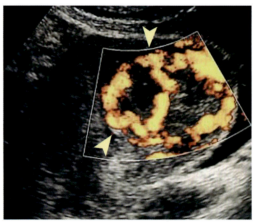

Figure 1-28. A Sagittal transabdominal image demonstrating a large, complex mass (uterine choriocarcinoma) filling the uterine cavity (arrow). **B** Power Doppler imaging demonstrates hypervascularization (arrowheads) of the mass in Figure 1-28A. Courtesy of South African Society of Obstetrics & Gynecology.

CHAPTER 1 REVIEW QUESTIONS

1. Laboratory evaluation for the diagnosis of pregnancy typically centers on measuring maternal serum levels of all of the following EXCEPT:
   A. Beta-hCG
   B. Early pregnancy factor
   C. Luteinizing hormone
   D. Progesterone

2. Human chorionic gonadotropin is actively secreted by:
   A. Trophoblastic tissue
   B. Ovaries
   C. Pituitary gland
   D. Adrenal gland

3. In measuring serum levels of beta-hCG, the Second International Standard (2IS) is generally:
   A. Equal to the First International Reference Preparation (1st IRP) level
   B. Half the 1st IRP level
   C. Twice the 1st IRP level
   D. Three times greater than the 1st IRP level

4. What is the name of the conceptus when it implants in the uterine lining?
   A. Zygote
   B. Morula
   C. Blastocyst
   D. Yolk sac

5. When does the trilaminar disc form?
   A. During implantation
   B. During neurulation
   C. During gastrulation
   D. During transit through the fallopian tube

6. The earliest sonographic sign of the presence of an intrauterine pregnancy is:
   A. Decidual thickening
   B. Double bleb sign
   C. Double sac sign
   D. Yolk sac

7. How does conceptual age relate to menstrual age?
   A. Conceptual age is 7 days greater than menstrual age.
   B. Conceptual age is 14 days greater than menstrual age.
   C. Conceptual age is 7 days less than menstrual age.
   D. Conceptual age is 14 days less than menstrual age.

8. The fluid-filled gestational sac is first visible sonographically at:
   A. 4.5–5.0 menstrual weeks
   B. 5.0–5.5 menstrual weeks
   C. 5.5–6.0 menstrual weeks
   D. 6.0–6.5 menstrual weeks

9. A normal gestational sac grows at the rate of approximately:
   A. 0.5 mm per day
   B. 1.0 mm per day
   C. 1.5 mm per day
   D. 2.0 mm per day

10. The sonographic presence of a small fluid-filled sac contained within the decidua at approximately 4–4.5 weeks is known as the:
    A. Double bleb sign
    B. Double sac sign
    C. Intradecidual sign
    D. Pseudogestational sac sign

11. All of the following are sonographic characteristics of a normal intrauterine gestational sac EXCEPT:
    A. Round, well-defined borders
    B. Irregular, echogenic borders
    C. Positioned in the mid portion of the uterine cavity
    D. Echogenic, intact borders

12. What is the name of the sonographic sign when the yolk sac is immediately adjacent to a similarly sized amnion?
    A. Secondary yolk sac
    B. Double bleb sign
    C. Double decidual sac sign
    D. Seagull sign

13. The echogenic ring formed by the decidua vera and decidua capsularis is called the:
    A. Double bleb sign
    B. Double decidual sac sign
    C. Intradecidual sign
    D. Pseudogestational sac sign

14. The double decidual sac sign is typically demonstrated by:
    A. 4.5–5.0 weeks
    B. 5.0–5.5 weeks
    C. 5.5–6.0 weeks
    D. 6.0–6.5 weeks

15. The yolk sac is typically demonstrated by:
    A. 3–4 weeks
    B. 4–5 weeks
    C. 5–6 weeks
    D. 6–7 weeks

16. What is the mean sac diameter at the earliest point that the normal yolk sac becomes visible?
    A. 4.0 mm
    B. 4.5 mm
    C. 5.0 mm
    D. 5.5 mm

17. A normal yolk sac will always be visualized when the mean sac diameter measures:
    A. ≥5.0 mm
    B. ≥6.0 mm
    C. ≥7.0 mm
    D. ≥8.0 mm

18. Embryonic cardiac activity may be visualized when the crown-rump length is approximately:
    A. 1–3 mm
    B. 2–4 mm
    C. 3–5 mm
    D. 4–6 mm

19. When does normal embryonic midgut herniation occur?
    A. 6 menstrual weeks
    B. 7 menstrual weeks
    C. 8 menstrual weeks
    D. 10 menstrual weeks

20. By when does normal embryonic midgut herniation regress back into the abdominal cavity?
    A. 11 menstrual weeks
    B. 12 menstrual weeks
    C. 13 menstrual weeks
    D. 14 menstrual weeks

21. The arrow in this image points to:

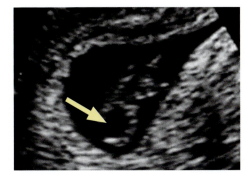

A. Hydrocephalus
B. Cisterna magna
C. Embryonic rhombencephalon
D. Nuchal translucency

22. All of the following sonographic findings are reliable indicators of abnormal early pregnancy EXCEPT:
    A. Mean sac diameter < 8 mm without a yolk sac
    B. Crown-rump length > 16 mm without an embryo
    C. Embryo > 5 mm without cardiovascular activity
    D. Amniotic sac noted without an embryo

23. All of the following sonographic findings are indicators of a failed first trimester gestation EXCEPT:
    A. Irregular shape of gestational sac
    B. Double sac sign
    C. Eccentric position of sac in uterine cavity
    D. Mean sac diameter growth rate < 0.6 mm per day

24. Physiologic termination of pregnancy prior to 20 weeks' gestation is called:
    A. Blighted ovum
    B. Anembryonic pregnancy
    C. Spontaneous abortion
    D. Therapeutic abortion

25. All of the following sonographic findings are consistent with a spontaneous complete abortion EXCEPT:
    A. Complex echogenic material in the uterine cavity
    B. Empty uterus with "clean" endometrial stripe
    C. Moderate to bright endometrial echoes
    D. Uterine enlargement

26. All of the following sonographic findings are consistent with an incomplete abortion EXCEPT:
    A. Complex echogenic material in the uterine cavity
    B. Acoustic shadowing from air bubbles in the uterine cavity
    C. Persistent trophoblastic Doppler waveforms near the endometrial cavity
    D. Empty uterus with "clean" endometrial stripe

27. What is the name for the presence of an intact gestational sac in the endometrial cavity measuring ≥ 25 mm without an accompanying embryo?
    A. Complete spontaneous abortion
    B. Anembryonic pregnancy
    C. Incomplete abortion
    D. Fetal demise

28. Implantation of a conceptus anywhere outside the central portion of the endometrial cavity is called:
    A. Ectopic pregnancy
    B. Incomplete abortion
    C. Missed abortion
    D. Blighted ovum

29. Approximately 80% of ectopic pregnancies implant in the:
    A. Uterine cornu
    B. Cervix
    C. Ampullary portion of the fallopian tube
    D. Interstitial portion of the fallopian tube

30. What sonographic finding is pathognomonic for ectopic pregnancy?
    A. Empty uterus in a patient with a positive pregnancy test
    B. Identification of an extrauterine gestational sac with live embryo
    C. Free fluid in the cul-de-sac
    D. Complex adnexal mass in a patient with a positive pregnancy test

31. What is the term for the concomitant implantations of both an intrauterine and an extrauterine conceptus?
    A. Ectopic pregnancy
    B. Heterotopic pregnancy
    C. Supernumerary pregnancy
    D. Twin pregnancy

32. All of the following sonographic findings are non-specific indicators of ectopic pregnancy EXCEPT:
    A. Free fluid in the cul-de-sac
    B. Empty uterus in a patient with a positive pregnancy test
    C. Identification of an extrauterine gestational sac with yolk sac
    D. Doppler "ring of fire" sign around a complex adnexal mass

33. All of the following are clinical signs associated with gestational trophoblastic disease EXCEPT:
    A. Beta-hCG levels less than expected for dates
    B. Beta-hCG levels greater than expected for dates
    C. First trimester vaginal bleeding
    D. Hyperemesis gravidarum

34. Which of the following ovarian pathologies is associated with hydatidiform mole?
    A. Corpus luteum cysts
    B. Follicular cysts
    C. Paraovarian cysts
    D. Theca-lutein cysts

35. What term refers to the pathologic entity in which an intrauterine gestation is composed completely of multisized hydropic villi?
    A. Hydatidiform mole
    B. Cornual pregnancy
    C. Anembryonic pregnancy
    D. Hydropic degeneration of placenta

36. A rare form of gestational trophoblastic disease in which molar tissue invades the myometrium or adjacent anatomic structures is called:
    A. Chorioadenoma destruens
    B. Uterine choriocarcinoma
    C. Placenta accreta
    D. Placenta percreta

37. A patient presents with a serum beta-hCG titer at discriminatory levels. She complains of lower-quadrant pain and vaginal spotting. Sonographic examination of the adnexa produces the results shown in this image. The most likely diagnosis is:

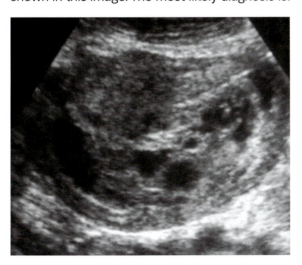

A. Complete abortion
B. Invasive mole
C. Ectopic pregnancy
D. Hydatidiform mole

38. A patient presents at a firm 8 weeks post LMP. Her beta-hCG titers are consistent with 5.5 weeks. She complains of mild vaginal bleeding and lower midline pain. Endovaginal sonography yields this image. The most likely diagnosis is:

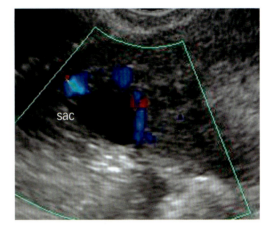

A. Interstitial ectopic pregnancy
B. Missed abortion
C. Pelvic inflammatory disease
D. Hydrocolpos

39. Five days following an episode of brisk vaginal bleeding accompanied by clots and tissue, this patient returns to her practitioner with complaints of continued bleeding, pain, and a mild fever. Her beta-hCG levels are low positive. Sonographic examination of the uterus yields this image. This patient probably has a(n):

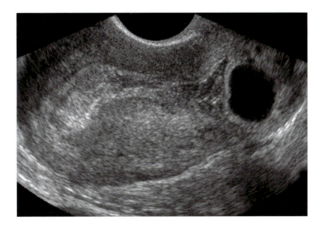

A. Ectopic pregnancy
B. Incomplete abortion

C. Persistent trophoblastic neoplasia
D. Choriocarcinoma

40. The sonographic findings in these images are most consistent with:

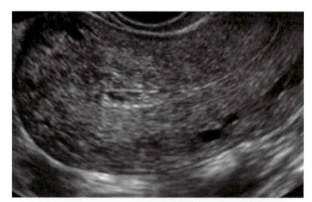

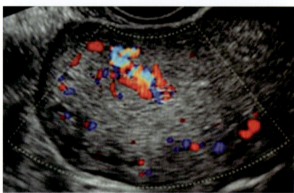

A. Complete hydatidiform mole
B. Partial hydatidiform mole
C. Chorioadenoma destruens
D. Placental abruption

41. The arrow in this image of a 10-week fetus is pointing to:

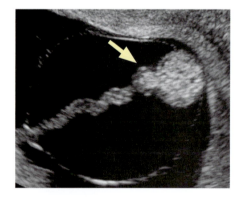

A. Gastroschisis
B. Normal embryonic midgut herniation
C. Omphalocele
D. Umbilical vein thrombosis

42. A patient presents with a positive pregnancy test, vaginal bleeding, and mid-pelvic pain. A coronal section through the uterus is presented in this image. The most likely diagnosis is:

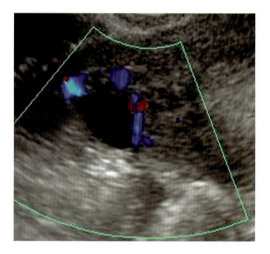

A. Missed abortion
B. Normal intrauterine pregnancy
C. Interstitial ectopic pregnancy
D. Gestational trophoblastic disease

43. A patient presents with a history of a hydatidiform mole evacuated 3 months prior. Routine serum surveillance demonstrates a sudden increase in beta-hCG levels. This image raises the suspicion of:

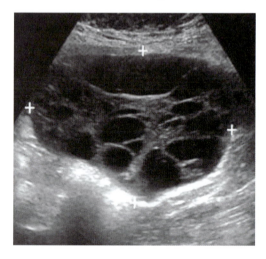

A. Stein-Leventhal syndrome
B. Retained molar tissue
C. Recurrent trophoblastic disease
D. Abdominal abscess

ANSWERS

See Appendix A on page 477 for answers.

REFERENCES

1. Fan XG, Zheng ZQ: A study of early pregnancy factor activity in preimplantation. Am J Reprod Immunology 37:359–364, 1977.

2. Bangham DR, Woodward PM: The Second International Standard for serum gonadotropin. Bull World Health Organ 35:761–773, 1966.

3. Connolly A, Ryan DH, Stuebe AM, et al: Reevaluation of discriminatory and threshold levels for serum β-hCG in early pregnancy. Obstet Gynecol 121:65–70, 2013.

4. Kaur A, Kaur A: Transvaginal ultrasonography in first trimester of pregnancy and its comparison with transabdominal ultrasonography. J Pharm Bioallied Sci 3:329–338, 2011.

5. Yeh HC: Sonographic signs of early pregnancy. Crit Rev Diagn Imaging 28:181–211, 1988.

6. The ALARA principle stipulates that exposure to ultrasound waves should be kept "as low as reasonably achievable."

7. Atrash HK, Hogue CJ, Grimes DA: Epidemiology of hydatidiform mole during early gestation. Am J Obstet Gynecol 154:906–909, 1986.

8. Chen FP: Molar pregnancy and living normal fetus coexisting until term: prenatal biochemical and sonographic diagnosis. Hum Reprod 12:853–856, 1997.

9. Buschi AJ, Brenbridge AN, Cochrane JA, et al: Hydropic degeneration of the placenta simulating hydatidiform mole. J Clin Ultrasound 7:60–61, 1979.

10. Kuyumcuoglu Y, Guzel A, Redemoglu M, et al: Risk factors for persistent trophoblastic neoplasia. J Exp Ther Oncol 9:81–84, 2011.

11. Smith HO, Kohorn E, Cole LA: Choriocarcinoma and gestational trophoblastic disease. Obstet Gynecol Clin North Am 32:661–684, 2005.

12. Vitellas KM, Bennett WF, Bova JG: Case 2: placental site trophoblastic tumor. Am J Roentgenol 175:896, 2000.

SUGGESTED READINGS

Callen PW: The obstetric ultrasound examination. In Callen PW (ed): *Ultrasonography in Obstetrics and Gynecology*, 5th edition. Philadelphia, Saunders Elsevier, 2008.

Fielding JR, Brown DL, Thurmond AS: *Gynecologic Imaging*. Philadelphia, Elsevier Saunders, 2011.

Goldstein C, Hagen-Ansert SL: First-trimester complications. In Hagen-Ansert SL (ed): *Textbook of Diagnostic Ultrasonography*, 7th edition. St. Louis, Elsevier Mosby, 2012, pp 1081–1102.

Levi CS, Lyons EA: The first trimester. In Rumack CM, Wilson SR, Charboneau JW, et al (eds): *Diagnostic Ultrasound*, 4th edition. Philadelphia, Elsevier Mosby, 2011, pp 1072–1118.

Malone FD: First trimester screening for aneuploidy. In Callen PW (ed): *Ultrasonography in Obstetrics and Gynecology*, 5th edition. Philadelphia, Saunders Elsevier, 2008.

Moore KL, Persaud TVN: *Before We Are Born*, 8th edition. Philadelphia, Saunders Elsevier, 2011, pp 29–70.

Scharf JH: *Essentials of Obstetrics and Gynecology: A Comprehensive Sonographer's Guide*, 2nd edition. Forney, TX, Pegasus Lectures, 2008.

Spitz JL: The normal first trimester. In Hagen-Ansert SL (ed): *Textbook of Diagnostic Ultrasonography*, 7th edition. St. Louis, Elsevier Mosby, 2012, pp 1064–1080.

CHAPTER 2

The Placenta

Embryology

Placental Anatomy and Physiology

Placental Variants and Abnormalities

The *placenta* is the life-giving link between the fetus and the mother. Anatomically, it is a highly vascularized, discoid organ occupying the same intrauterine space as the fetus. Its size, position, and attachment to the uterine wall—abnormalities and variations of which are reliably demonstrable sonographically—have a significant impact on the normal progression of a pregnancy. Physiologically, the placenta provides oxygen and nutrition to the fetus and carries away byproducts of fetal metabolism via the mother's vascular system. Hemodynamically, the placenta is a perfusional powerhouse, with increasingly high-volume, low-resistance flow on the maternal side and pulsatile output of the baby's circulation entering the fetal side as the pregnancy progresses to term. The complex hemodynamic patterns produced by the apposition of these two separate circulatory systems are amenable to interrogation with all the Doppler modalities available on contemporary ultrasound imaging systems.

EMBRYOLOGY

Approximately 1 week after conception (3 menstrual weeks), the developing conceptus or blastocyst burrows into the uterine wall (*endometrium*) and the placenta begins to develop (Figure 2-1). The blastocyst's outer layer, the *trophoblast*, is composed of the *cytotrophoblast* (underlying layer of cells) and the *syncytiotrophoblast*, which will become the surface layer of the placenta. By approximately 3.5 menstrual weeks, the syncytiotrophoblast has eroded the endometrial tissues (capillaries, glands, and connective tissue), allowing maternal blood to seep out and surround implanted villous tissue and establishing a primitive *uteroplacental circulation*. By approximately 4.5 menstrual weeks, the gestational sac is visible transvaginally and is surrounded by an echogenic rim of tissue that represents the developing placenta.

DECIDUAL LAYERS

By 4.5 menstrual weeks, the placental tissue—which will grow throughout the pregnancy—has developed numerous *villi* (singular, *villus*), fingerlike vascular projections that surround the site of implantation. As the implanted blastocyst begins to grow out into the uterine cavity, it pushes the surrounding layer of decidua out into the cavity, resulting in three layers of decidua (Figures 2-2A and B):

- *Decidua basalis* (also called *decidua serotina*): the layer that develops where the blastocyst implants and contributes to the maternal portion of the placenta; the villi adjacent to the myometrium extend into this layer to form the *chorion frondosum*.

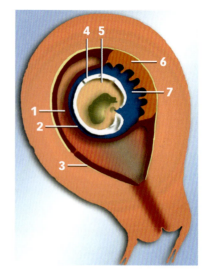

Figure 2-1. Early placentation: schematic representation of the decidual layers, membranes, and cavities. 1 = decidua capsularis, 2 = chorion laeve, 3 = decidua parietalis, 4 = chorionic cavity, 5 = amniotic cavity, 6 = decidua basalis, 7 = chorion frondosum.

- *Decidua parietalis* (also called *decidua vera*): the nonplacental lining of the uterine cavity.
- *Decidua capsularis* (also called *decidua reflexa*): the layer overlying the blastocyst that closes over and surrounds it and progressively diminishes as the chorionic sac grows.

During first trimester sonographic examination, the chorion frondosum can be seen as a thickened, echogenic area adjacent to the gestational sac at the site of implantation, usually opposite the "double sac sign." By 10–12 menstrual weeks, the thickened portion of the placenta adjacent to the myometrium is visible sonographically. By 12–13 weeks (end of the first trimester),

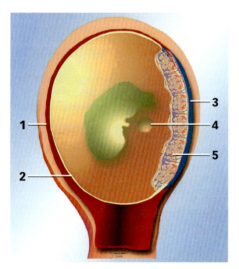
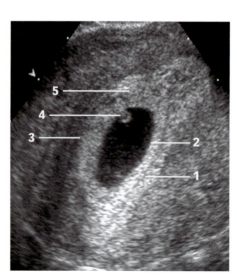

Figure 2-2. **A** Illustration and **B** sonogram of decidual layers. 1 = decidua parietalis, 2 = decidua capsularis, 3 = decidua basalis, 4 = yolk sac, 5 = chorion frondosum.

A B

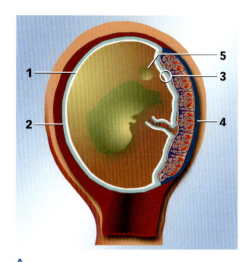
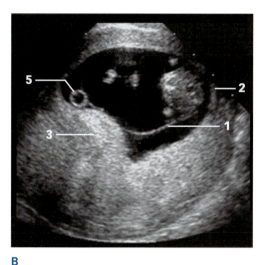

Figure 2-3. A Illustration and **B** sonogram of membranes and yolk sac. 1 = amniotic membrane, 2 = chorionic membrane, 3 = chorionic plate, 4 = basal plate (not visualized in sonogram), and 5 = yolk sac.

the maternal blood supply to the placenta is completely established and blood flow can be observed within the placenta by color and power Doppler.

FORMATION OF MEMBRANES

As mentioned in Chapter 1, the *secondary yolk sac* forms toward the end of menstrual week 4. It is a membranous sac forming along the ventral aspect of an embryo that provides for its early development and is a source for early blood cells. It is considered one of the three embryonic membranes that can be identified sonographically in the first trimester (the others are the chorion and the amnion). Identification of a normal secondary yolk sac with endovaginal ultrasound is one of several critical findings in the normal first trimester (see Figures 2-3A and B).

The *chorion* (*chorion laeve*) arises from extraembryonic mesoderm and the trophoblast. As the pregnancy grows, this chorionic membrane surrounds the non-placental portion of the uterine cavity. The *chorionic plate* consists of the amnion, some extraembryonic tissue, and the chorionic villi, which arise from cyto- and syncytiotrophoblastic tissue. The *basal plate* is the peripheral region on the maternal side of the placenta that is in contact with the uterine wall. Its two tissue layers derive from the cyto- and syncytiotrophoblastic layers on the embryonic side and the decidua basalis on the maternal side (Figure 2-4).

The *amnion* arises from the embryonic epiblast and forms a membranous sac that surrounds the embryo and, later in pregnancy, the fetus. It also forms the epithelial surface of the umbilical cord.

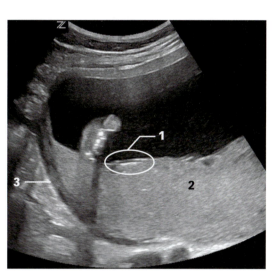

Figure 2-4. Sonogram demonstrating the appearance and relational anatomy between the chorionic plate (1), placenta (2), and basal plate (3).

PLACENTAL ANATOMY AND PHYSIOLOGY

The highly vascular, discoid placenta provides for the nutritional needs of the fetus. Histologically it can be described as the apposition, or fusion, of fetal organs to maternal tissue for the purpose of physiologic exchange. This exchange occurs at the level of the *villus*, which is the basic functional unit of the placenta. There are an estimated 120 villi in a normal placenta at term.[1] Each villus is an extension of the chorionic tissue of the embryo that anastomosed itself to the maternal decidua during implantation.

One or several stem villi, which are anchored to the chorion, arborize into floating villi that project into the pool of maternal blood filling an intervillous space, creating the 15–28 cotyledons typically found in a normal placenta. A *cotyledon* is a separation of the decidua basalis by a placental septum and contains one stem villus. The cotyledon receives fetal blood from the chorionic vessels branching off cotyledon vessels; those vessels in turn arborize into a richly supplied capillary bed. The cotyledons are surrounded by maternal blood, which comes in direct contact with the fetal chorion; there is no direct fluid exchange between the two sides of placental circulation. It is this bathing of fetal tissue by maternal blood at the capillary level that provides for the physiologic exchange of oxygen, nutrients, and metabolites.

Functionally and anatomically, the placenta is divided into two portions, maternal and fetal.

MATERNAL PORTION OF THE PLACENTA

The maternal portion of the placenta (Figure 2-5A) constitutes less than one-fifth (20%) of total placental weight. During the first trimester, it is composed of compressed sheets of decidua basalis and tongue-like projections called *placental septa*, which partition the placenta into the cotyledons.

Maternal blood flow into the cotyledons takes place via the *spiral arteries* that initially perfuse the decidua. The spiral arteries are branches of the basal plate endometrial arteries, which are terminal branches of the bilateral uterine arteries. As the gestation advances, these arteries enlarge and straighten to increase the volume of blood flow into the placenta and to provide for the increased physiologic demands of the conceptus. Blood flows out of the placenta by way of venous conduits in the cotyledons that drain through orifices in the basal plate to the endometrial veins, finally returning to maternal circulation via the uterine veins.

The extensive network of *retroplacental vasculature*, which is the main source of arterial supply and venous drainage of the placenta, carries up to 700 milliliters per minute.[2] Sonographically, the retroplacental vasculature appears as a complex hypoechoic space between the placental body and the uterine wall. With the use of color Doppler imaging, this area lights up with the high-amplitude, high-volume blood flow coursing through the multiple tortuous and intertwined arterial and venous structures (Figure 2-5B).

FETAL PORTION OF THE PLACENTA

The fetal portion of the placenta (Figure 2-6A), which is derived from the syncytiotrophoblastic portion of the conceptus, is the greatest contributor to placental mass, accounting for more than 80% of its total. It is composed of multiple villi, which project into the pools of maternal blood circulating in the intervillous spaces. Each villus receives its blood supply from a stem artery that branches from the eight or more terminal chorionic plate arteries, arborizing from the paired umbilical arteries. The stem artery branches farther into an arteriovenous capillary network that brings fetal blood in close apposition to maternal blood. Relieved of carbon dioxide and waste products carried into the placenta, blood exits the placenta revitalized with oxygen and nutrients and returns to the fetus via the single umbilical vein (Figure 2-6B).

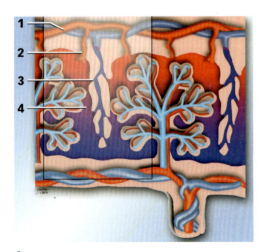

A

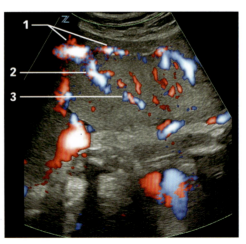

B

Figure 2-5. **A** Illustration and **B** sonogram demonstrating the major vascular components of the maternal side of fetoplacental circulation. 1 = retroplacental vasculature, 2 = spiral artery, 3 = maternal vein, 4 = intervillous spaces (not visualized in the sonogram).

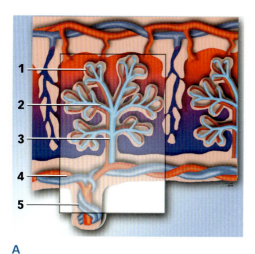
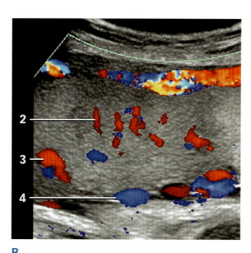

Figure 2-6. **A** Illustration and **B** sonogram demonstrating the major vascular components of the fetal side of fetoplacental circulation. 1 = terminal villi (not visible in the sonogram), 2 = intermediate villi, 3 = main stem villus, 4 = subchorionic umbilical vasculature, 5 = umbilical vessels (not visible in the sonogram).

NORMAL SONOGRAPHIC SIGNS

The following are the characteristic sonographic signs of the normal placenta (Figures 2-7 and 2-8):

- Discoid shape.
- Homogeneous, granular texture.
- Chorionic membrane seen as a bright, smooth, specular reflection covering the fetal surface of the placenta.
- Subchorionic space that appears smooth and uninterrupted except at the site of cord insertion on the placenta. As gestation continues, the presence of fetal subchorionic blood vessels becomes more apparent.
- Retroplacental space that appears hypoechoic, with irregular, linear echogenic areas interspersed throughout. This represents the maternal vasculature portion of the placenta derived from the decidua basalis. As the gestation continues, large venous structures may be identified.
- Measures 2–4 cm in thickness throughout the second and third trimesters.

PLACENTAL VARIANTS AND ABNORMALITIES

Placental variants and abnormalities that may emerge from sonographic evaluation over the course of the pregnancy may include abnormalities of size, abnormal placental aging, extrachorial variants, accessory variations, intraplacental lesions, placenta previa, placental abruption, abnormal adherence, chorioangioma, or placental hydrops. (See Table 2-1.)

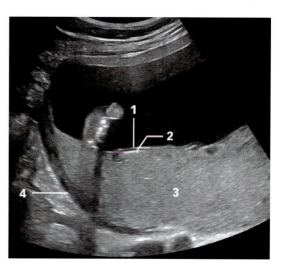

Figure 2-7. Normal placental sonographic appearance. 1 = chorionic membrane, 2 = subchorionic space, 3 = homogeneous, granular texture, 4 = retroplacental space.

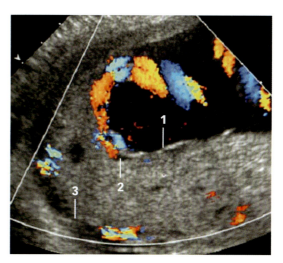

Figure 2-8. Color Doppler image demonstrating placental layers. 1 = chorionic plate, 2 = subchorionic layer (fetal vascular), 3 = retroplacental layer (maternal vascular).

Table 2-1.	Summary of placental variants and abnormalities.
Type	Anomaly
Size abnormalities	Abnormally thin Abnormally thick
Aging abnormalities	—
Extrachorial variants	Circummarginate placenta Circumvallate placenta Placenta membranacea
Accessory variations	Succenturiate lobe Bipartite placenta Annular placenta
Intraplacental lesions	Placental calcifications Hypoechoic/cystic lesions
Placenta previa	Complete previa Partial previa Marginal previa Low-lying placenta Vasa previa
Placental abruption	Concealed abruption External abruption Chronic retroplacental submembranous hematoma Marginal and subchorionic hemorrhage
Abnormal adherence	Placenta accreta Placenta increta Placenta percreta
Chorioangioma	—
Placental hydrops	—

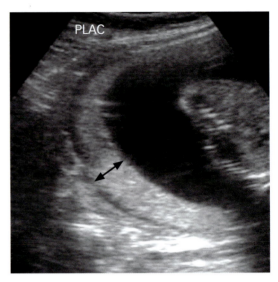

Figure 2-9. Sagittal sonogram through an abnormally thin fundal placenta (PLAC) at 28 weeks. Double arrow = placental thickness of 1.5 cm.

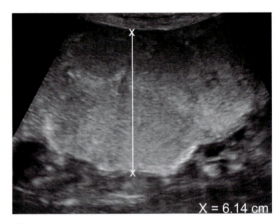

Figure 2-10. Enlarged placenta, with calipers showing a measurement of 6.14 cm—greater than the normal upper limit of thickness of 4 cm.

ABNORMAL PLACENTAL SIZE

As noted above, throughout the second and third trimesters a normal placenta measures 2–4 cm in thickness. As the placenta is a fetal organ, significant abnormalities in its size can reflect concomitant abnormalities with the fetus.

A thin placenta (Figure 2-9) may be associated with the following:

- A small-for-dates fetus or intrauterine growth restriction (IUGR)
- Chromosomal abnormalities
- Severe intrauterine infection
- Severe maternal diabetes mellitus
- Maternal hypertension
- Maternal toxemia

A full-term placenta should not exceed 4 cm in thickness. An abnormally thick placenta (Figure 2-10) may be associated with the following:

- Triploidy
- Diabetes mellitus
- Maternal anemia
- Blood group incompatibilities

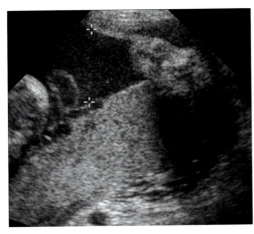
Grade 0

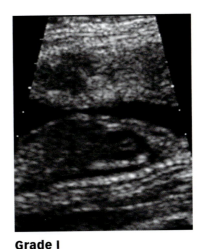
Grade I

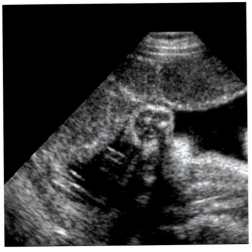
Grade II

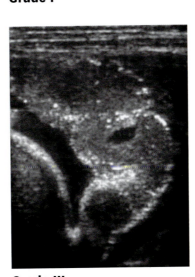
Grade III

Figure 2-11. Grannum's placental grading system: Grade 0 = smooth echo pattern of parenchyma with no calcifications and no indentations; grade I = diffuse, randomly distributed calcifications (2–4 mm); grade II = dot-dash calcifications parallel to the basal plate and larger indentations of the chorionic plate; grade III = larger calcifications and indentations of the basal plate.

- Placental hemorrhage
- Hydrops
- Infection
- Aneuploidy

GRADING FOR PLACENTAL AGE ABNORMALITIES

The primary utility of placental grading is in identifying a prematurely aged placenta, particularly in a patient with underlying comorbidities. The use of grading as an indicator of fetal age or predictor of fetal lung maturity is not reliable. Identification of a grade III placenta in the second or early third trimester may indicate impending placental insufficiency, especially in the presence of underlying maternal medical complications. However, early aging and calcium accumulation can also be related to maternal factors such as cigarette smoking, advanced maternal age (≥35 years), and advanced parity (i.e., the woman's status resulting from the prior delivery of at least two pregnancies).

The traditional sonographic method, Grannum's placental grading system, uses four grades based on structural changes identified in the placenta (Figure 2-11):

- *Grade 0*: Homogeneous placenta with a smooth chorionic plate (late first to early second trimester).
- *Grade I*: Scattered echogenic calcifications throughout the placenta (mid second to early third trimester).
- *Grade II*: Scattered echogenic calcifications throughout the placenta and subtle comma-like densities at the chorionic plate (late third trimester to term).
- *Grade III*: Scattered echogenic calcifications throughout the placenta and at the base, increased comma-like densities at the chorionic plate, and cystic areas within the placenta (39 weeks to post delivery).

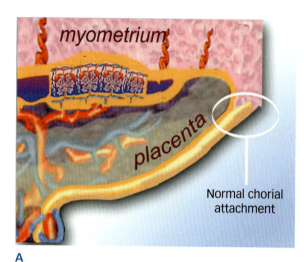

A

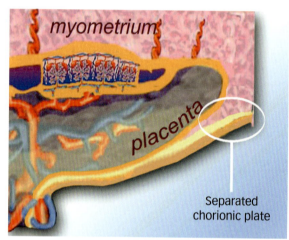

B

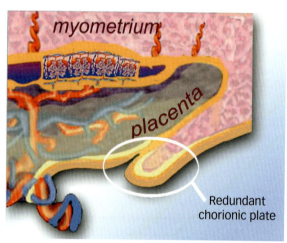

C

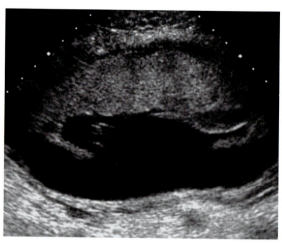

D

Figure 2-12. **A** Normal chorial attachments—extrachorial placental variants. **B** Normal chorial attachments—circummarginate placenta. **C** Circumvallate placenta. **D** Transverse sonographic section through an anterior placenta at 32 weeks, demonstrating a redundant chorionic plate in a circumvallate placenta.

EXTRACHORIAL PLACENTAL VARIANTS

Extrachorial placental variants arise from an abnormal relationship between the outer rim of the placenta and the takeoff of the chorionic membrane. In a normal configuration (Figure 2-12A), the chorionic membrane extends to the very outer edge of the placenta before taking off to envelop the remainder of the uterine cavity.

Circummarginate Placenta

In a *circummarginate placenta* (Figure 2-12B), the short, tight chorionic membrane takes off early and does not extend to the periphery of the placenta. Identification of a circummarginate placenta has been reported in the literature but is not routinely demonstrable sonographically.

Circumvallate Placenta

A *circumvallate placenta* (Figure 2-12C) is characterized by a loose, redundant ring of chorionic membrane encircling its fetal surface. As with the circummarginate variant, the chorion does not extend to the outer edge of the placenta. A circumvallate placenta may be predisposed to early separation from the uterine wall and is associated with antepartum bleeding, intrauterine growth restriction, fetal anomalies, and perinatal death. It has also been implicated as a cause of amniotic band syndrome.

A circumvallate placenta has a unique sonographic appearance and can be identified during imaging of the chorionic plate by visualizing infolding of the fetal membrane onto the placental surface (Figure 2-12D). A circumvallate placenta is demonstrable only during the mid second trimester.

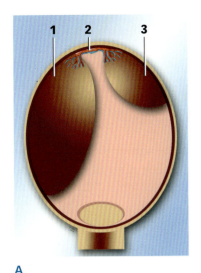 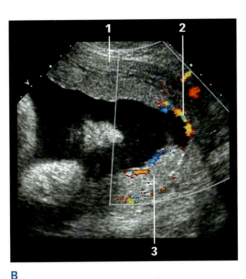

Figure 2-13. A Illustration and **B** sonogram demonstrating a succenturiate lobe of the placenta. 1 = main placental body, 2 = connecting vasculature, 3 = succenturiate (accessory) lobe.

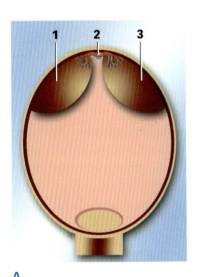 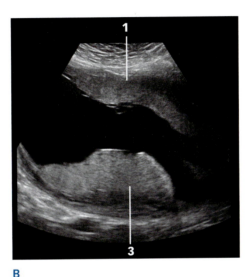

Figure 2-14. A Illustration and **B** sonogram demonstrating a bipartite placenta. 1 = lobe 1, 2 = connecting vasculature (not visualized in the sonogram), 3 = lobe 2.

Placenta Membranacea

Early in pregnancy, the entire surface of the gestational sac is covered with villi; as the pregnancy progresses, the villi usually regress over most of the surface of the sac, and what remains becomes the placenta. If this regression does not occur, the placenta may cover the entire surface of the sac; if it is patchy, there may be two or more separate areas of placental formation. In either case, this condition is called *placenta membranacea*. In this condition, the placenta is thin and is not localized to a specific area. Identification of placenta membranacea is not routinely demonstrable sonographically.

ACCESSORY TYPES OF VARIATION

Alterations in the mechanism of early placentation can create three accessory types of variation, which are characterized by a lobe of the placenta situated distant from the main body of the placenta. As the accessory lobe is fully functional and robustly vascularized, its presence in the lower uterine segment could create catastrophic results should a vaginal delivery be attempted.

Succenturiate Lobe

A *succenturiate lobe* (Figures 2-13A and B) is an accessory cotyledon located away from the main placental body. It is connected to the main placental circulation via large blood vessels that course through the membranes that accompany it.

Bipartite Placenta

A *bipartite placenta* (Figures 2-14A and B) is one that is divided into two approximately equal-sized lobes and is sometimes called a bilobed placenta.

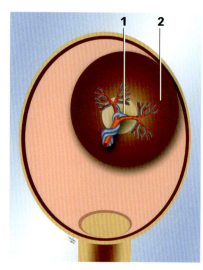

Figure 2-15. Illustration demonstrating the central insertion of the umbilical vessels on a disc-shaped annular placenta. 1 = central insertion of vessels, 2 = disc-shaped placenta.

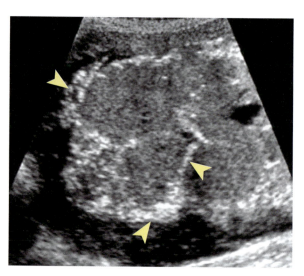

Figure 2-16. Calcifications in a grade III placenta deposited around the periphery of several cotyledons. Arrowheads = calcifications.

Annular Placenta

An *annular placenta* (Figure 2-15) is a ring-shaped placenta that attaches circumferentially to the myometrium. This type of placental variant is rarely diagnosed sonographically.

Sonographic Signs

The primary role of sonography in the evaluation of accessory placental lobes is to rule out vasa previa overlying the internal cervical os.

- Succenturiate lobes and bipartite placentas are identifiable on sonographic examination. Two-dimensional imaging will demonstrate two masses of placental tissue that appear unconnected. Color Doppler imaging will show robust flow in the blood vessels that vascularize the accessory lobe. When the lobes are of almost equal size, the primary lobe can be identified by the presence of the umbilical cord insertion on its chorionic surface.
- Annular placenta is rare, and sonographic detection has not been reported in the recent medical literature.

INTRAPLACENTAL LESIONS

Placental Calcifications

Calcification is a normal part of placental aging (see page 37). After 33 weeks, more than 50% of placentas contain some degree of calcification.[3,4] Calcifications are usually found at the base of the placenta, in the septa, and in the subchorionic and perivillous spaces. Calcification is more common in women of low parity, in those who smoke cigarettes, and in mothers who have thrombotic disorders and are on anticoagulants such as heparin or aspirin therapy. (The anticoagulant warfarin [brand name, Coumadin] crosses the placenta and is associated with embryologic abnormalities; it is usually discontinued in the first trimester. Hence there is no literature on the association of warfarin with placental calcifications.)

Sonographic Signs

The following sonographic signs are associated with placental calcifications:

- Punctate hyperechoic foci are scattered throughout the placenta.
- Calcifications may be localized to basal or subchorionic layers or the placental parenchyma (Figure 2-16).

Hypoechoic/Cystic Lesions

Cystic or *hypoechoic lesions* in the placenta are observed fairly commonly, particularly after 25 weeks' gestation. Most are not clinically significant. From a sonographic perspective, these cystic or hypoechoic lesions can be divided into three general groups: those that are subchorionic, those in the mid-placental region, and those identified near the basal plate.

Subchorionic Lesions

Subchorionic lesions and cystic or hypoechoic areas immediately under the chorionic membrane adjacent to the fetal surface of the placenta are typically acute

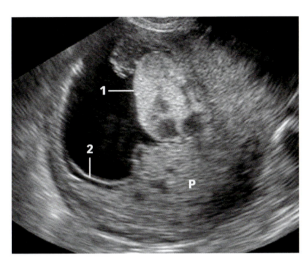

Figure 2-17. Endovaginal sonogram demonstrating a focal, echogenic subchorionic hematoma in a first trimester pregnancy. 1 = subchorionic hematoma, 2 = chorionic membrane, P = placenta.

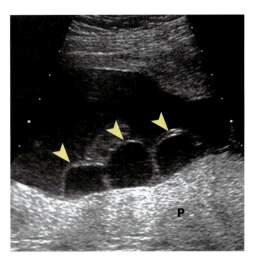

Figure 2-18. Sonographic demonstration of three subchorionic cysts. Arrowheads = subchorionic cysts, P = placenta.

or chronic areas of thrombus. Rarely, well-defined subchorionic cysts may be observed. Such cysts do not represent hemorrhagic areas and are insignificant clinically.

Sonographic Signs

The following are the characteristic sonographic signs of subchorionic lesions:

- *Subchorionic thrombotic lesions*: echogenic focus beneath the chorionic plate (Figure 2-17)
- *Subchorionic cystic lesions*: well-circumscribed, anechoic areas beneath the chorionic plate (Figure 2-18)

Mid-Placental Lesions

Most hypoechoic or cystic areas in the mid placenta are due to intervillous thrombus in the space between the fetal and the maternal sides of the placenta. Early in the hemorrhagic process, flow may be observed within these spaces as hypoechoic areas, and therefore these areas are sometimes termed *maternal lakes*. A *septal cyst* is a rare mid-placental cystic structure; it is a cyst that forms between cotyledons of the placenta.

The deposition of fibrinous material in intervillous spaces is another common cause of focal hypoechoic lesions identified during routine sonographic examination of the placenta. Unless these lesions are massive and associated with concomitant placental hemorrhagic pathology, they are of no clinical significance. Differentiation between intervillous thrombosis and fibrin deposition is not possible sonographically.

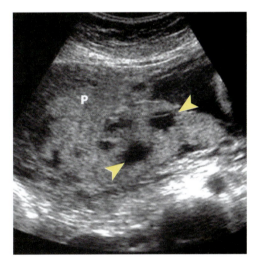

Figure 2-19. Several irregularly marginated, hypoechoic maternal lakes in a placenta at 16 weeks. Arrowheads = maternal lakes, P = placenta.

Sonographic Signs

Primary sonographic signs of mid-placental lesions are:

- Maternal lakes (Figure 2-19)
- Intervillous thrombosis (Figure 2-20)

Basal Plate Lesions

Hypoechoic or cystic areas at the placental myometrial interface are more significant. These may represent retroplacental hematomas or areas of abruption. A rare condition called *maternal basal plate infarction* produces massive blood and fibrin deposition that extends into the intervillous space. If blood collections deep to the placenta are large enough, covering 30%–40% of

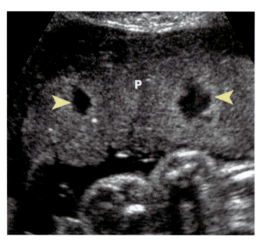

Figure 2-20. Two irregularly marginated, hypoechoic thrombotic lesions in intervillous spaces in a 24-week placenta. Arrowheads = intervillous thrombosis, P = placenta.

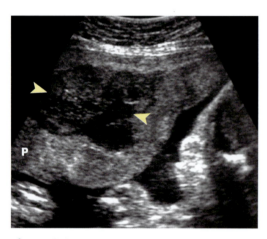

Figure 2-21. A large basal plate hematoma extending into the intervillous spaces in a 28-week placenta. Arrowheads = basal plate hematoma, P = placenta.

the placenta, intrauterine growth restriction or fetal death may occur. In some cases, associated infarction of the deep portion of the placenta may also occur.

Sonographic Signs
- Placental infarctions are not usually visible sonographically, but occasionally a portion of infarcted placenta may appear echogenic.
- Basal plate hematoma (Figure 2-21) and retroplacental hematoma associated with placental abruption may not be differentiated sonographically.

PLACENTA PREVIA

Early in pregnancy, the placenta is less localized and often covers the internal os. As the placenta localizes, it usually migrates away from the os. Even if the

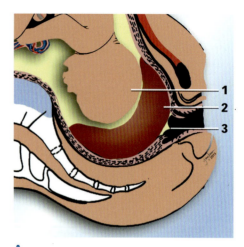

A

Figure 2-22. A Illustration demonstrating a centrally implanted complete placenta previa. 1 = presenting fetal part, 2 = central placenta implantation, 3 = internal cervical os. (Figure continues . . .)

placental margin covers the os at 15–17 weeks, it is likely to migrate away later as the lower uterine segment elongates. *Placenta previa* is the implantation of the placenta with complete or partial covering of the internal os. The typical clinical presentation of placenta previa is painless vaginal bleeding. Clinical complications of the pregnancy relate to potential rupture of the large retroplacental blood vessels and subsequent hemorrhage at the time of labor and delivery.

The incidence of placenta previa is increased in older mothers and in women who have a history of prior abortion, smoking, multiparity, or previous cesarean section. In the older or multiparous patient, the decidua is thinner, so less is available for implantation. Prior cesarean section may result in scarring at the lower uterine segment, preventing the normal upward migration of the placenta. The incidence of a placenta previa at term is 5% if the placenta extends more than 15 mm over the internal os at 12–16 weeks; thus, 95% of placentas covering the os in the first trimester will no longer be previa by the third trimester. When the placenta is visualized 2 cm or less from the internal os near term, the patient may require a cesarean section.

Placenta previa is classified as complete, partial, marginal, low-lying, or vasa previa.

Complete Previa

Complete previa is the complete covering of the internal cervical os by the placenta, membranes, or placental vasculature. A *centrally implanted previa* (Figures 2-22A and B) refers to a placenta that has implanted

The Placenta | CHAPTER 2

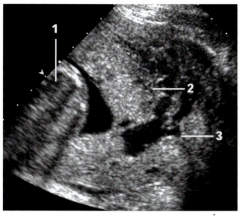

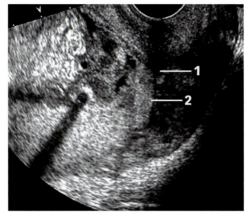

Figure 2-22, continued. **B** Sonogram demonstrating a centrally implanted complete placenta previa. 1 = presenting fetal part, 2 = central placenta implantation, 3 = internal cervical os. **C** Endovaginal sonographic demonstration of a noncentrally implanted, posterior complete placenta previa. 1 = internal cervical os, 2 = lower edge of posterior placenta.

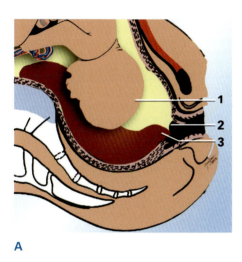

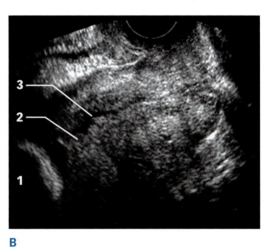

Figure 2-23. **A** Illustration and **B** sonogram demonstrating a partial placenta previa. 1 = presenting fetal part (head), 2 = internal cervical os, 3 = placenta partially covering os.

on the internal cervical os and lower uterine segment. A placenta that implants on the anterior, posterior, or lateral uterine walls may also extend inferiorly to completely cover the internal os (Figure 2-22C). In neither case are patients with complete placenta previa candidates for vaginal delivery.

Sonographic Signs
- All or part of the placenta covers the internal cervical os.

Partial Previa

Partial previa is the incomplete covering of the internal cervical os by the placenta (Figures 2-23A and B, 2-24A). While of academic interest, clinically it bears little significance, as the patient with a partial previa is similarly not a candidate for vaginal delivery. The presence of placental tissue, retroplacental vasculature, and membranes in close proximity to the birth canal poses great risk of hemorrhagic catastrophe during labor and

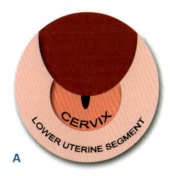

Figure 2-24. **A** Illustration demonstrating relational anatomic differences between the lower edge of the placenta and internal cervical os in partial previa. (Figure continues . . .)

delivery. Differentiation of complete from partial previa is usually not possible sonographically.

Sonographic Signs
- Identification of placental tissue, retroplacental vasculature, and/or membranes partially covering the internal cervical os.
- Differentiation of complete from partial previa is usually not possible sonographically.

Marginal Previa

Marginal previa refers to cases in which the placenta encroaches on the internal cervical os but does not cover it (Figure 2-24B). Sonographically, the placenta may be observed close to the internal os but with the opening itself clear of any placental tissue, retroplacental vasculature, or membranes preceding the fetal presenting part (Figures 2-25A and B). Translabial imaging is useful in differentiating marginal from complete or partial placenta previa.

Sonographic Signs
- Identification of the placenta close to but not covering the internal cervical os.

Low-Lying Placenta

Low-lying placenta occurs when the lower edge of the placenta extends to within 2 cm of the internal cervical os (Figures 2-26A and B). This condition is commonly observed, especially during the first and early second trimesters. As mentioned above, more than 90% of low-lying placentas identified early in pregnancy will migrate away from the internal cervical os by the third trimester.

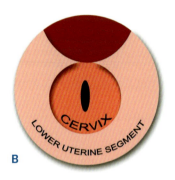

Figure 2-24, continued. B Illustration demonstrating relational anatomic differences between the lower edge of the placenta and internal cervical os in marginal previa.

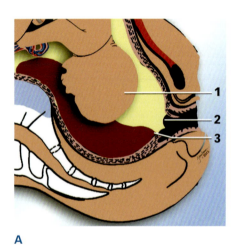
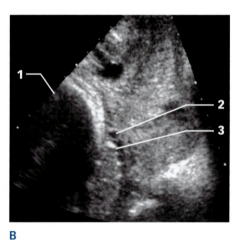

Figure 2-25. A Illustration and **B** sonogram demonstrating a marginal placenta previa. 1 = presenting fetal part, 2 = internal cervical os, 3 = placenta encroaching on the os.

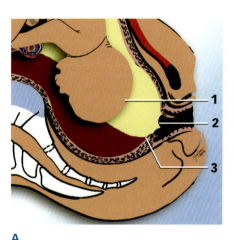
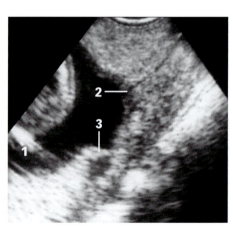

Figure 2-26. A Illustration and **B** sonogram demonstrating a low-lying placenta. 1 = presenting fetal part, 2 = internal cervical os, 3 = inferior placental edge.

Sonographic Signs

- Identification of the placenta in the lower uterine segment more than 2 cm above the internal cervical os.

Vasa Previa

Vasa previa is a clinically serious condition in which velamentously inserted cord vessels precede the fetal presenting part (Figures 2-27A and B). The body of the placenta may be well away from the os, but the membranes lining the uterine cavity and the accompanying cord vessels cover the internal cervical os. Prenatal sonographic identification of vasa previa is critical clinical information, as a patient going into active labor risks tearing of the large umbilical vessel and certain catastrophic hemorrhagic sequelae unless surgical intervention is initiated immediately.

Sonographic Signs

- Identification of umbilical cord vasculature preceding the presenting fetal parts.
- Color Doppler is a useful diagnostic aid.

Sonographic Tips and Pitfalls

- Transvaginal and translabial scanning are the methods of choice in demonstrating the relationship between the internal cervical os and the lower edge of the placenta.
- True placenta previa cannot be diagnosed sonographically prior to 34–36 weeks unless more than one-third of the placental mass covers the os.
- Overdistended urinary bladder may compress the lower uterine segment (LUS), creating the appearance of previa where it does not exist.
- Focal LUS myometrial contractions may mimic previa. Repeat scanning after 30 minutes may resolve this.

PLACENTAL ABRUPTION

Placental abruption (also known as *placenta abruptio* or *abruptio placentae*) is the premature separation of the normally implanted placenta from the uterus. The retroplacental myometrium containing uteroplacental vessels should not exceed 1–2 mm in thickness unless there is a uterine contraction in the area. Usually placental abruption starts at the edge of the placenta and extends both ways from the margin.

Abruption is more likely in patients who have hypertension, who have experienced trauma, or who use cocaine. Women who have extensive abruption may experience pain, extensive bleeding, and hypovolemic shock. Immediate delivery is usually necessary, and there is no time for a sonogram as fetal demise and maternal clinical sequelae are likely. With chronic abruptions, if more than 30%–40% of the placenta separates, intrauterine growth restriction may occur.

Placental abruption may present in several ways: as concealed abruption, external abruption, chronic retroplacental submembranous hematoma, or marginal and subchorionic hemorrhage.

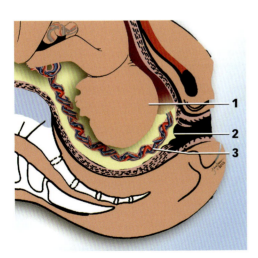

A

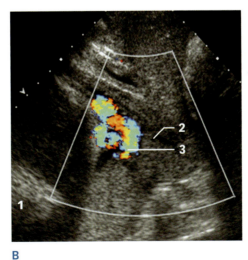

B

Figure 2-27. A Illustration and **B** sonogram demonstrating a vasa previa. 1 = presenting fetal part, 2 = internal cervical os, 3 = umbilical cord.

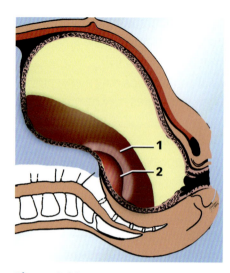

Figure 2-28. A Illustration demonstrating retroplacental bleeding contained within the uterine cavity in a concealed placental abruption. 1 = elevated placenta, 2 = retroplacental bleeding.

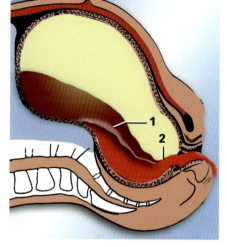

Figure 2-29. Illustration demonstrating bleeding *per vaginam* in an external placental abruption. 1 = elevated placenta, 2 = bleeding *per vaginam*.

Concealed Abruption

Concealed abruption, which may be diagnosed sonographically, occurs in about 20% of cases, and the hemorrhage is confined to the uterine cavity. The detachment of the placenta may be complete, and the consequences are severe (Figure 2-28).

External Abruption

With *external abruption*, blood drains through the cervical os. Detachment is usually not as severe. If no blood remains concealed in the retroplacental space, sonographic diagnosis is not possible (Figure 2-29).

Chronic Retroplacental Submembranous Hematoma

With *chronic retroplacental submembranous hematoma*, the persistence of an unresolved blood clot in the retroplacental space is the result of a small placental abruption. There is usually no association with clinical problems or poor outcome; these hematomas typically resolve spontaneously. However, they may result in maternal disseminated intravascular coagulopathy (DIC), a complex pathologic activation of blood-clotting mechanisms.

Marginal and Subchorionic Hemorrhage

If a hemorrhage is located at the edge of the placenta but does not extend posterior to the placenta, it is called a *marginal hemorrhage* (Figure 2-30). In early pregnancy, hemorrhage outside the amniotic sac but not under the placenta is usually called *subchorionic hemorrhage*.

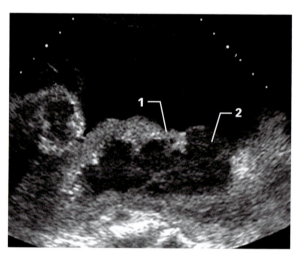

Figure 2-30. A large hypoechoic marginal hematoma elevating the placental edge from the uterine wall. 1 = elevated placental edge, 2 = marginal hematoma.

Sonographic Signs

The appearance of placental abruption varies depending on type, size, location, and age of the blood clot. Typically the hemorrhage from the abruption will appear hyperechoic initially (0–48 hours after abruption) and hypoechoic at 1–2 weeks. After 2 weeks, portions of the clot may become anechoic. Typical findings include the following:

- Placenta elevated from the uterine wall (Figure 2-31A)
- Retroplacental sonolucent or complex mass representing blood and hematoma (Figure 2-31B)
- Normal, thickened, or heterogeneous appearance of the placenta

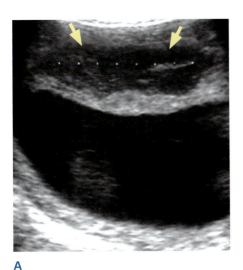 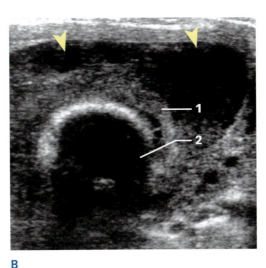

Figure 2-31. A Transverse sonogram in a 14-week pregnancy demonstrating a hypoechoic retroplacental hematoma elevating the placenta from the uterine wall. Arrows = hematoma. **B** Sonographic demonstration of a large retroplacental hematoma in a demised pregnancy at 18 weeks. Arrowheads = retroplacental hematoma, 1 = placenta elevated from uterine wall, 2 = fetal head.

ABNORMAL ADHERENCE

Deficiency of the decidua during implantation may cause placental villi to adhere to the myometrium. These adhesions are referred to as *placenta accreta*, *placenta increta*, and *placenta percreta*:

- *Placenta accreta* is the condition in which placental villi penetrate the decidua but do not invade the myometrium. It is usually the result of a defect in or the absence of the decidua basalis. It is the most common abnormality of adherence (accounting for 60% of cases) and the least severe (Figure 2-32A).
- *Placenta increta* involves further penetration of the villi into the myometrium but not into the serosal layer (Figure 2-32B).
- *Placenta percreta*, a condition in which the villi penetrate through both the myometrium and the serosa, may result in uterine rupture and invasion of nearby pelvic structures (Figure 2-32C).

There are variable degrees of abnormal adherence, classified as focal, partial, or complete. *Focal adherence* indicates that only a small, localized area of the placenta is invasive, while *partial* and *complete* adherence, respectively, indicate that most or all of the retroplacental area is affected. In cases of percreta, the placenta may invade other pelvic organs, such as the bladder, parauterine musculature, bowel, or rectum.

Although these conditions are considered rare, there appears to be increased incidence in patients with

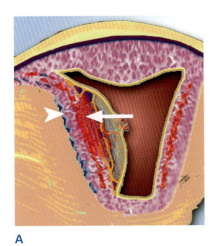 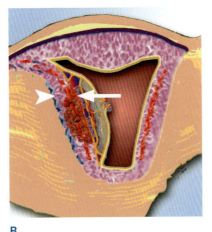 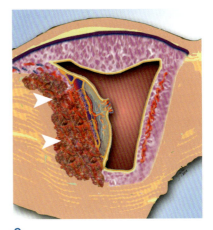

Figure 2-32. Abnormal adherence. **A** Illustration of placenta accreta, with villi penetrating the decidua but not invading the myometrium. Arrowhead = myometrium, arrow = villi. **B** Illustration of placenta increta. Villi penetrate the myometrium. Arrowhead = myometrium, arrow = villi. **C** Illustration of placenta percreta. Villi penetrate through both the myometrium and the serosa. Arrowheads = villi penetrating through uterine wall.

a history of multiple cesarean sections. In addition to prior cesarean sections, predisposing factors for placenta accreta, increta, and percreta include the following:

- Concomitant placenta previa (10% of cases)
- Prior dilatation and curettage
- Grand multiparity
- Endometritis
- Submucosal fibroids
- Synechiae (Asherman syndrome)
- Advanced maternal age (≥35 years)
- Adenomyosis
- Smoking
- Hypertension

This tenacious attachment of highly vascularized placental tissue to the myometrium creates the potential for significant morbidity and mortality at the time of delivery, as the placenta cannot be delivered in the usual fashion, if at all. Hemorrhage, retained products of conception, and uterine rupture can occur. Emergent hysterectomy may be required.

Sonographic Signs

Placenta Accreta

Antenatal diagnosis of placenta accreta is difficult; one study demonstrated a 2.5% detection rate using both sonography and magnetic resonance imaging (MRI).[5] A careful examination of the retroplacental space with attention to the presence and contiguity of normal vasculature may yield useful sonographic observations, including the following:

- Focal basal plate thinning (<2 mm) or absence (Figure 2-33A)
- Loss of myometrial/placental interface (Figure 2-33B)
- Multiple hypoechoic/anechoic spaces in the placenta, sometimes termed "Swiss cheese appearance"
- Increased color Doppler flow in the underlying area, especially at the edges of the area of accreta (Figure 2-33C)

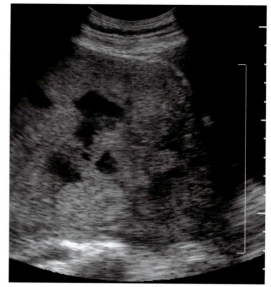

A

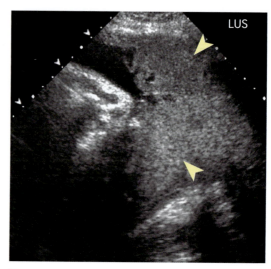

B

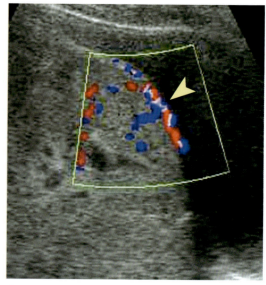

C

Figure 2-33. A Placenta accreta: sonographic demonstration of focal thinning of the basal plate (cursors). **B** Placenta accreta: sonographic demonstration of a homogeneous placental/myometrial interface (arrowheads); LUS = lower uterine segment. **C** Placenta accreta: color Doppler demonstration of increased blood flow at the edge of the invading villi.

Placenta Increta and Percreta

Placenta increta and placenta percreta have a similar sonographic appearance. While it is frequently impossible to differentiate the two pathologic subtypes of abnormal placental adherence, the sensitivity and specificity of sonographic detection, particularly using color and power Doppler methods, is upwards of 90%.[6] Signs include the following:

- Loss of hypoechoic space between bladder and placenta
- Invasion of bladder by infiltrating placental tissue
- Disruption of normal bladder wall architecture
- Aberrant vasculature in the region of interest extending into the bladder or other parauterine structures (Figure 2-34)

CHORIOANGIOMA

Chorioangioma is the most common benign neoplasm of the placenta. It is a vascular tumor arising from chorionic tissue. The majority of chorioangiomas are clinically insignificant. Those larger than 5 cm are associated with a 30% rate of maternal or fetal complications, such as polyhydramnios, intrauterine growth restriction, placenta previa, placental abruption, congestive heart failure/cardiomegaly, pre-eclampsia, anemia, and congenital anomalies. Arteriovenous shunting associated with chorioangioma may cause fetal cardiac enlargement, which can lead to anemia and eventually high-output congestive heart failure. If the tumor mass compresses the umbilical vein, umbilical vein thrombosis may occur, resulting in fetal death. When a chorioangioma, or any large placental lesion, is identified during sonographic examination, care should be taken to examine the fetus for evidence of hydrops or fluid overload.

Sonographic Signs

The following are the characteristic sonographic signs of chorioangioma:

- Hypoechoic, well-circumscribed mass near the chorionic surface of the placenta, often close to the cord insertion (Figure 2-35A)
- Frequent location near the site of umbilical cord insertion
- Hemodynamic abnormalities visualized with color or power Doppler (Figure 2-35B)

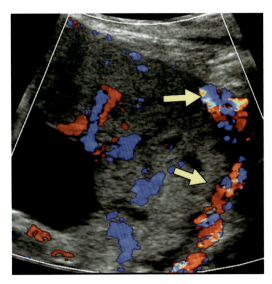

Figure 2-34. Placenta percreta: color Doppler demonstration of aberrant vasculature extending into adjacent soft tissue structures (arrows).

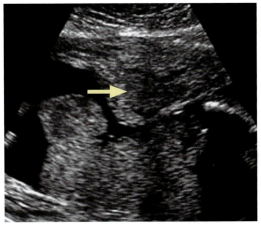

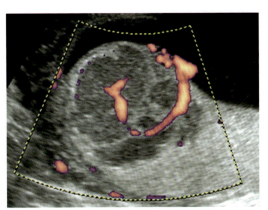

Figure 2-35. Chorioangioma. **A** Focal, hypoechoic solid lesion reflecting the chorionic plate away from the placental body (arrow). **B** Power Doppler image of a lobulated chorioangioma demonstrating vasculature typical of a chorioangioma.

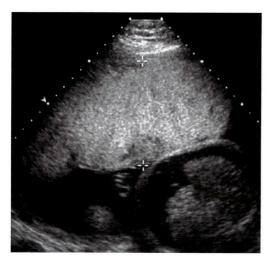

Figure 2-36. Placental hydrops: large, edematous placenta measuring > 5 cm in hydrops fetalis. The accompanying fetal ascites is consistent with the diagnosis of hydrops.

PLACENTAL HYDROPS

Placental hydrops is an edematous condition of the placenta typically caused by fetal cardiac failure. It is frequently found in association with hydrops fetalis (see Chapter 12, pages 302–304), which may result from Rh isoimmunization, ABO incompatibility, and other nonimmune causes.

Sonographic Signs

The following are the characteristic sonographic signs of placental hydrops:

- Abnormally thickened (≥5 cm) placenta[3] (Figure 2-36)
- Rigid, bulbous appearance
- Loss of normal placental architecture, replaced by a "ground-glass" appearance

CHAPTER 2 REVIEW QUESTIONS

1. The placenta develops from embryonic tissue called the:
   A. Cytotrophoblast
   B. Decidua vera
   C. Syncytiotrophoblast
   D. Decidua capsularis

2. Fetal/maternal metabolic exchange in the placenta occurs at the level of the:
   A. Decidua
   B. Villi
   C. Cotyledons
   D. Lobes

3. A thicker than expected placenta may be associated with all of the following medical conditions EXCEPT:
   A. Diabetes mellitus
   B. Intrauterine growth restriction (IUGR)
   C. Hydrops fetalis
   D. Maternal anemia

4. As a rule of thumb, the anteroposterior (AP) diameter of a full-term placenta should not exceed:
   A. 3 cm
   B. 4 cm
   C. 5 cm
   D. 6 cm

5. Scattered echogenic calcifications and focal cystic spaces within a placenta are consistent with:
   A. Grade 0
   B. Grade I
   C. Grade II
   D. Grade III

6. A placenta in which a loose chorionic membrane folds back upon itself and encircles the fetal surface is called:
   A. Circumvallate
   B. Circummarginate
   C. Succenturiate
   D. Annular

7. An accessory cotyledon located away from the main placental body is called:
   A. Circumvallate
   B. Circummarginate
   C. Succenturiate
   D. Annular

8. A ring-shaped placenta that attaches circumferentially to the myometrium is called:
   A. Circumvallate
   B. Circummarginate
   C. Succenturiate
   D. Annular

9. Incomplete covering of the internal cervical os by the lower edge of the placenta is called:
   A. Complete previa

B. Partial previa
C. Marginal previa
D. Low-lying placenta

10. A clinically serious condition in which velamentously inserted cord vessels precede the fetal presenting part is called:
    A. Complete previa
    B. Partial previa
    C. Prolapsed cord
    D. Vasa previa

11. Premature separation of the placenta from the myometrium is called:
    A. Placenta previa
    B. Placenta percreta
    C. Placental abruption
    D. Placenta accreta

12. The condition characterized by the deep invasion of placental villi into the myometrium but not the serosal layer is called:
    A. Placenta percreta
    B. Placenta increta
    C. Chorioangioma
    D. Placental abruption

13. Invasion and perforation of the uterine wall by placental villi is called:
    A. Placenta accreta
    B. Placenta increta
    C. Placenta percreta
    D. Placental abruption

14. A patient presents with a recent history of bright red vaginal bleeding. A transabdominal sagittal sonogram is presented in this image. The most likely diagnosis is:

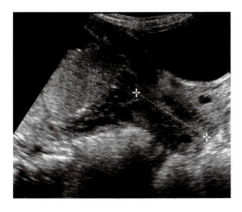

    A. Placenta percreta
    B. Partial placenta previa
    C. Complete placenta previa
    D. Placental abruption

15. A multiparous patient with a history of cesarean section presents with mid-pelvic pain and sudden onset of vaginal bleeding. This image is a sagittal section through the lower uterine segment. These findings are most consistent with:

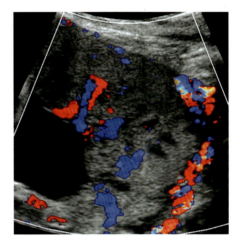

    A. Placenta previa
    B. Placental rupture
    C. Placenta increta
    D. Placental abruption

ANSWERS

See Appendix A on page 478 for answers.

REFERENCES

1. Cunningham FG, Leveno KJ, Bloom SL, et al: Implantation, embryogenesis, and placental development. In Cunningham FW, Leveno KJ, Bloom SL, et al (eds): *Williams Obstetrics*, 23rd edition. New York, McGraw-Hill, 2009, ch 3.

2. Ellery PM, Cindrova-Davies T, Jauniaux E, et al: Evidence for transcriptional activity in the syncytiotrophoblast of the human placenta. Placenta 30:329–334, 2009.

3. Spirt BA, Cohen WN, Weinstein HM: The incidence of placental calcification in normal pregnancies. Radiology 142:707–711, 1982.

4. Tindall VR, Scott JS: Placental calcification: a study of 3,025 singleton and multiple pregnancies. J Obstet Gynaecol Br Commonw 72:356–373, 1965.

5. Gielchinsky Y, Rojansky N, Fasouliotis SJ, et al: Placenta accreta—summary of 10 years: a survey of 310 cases. Placenta 23:210–214, 2002.

6. Obaidly SA, Kurjak A: Prenatal diagnosis of morbidly adherent placenta with 2D ultrasonography, 3D color power Doppler and magnetic resonance imaging. Donald School J Obstet Gynecol 4:199–204, 2010.

SUGGESTED READINGS

Baun J, Gill KA: The placenta and umbilical cord. In Gill KA: *Ultrasound in Obstetrics and Gynecology: A Practitioner's Guide*. Pasadena, CA, Davies Publishing, 2014.

Benirschke K: Normal early development. In Creasy RK, Resnick R (eds): *Maternal-Fetal Medicine: Principles and Practice*, 7th edition. Philadelphia, Elsevier Saunders, 2014, pp 37–46.

Cunningham FG, Leveno KJ, Bloom SL, et al: Implantation and placental development. In Cunningham FW, Leveno KJ, Bloom SL, et al (eds): *Williams Obstetrics*, 24th edition. New York, McGraw-Hill, 2014, pp 80–115.

Feldstein VA, Harris RD, Machin GA: Ultrasound evaluation of the placenta and umbilical cord. In Callen PW (ed): *Ultrasonography in Obstetrics and Gynecology*, 5th edition. Philadelphia, Saunders Elsevier, 2008, pp 721–757.

Fleischer AC, Toy E, Lee W, et al (eds): *Sonography in Obstetrics and Gynecology: Principles and Practice*, 7th edition. New York, McGraw-Hill, 2011, ch 7.

Foy PM: The placenta. In Hagen-Ansert SL (ed): *Textbook of Diagnostic Ultrasonography*, 7th edition. St. Louis, Elsevier Mosby, 2012, pp 1220–1237.

Moore KL, Persuad TVN, Torchia MG: *The Developing Human: Clinically Oriented Embryology*, 9th edition. Philadelphia, Elsevier Saunders, 2012.

Nelson LH: *Ultrasonography of the Placenta: A Review*. Laurel, MD, American Institute of Ultrasound in Medicine, 1994.

Shipp TD: Sonographic evaluation of the placenta. In Rumack CM, Wilson SR, Charboneau JW, et al (eds): *Diagnostic Ultrasound*, 4th edition. Philadelphia, Elsevier Mosby, 2011, pp 1499–1526.

CHAPTER 3

The Umbilical Cord

Embryology

Cord Anatomy and Physiology

Cord Abnormalities

The umbilical cord is the pipeline of the maternal-fetal circulatory system, physiologically linking the hemodynamic powerhouse of the placenta to the cardiovascular system of the fetus.

EMBRYOLOGY

The umbilical cord begins its development at about 4 menstrual weeks, when the body stalk and the omphalomesenteric duct are enveloped by the growing amnion. By about 8 weeks, the amnion and chorion have fused with the extraembryonic mesoderm associated with each membrane to form the early umbilical cord. Wrapped within this emerging tubular connection with the primitive placenta are nascent vascular structures that will develop into the two umbilical arteries and the single umbilical vein. By 12 weeks, the cord has assumed its final form, and it continues to grow until it reaches its full length at term, averaging 50–60 cm.

CORD ANATOMY AND PHYSIOLOGY

The normal umbilical cord contains two arteries and one vein. The arteries are extensions of the fetal internal iliac arteries and course along the inferolateral aspect of the fetal urinary bladder, exiting the anterior abdominal wall at the level of the dome of the bladder. While they are anatomically designated as arteries, they in fact behave as veins, carrying waste-laden and deoxygenated blood from the fetus to the placenta.

After entering the base of the cord, the arteries are twisted by rotational fetal movements around the single umbilical vein, giving it its characteristic helical appearance. The umbilical vein is formed by myriad anastomosing subchorionic tributaries moving oxygenated and nutrient-rich blood from the surface of the placenta to the fetus. It enters the fetal abdomen, courses cephalad toward the undersurface of the liver, and empties into the right-sided fetal circulation via large portal and hepatic venous shunts (Figure 3-1).

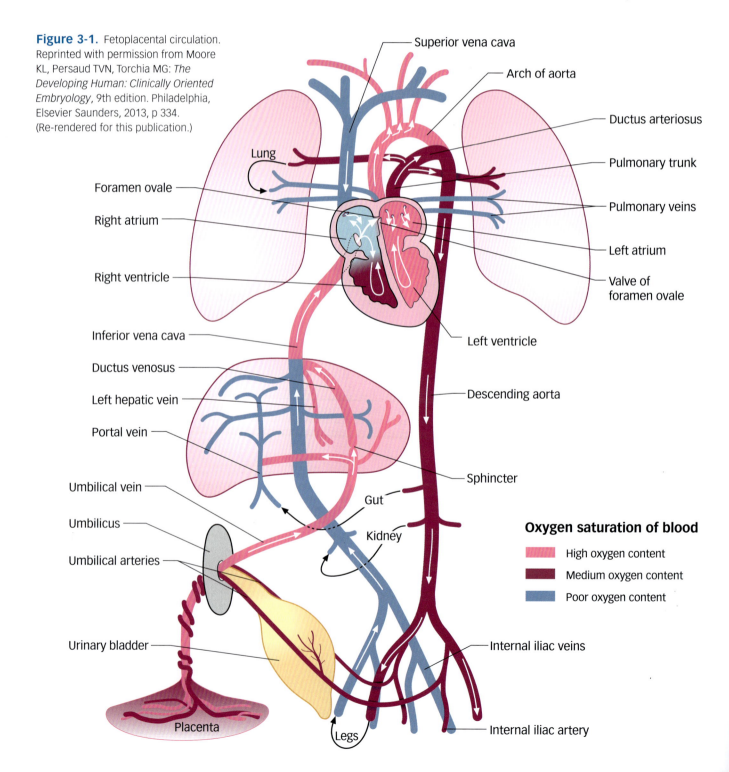

Figure 3-1. Fetoplacental circulation. Reprinted with permission from Moore KL, Persaud TVN, Torchia MG: *The Developing Human: Clinically Oriented Embryology*, 9th edition. Philadelphia, Elsevier Saunders, 2013, p 334. (Re-rendered for this publication.)

The vessels within the cord are surrounded by Wharton's jelly, a gelatinous connective tissue that protects the umbilical vessels from compression. In some cords, a generous amount of Wharton's jelly can be identified as homogeneously echogenic material surrounding the relatively echopenic lumina of the umbilical blood vessels. This finding is a normal variant and is not cause for concern (Figure 3-2).

The length of the cord depends on the force placed on it by the pull of fetal movement. Adequate amniotic fluid facilitates the fetal activity necessary for normal length and coiling of the cord. (See Chapter 7, pages 153–156.)

NORMAL SONOGRAPHIC SIGNS

The umbilical cord is first visible sonographically at approximately 8 menstrual weeks and appears as a straight, thick structure. At this time the length of the umbilical cord is approximately the same as the crown-rump length (CRL). The cord diameter during gestation is normally less than 2 cm.

Assessment of cord vessels is an integral component of any complete obstetric ultrasound examination. The three vessels in the cord can be routinely visualized sonographically. Color Doppler imaging is an excellent adjunct to 2D sonographic imaging in identifying the number of cord vessels, their patency, and the hemodynamic characteristics of each. A normal three-vessel cord can be demonstrated in three different ways:

- Long axis: Two smaller arteries are seen wrapping around a single larger vein (Figure 3-3A).
- Short axis: Two smaller arteries are seen lying obliquely to a single umbilical vein (Figure 3-3B).
- In the fetal pelvis: Two paired iliac arteries can be identified coursing along the lateral aspect of the fetal bladder, exiting the fetus as the umbilical arteries (Figures 3-4A and B).

Insertion sites on both the fetal abdominal wall (Figures 3-5A and B) and the surface of the placenta (Figures 3-6A and B) are readily visible on sonographic evaluation.

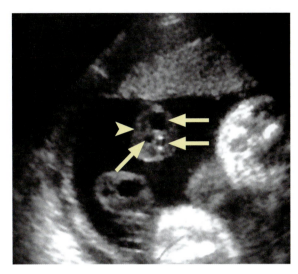

Figure 3-2. Cross section through a three-vessel umbilical cord with a generous amount of Wharton's jelly. Arrowhead = jelly, arrows = umbilical vessels.

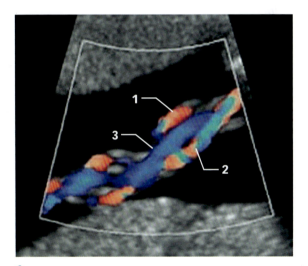

A

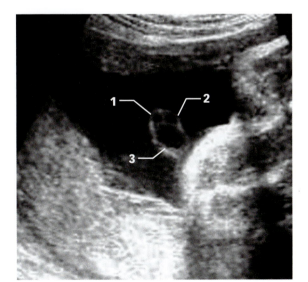

B

Figure 3-3. A Long-axis (longitudinal) view through a normal three-vessel umbilical cord using color Doppler imaging. **B** Short-axis (transverse) view through a normal three-vessel umbilical cord. 1 and 2 = umbilical arteries, 3 = umbilical vein.

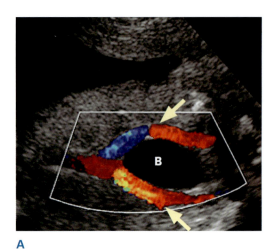
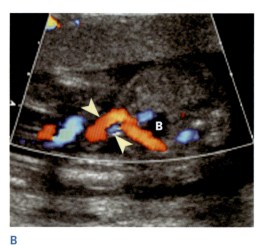

Figure 3-4. A Bilateral iliac arteries (arrows) coursing along the lateral aspect of the fetal bladder. **B** Additional color Doppler imaging of bilateral umbilical arteries (arrowheads) seen in Figure 3-4A. B = fetal bladder.

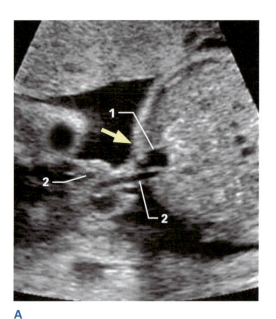
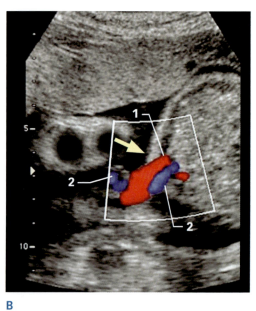

Figure 3-5. Cord insertion on the fetal anterior abdominal wall. **A** 2D demonstration of the larger umbilical vein between the two smaller umbilical arteries. **B** Correlative color Doppler imaging of cord insertion seen in Figure 3-5A. 1 = umbilical vein, 2 = umbilical arteries, arrow = anterior abdominal wall.

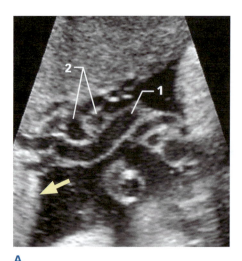
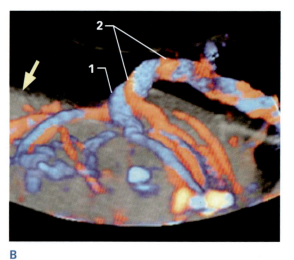

Figure 3-6. Cord insertion on the surface of the placenta. **A** 2D demonstration of cord vasculature inserting on the surface of the placenta. **B** Correlative color Doppler imaging of cord insertion seen in Figure 3-6A. 1 = umbilical vein, 2 = umbilical arteries, arrow = placental surface.

CORD ABNORMALITIES

Umbilical cord abnormalities that may emerge from sonographic evaluation over the course of the pregnancy include vascular cord abnormalities, structural cord abnormalities, cord insertion abnormalities, cord cysts, and cord masses. (See Table 3-1.)

VASCULAR CORD ABNORMALITIES

Vascular cord abnormalities are those related to the two umbilical arteries and the single umbilical vein present in a normal cord. These anomalies may be variations in the number or anatomic integrity of these vascular structures.

Single Umbilical Artery

The most common vascular abnormality of the umbilical cord is *single umbilical artery* (SUA), also called the *two-vessel cord*, which is seen in approximately 1% of all pregnancies. Causes of single umbilical artery include primary agenesis of one of the arteries, secondary atrophy of a previously present artery, and persistence of the original single embryonic artery.

The most common cause is believed to be secondary atrophy of a previously normal vessel.[1]

There is a 20%–60% incidence of concomitant fetal anomalies in the presence of a single umbilical artery.[2,3] Single umbilical artery may be associated with malformations of any of the major organ systems and may be identified in fetuses with chromosomal abnormalities. Even in the absence of associated anomalies, there is an increased risk of intrauterine growth restriction in these pregnancies.

Associated Conditions

Conditions associated with single umbilical artery include:

- Chromosomal abnormalities (trisomies 13, 18)
- Multiple gestations
- Maternal diabetes
- Persistent right umbilical vein
- Congenital renal anomalies
- Sirenomelia
- Velamentous insertion of cord

Sonographic Signs

The following are the characteristic sonographic signs of single umbilical artery:

- Only two vessels demonstrated in a true cross section through the cord (Figure 3-7A)
- Absence of one of the two umbilical arteries emptying into the fetal internal iliac artery demonstrated with color Doppler imaging (Figure 3-7B)

Table 3-1. Summary of umbilical cord abnormalities.

Type of Abnormality	Anomaly
Vascular cord abnormalities	Single umbilical artery (SUA)
	Cord stricture
	Umbilical vein thrombosis
Structural cord abnormalities	Short cord
	Long cord
	Nuchal cord
	Cord knots
	Cord prolapse
	Cord entanglement
Cord insertion abnormalities	Battledore placenta
	Velamentous insertion
Cord cysts	Omphalomesenteric cysts
	Allantoic cysts
Cord masses	Hemangiomas
	Varices/aneurysms
	Teratomas
	Hematomas

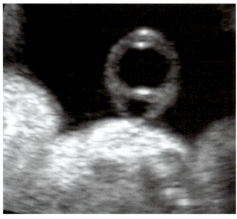

A

Figure 3-7. Single umbilical artery. **A** Cross section through an anomalous cord demonstrates a single artery and vein. (Figure continues . . .)

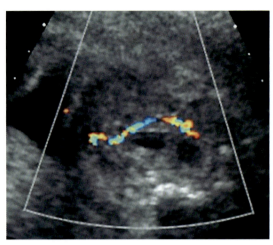

B

Figure 3-7, continued. B Color Doppler demonstrates the absence of one of the paired umbilical arteries in the fetal pelvis.

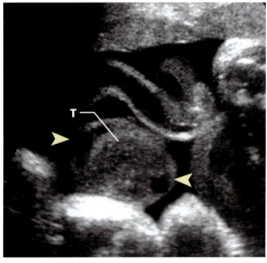

Figure 3-8. Umbilical vein thrombosis: Cross section through the umbilical cord demonstrates echogenic filling of the venous lumen (T) located between the paired umbilical arteries (arrowheads).

Cord Stricture

Mechanical constriction of the umbilical cord may cause a hemodynamically significant reduction of blood flow to the fetus or placenta. In its most severe manifestation, complete occlusion of the umbilical vessels occurs, resulting in fetal demise. In fact, cord stricture has been implicated in 19% of all cases of fetal demise.[4]

The etiology of umbilical cord stricture is unknown, although a deficiency in Wharton's jelly in the umbilical cord at the level of the stricture has been observed in these fetuses. This could, however, be a postmorbid change.

Sonographic Signs

Prenatal diagnosis of cord stricture cannot be made sonographically.

Umbilical Vein Thrombosis

Torsion, knotting, or compression of the umbilical cord may cause venostasis and subsequent occlusive thrombosis of the umbilical vein. As the umbilical vein is the only source of perfusion to the fetus, demise virtually always occurs in the presence of complete occlusion. This condition occurs most frequently in infants born to diabetic mothers and in fetuses with nonimmune hydrops.

Associated Conditions

Conditions associated with umbilical vein thrombosis include:

- Long umbilical cord
- Velamentous insertion of the cord
- Cord knots

Sonographic Signs

The following are the characteristic sonographic signs of umbilical vein thrombosis:

- Increased echogenicity in the lumina of umbilical vessels (Figure 3-8)
- Absence of Doppler signals within an umbilical vessel
- Absence of color flow within an umbilical vessel

STRUCTURAL CORD ABNORMALITIES

Structural abnormalities are those that pertain to variations in size, shape, and configuration of the umbilical cord. Abnormally long cords may become knotted, entangled, or prolapsed; short cords may restrict fetal movement and normal hemodynamic exchange in utero and present problems at delivery. Enlarged cords have been reported with diabetes, hydrops, and diffuse hematoma. Twin-to-twin transfusion can result in diffuse enlargement of the cord of the recipient twin because of the increased flow through the vessels and superimposed edema of Wharton's jelly.

Short Cord

A *short cord* can occur as a primary phenomenon due to failure of embryonic infolding. A short umbilical cord may cause a predisposition toward inadequate fetal descent during labor, fetal heart-rate abnormalities related to cord compression, and placental abruption.

Associated Conditions

Conditions that restrict or reduce fetal movements that can also result in a short cord include:

- Oligohydramnios
- Multiple gestations
- Tethering of the fetus by an amniotic band
- Intrinsic fetal anomalies
- Musculoskeletal abnormalities
- Central nervous system abnormalities

Sonographic Signs

Cord length cannot be reliably assessed prenatally.

Long Cord

An excessively *long umbilical cord* may lead to cord compression and decreased perfusion by mechanical obstruction of venous return. Vascular compromise is more likely if the cord becomes kinked or obstructed, as may be the case with knots, prolapse, or entanglement of the cord (see below).

Associated Conditions

Conditions that may be associated with a long cord include:

- Cord knots, kinking
- Cord entanglement in twin pregnancies
- Cord prolapse

Sonographic Signs

Cord length cannot be reliably assessed prenatally.

Nuchal Cord

Nuchal cords are present in 25% of pregnancies and are of clinical significance when there are two or more loops around the fetal neck. A single loop of umbilical cord seen near the fetal neck is most often an incidental finding. Pregnancies complicated by multiple nuchal loops, however, have been associated with significantly increased risk of meconium in the amniotic fluid, abnormal heart-rate patterns in advanced labor, operative vaginal delivery, and mild acidosis at birth.[5] Nuchal cords rarely cause fetal demise and are not intrinsic reasons for intervention.

Associated Conditions

Conditions that may be associated with a nuchal cord include:

- Long umbilical cord
- Fetal heart-rate anomalies

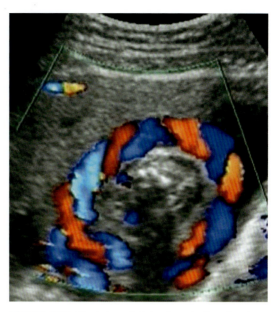

Figure 3-9. Nuchal cord: Color Doppler imaging demonstrates complete encirclement of the fetal neck by a loop of umbilical cord.

Sonographic Signs

The following sonographic signs are associated with nuchal cord:

- Two adjacent loops of cord in cross section seen posterior to the fetal neck in sagittal section
- Loops of cord seen circumferentially around the neck in transverse section (Figure 3-9)

Cord Knots

Knots of the umbilical cord are classified as true and false knots. *True knots* occur in 1% of singleton pregnancies. They may result from torsion of the cord, which forms a loop through which the fetus may slip to form a knot. *False knots* are so named because they simply represent a focal redundancy of the vessels, which appear as vascular protrusions not present in all sonographic planes.

Sonographic Signs

Cord knots are rarely visualized on ultrasound and therefore cannot be adequately assessed prenatally with sonography.

Cord Prolapse

A prolapsed umbilical cord is one that protrudes into the dilated cervical canal. When the cord precedes the fetal presenting part and the membranes rupture, there is a significant risk that the cord will prolapse, creating a potential obstetric emergency necessitating an expeditious delivery.

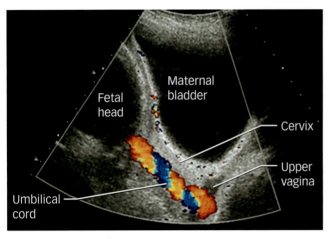

Figure 3-10. Cord prolapse: Sagittal section through the birth canal using color Doppler imaging demonstrates a segment of cord present in the dilated cervix.

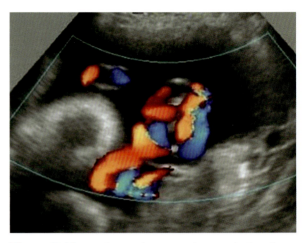

Figure 3-11. Cord entanglement: Color Doppler imaging demonstrates an entangled mass of umbilical cord vessels.

Associated Conditions

Concomitant conditions associated with cord prolapse include:[6]

- Multiple gestations
- Breech or transverse presentation
- Low birth weight (<2500 g at term)
- Polyhydramnios
- Premature rupture of membranes (PROM)
- Long umbilical cord (>90 cm)

Sonographic Signs

Cord prolapse is a critical clinical condition not typically demonstrated in patients referred for obstetric sonography. However, when it is identified during prenatal examination, the imaging findings include:

- Presence of the cord in a dilated cervix/vagina (Figure 3-10)
- Hemodynamic activity within the cord upon Doppler color imaging

Cord Entanglement

Entanglement of the umbilical cord is another potential complication related to an excessively long cord in which one or more loops of cord encircle fetal body parts or the cord becomes intertwined with itself. It is a classic feature of monochorionic/monoamniotic pregnancy but can be observed in diamniotic and singleton pregnancies as well. Entanglement of the cord is often considered a normal sonographic finding in the first trimester and becomes clinically problematic only if hemodynamic compromise occurs.

Associated Conditions

Conditions that can also result in an entangled cord include:

- Long cord
- Monochorionic/monoamniotic twin pregnancy

Sonographic Signs

The identification of a mass of tangled cord as an isolated finding (Figure 3-11) rarely bodes ill for a fetus. However, if hemodynamic compromise has occurred, the Doppler findings typically include:

- Abnormal resistivity indices (RIs) and systolic/diastolic (S/D) ratios
- Presence of diastolic notching
- Reduction in end-diastolic flow in umbilical arteries
- Pulsatile waveforms in the umbilical vein

CORD INSERTION ABNORMALITIES

During early development, the embryo rotates so that the yolk sac and adjacent connecting stalk are positioned opposite the implantation site, allowing for the central insertion of the umbilical cord onto the placenta (Figure 3-12A). As the placenta develops, it tends to grow more freely in areas where myometrial perfusion is robust and less freely in areas where perfusion is weaker. As a result, the cord may insert eccentrically on the placenta. This process is called *trophotropism*—the two most common clinical manifestations being battledore placenta and velamentous insertion of the cord (Figures 3-12B and C).

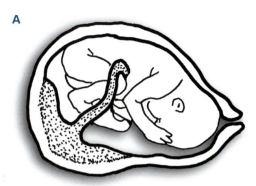
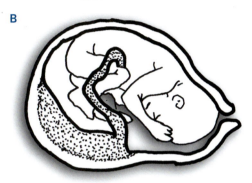
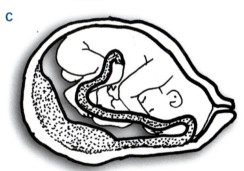

Figure 3-12. Illustration of cord insertion variants. **A** Normal implantation of the cord on the central portion of the placenta. **B** Battledore placenta, in which the cord inserts along the placental margin. **C** Velamentous insertion, with cord attaching to the membranes distant to the placental body.

Battledore Placenta

A *battledore placenta* is one in which the cord inserts along the margin of the placenta. This condition is also called a *marginal insertion of the cord* and is usually of no clinical significance.

Sonographic Signs

Sonography plays a role in identifying battledore placenta:

- Insertion of the umbilical cord is at the periphery of the placenta (Figure 3-13).
- Color Doppler imaging is useful in confirmation of the vascular insertion site.

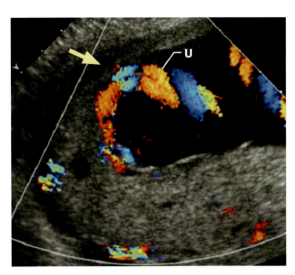

Figure 3-13. Marginal cord insertion of battledore placenta. Color Doppler demonstrates the umbilical vessels inserting along the lateral margin of a posterior placenta, in transverse section. U = umbilical vessels, arrow = placental body.

Velamentous Insertion

A *velamentously inserted cord* attaches beyond the placental edge and into the free membranes of the placenta. Velamentous insertion may be complicated by rupture or thrombosis of the umbilical vessels because they are not protected by Wharton's jelly. The fetus may also experience intrauterine growth restriction as a result of diminished blood flow and systemic perfusion. In twin pregnancy, there is an increased risk of twin-to-twin transfusion syndrome.

A rare form of velamentous insertion, where the umbilical vessels lie across the internal cervical os, is called a *vasa previa*. It may be difficult to detect on routine obstetric sonography, but color Doppler imaging can demonstrate it. If vasa previa goes undetected before birth, the risk of catastrophic outcome for both fetus and mother is great. Rupture of the ectopically located umbilical vasculature can be fatal. (See also Chapter 2, pages 42–45.)

Associated Conditions

Conditions associated with a velamentously inserted cord include:[7]

- Bilobed placenta
- Twin pregnancy
- Uterine anomalies
- Presence of an intrauterine contraceptive device
- Single umbilical artery

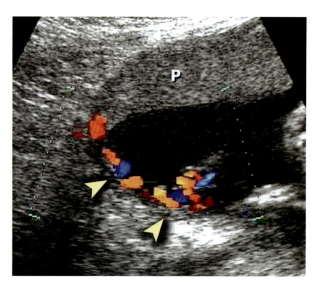

Figure 3-14. Velamentous insertion. Color Doppler demonstrates umbilical vessels inserting on membranes distant from the body of the placenta. Arrowheads = umbilical vessels, P = placenta.

Sonographic Signs

The following are characteristic sonographic signs and tips when encountering velamentous insertion:

- Umbilical vasculature in the chorioamniotic membrane is distant to the placental body.
- Color Doppler imaging is useful in confirmation of the vascular insertion site (Figure 3-14).

CORD CYSTS

Umbilical cord cysts may arise from the omphalomesenteric duct or allantois, distinguishable only by histologic examination. The *allantois* is an embryologic fluid-filled structure that extends from the developing bladder into the base of the umbilical cord. The *omphalomesenteric duct* is a connection from the gastrointestinal tract to the yolk sac. These cysts tend to be closer to the fetal end of the cord, and most are small, typically 1–2 cm in diameter. They may be seen in association with anomalies of the gastrointestinal and genitourinary tracts because they are developmentally related.

For instance, *allantoic duct cysts* have been reported in association with omphalocele, patent urachus, and possibly obstructive uropathy.[8,9] Amorphous cystic areas in the umbilical cord may be observed if a small hemangioma exists in the umbilical cord. The condition is sometimes called *mucinous degeneration of the umbilical cord*. The cystic areas are caused by fluid oozing from the hemangioma, and the cysts may enlarge during pregnancy. Several studies have shown association of second and third trimester umbilical cord cysts with fetal anomalies and aneuploidy in up to 50% of cases.[10,11] Thus, karyotyping is recommended when an umbilical cyst is detected. Cysts of the umbilical cord detected in the first trimester more likely represent normal variants.

Associated Conditions

Conditions associated with cord cysts include:

- Trisomy 18 (Edwards syndrome)
- Trisomy 21 (Down syndrome)

Sonographic Signs

The following are the characteristic sonographic signs of umbilical cord cysts:

- A well-circumscribed, nonvascular, anechoic cystic mass is visualized on the cord (Figure 3-15A).
- Color Doppler demonstrates blood flow in adjacent vascular structures.
- Masses close to the fetal end are more commonly omphalomesenetric cysts (Figure 3-15B).
- Masses close to the placental end are more commonly allantoic cysts (Figure 3-15C).

CORD MASSES

Umbilical cord masses are uncommon prenatal sonographic findings. Pathologic possibilities include hemangiomas, vascular anomalies such as venous varices and arterial aneurysms, teratomas, and hematomas.

Hemangiomas

While still rare, the most common tumor of the umbilical cord is a benign vascular tumor called a *hemangioma*. Cord hemangiomas have been associated with increased alpha-fetoprotein (AFP) levels, polyhydramnios, some congenital anomalies, and increased perinatal mortality. Impaired umbilical circulation has been proposed as the predisposing factor for fetal compromise.[12]

Associated Conditions

Conditions associated with hemangiomas include:

- Polyhydramnios
- Fetal hydrops
- Elevated AFP levels

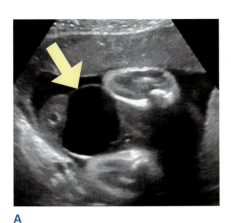 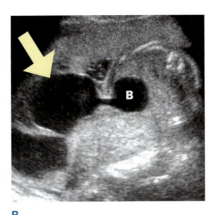 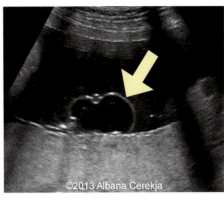

Figure 3-15. A A well-circumscribed, anechoic cystic mass (arrow) on the umbilical cord. **B** Omphalomesenteric cyst (arrow) originating at the fetal end of the cord. B = fetal urinary bladder. **C** Allantoic cyst (arrow) originating closer to the placental end of the cord. © 2013 Albana Cerekja; reprinted with permission from TheFetus.net.

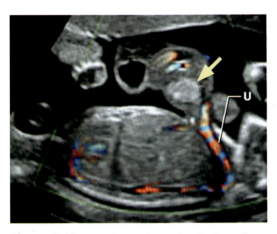

Figure 3-16. Cord hemangioma: focal echogenic mass (arrow) contained within the umbilical cord. U = umbilical vessels.

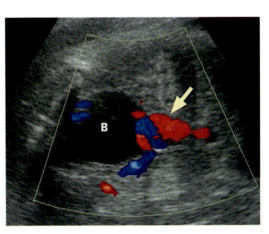

Figure 3-17. Umbilical venous varix: color Doppler demonstrates a dilated umbilical vein (arrow) adjacent to the fetal urinary bladder. B = fetal urinary bladder.

Sonographic Signs

The primary sonographic sign of hemangioma is an echogenic or multicystic mass located near the placental insertion of the cord (Figure 3-16).

Varices/Aneurysms

Focal dilatation of an umbilical artery or vein, while rare, has been reported in the literature. Focal dilatation of a vein is termed a *varix*, while dilatation of an artery is called an *aneurysm*. Either may thrombose and cause fetal death.

Associated Conditions

Conditions associated with varices and aneurysms may include:[13]

- Poor fetal outcomes
- Other fetal anatomic abnormalities

Sonographic Signs

In nonoccluded lesions, color Doppler imaging is useful in differentiating arterial from venous pathology (Figure 3-17).

Teratomas

Teratomas are neoplastic lesions containing tissue from all three germ cell layers. Their appearance in the umbilical cord is rare but has been reported in the literature. Depending on the gross pathologic composition of the tumor, it may appear predominantly cystic, solid, or complex.

Associated Conditions

Poor fetal outcomes are associated with teratomas. The clinical concern is that the mass may compress umbilical blood vessels, resulting in adverse fetal sequelae.

Sonographic Signs

A teratoma is visualized as a cystic, solid, or complex umbilical cord mass.

Hematomas

Hematomas are caused by bleeding into the umbilical cord. A mural tear of one of the cord vessels or continued bleeding after a cordocentesis or other needle procedure permits blood to seep into the cord. The mass effect of the confined blood can mechanically compress the vessels, causing vascular compromise to the fetus and raising the specter of fetal distress, asphyxia, and death. Hematomas are most commonly focal lesions but can dissect beneath the membranes diffusely, affecting a long portion of the cord.

Associated Conditions

Cord hematomas may result in acute fetal distress.

Sonographic Signs

The following are the characteristic sonographic signs of hematoma:

- Focal, hyperechoic mass confined to the umbilical cord
- Echogenicity that may vary with the age of the hematoma

CHAPTER 3 REVIEW QUESTIONS

1. The umbilical cord consists of:
   A. One artery and two veins
   B. Two arteries and one vein
   C. One artery and one vein
   D. Two arteries and two veins

2. The umbilical vein carries:
   A. Oxygenated blood from the placenta to the fetus
   B. Deoxygenated blood from the placenta to the fetus
   C. Oxygenated blood from the fetus to the placenta
   D. Deoxygenated blood from the fetus to the placenta

3. The umbilical cord is sonographically visible starting at which menstrual week?
   A. 6
   B. 8
   C. 10
   D. 12

4. Which fetal vessel(s) in the fetal pelvis help identify the umbilical cord?
   A. Umbilical arteries
   B. Umbilical vein
   C. Iliac arteries
   D. Hepatic vein

5. All of the following conditions may be associated with a short umbilical cord EXCEPT:
   A. Oligohydramnios
   B. Polyhydramnios
   C. Amniotic band syndrome
   D. Multiple gestations

6. Which of the following is the most common vascular abnormality of the umbilical cord?
   A. Single umbilical artery (SUA)
   B. Four-vessel cord
   C. Cord cyst
   D. Short cord

7. This image was obtained in a healthy, asymptomatic patient at 28 weeks' gestation and represents:

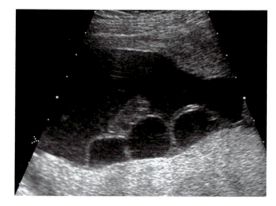

   A. Cystic hygroma
   B. Umbilical cord cysts
   C. Placental teratoma
   D. Uterine synechiae

8. This power Doppler image demonstrates:

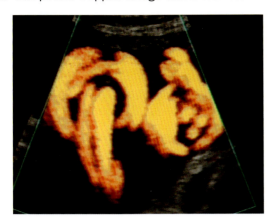

   A. Normal cord
   B. Nuchal cord
   C. Tethered cord
   D. Cord entanglement

9. Which of the following are the two most common clinical manifestations of trophotropism?
   A. Battledore placenta and velamentous insertion
   B. Battledore placenta and two-vessel cord
   C. Battledore placenta and single umbilical vein
   D. Battledore placenta and single umbilical artery

10. The sonographic finding demonstrated in this image is associated with all of the following EXCEPT:

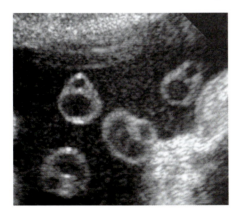

   A. Placenta previa
   B. Maternal diabetes
   C. Chromosomal abnormalities
   D. Multiple gestations

11. Cord entanglement is most often seen in:
   A. Diamniotic/monozygotic pregnancies
   B. Singleton pregnancies
   C. Monoamniotic/dizygotic pregnancies
   D. Monochorionic/monoamniotic pregnancies

12. The sonographic findings demonstrated in this image are most consistent with:

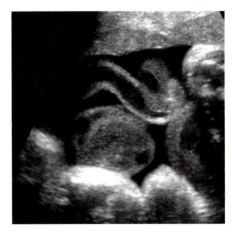

   A. Umbilical vein thrombosis
   B. Allantoic cyst
   C. Omphalomesenteric cyst
   D. Cord teratoma

13. Which of the following umbilical cord conditions may cause fetal death?
   A. Cord stricture
   B. Excessive Wharton's jelly
   C. Short cord
   D. Long cord

14. What is the most common cause of single umbilical artery?
   A. Primary agenesis of one of the umbilical arteries
   B. Persistence of the original single embryonic artery
   C. Secondary atrophy of a previously normal vessel
   D. Chromosomal abnormalities

ANSWERS

See Appendix A on page 478 for answers.

REFERENCES

1. Spirt BA, Cohen WN, Weinstein HM: The incidence of placental calcification in normal pregnancies. Radiology 142:707–711, 1982.

2. Benirsche K, Kaufman P: *Pathology of the Human Placenta*, 2nd edition. New York, Springer, 1990.

3. Jassani MN, Brennan JN, Merkatz IR: Prenatal diagnosis of umbilical artery by ultrasound. J Clin Ultrasound 8:447–448, 1980.

4. Peng HQ, Levittin-Smith M, Rochelson B, et al: Umbilical cord stricture and overcoiling are common causes of fetal demise. Pediatr Dev Pathol 9:14–19, 2006.

5. Larson JD, Rayburn WF, Crosby S, et al: Multiple nuchal cord entanglements and intrapartum complications. Am J Obstet Gynecol 173:1228–1231, 1995.

6. Dilbaz B, Ozturkoglu E, Dilbaz S, et al: Risk factors and perinatal outcomes associated with umbilical cord prolapse. Arch Gynecol Obstet 274:104–107, 2006.

7. Dudiak CM, Salomon CG, Posniak HV, et al: Sonography of the umbilical cord. RadioGraphics 15:1035–1050, 1995.

8. Fink IJ, Filly RA: Omphalocele associated with umbilical cord allantoic cyst: sonographic evaluation in utero. Radiology 149:473–476, 1983.

9. Frazier HA, Guerrieri JP, Thomas RL, et al: The detection of a patent urachus and allantoic cyst of the umbilical cord on prenatal ultrasonography. J Ultrasound Med 11:117–120, 1992.

10. Weissman A, Jakobi P, Bronshtein M, et al: Sonographic measurements of the umbilical cord and vessels during normal pregnancies. J Ultrasound Med 13:11–14, 1994.

11. Skibo LK, Lyons C, Levi CS: First-trimester umbilical cord cysts. Radiology 182:719–722, 1992.

12. Papadopoulos VG, Kourea HP, Adonakis GL, et al: A case of umbilical cord hemangioma: Doppler studies and review of the literature. Eur J Obstet Gynecol Reprod Biol 144:8–14, 2009.

13. Rahemtullah A, Lieberman E, Benson C, et al: Outcome of pregnancy after prenatal diagnosis of umbilical vein varix. J Ultrasound Med 2001:135–139.

SUGGESTED READINGS

Baun J, Gill KA: The placenta and umbilical cord. In Gill KA: *Ultrasound in Obstetrics and Gynecology: A Practitioner's Guide*. Pasadena, CA, Davies Publishing, 2014.

Feldstein VA, Harris RD, Machin GA: Ultrasound evaluation of the placenta and umbilical cord. In Callen PW (ed): *Ultrasonography in Obstetrics and Gynecology*, 5th edition. Philadelphia, Saunders Elsevier, 2008, pp 721–757.

Finberg HJ: Umbilical cord and amniotic membranes. In McGahan JP, Porto M (eds): *Diagnostic Obstetrical Ultrasound*. Philadelphia, Lippincott, 1994, pp 104–133.

Fleischer AC, Finberg HJ, Graham DF: Sonography of the umbilical cord and intrauterine membranes. In Fleischer AC, Toy E, Lee W, et al (eds): *Sonography in Obstetrics and Gynecology: Principles and Practice*, 7th edition. New York, McGraw-Hill, 2011, ch 7.

Hagen-Ansert SL: The umbilical cord. In Hagen-Ansert SL (ed): *Textbook of Diagnostic Ultrasonography*, 7th edition. St. Louis, Elsevier Mosby, 2012, pp 1238–1248.

Klatt TE, Cruikshank DP: Breech, other malpresentations, and umbilical cord complications. In Gibbs RS, Danforth DN (eds): *Danforth's Obstetrics and Gynecology*, 10th edition. Baltimore, Lippincott Williams & Wilkins, 2008, pp 400–416.

CHAPTER 4

Fetal Biometry

Biometric Parameters

Measuring Gestational Age

First Trimester Measurements

Second and Third Trimester Measurements

Fetal Biophysical Profile

Fetal biometry refers to the entire gamut of quantitative measurements of various body parts taken during the course of second and third trimester obstetric ultrasound examinations. By contrast, measurements during the first trimester are limited to gestational sac size and embryonic length. Although these first trimester measurements fall short of true fetal biometry, they are addressed here both as a matter of organizational convenience and because they provide accurate and critical information about gestational age in early pregnancy.

Measurements of various fetal anatomic structures—as single absolute values or as mathematically calculated ratios and weighted averages—provide important information about the gestational age, size, weight, and growth of a fetus. Over many decades, virtually every fetal soft tissue and skeletal structure has been measured and correlated with one or more parameters of fetal age and size.

BIOMETRIC PARAMETERS

BASIC PARAMETERS

By far, the most common and routinely employed biometric measurements during the first trimester include crown-rump length (CRL) and mean sac diameter (MSD). During the second and third trimesters, the following measurements are the basic ones employed:

- Biparietal diameter (BPD)
- Head circumference (HC)
- Abdominal circumference (AC)
- Femur length (FL)

ADDITIONAL PARAMETERS

Once the basic second and third trimester parameters have been measured, they can then be related mathematically to generate other common, clinically relevant data points, which include:

- Cephalic index (CI)
- HC/AC ratio
- FL/BPD ratio
- FL/AC ratio
- FL/HC ratio

Other biometric measurements that may be used either routinely or as components in a more targeted sonographic assessment of fetal age, growth, and well-being include:

- Other fetal long bones
- Thoracic circumference
- Nasal length
- Renal length
- Spleen, liver, and lung length

PARAMETERS FOR MULTIPLE GESTATIONS

Most of the biometric data gathered over the decades have been obtained from singleton pregnancies. In multiple gestations, measurements of crown-rump length taken in the first trimester are as accurate as they are in singleton pregnancies and are the preferred method of dating.[1] Although growth charts have been established for twins and triplets in the second and third trimesters, singleton nomograms are frequently used and have been found to be accurate.[2] For the most part, twins grow at the same rate as singletons at least up to 30 weeks' gestation. However, after 30 weeks fetal growth rates of singletons and multiples begin to deviate, and by term the 50th percentile birth weight of neonates in multiple gestations is equivalent to a singleton's 10th percentile birth weight. Serial biometric assessment of each fetus in a multiple gestation is useful for detecting growth abnormalities that may impact the management of the pregnancy.

MEASURING GESTATIONAL AGE

As discussed in Chapter 1, *menstrual age* refers to the number of weeks' gestation measured from the first day of the last menstrual period (LMP). Clinicians usually measure the duration of a pregnancy in menstrual weeks and may use the term *gestational age* to refer to it; in fact, in clinical obstetric practice, *menstrual age* and *gestational age* are used interchangeably. In embryology, by contrast, gestational age is calculated from the time of conception, which occurs approximately two weeks *after* the beginning of the last menstrual period and therefore is two weeks (14 days) *less than* menstrual age; this is more commonly referred to as *conceptual age*. Throughout this book, unless otherwise specified, *menstrual age* is used when referring to the "gestational age" or the age of an embryo or a fetus.

Determining gestational age is a necessary and routine component of a complete sonographic examination of pregnancy. Because genetic and biologic variations in the size of an embryo are virtually nil, the most accurate assessment of gestational age is done during the first trimester, when statistical deviation (±3–5 days) is the lowest it is at any point throughout gestation. As the pregnancy enters the mid second trimester, the sonographically derived age of the fetus varies by about two weeks (i.e., one week plus or minus the true gestational age), and by the third trimester the variance is a full four weeks (±2 weeks). Clearly, the ideal time to date a pregnancy is during the first trimester, when high-resolution endovaginal scanning methods can be used to measure the embryo's size with the greatest accuracy.

Accurate determination of menstrual age is important, as it affects clinical management of the pregnancy in several significant ways:

- Menstrual age is used to schedule invasive procedures such as chorionic villus sampling and genetic amniocentesis, which, if not timed properly, can yield suboptimal karyotype results.
- Accurate menstrual age is also important when interpreting biochemical tests, such as maternal serum alpha-fetoprotein and triple-screen testing, as the range of normal values varies with stage of gestation.
- Knowledge of menstrual age allows the obstetrician to anticipate normal spontaneous delivery or to assist in planning elective cesarean delivery.
- This knowledge also allows the physician to manage the pregnancy and optimize fetal outcome in case of early or post-term labor.
- In a fetus that is growth restricted, an early sonographic determination of fetal age is essential in interpreting serial follow-up studies of fetal growth.
- When an anomaly is discovered sonographically, the mother's choices regarding therapy or termination are heavily influenced by menstrual age.
- Essentially, all important clinical decisions require an accurate knowledge of menstrual age.

Prior to the use of sonography, gestational age of a pregnancy was determined solely by clinical observations, i.e., the reported date of the patient's last menstrual period and the size of the uterus as calculated from fundal height measurements. In a patient with a firm menstrual history and an easily palpable uterine fundus, clinical assessment of gestational age is usually accurate enough for management of an uncomplicated pregnancy. However, inaccuracies in the clinical assessment of gestational age can arise from many sources, including:

- The patient's inability to recall, or her inaccurate recall, of the first day of the last menstrual period
- The patient's misunderstanding of the question posed and consequent reporting of the *last day* of the last menstrual period as opposed to the *first day*
- Variation in menstrual patterns such as oligomenorrhea, abnormal bleeding events, and the use of oral contraceptives, making identification of the true beginning of the last menstrual period unreliable
- Pregnancy occurring in the first ovulatory cycle after a prior delivery

Sonographic methods used in assessing the duration of pregnancy are based on measurements of the embryo or the fetus as an indirect indicator of menstrual age. The American Institute of Ultrasound in Medicine recommends using crown-rump length (CRL) in the first trimester and, in the second and third trimesters, biparietal diameter (BPD), head circumference (HC), abdominal circumference (AC), and femur length (FL) to estimate menstrual age and to estimate fetal weight. (See Appendix C for guidelines on the performance of routine obstetric ultrasound examinations.[3])

FIRST TRIMESTER MEASUREMENTS

As mentioned above, biometric measurements obtained during the first trimester using an endovaginal approach provide the most accurate estimates of gestational age through all of pregnancy. During the first 10 weeks, appropriately obtained crown-rump length measurements are fully adequate in establishing gestational age and calculating an *estimated date of confinement* (EDC, also known as the *expected date of delivery* or the *estimated due date*) in virtually all normal pregnancies. Even when fetal biometric assessment is performed as part of a routine second trimester ultrasound examination, the expected statistical variance on these measurements precludes them from overriding the first trimester EDC except in cases of maternal or fetal complication.

MEAN SAC DIAMETER

The earliest unequivocal sonographic sign of pregnancy is the demonstration of a gestational sac in the central portion of the uterine cavity. A more precise term may be *chorionic sac*, as it is the developing chorionic villi that create the bright echogenic ring noted within the endometrial cavity. The fluid contained within the sac is essentially all chorionic fluid during very early development. A gestational sac may be seen using high-resolution endovaginal scanning methods as early as 4.5 weeks but can reliably be imaged by 5 weeks. When correlated with serum alpha-fetoprotein levels, an intrauterine pregnancy will always be identifiable when beta-hCG titers reach the discriminatory level. (See Chapter 1, Table 1-1.)

Protocols and Techniques

The mean diameter of a gestational sac is the earliest measure of sonographically obtainable gestational age. Because several extrinsic factors can alter sac dimensions, sac size, as an indicator of gestational age, is best used prior to the identification of a crown-rump length. Crown-rump measurements can be obtained almost as soon as a sac is seen in the uterine cavity, so practical use of mean sac diameter (MSD) for gestational dating is limited to 6 weeks or less.

Endovaginal ultrasound is the imaging method of choice throughout the first trimester and is particularly important in producing accurate biometric results. The following criteria are used in the sonographic study of mean sac diameter:

- MSD is calculated from three planar sections.
- When measuring the gestational sac diameter, the sonographer should measure across the sac to the interface of the chorionic villi and chorionic fluid (Figure 4-1).
- MSD = (anteroposterior + longitudinal + transverse diameter [mm]) ÷ 3.
- MSD is first observable when it measures 2–3 mm, when the menstrual age is 4 weeks, 3–4 days.[4]

Diagnostic Criteria

- As a rule of thumb, at 5 weeks MSD = 5 mm.
- Sac size increases approximately 1 mm per day.
- When MSD − CRL < 5 mm, there is an associated high risk of spontaneous abortion.

Tips and Pitfalls

- Transabdominal measurements, while obtainable in most gestations, are not usually adequate for biometric accuracy and for establishing viability.
- A pseudogestational sac, frequently associated with ectopic pregnancy, may mimic an early gestational sac.

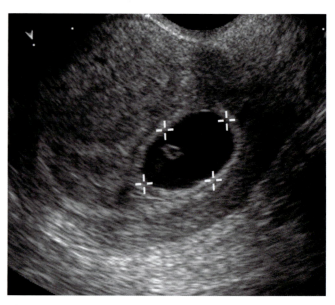

Figure 4-1. Gestational sac measurements: The cursors (+) are placed on the inner edge of the chorionic villi and the measurement is to the outer edge of the chorionic fluid.

CROWN-RUMP LENGTH

The crown-rump length (CRL) between 7 and 10 weeks is the most accurate of all sonographic measures of menstrual age. The developing embryo may be seen when it is as small as 2 mm at 4.5 menstrual weeks (Figure 4-2A). In a normal pregnancy it can reliably be visualized when the crown-rump length reaches 5 mm at 5 menstrual weeks (Figure 4-2B). If the embryo can be measured, then the mean sac diameter is no longer the most accurate measurement of gestational age. By the 5th to 6th menstrual week, the early embryo and cardiac activity will be seen routinely with endovaginal sonography. By 7 weeks, more anatomic and structural detail becomes visible, allowing for a more accurate placement of measurement calipers at the rostral (crown) and caudal (rump) ends of the embryo (Figure 4-2C).

As gestation continues into the early second trimester, normal flexion and extension of the fetus can skew the accuracy of the linear crown-rump length measurement. It is also possible, by as early as 10 weeks, to obtain other biometric data, such as biparietal diameter, head circumference, abdominal circumference, and femur length. For these reasons, crown-rump length should not be relied upon to date a pregnancy after 10 weeks.

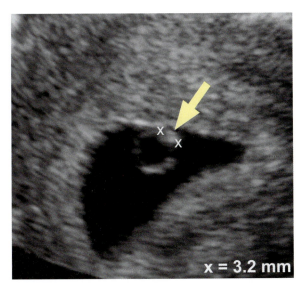
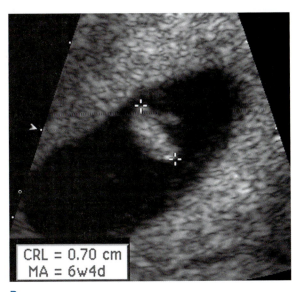
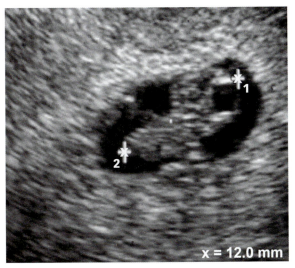

Protocols and Techniques

There are several rules of thumb for estimating gestational age based on crown-rump length imaging parameters. Although these are simple visual estimates, their accuracy is remarkable.

- If a chorionic sac with no yolk sac or embryo is seen, estimate the age at 5 menstrual weeks.
- If a chorionic sac with a tiny embryo (≤5 mm) adjacent to the yolk sac is seen, estimate the age at 6 menstrual weeks.[5]

There are also two rules of thumb for estimating gestational age based on calculations made from the crown-rump length:

- Size in cm + 6 = gestational age in weeks

  Example:

  CRL = 4.0 mm (0.4 cm)

  0.4 + 6.0 = 6.4 weeks

- Size in mm + 42 = gestational age in days

  Example:

  CRL = 4 mm

  4 mm + 42 = 46 days

Tips and Pitfalls

As noted above, after 10 weeks normal flexion and extension of the fetus can skew the linear crown-rump length measurements. Therefore crown-rump length should not be the measure of gestational age after this time.

Figure 4-2. **A** An embryo (arrow) at less than 5 menstrual weeks, measuring 3.2 mm (calipers). **B** The crown-rump length (calipers) of this 6.7-week embryo measures 7 mm. CRL = crown rump length, MA = menstrual age. **C** At 7.2 weeks, this embryo measures 1.2 cm, with cursors placed at the rostral (crown, cursor #1) and caudal (rump, cursor #2) ends.

SECOND AND THIRD TRIMESTER MEASUREMENTS

BIPARIETAL DIAMETER

The biparietal diameter (BPD) is as accurate as the first trimester crown-rump length in estimating gestational age if obtained between 14 and 24 weeks. The measurement is obtained using an axial section through the fetal head at the level of the thalami and cavum septi pellucidi. (See Table 4-1.)

Protocols and Techniques

General rules for measuring the biparietal diameter include the following:

- Use a true axial section. The transducer must transect the parietal bones at 90° at the level of the third ventricle and thalami (Figures 4-3A and B).
- The calvaria should appear smooth and symmetric.
- Cursors should be placed "leading edge to leading edge," i.e., outer edge of the near calvarial wall to inner edge of the far calvarial wall (Figure 4-4).

Table 4-1. Multiple fetal parameters in assessment of menstrual age during the second and third trimesters.

Mean Menstrual Age (Weeks)	Mean Biparietal Diameter (mm)	Mean Head Circumference (mm)	Mean Abdominal Circumference (mm)	Mean Femur Length (mm)
12	17	68	46	7
13	21	82	60	11
14	25	97	73	14
15	29	110	86	17
16	32	124	99	20
17	36	138	112	24
18	39	151	125	27
19	43	164	137	30
20	46	177	150	33
21	50	189	162	35
22	53	201	174	38
23	56	213	185	41
24	59	224	197	44
25	62	235	208	46
26	65	246	219	49
27	68	256	230	51
28	71	266	240	54
29	73	275	251	56
30	76	284	261	58
31	78	293	271	60
32	81	301	281	62
33	83	308	291	64
34	85	315	300	66
35	87	322	309	68
36	89	328	318	70
37	90	333	327	72
38	92	338	336	74
39	93	342	344	75
40	94	346	353	77

Source: Reprinted by permission from Hadlock FP, Deter RL, Harrist RB, et al: Estimating fetal age: computer-assisted analysis of multiple fetal growth parameters. Radiology 152:497, 1984.

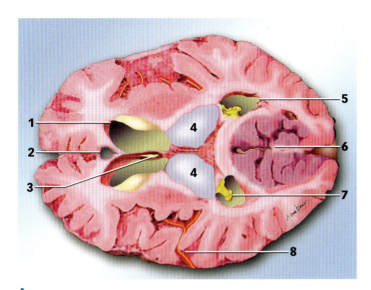 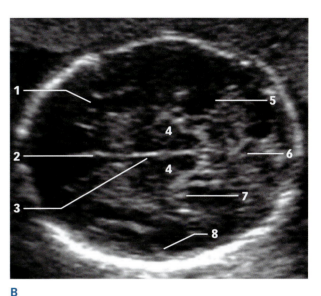

Figure 4-3. A Illustration of the fetal brain at the biparietal diameter (BPD) level, based on a gross anatomic section. **B** Corresponding sonographic image. 1 = lateral ventricle—frontal horn, 2 = cavum septi pellucidi, 3 = third ventricle, 4 = thalamus, 5 = lateral ventricle—atrium, 6 = cerebellum, 7 = choroid plexus, 8 = Sylvian fissure.

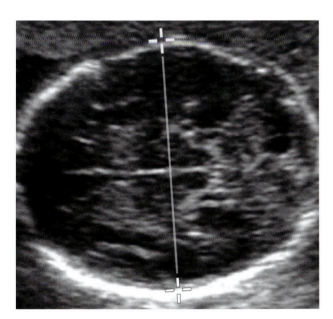

Figure 4-4. Proper cursor placement for measuring biparietal diameter: leading edge to leading edge.

- Gain controls should be adjusted to minimize the loud ring-down artifact emanating from the calvarial wall closest to the transducer. The width of the parietal skull echo should be no greater than 5 mm.
- Minimal pressure with a real-time transducer is often sufficient to change an obliquely oriented fetal head to an occiput transverse position for a better true axial section.

Tips and Pitfalls
- Measurement error inherent in caliper placement is 1–2 mm.
- An eccentric fetal position (such as breech presentation) or a significant reduction in amniotic fluid can affect the shape of the calvaria, thereby reducing the reliability of the biparietal diameter for assessing gestational age.
- The head circumference, rather than biparietal diameter, should be used for gestational age assessment whenever dolichocephaly or brachycephaly occurs.
- With oligohydramnios, the fetal head molds to the contour of the uterus, resulting in a reduced biparietal diameter that may affect occipitofrontal diameter (OFD). Consequently, the biparietal diameter or the head circumference measurement will be more variable in the presence of oligohydramnios than when the amniotic fluid volume is normal.

HEAD CIRCUMFERENCE

The head circumference (HC) measurement is obtained from an axial section of the head at the same level as that used for the biparietal diameter. Anatomic landmarks at the proper plane of section include the cavum septi pellucidi, thalamic nuclei, falx cerebri, and choroid plexus.[6,7] The variability inherent in estimating fetal age from the biparietal diameter is generally greater than with the head circumference. The variability is not constant throughout pregnancy but increases with gestational age. (See Tables 4-1 and 4-2.)

The formula for measuring head circumference is as follows:

$$HC = (BPD + OFD) \times 1.57$$

where 1.57 is the factor that corrects for an ellipsoid.

The head circumference is part of several formulas used to estimate fetal weight and is also used to monitor growth between examinations. Finally, the head circumference can be compared with other measurements, such as abdominal circumference and femur length, to assess the possible effects on the fetus of growth disturbances (e.g., macrosomia and growth restriction).

Table 4-2. Values for fetal head circumference by gestational age and percentile.

Menstrual Weeks	Head Circumference (cm)				
	3rd	10th	50th	90th	97th
14	8.8	9.1	9.7	10.3	10.6
15	10.0	10.4	11.0	11.6	12.0
16	11.3	11.7	12.4	13.1	13.5
17	12.6	13.0	13.8	14.6	15.0
18	13.7	14.2	15.1	16.0	16.5
19	14.9	15.5	16.4	17.4	17.9
20	16.1	16.7	17.7	18.7	19.3
21	17.2	17.8	18.9	20.0	20.6
22	18.3	18.9	20.1	21.3	21.9
23	19.4	20.1	21.3	22.5	23.2
24	20.4	21.1	22.4	23.7	24.3
25	21.4	22.2	23.5	24.9	25.6
26	22.4	23.2	24.6	26.0	26.8
27	23.3	24.1	25.6	27.1	27.9
28	24.2	25.1	26.6	28.1	29.1
29	25.0	25.9	27.5	29.1	30.0
30	25.8	26.8	28.4	30.0	31.0
31	26.7	27.6	29.3	31.0	31.9
32	27.4	28.4	30.1	31.8	32.8
33	28.0	29.0	30.8	32.6	33.6
34	28.7	29.7	31.5	33.3	34.3
35	29.3	30.4	32.2	34.1	35.1
36	29.9	30.9	32.8	34.7	35.8
37	30.3	31.4	33.3	35.2	36.3
38	30.8	31.9	33.8	35.8	36.8
39	31.1	32.2	34.2	36.2	37.3
40	31.5	32.6	34.6	36.6	37.7

Source: Reprinted by permission from Callen PW: *Ultrasonography in Obstetrics and Gynecology*, 4th edition. Philadelphia, Saunders Elsevier, 2000, Table A-10, p 1025. Adapted from Hadlock FP, Deter RL, Harrist RB, et al: Estimating fetal age: computer-assisted analysis of multiple fetal growth parameters. Radiology 152:497, 1984.

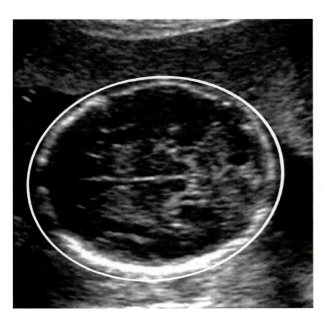

Figure 4-5. Proper cursor placement for measuring fetal head circumference. The ellipse caliper encompasses the bony calvaria.

Protocols and Techniques

General rules for measuring fetal head circumference include the following:

- Measure at same level as that used for biparietal diameter (page 72).
- Fit ellipse tight to bony calvaria (Figure 4-5).
- When occipitofrontal diameter (OFD) measurements are used in conjunction with the biparietal diameter to calculate head circumference, the OFD should be measured from the outer edge of the frontal bone to the outer edge of the occipital bone.

Tips and Pitfalls

- It can be difficult to accurately fit an ellipse trace to an eccentrically shaped head.
- Measurement error inherent in caliper placement is 1–2 mm when two linear measurements are used.

CEPHALIC INDEX (CI)

When the normocephalic shape of the fetal head is distorted by oligohydramnios, breech presentation, or crowded twinning, cephalic biometric values will be skewed from their normal patterns. A dolichocephalic head will yield biparietal diameter values significantly lower than those appropriate for gestational age, while a brachycephalic head will produce values that are greater than expected. The *cephalic index* (CI) is a useful measure of the reliability of standard biparietal diameter and head circumference measurements.

Protocols and Techniques

The cephalic index is calculated using the biparietal diameter and the occipitofrontal diameter (which, as mentioned above, is measured from the outer edge to outer edge of the calvaria), according to the following formula:

$$CI = BPD/OFD \times 100$$

If the cephalic index varies by more than one standard deviation (SD) above or below the expected value (i.e., if CI is either ≤ 74 or ≥ 83), then the head circumference is a more reliable indicator of gestational age than is the biparietal diameter.[8]

Tips and Pitfalls

The cephalic index is subject to the same difficulties as measurement of head circumference:

- It can be difficult to accurately fit an ellipse trace to an eccentrically shaped head.
- Measurement error inherent in caliper placement is 1–2 mm when two linear measurements are used.

ABDOMINAL CIRCUMFERENCE

Abdominal circumference (AC) measurements are most useful in assessing the normal somatic growth of a fetus and less useful as absolute indicators of gestational age. This is partly because the abdominal circumference is more acutely affected by growth disturbances than are the other basic parameters. Some believe that the variability is probably due to measurement error more than to biologic variability; however, the abdomen is not rigid like the head, but soft and flexible, so it is more variable in size and shape.

Abdominal circumference measurements are obtained at the level where the transverse diameter of the liver is greatest, as it is the largest organ in the fetal torso, and its size reflects variations of growth in the fetus, particularly growth restriction and macrosomia. Sonographic landmarks at this level include the portal sinus and the fluid-filled stomach (Figures 4-6A and B). Values for fetal abdominal circumference are summarized in Tables 4-1 and 4-3.

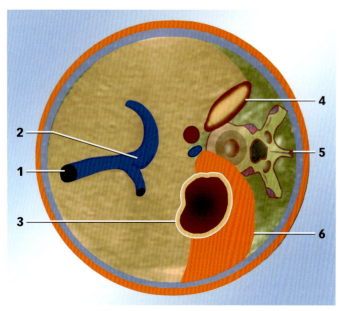
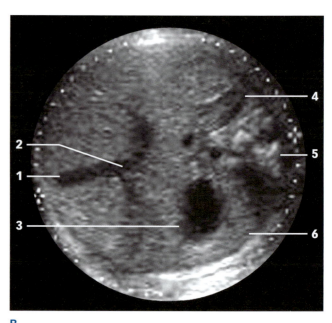

Figure 4-6. A Illustration and **B** correlative sonographic image of abdominal circumference measurements, which are obtained at the level where the transverse diameter of the liver is greatest. 1 = umbilical vein, 2 = portal sinus, 3 = stomach, 4 = adrenal gland, 5 = spine, 6 = spleen.

Protocols and Techniques

General rules for measuring the abdominal circumference include the following:

- Measure at the level of the portal sinus and stomach.
- Include all soft tissues beneath the skin line.
- The appearance of the lower ribs should be symmetric.

Abdominal circumference is typically obtained using software that calculates area using a computer-generated ellipse tracing, available on most of today's sonographic instruments. However, circumference can also be calculated using two linear measurements, i.e., the transverse (D1) and anteroposterior (D2) diameters of the abdomen, using the following formula:

$$AC = (D1 + D2) \times 1.57$$

Tips and Pitfalls

- Abdominal circumference measurements are the least reliable indicator of gestational age, because of possible genetic and physiologic variations in size after 25 weeks. The primary use of abdominal circumference measurements is in algorithms that estimate fetal weight and growth.
- In patients who present an imaging challenge, the "round" rule is helpful. When the anatomic landmarks are difficult to demonstrate, use an image in which the anteroposterior and transverse diameters approximate each other; that is, if the fetal abdomen appears round, reasonable measurements can be obtained.
- Excessive pressure with the transducer should be avoided because it can distort the shape of the fetal abdomen.

FEMUR LENGTH

Femur length (FL), like biparietal diameter, is as accurate as crown-rump length in estimating gestational age in an anatomically normal fetus. Only the ossified portion of the femoral diaphysis is included in the measurement of the femur; the cartilaginous epiphyses at each end of the bone are excluded (see "Epiphyseal Appearance" on pages 79–80). A true long-axis view will demonstrate the femoral and one of the distal femoral condyles in a single image.

The cursors are positioned at the junction of the bone with the cartilage (Figures 4-7A and B). The most accurate measurements are obtained from an image that is

Table 4-3. Values for fetal abdominal circumference by gestational age and percentile.

Menstrual Weeks	Abdominal Circumference (cm)				
	3rd	10th	50th	90th	97th
14	6.4	6.7	7.3	7.9	8.3
15	7.5	7.9	8.6	9.3	9.7
16	8.6	9.1	9.9	10.7	11.2
17	9.7	10.3	11.2	12.1	12.7
18	10.9	11.5	12.5	13.5	14.1
19	11.9	12.6	13.7	14.8	15.5
20	13.1	13.8	15.0	16.3	17.0
21	14.1	14.9	16.2	17.6	18.3
22	15.1	16.0	17.4	18.8	19.7
23	16.1	17.0	18.5	20.0	20.9
24	17.1	18.1	19.7	21.3	22.3
25	18.1	19.1	20.8	22.5	23.5
26	19.1	20.1	21.9	23.7	24.8
27	20.0	21.1	23.0	24.9	26.0
28	20.9	22.0	24.0	26.0	27.1
29	21.8	23.0	25.1	27.2	28.4
30	22.7	23.9	26.1	28.3	29.5
31	23.6	24.9	27.1	29.4	30.6
32	24.5	25.8	28.1	30.4	31.8
33	25.3	26.7	29.1	31.5	32.9
34	26.1	27.5	30.0	32.5	33.9
35	26.9	28.3	30.9	33.5	34.9
36	27.7	29.2	31.8	34.4	35.9
37	28.5	30.0	32.7	35.4	37.0
38	29.2	30.8	33.6	36.4	38.0
39	29.9	31.6	34.4	37.3	38.9
40	30.7	32.4	35.3	38.2	39.9

Source: Reprinted by permission from Callen PW: *Ultrasonography in Obstetrics and Gynecology*, 4th edition. Philadelphia, Saunders Elsevier, 2000, Table A-12, p 1026. Adapted from Hadlock FP, Deter RL, Harrist RB, et al: Estimating fetal age: computer-assisted analysis of multiple fetal growth parameters. Radiology 152:497, 1984.

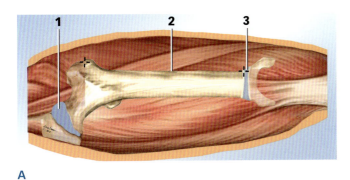
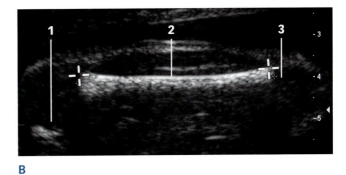

A

B

Figure 4-7. **A** Illustration and **B** correlative sonographic image of femur length measurements: To measure femur length, place the cursors (see sonogram) at the junction of the bone with the cartilage. 1 = proximal femoral epiphysis, 2 = ossified diaphysis, 3 = distal femoral epiphysis. (Figure continues on page 79 . . .)

produced when the acoustic beam strikes the long axis of the femur at 90°. Because the femur is a strongly reflective linear acoustic interface, oblique incidence of the beam will cause artifactual distortion at both ends of the long bone and reduce the accuracy of any measurements taken. A femur imaged vertically can be significantly shorter than one imaged horizontally, with up to a 2.6-week difference in gestational age prediction. Values for fetal femur length are summarized in Tables 4-1 and 4-4.

Protocols and Techniques

General rules for measuring the femur length include the following:

- Position cursors at the junction of the bone with the cartilage.
- Include only the ossified diaphysis; exclude epiphyseal cartilage.
- A linear array transducer is preferred to minimize errors related to beam-distortion artifacts.

Table 4-4. Values for fetal femur length by gestational age and percentile.

Menstrual Weeks	Femur Length (cm)				
	3rd	10th	50th	90th	97th
14	1.2	1.3	1.4	1.5	1.6
15	1.5	1.6	1.7	1.9	1.9
16	1.7	1.8	2.0	2.2	2.3
17	2.1	2.2	2.4	2.6	2.7
18	2.3	2.5	2.7	2.9	3.1
19	2.6	2.7	3.0	3.3	3.4
20	2.8	3.0	3.3	3.6	3.8
21	3.0	3.2	3.5	3.8	4.0
22	3.3	3.5	3.8	4.1	4.3
23	3.5	3.7	4.1	4.5	4.7
24	3.8	4.0	4.4	4.8	5.0
25	4.0	4.2	4.6	5.0	5.2
26	4.2	4.5	4.9	5.3	5.6
27	4.4	4.6	5.1	5.6	5.8
28	4.6	4.9	5.4	5.9	6.2
29	4.8	5.1	5.6	6.1	6.4
30	5.0	5.3	5.8	6.3	6.6
31	5.2	5.5	6.0	6.5	6.8
32	5.3	5.6	6.2	6.8	7.1
33	5.5	5.8	6.4	7.0	7.3
34	5.7	6.0	6.6	7.2	7.5
35	5.9	6.2	6.8	7.4	7.8
36	6.0	6.4	7.0	7.6	8.0
37	6.2	6.6	7.2	7.9	8.2
38	6.4	6.7	7.4	8.1	8.4
39	6.5	6.8	7.5	8.2	8.6
40	6.6	7.0	7.7	8.4	8.8

Source: Reprinted by permission from Callen PW: *Ultrasonography in Obstetrics and Gynecology*, 4th edition. Philadelphia, Saunders Elsevier, 2000, Table A-15, p 1027. Adapted from Hadlock FP, Deter RL, Harrist RB, et al: Estimating fetal age: computer-assisted analysis of multiple fetal growth parameters. Radiology 152:497, 1984.

- If femur length falls two standard deviations below the mean femur length, short limb dysplasia may be present. Other long bones should be measured.
- The femur closest to the transducer should be measured to minimize the variation associated with measuring at different depths.

Tips and Pitfalls
- The use of mechanical and some phased sector probes may result in artifactual "bowing."
- Correct placement of the measurement calipers should exclude epiphyseal cartilage.
- Inclusion of the "distal femur point" will result in a specular reflection from the lateral surface of the distal epiphysis and should not be included in the measurement[9] (Figure 4-7C).
- In an obliquely obtained image, true femur length can be underestimated.

EPIPHYSEAL APPEARANCE

Ossification of the human skeletal system begins in the embryonic period and continues throughout the individual's childhood. Bone measurements—especially of femur length but also of other bones (see "Miscellaneous Measurements," pages 81–82)—have been used for determining the age of an individual and are based on the appearance of ossification in the cartilaginous scaffolding of bones. Long bones begin to ossify from the *diaphysis* (shaft) outward toward both ends. The junction of the calcified shaft with the cartilaginous ends of the bones is called the *epiphysis*. Within each epiphysis is a separate ossification center, which appears at a predictable chronological moment in the growth of the fetus. Observation of these epiphyseal ossification centers can, therefore, be useful in determining the age of the gestation (Table 4-5).

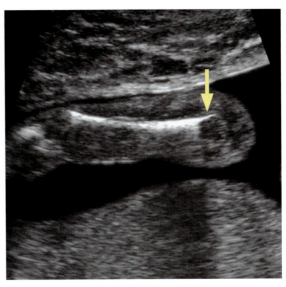

C

Figure 4-7, continued. C Distal femur point (arrow): A specular reflection from the lateral surface of the distal epiphysis in the measurement should not be included in a femur length measurement.

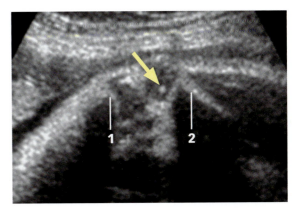

A

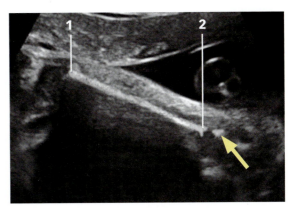

B

Figure 4-8. A Distal femoral epiphysis (arrow) at 33 weeks. 1 = proximal tibia, 2 = distal femur. **B** Proximal tibial epiphysis (arrow) at 35 weeks. 1 = distal tibia, 2 = proximal tibia.

Table 4-5.	Epiphyseal appearance.
Menstrual Age (Weeks)	Appearance
33	Distal femoral epiphysis (Figure 4-8A)
35	Proximal tibial epiphysis (Figure 4-8B)
38	Proximal humeral epiphysis

Protocols and Techniques

Sagittal imaging through the fetal knee can demonstrate both distal femoral and proximal tibial epiphyses in a single view. The maximum dimension of each epiphysis is measured.

Tips and Pitfalls

A fetus with its legs tucked under its abdomen and in a face-down position may preclude adequate imaging of the legs.

ORBITAL MEASUREMENTS

Several measurements of the fetal orbits can be made that are useful adjuncts to other biometric parameters in assessing fetal age. Measurements of binocular distance, interorbital distance, and orbital diameter are particularly useful when the fetal head is in a direct occiput posterior position and getting accurate biparietal diameter and head circumference measurements is impossible. (See Table 4-6.)

Protocols and Techniques

- *Binocular distance* is measured from the lateral edge of one orbit to the lateral edge of the other orbit (Figure 4-9A).
- *Interorbital distance* is the distance between the two orbits measured between the two medial inner bony surfaces (Figure 4-9B).
- *Orbital diameter* is the measurement of a single orbit from medial inner bony surface to lateral inner bony surface (Figure 4-9C).

Table 4-6. Mean values for fetal orbital measurements by gestational age.

Menstrual Weeks	Mean OD (mm)	Mean BOD (cm)	Mean IOD (mm)
14	5.2	1.91	n/a
15	6.1	2.15	10
16	6.6	2.24	10
17–18	7.3	2.55–2.78	11
19–20	9.8	2.97–3.07	12
21	10.5	3.29	12
22	10.4	3.46	13
23	10.7	3.67	13
24	11.6	3.77	14
25	11.2	4.03	15
26	12.7	4.16	15
27	13.0	4.33	16
28	13.0	4.49	16
29	13.9	4.67	17
30–31	14.2	4.76–4.98	17–18
32–33	14.4	5.05–5.17	18–19
34–36	15.8	5.39–5.56	19–20
37–40	n/a	5.7–5.9	21–22

Notes: OD = orbital diameter; BOD = binocular distance; IOD = interorbital distance.

Source: Data for binocular distance are from Tongsong T, Wanapitrak C, Jesadapornchai S, et al: Fetal binocular distance as a predictor of menstrual age. Int J Gynaecol Obstet 38:87–91, 1992. Data for orbital diameter are from Goldstein I, Tamir A, Zimmer EZ, et al: Growth of the fetal orbit and lens in normal pregnancies. Ultrasound Obstet Gynecol 12:175–179, 1998. IOD value for 37–40 weeks from Sukonpan K, Phupong V: Fetal orbital distance in normal pregnancies. J Med Assoc Thai 91:1318–1322, 2008.

TRANSCEREBELLAR DIAMETER

Similarly, when a head circumference measurement is difficult to obtain, the transcerebellar diameter may be useful in determining fetal age. Between 14 and 20 weeks' gestation, the transverse cerebellar diameter in millimeters is roughly equivalent to the gestational age in weeks. It is measured from the right to left lateral aspects of the cerebellum in an axial plane of section (Figure 4-10). These measurements are compared to an established nomogram that relates the diameter to fetal gestational age (Table 4-7).

MISCELLANEOUS MEASUREMENTS

In addition to the standard measures used during routine sonographic examination of a pregnancy, many other biometric tables have been assembled over the years that correlate various fetal anatomic parts with gestational age. Tibia, fibula, radius, ulna, clavicle, foot, mandible, nasal, renal, spleen, liver, and lung lengths, as well as thoracic circumference, have all been used. However, these additional biometric measures are more useful in diagnosing fetal skeletal dysplasias than in contributing to the final estimate of fetal age.

Nasal Bone

Nasal bone length, measured from the ossified proximal endpoint to the distal endpoint, can be correlated with gestational age. The observation of the absence

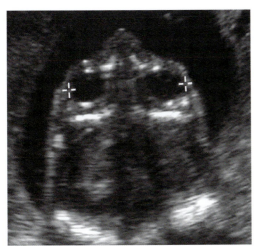

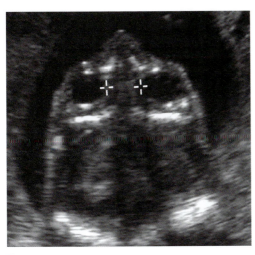

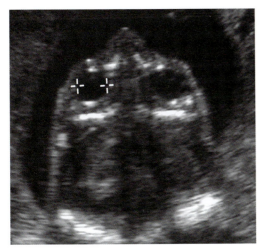

Figure 4-9. A Binocular distance is measured from the lateral edge of one orbit to the lateral edge of the other. **B** Interorbital distance is measured between the two medial inner bony surfaces of the orbits. **C** Orbital diameter (distance) is measured from the medial inner bony surface to the lateral inner bony surface of each orbit individually.

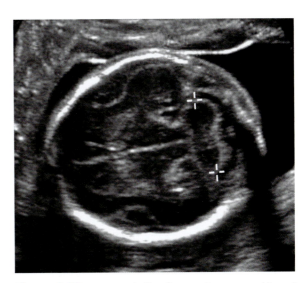

Figure 4-10. Transcerebellar diameter is measured from the right to left lateral aspects of the cerebellum in an axial plane of section.

Table 4-7. Transverse cerebellar diameter by gestational age and percentile.

Menstrual Age (Weeks)	Cerebellum Diameter (mm) Percentile				
	10th	25th	50th	75th	90th
15	10	12	14	15	16
16	14	16	16	16	17
17	16	17	17	18	18
18	17	18	18	19	19
19	18	18	19	19	22
20	18	19	20	20	22
21	19	20	22	23	24
22	21	23	23	24	24
23	22	23	24	25	26
24	22	24	25	27	28
25	23	21.5	28	28	29
26	25	28	29	30	32
27	26	28.5	30	31	32
28	27	30	31	32	34
29	29	32	34	36	38
30	31	32	35	37	40
31	32	35	38	39	43
32	33	36	38	40	42
33	32	36	40	43	44
34	33	38	40	41	44
35	31	37	40.5	43	47
36	36	29	43	52	55
37	37	37	45	52	55
38	40	40	48.5	52	55
39	52	52	52	55	55

Source: Reprinted with permission from Goldstein I, Reece A, Pilu G, et al: Cerebellar measurements with ultrasonography in the evaluation of fetal growth and development. Am J Obstet Gynecol 156:1065, 1987.

of nasal bone calcification has also proven useful in increasing the accuracy of sonographic identification of trisomy conditions, particularly trisomy 21. Absence of a sonographically identifiable nasal bone during the first trimester has been associated with an increased risk of aneuploidy.[10]

Renal Length
Both kidneys are measured in long axis, and the greatest value is compared to standardized charts for determination of gestational age. Renal length measurements are most accurate between 24 and 38 weeks.[11]

Spleen, Liver, and Lung Lengths
Spleen, liver, and lungs can also be measured in long axis and the obtained values compared to standardized charts to provide adjunctive data in the assessment of gestational age.

Thoracic Circumference
Similar to abdominal circumference measurements, the cross-sectional diameter or area of the fetal chest can be obtained and compared to standardized charts to provide adjunctive data in the assessment of gestational age.

Table 4-8. Fetal biophysical profile scores.

Parameter	Normal (2 Points)	Abnormal (0 Points)
Nonstress test (NST)	At least 2 accelerations in 20 minutes	<2 accelerations in 20 minutes
Fetal breathing	At least 1 episode ≥20 seconds over 30 minutes	<20 seconds over 30 minutes
Fetal muscle tone	At least 1 episode as described	Absent or slow and incomplete movements
Fetal activity	At least 2 movements of the torso and limbs over 30 minutes	<2 movements over 30 minutes
Amniotic fluid volume (maximum vertical pocket)	At least 1 pocket >2 cm	Largest pocket ≤2 cm

FETAL BIOPHYSICAL PROFILE

The *biophysical profile* (BPP) is a prenatal method of evaluating fetal well-being, normally assessed only during the late second trimester and third trimester. BPPs are indicated when concerns arise about the overall health of the pregnancy, usually as a result of a nonreactive stress test or other clinical complications during pregnancy.

Five parameters are measured in a BPP: four observed sonographic assessments and a nonstress test (NST). The NST monitors fetal heart rate (FHR) and its response to fetal movement. The results are generally categorized as *reactive*, in which the fetal heart rate accelerates to at least 15 beats per minute for at least 15 seconds within a 20-minute window, or *nonreactive*, in which the heart rate fails to meet this criterion.

The sonographic parameters assessed during a biophysical profile are observed over a 30-minute period and include the following:

- *Fetal breathing motion*, considered abnormal if breathing activity is absent or lasts 20 seconds or less over 30 minutes of observation.
- *Fetal tone*, as evidenced by flexion/extension of the limbs or by bending and straightening of the trunk. Tone is considered abnormal if fetal movement is absent or slow and flexion/extension are incomplete.
- *Fetal activity*, as evidenced by gross body movements of the torso and/or limbs. Activity is considered abnormal if there are fewer than two episodes of limb/body movement over the 30 minutes of observation.
- *Amniotic fluid volume*, as determined by measuring the largest vertical pocket. Fluid volume is considered abnormal if the largest pocket is ≤ 2 cm. (For more on measuring amniotic fluid, see Chapter 7.)

The observed presence of these biophysical parameters provides indirect evidence of adequate fetal oxygenation; their absence implies hypoxemia. Oxygen-compromised fetuses typically exhibit diminished accelerations of fetal heart rate, decreased body movement and breathing, hypotonia, and, less acutely, decreased amniotic fluid volume.

In the scoring of a biophysical profile, each of these parameters is assigned a value of either 2 or 0 points—2 indicating that the observed parameter meets normal standards and 0 indicating a parameter that falls below the standard (Table 4-8). The maximum total score for the sonographic components of a biophysical profile is 8. When added to the score for a normal nonstress test, the maximum score can be 10.

The biophysical profile provides useful information in managing a pregnancy that may be at risk. Guidelines have been established for recommended management of a patient based on the biophysical profile score (Table 4-9).

Table 4-9. Recommended management based on biophysical profile (BPP) score.

Score	Management
≤2	Labor induction
4	Labor induction if gestational age >32 weeks
<6	Repeat BPP on same day if <32 weeks, then deliver if the score is the same or less
8	Labor induction if oligohydramnios is present

CHAPTER 4 REVIEW QUESTIONS

1. Using an endovaginal approach, the sonographer can identify a gestational sac within the uterine cavity as early as:
   A. 3.5 weeks
   B. 4.0 weeks
   C. 4.5 weeks
   D. 5.0 weeks

2. The earliest measure of sonographically demonstrable gestational age is:
   A. Biparietal diameter
   B. Mean sac diameter
   C. Yolk sac size
   D. Crown-rump length

3. A normal intrauterine gestational sac grows at the rate of approximately:
   A. 1 mm per day
   B. 2 mm per day
   C. 3 mm per day
   D. 4 mm per day

4. There is an increased risk of spontaneous abortion when the mean sac diameter (MSD) minus the crown-rump length (CRL) is:
   A. < 5 mm
   B. < 7 mm
   C. < 10 mm
   D. < 12 mm

5. Anatomic landmarks identified at a proper plane of section for head circumference include:
   A. Cavum septi pellucidi, falx cerebri, and thalamic nuclei
   B. Cavum septi pellucidi, cerebellar hemispheres, and thalamic nuclei
   C. Falx cerebri, interhemispheric fissure, and thalamic nuclei
   D. Falx cerebri, Sylvian fissure, and cerebellar hemispheres

6. The most accurate sonographic estimation of gestational age in a dolichocephalic fetus may be obtained by measuring the:
   A. Biparietal diameter
   B. Head circumference
   C. Cephalic index
   D. BPD/AC ratio

7. Abdominal circumference measurements are most useful in assessing:
   A. Gestational age
   B. Estimated date of confinement (EDC)
   C. Normal somatic growth of the fetus
   D. Fetal oxygenation

8. The least reliable indicator of gestational age is:
   A. Crown-rump length
   B. Biparietal diameter
   C. Mean sac diameter
   D. Abdominal circumference

9. The distal femoral epiphysis is demonstrable sonographically at:
   A. 32 weeks
   B. 33 weeks
   C. 34 weeks
   D. 36 weeks

10. All of the following parameters are assessed in a fetal biophysical profile EXCEPT:
    A. Fetal femur length
    B. Fetal breathing
    C. Amniotic fluid volume
    D. Fetal tone

11. A perfectly normal score from the sonographic parameters assessed during a fetal biophysical profile is:
    A. 5
    B. 6
    C. 7
    D. 8

12. In a normal fetal biophysical profile, the maximum vertical pocket of amniotic fluid should measure:
    A. >2 cm
    B. >4 cm
    C. >6 cm
    D. >8 cm

ANSWERS

See Appendix A on page 478 for answers.

REFERENCES

1. Kalish RB, Chervenak FA. Sonographic determination of gestational age. Ultrasound Rev Obstet Gynecol 5:254–258, 2005.

2. Lynch L, Lapinski R, Alvarez M, et al: Accuracy of ultrasound estimation of fetal weight in multiple pregnancies. Ultrasound Obstet Gynecol 6:349–352, 1995.

3. Wax J, Minkoff H, Johnson A, et al: Consensus report on the detailed fetal anatomic ultrasound examination: indications, components, and qualifications. J Ultrasound Med 33:189–195, 2014.

4. de Crespigny LC, Cooper D, McKenna M: Early detection of intrauterine pregnancy with ultrasound. J Ultrasound Med 7:7–10, 1988.

5. Benson CB, Doubilet PM: Fetal measurements: normal and abnormal fetal growth. In Rumack CM, Wilson SR, Charboneau JW (eds): *Diagnostic Ultrasound*, 2nd edition. Philadelphia, Elsevier Mosby, 1994, p 1014.

6. Hadlock FP: Ultrasound evaluation of fetal growth. In Callen PW (ed): *Ultrasonography in Obstetrics and Gynecology*, 3rd edition. Philadelphia, Saunders Elsevier, 1994, p 132.

7. DuBose TJ, Hagen-Ansert SL: Obstetric measurements and gestational age. In Hagen-Ansert SL (ed): *Textbook of Diagnostic Sonography*, 7th edition. St. Louis, Elsevier Mosby, 2012, pp 1147–1149.

8. Gray DL, Songster GS, Parvin CA, et al: Cephalic index: a gestational age–dependent biometric parameter. Obstet Gynecol 74:600–603, 1989.

9. Goldstein RB, Filly RA, Simpson G: Pitfalls in femur length measurements. J Ultrasound Med 6:203–207, 1987.

10. Rossen T, D'Alton ME, Platt LD, et al: First-trimester ultrasound assessment of the nasal bone to screen for aneuploidy. Obstet Gynecol 110:399–404, 2007.

11. Konje JC, Abrams KR, Bell SC, et al: Determination of gestational age after the 24th week of gestation from fetal kidney length measurements. Ultrasound Obstet Gynecol 19:592–597, 2002.

SUGGESTED READINGS

Benson CB, Doubilet PM: Fetal measurements: normal and abnormal fetal growth. In Rumack CM, Wilson SR, Charboneau JW, et al (eds): *Diagnostic Ultrasound*, 4th edition. Philadelphia, Elsevier Mosby, 2011, pp 1455–1471.

Galan HL, Panipati S, Filly RA: Ultrasound evaluation of fetal biometry and normal and abnormal fetal growth. In Calen PW (ed): *Ultrasonography in Obstetrics and Gynecology*, 5th edition. Philadelphia, Saunders Elsevier, 2008, pp 225–265.

Rodriguez J, Gill KA, Sliman MH: The second and third trimesters: basic and targeted scans. In Gill KG, *Ultrasound in Obstetrics and Gynecology: A Practitioner's Guide*. Pasadena, Davies, 2014, pp 119–178.

CHAPTER 5

The Fetal Face and Neck

Embryology

Face and Neck Abnormalities

Evaluation of the fetal face and neck provides detailed information about the morphologic integrity of the fetus. Both the overlying soft tissue and the underlying bony structures of the face yield information that can be valuable in detecting anomalous fetal conditions and syndromes. Newer applications of diagnostic sonography, particularly three-dimensional (3D) surface rendering, permit imaging of the fetal face and neck at a new level of detail and accuracy.

EMBRYOLOGY

FACE

By 6 menstrual weeks, the components of the embryonic face are gathered around the primordial mouth and nasal cavity, the stomodeum. Three facial prominences (Figure 5-1) evolve into the several areas of the face:

- The single *frontonasal prominence*, which surrounds the forebrain, gives rise to the forehead, nose, and eyes.
- The paired *maxillary* and *mandibular prominences* grow to create the boundaries of the primitive mouth.

The bony structures of the face begin to form at 6–7 menstrual weeks. By 8–9 weeks ossification of the mandible, maxilla, and orbits has begun, and by 11–12 weeks the bony structures of the face are routinely visible sonographically. By 14–16 weeks the structures are more completely formed and are more amenable to a detailed sonographic examination. The calcification present in the facial bones produces the high-amplitude echoes that permit early examination of the fetal face.

The developmental mechanism of the hard and soft palates begins at the end of the 7th menstrual week and is completed at the beginning of 11th menstrual week. The palate develops from bits and pieces of both nasal and maxillary prominences that grow symmetrically toward the midline from each side. As they fuse, they form the *primary palate*, which will become the *premaxillary portion* of the maxilla, the small segment of the maxilla that holds the four incisor teeth (Figure 5-2). The *philtrum* is also formed by the merging nasal prominences. The *secondary palate*, arising from mesenchymal tissue projecting from the maxillary prominences, will form the hard and soft palates. These projections, known as the *lateral palatine processes*, grow horizontally to form the roof of the oral cavity (Figure 5-3). Development of the palate is complete by the end of the first trimester (Figure 5-4) and marks the completion of facial development as well.

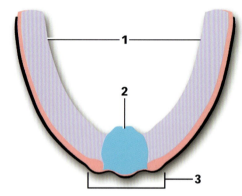

Figure 5-2. Embryology of the primary palate. 1 = developing maxilla (maxillary prominences), 2 = primary palate (fused nasal prominences), 3 = philtrum of lip.

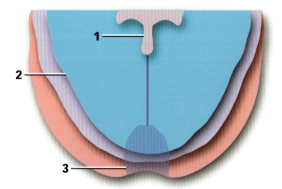

Figure 5-3. Embryology of the hard and soft palates. 1 = lateral palatine process, 2 = secondary palate, 3 = philtrum of lip.

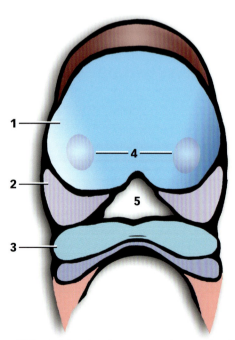

Figure 5-1. Facial embryology at 6 weeks. Anterior view of the embryonic face at 6 conceptual (8 menstrual) weeks demonstrating primitive eyes and mouth (stomodeum). 1 = frontonasal prominence, 2 = maxillary prominence, 3 = mandibular prominence, 4 = primitive eyes, 5 = stomodeum.

NECK

The *pharyngeal arches* and *grooves* are outpouchings of embryonic connective tissue (mesenchyme) that, by the 12th menstrual week, have metamorphosed into face, nasal cavities, mouth, tongue, larynx, pharynx, and neck fascia. The adenomatous tissues in the neck—i.e., salivary and thyroid glands—develop from thickened swatches of endoderm lining the stomodeum, while the skeletal, neural, muscular, and vascular structures of the neck arise from simple mesenchyme in the arches. *Somites*—bilaterally paired blocks of mesoderm that form along the anterior-posterior axis of the developing embryo—give rise to axial skeletal muscle, cartilage, tendons, endothelial cells, and dermis (Figure 5-5).

During routine sonographic examination of the fetal face, which includes a real-time survey of both bony and soft tissue structures, most clinically significant anomalies can be identified, prompting a targeted and detailed assessment of facial anatomy. Fetal facial anatomy can be visualized with great clarity using high-resolution sonographic imaging methods, particularly when 3D surface rendering techniques are used by 10 weeks' gestation (Figure 5-6).

The protocol for a targeted and detailed examination of the fetal face includes the following:

- Sagittal views of the orbits, nose, lips, maxilla, and anterior portion of the mandible (Figures 5-7A and B).
- Profile view of the soft tissues of the mouth and nasopharynx (Figure 5-8).
- Views of the brow, cheeks, and eyelids (Figures 5-9A and B).
- Views of the lenses and nasal septum (Figure 5-10).

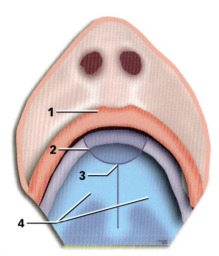

Figure 5-4. Complete palate anatomy. 1 = lip, 2 = primary palate, 3 = incisive foramen, 4 = secondary palate.

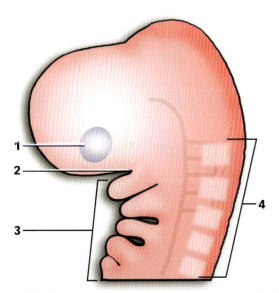

Figure 5-5. Pharyngeal arches, which metamorphose into the eye (1), stomodeum (2), and other aspects of the face and neck, such as the nasal cavities, larynx, pharynx, and neck fascia (3). The somites (4) will give rise to skeletal muscle, cartilage, tendons, endothelial cells, and dermis.

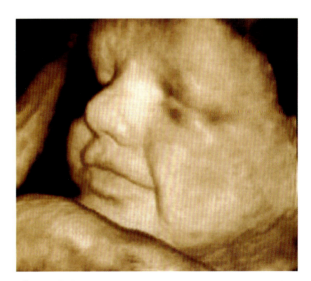

Figure 5-6. 3D facial surface rendering of an 18-week fetus.

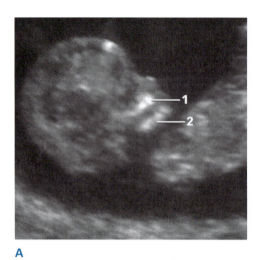

A

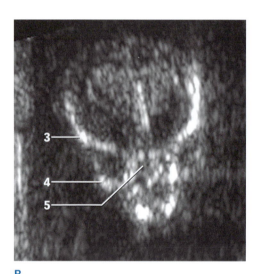

B

Figure 5-7. Facial skeletal embryology at 10 weeks. **A** Sagittal section. **B** Coronal section. 1 = maxilla, 2 = mandible, 3 = frontal bone, 4 = zygoma, 5 = nasal apparatus.

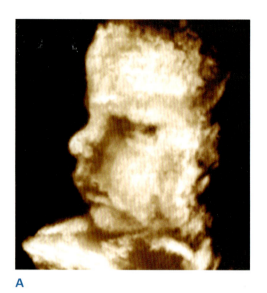

A

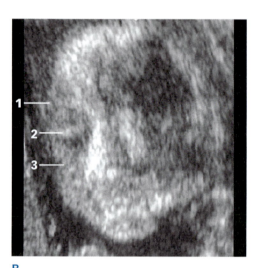

B

Figure 5-9. **A** 3D (profile) and **B** 2D (obllique) coronal views of fetal brow, cheeks, and eyelids. 1 = brow, 2 = eyelid, 3 = cheek.

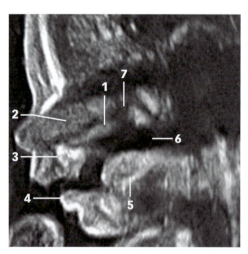

Figure 5-8. Profile view of the soft tissues of the mouth and nasopharynx. 1 = soft palate, 2 = nasal apparatus, 3 = hard palate, 4 = lower lip, 5 = tongue, 6 = oral pharynx, 7 = nasal pharynx.

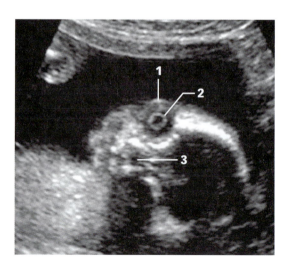

Figure 5-10. Coronal section through the fetal face demonstrating a lens and nasal septum. 1 = orbital rim, 2 = lens, 3 = nasal septum.

- Detailed imaging of the nose and lips, necessary to exclude cleft lip (Figure 5-11).
- In the early second trimester fetus, details of the maxilla, mandible, and (after about 20 weeks) tooth buds (Figure 5-12).
- Views of the fetal tongue, identified most easily during swallowing movements; in some second trimester fetuses, the hard palate can also be evaluated if the fetal position is favorable (Figure 5-13).
- Views of the ears (Figure 5-14).

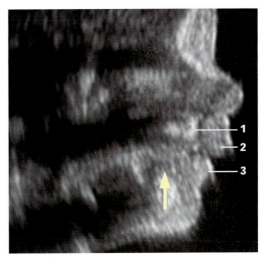

A

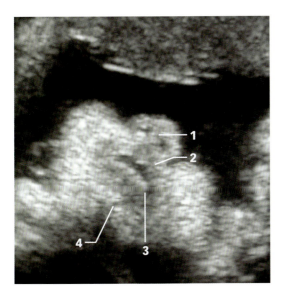

Figure 5-11. Coronal oblique view of the nose and lips to rule out cleft lip in a normal fetus. 1 = median nasal septum, 2 = upper lip, 3 = lower lip, 4 = chin.

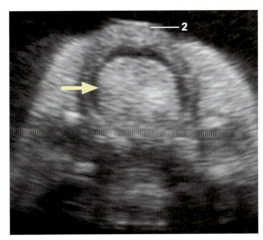

B

Figure 5-13. Two views of the tongue in a second trimester fetus: **A** sagittal and **B** axial. Arrows = tongue, 1 = hard palate, 2 = upper lip, 3 = lower lip.

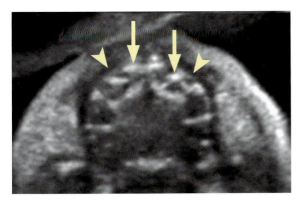

Figure 5-12. Maxilla (arrowheads) and tooth buds (arrows) in this axial section of a 20-week fetus.

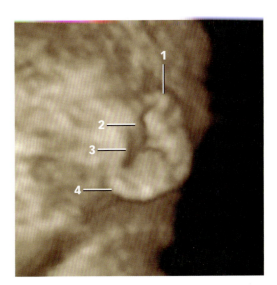

Figure 5-14. 3D surface rendering of a fetal ear at 14 weeks. 1 = helix, 2 = concha, 3 = tragus, 4 = lobule.

- Views of the orbits (Figure 5-15): The orbits are optimally imaged in the axial plane slightly below the plane used for the biparietal diameter (BPD) and head circumference (HC). Subjective assessment of normal orbits will demonstrate them to be of reasonable size and approximately equal in dimension. The *interocular* (also called the *interorbital*) *distance*—i.e., the distance between orbits, measured from the medial or inner canthus of one orbit to the medial or inner canthus of the other—should be approximately equal to the *orbital diameter*, i.e., the distance from the medial to the lateral canthus of one orbit (Figure 5-16). Orbital measurement tables have been established.[1] (See Tables 5-1 and 5-2; for the use of orbital measurements in assessing gestational age, see Chapter 4, page 80.)

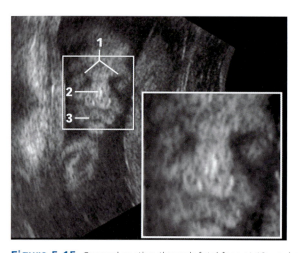

Figure 5-15. Coronal section through fetal face at 18 weeks demonstrating fetal orbits (1), nose (2), and upper lip (3). Inset demonstrates a high-resolution magnification of normal soft tissue structures.

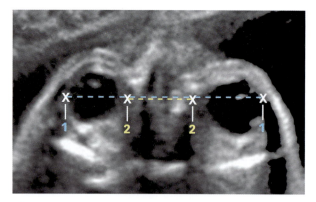

Figure 5-16. Normal orbital distances. 1 (blue) = binocular distance, 2 (yellow) = interocular distance. The orbital diameter is measured from the medial edge to the lateral edge of a single orbit (1 to 2) and should approximate the interocular distance.

FACE AND NECK ABNORMALITIES

Face and neck abnormalities that may emerge from sonographic evaluation over the course of the pregnancy may include clefting anomalies of the lip and palate, orbital/ocular abnormalities, and chin/neck abnormalities. (See Table 5-1.)

CLEFTING ANOMALIES

The category *cleft lip and palate* covers a broad spectrum of relatively common congenital facial anomalies ranging from a simple, unilateral, minor lip defect to severe craniofacial anatomic abnormalities. Cleft lip and palate are especially conspicuous in both gross and sonographic appearance because they result in an abnormal facial appearance and defective speech.

Pathology

Despite the fact that these anomalies are often discussed in the same breath, cleft lip and cleft palate are two separate anomalous entities, each arising at a different moment in the embryologic development of the face. Disruption during the formation of the primary palate, early in the 8th menstrual week, yields anterior cleft anomalies. Failure of proper development of the secondary palate during the 8th–11th weeks produces posterior cleft anomalies as described below.

Table 5-1. Summary of fetal face and neck abnormalities.

Type of Abnormality	Anomaly
Clefting anomalies	Anterior
	Posterior
	Median
Orbital/ocular abnormalities	Hypertelorism
	Hypotelorism
	Cyclopia
	Microphthalmia
	Anophthalmia
Chin/neck abnormalities	Micrognathia
	Macroglossia
	Neck cysts
	Neck teratomas
	Epignathus
	Cystic hygroma

While the exact pathologic appearance of a complex facial cleft varies, the sonographic examination of the fetal face can be simplified by imaging the upper lip, the anterior primary palate, and the posterior secondary palate simultaneously or individually. Two major groups of clefting abnormalities are anterior and posterior cleft anomalies; a third, median cleft facial syndrome, is rare.

Anterior Cleft Palate Anomalies

Clefts of the primary palate include the following:

- Simple cleft lip without premaxillary cleft: incomplete unilateral cleft lip (Figure 5-17A)
- Clefts of the upper lip with premaxillary cleft: complete unilateral cleft lip (Figure 5-17B) and complete bilateral cleft lip (Figure 5-17C)
- Complete anterior cleft extending through lip and maxilla to the incisive fossa: bilateral (Figure 5-17D) and unilateral

Posterior Cleft Palate Anomalies

The landmark for distinguishing anterior from posterior cleft anomalies is the *incisive fossa*. Clefts of the secondary palate through the hard and soft palates include the following:

- Simple cleft palate (Figure 5-18A)
- Unilateral cleft lip and palate (Figure 5-18B)
- Complete (bilateral) cleft palate extending from the posterior soft palate anteriorly to the incisive fossa (Figure 5-18C)

Median Cleft Facial Syndrome

Median cleft facial syndrome, also called *frontonasal dysplasia sequence*, is an extremely rare mesenchymal developmental defect. A median cleft is characterized by derangement of the normal internal anatomic relationships between the nasal cavity and frontal bones in the midline of the skull. It is rarely associated with lip or external facial clefts. The exact pathologic appearance varies widely (Figure 5-19).

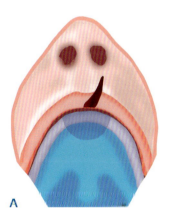
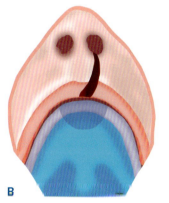
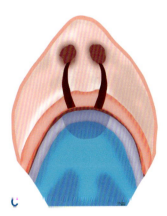
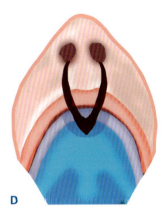

Figure 5-17. Cleft variants of the primary palate. **A** Incomplete unilateral cleft lip. **B** Complete unilateral cleft lip. **C** Complete bilateral cleft lip. **D** Complete anterior cleft extending through lip and maxilla to the incisive fossa: bilateral.

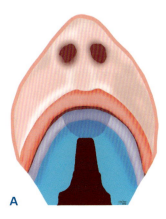
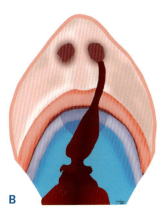
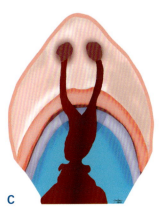

Figure 5-18. Cleft variants of the secondary palate. **A** Simple cleft palate. **B** Unilateral cleft lip and palate. **C** Bilateral cleft lip and palate.

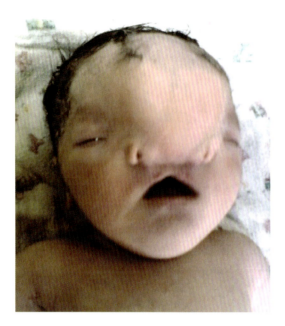 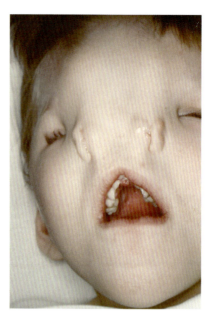

Figure 5-19. Median facial clefting. These two photos of newborns with this rare syndrome demonstrate the wide variation in appearance resulting from the disorder.

Prevalence

- Cleft lip without cleft palate has a prevalence of 0.42 per 1000 live births.
- Cleft palate combined with cleft lip has a prevalence of 0.51 per 1000 live births and accounts for 50% of all facial clefts.[2]
- Cleft palate without cleft lip has a prevalence of 0.47 per 1000 live births and accounts for 30% of all facial clefts.
- Median facial clefting is rare, occurring in only 1 per 10,000 live births.[3]

Sonographic Signs

As mentioned above, evaluation of the soft tissue of the fetal face has been enhanced in the past several years with the introduction of 3D surface rendering methods. The ability to see distinctly and in high resolution the soft tissues of the fetal face in apposition to amniotic fluid is a major advantage of 3D ultrasound, from the perspectives of both patient satisfaction and diagnostic accuracy. By altering the gray-scale assignment curve, the sonographer can create an image that is tinted using various pre- and post-processing methods to produce a skin-tone prenatal portrait that astounds parents and that adds great confidence to the final diagnostic product. Two-dimensional (2D) gray-scale sonographic imaging of the fetal face, while not always as aesthetically dramatic as its 3D adjunct, is equally efficacious in facilitating examination of the fetal face for the types of abnormalities reviewed here.

The following are the characteristic sonographic signs of anterior cleft anomalies:

- The defect may be demonstrated sonographically as a groove extending from one nostril through the lip, usually best demonstrated in a coronal (Figure 5-20A) or axial oblique (Figure 5-20B) plane of section.
- The defect may be unilateral or bilateral (Figures 5-21A and B).
- Polyhydramnios resulting from swallowing difficulties may be present.

The following sonographic signs, tips, and diagnostic challenges are associated with cleft anomalies:

- Cleft palate in the absence of an associated cleft lip is a diagnostic challenge.
- Cleft palate with an associated cleft lip will demonstrate the contiguity of the lip defect with deeper facial structures (Figure 5-22A).
- Amniotic fluid creates excellent sonographic contrast in the oropharyngeal spaces.
- Cleft palate may be accompanied by an alveolar ridge (Figure 5-22B).

As they are rarely associated with concomitant external clefting anomalies of the face or lip, median cleft anomalies have not been reported in the medical literature as being demonstrable sonographically.

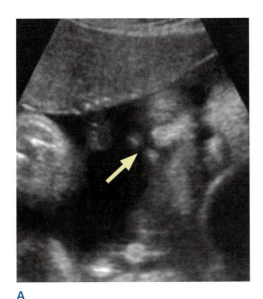
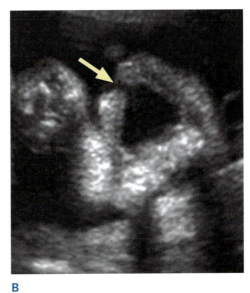

Figure 5-20. A Coronal image of a cleft lip, demonstrated as a groove (arrow) extending from one nostril. **B** Axial oblique image of a cleft (arrow) through the lip.

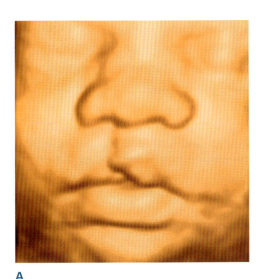
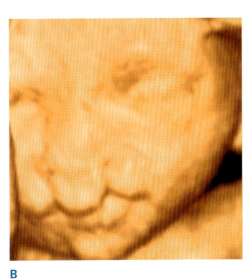

Figures 5-21. 3D surface–rendered images demonstrating **A** unilateral variant of a cleft lip and **B** bilateral variant of a cleft lip.

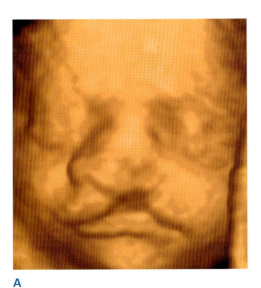
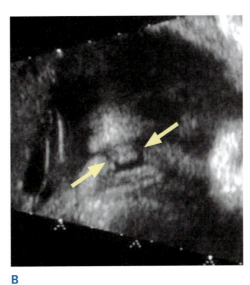

Figure 5-22. Cleft lip and palate variants demonstrated on coronal section: **A** Unilateral in 3D surface rendering. **B** B-mode demonstrating an alveolar ridge (arrows).

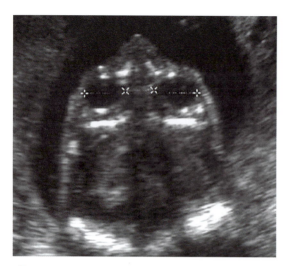

Figure 5-23. Axial oblique view demonstrating orbital symmetry in a normal 14-week fetus.

OCULAR AND ORBITAL ABNORMALITIES

Ocular and orbital malformations are often principal signs of a plethora of generalized syndromes. Hypertelorism, hypotelorism, cyclopia, microphthalmia, and anophthalmia, when identified during routine sonographic examination of fetal anatomy, should prompt the examiner to obtain orbital biometric measurements.

While an experienced sonographer can subjectively identify orbital symmetry in the normal fetus (Figure 5-23) and appreciate any significant asymmetry or disparity in normal orbital diameter, two objective measurements are useful in documenting and quantifying abnormalities.[4] There is a linear association between the size of the head, as measured by the biparietal diameter (BPD), and both *interocular distance* (IOD, also called *interorbital distance*) and *binocular distance* (BOD, also called *outer orbital distance* or OOD).

- Interocular distance is measured between the medial (inner) canthi of the eyes.
- Binocular distance is measured between the lateral (outer) canthi of the eyes (see Figure 5-16).

These values have been plotted on nomograms (Figures 5-24A and B) that are useful visual reference tools for determining normality or quantifying discordance. Tables listing standard measurements by gestational (menstrual) week have also been published (see Tables 5-2 and 5-3).

Orbital Hypertelorism

Orbital *hypertelorism* is identified as an increase in intraorbital distance above the 95th percentile. Subjectively, the orbits appear farther apart, with the interorbital distance visibly as well as measurably larger than the individual orbital diameter. The two conditions typically associated with hypertelorism are midline facial clefting syndrome and frontal encephalocele. In *midline facial clefting syndrome*, a rare condition (see page 92, "Clefting Anomalies"), the face retains its early embryologic appearance, with eyes located laterally on the head and with flanged nares (nostrils) widely separated from each other. With *frontal encephalocele*, neural tissue and meninges protrude through a bony defect on the anterior skull.

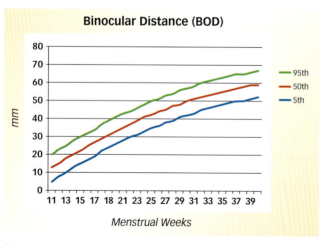

A

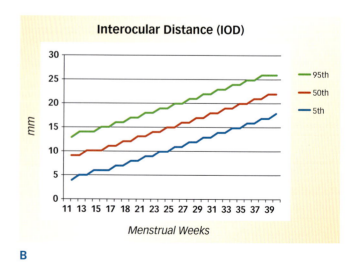

B

Figure 5-24. A Nomogram for binocular distance, based on data in Table 5-2. **B** Nomogram for interocular distance, based on data from Romero R, Pilu G, Jeanty P, et al: *Prenatal Diagnosis of Congenital Anomalies*. New York: Appleton, 1988, p 84. Available at TheFetus.net, http://www.sonoworld.com/Client/Fetus/Files/pcda/PDCA_Face.pdf.

Table 5-2. Mean fetal binocular distance with standard deviations and 5th, 50th, and 95th percentiles for gestational age.

Menstrual Weeks	Mean BOD (cm)	SD (cm)	Percentile 5th	Percentile 50th	Percentile 95th
14	1.91	0.25	1.60	1.90	2.30
15	2.15	0.25	1.70	2.10	2.35
16	2.24	0.24	1.71	2.31	2.69
17	2.55	0.21	2.10	2.51	2.80
18	2.78	0.27	2.30	2.81	3.24
19	2.97	0.25	2.56	3.00	3.53
20	3.07	0.21	2.70	3.10	3.54
21	3.29	0.23	2.85	3.25	3.74
22	3.46	0.19	3.02	3.50	3.80
23	3.67	0.22	3.21	3.66	4.01
24	3.77	0.27	3.48	3.75	4.27
25	4.03	0.23	3.60	4.06	4.40
26	4.16	0.21	3.82	4.15	4.58
27	4.33	0.24	3.95	4.31	4.75
28	4.49	0.22	4.10	4.52	5.03
29	4.67	0.24	4.30	4.61	5.19
30	4.76	0.21	4.41	4.79	5.23
31	4.98	0.26	4.50	5.04	5.40
32	5.05	0.20	4.71	5.12	5.40
33	5.17	0.23	4.73	5.20	5.63
34	5.39	0.26	4.85	5.41	5.82
35	5.46	0.23	4.95	5.60	6.05
36	5.56	0.24	5.02	5.62	5.95
37	5.65	0.27	5.09	5.70	6.10
38	5.81	0.28	5.31	5.80	6.24
39	5.82	0.27	5.32	5.90	6.29
40	5.95	0.27	5.40	6.00	6.40

*BOD = binocular distance; SD = standard deviation.

Source: Adapted from Tongsong T, Wanapitrak C, Jesadapornchai S, et al: Fetal binocular distance as a predictor of menstrual age. Int J Gynaecol Obstet 38:87–91, 1992.

Table 5-3. Values for the fetal orbital diameter (mm).

Menstrual Weeks	Mean	95th CI	Percentile				
			5th	25th	50th	75th	90th
14	5.2	4.8–5.7	4.5	5.0	5.3	5.7	5.7
15	6.1	5.9–6.3	5.4	5.5	6.2	6.5	6.7
16	6.6	6.3–6.9	5.8	6.2	6.5	7.0	7.6
17–18	7.3	6.7–7.8	6.2	6.5	6.7	9.0	9.0
19–20	9.8	9.3–10.2	8.6	9.0	10.0	10.1	11.3
21	10.5	10.0–10.9	9.4	9.9	10.0	11.0	12.0
22	10.4	10.0–10.7	9.5	9.6	10.5	11.0	11.3
23	10.7	10.4–11.1	9.6	10.0	10.5	11.4	11.5
24	11.6	11.3–11.8	10.7	11.0	11.5	12.0	12.5
25	11.2	11.4–12.4	10.3	11.0	12.2	12.5	12.8
26	12.7	12.0–13.4	11.0	11.0	12.7	13.8	14.5
27	13.0	12.4–13.5	11.9	12.0	12.9	13.4	14.8
28	13.0	12.7–13.3	12.1	12.0	13.1	13.3	14.1
29	13.9	13.4–14.4	12.6	13.0	13.7	14.6	15.7
30–31	14.2	13.8–14.5	13.3	13.0	13.9	14.7	15.4
32–33	14.4	13.7–15.1	12.2	13.0	14.1	14.8	17.5
34–36	15.8	15.4–16.2	14.6	15.0	15.7	16.5	16.9

CI = confidence interval.

Source: Adapted from Goldstein I, Tamir A, Zimmer EZ, et al: Growth of the fetal orbit and lens in normal pregnancies. Ultrasound Obstet Gynecol 12:175–179, 1998.

Associated Abnormalities

The following abnormalities are characteristically associated with hypertelorism:

- Trisomy 21 (Down syndrome)
- Trisomy 13 (Patau syndrome)
- Agenesis of the corpus callosum
- Turner syndrome
- Ehlers-Danlos syndrome
- Apert syndrome

Sonographic Signs

The following are the characteristic signs of hypertelorism:

- Orbits placed far apart (Figures 5-25A–C)
- Interocular distance and binocular distance at or above the 95th percentile for dates

Orbital Hypotelorism

Orbital *hypotelorism* is a reduction in the intraorbital distance to below the 5th percentile. When both inner and outer orbital measurements fall below two standard deviations of the mean, other fetal anatomic anomalies are certain to be present. Hypotelorism is most commonly seen in fetuses with concomitant holoprosencephaly (Figure 5-26B); however, it is associated with many other conditions as well.[5]

Associated Abnormalities

The following abnormalities are characteristically associated with hypotelorism:

- Trisomy 13
- Encephalocele (other than frontal encephalocele)
- Cleft palate
- Cardiac anomalies

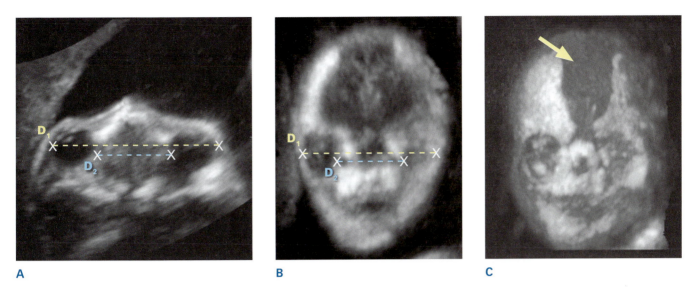

Figure 5-25. Hypertelorism demonstrated by increased transorbital (D_1) and interorbital (D_2) distances. **A** Axial section. **B** Coronal section. **C** 3D reconstruction, also demonstrating a large metopic suture (arrow).

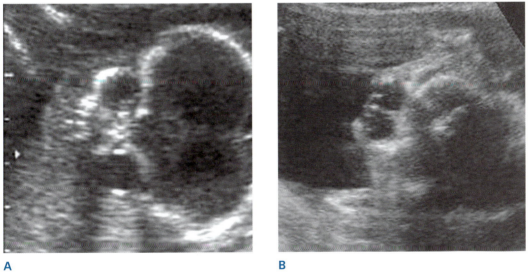

Figure 5-26. Hypotelorism. **A** Moderate hypotelorism, with the nasal apparatus separating the orbits. **B** Severe hypotelorism in a holoprosencephalic fetus.

- Imperforate anus
- Diaphragmatic hernia
- Meckel-Gruber syndrome

Sonographic Signs

The following are the characteristic signs of hypotelorism:

- Close-appearing orbits (Figures 5-26A and B)
- Interocular distance and binocular distance below the 5th percentile for dates

Cyclopia

Cyclopia, also called *cyclocephaly* or *synophthalmia*, is a rare congenital abnormality characterized by a single palpebral fissure and a single midline orbit (Figure 5-27). It results from a severe defect in the embryologic production of two orbits during the growth of the prosencephalon. While it is frequently associated with alobar holoprosencephaly, cyclopia can also be induced by genetic abnormalities or by exposure to certain teratogenic toxins. A single midline orbit can

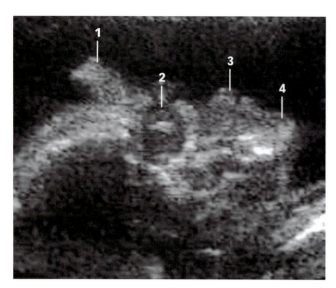

Figure 5-27. Cyclopia is demonstrated in this midline sagittal image. 1 = proboscis, 2 = single midline orbit, 3 = normal-appearing upper lip, 4 = normal-appearing chin.

be anophthalmic, monophthalmic, or synophthalmic (with fusion of the eyes in the latter case). In less severe forms there may be two separate eyes in a single median orbit or two separate orbits set very close together in the mid face. A proboscis is usually present and located above the orbit. Nasal structures are absent. The anterior part of the brain and the mesodermal midline structures are always abnormal in fetuses and infants with cyclopia or synophthalmia.

Associated Abnormalities

The following abnormalities are characteristically associated with cyclopia:

- Alobar holoprosencephaly
- Median facial clefting
- Trisomy 13
- Meckel-Gruber syndrome
- CHARGE association (coloboma of the eye, heart defects, atresia of the nasal choanae, retardation of growth and/or development, genital and/or urinary abnormalities, and ear abnormalities and deafness)

Sonographic Signs

The following are the characteristic sonographic signs of cyclopia:

- Single midline orbit
- Microcephaly associated with 64% of cases
- When associated with holoprosencephaly, additional sonographic findings may include proboscis and other intracranial abnormalities.

Microphthalmia

Microphthalmia is a reduction in orbital size. Subjectively, the affected orbit is disproportionately small in comparison with adjacent facial and cranial structures. This condition may be unilateral or bilateral, and it may occur as an isolated defect or in conjunction with a number of congenital conditions.

Associated Abnormalities

The following abnormalities are characteristically associated with microphthalmia:

- Holoprosencephaly
- In utero infection
- Fetal alcohol syndrome
- Triploidy
- Trisomy 13
- Treacher Collins syndrome

Sonographic Signs

The characteristic sonographic signs of microphthalmia are:

- Reduced orbital size (Figure 5-28)
- Characteristic sonographic findings associated with concomitant congenital conditions when present

Anophthalmia

Anophthalmia is the congenital absence of an eyeball within an orbit. Causes include the failure of primordial eye tissue to grow into the orbit, halted development of the optic vessel for unknown reasons, and degeneration of a developed eye secondary to a toxic or ischemic insult. What remains is a clump of vascularized connective tissue filling the orbit. It may occur unilaterally (Figure 5-29) or bilaterally. Sonography demonstrates complex, echogenic filling of the orbital cavity; the normal anechoic compartments of the eye are absent. Like microphthalmia, anophthalmia may occur in isolation or as part of a syndrome with complex genetic, chromosomal, and environmental factors implicated as causes.[6]

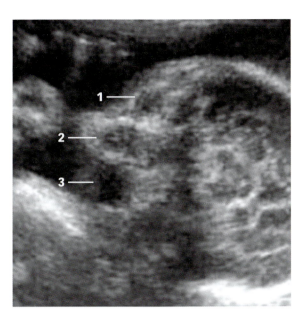

Figure 5-28. Microphthalmia. 1 = microphthalmic right eye (reduced orbital size), 2 = nasal apparatus, 3 = normal-appearing left eye.

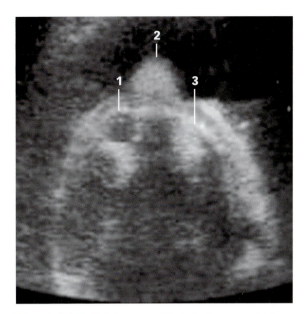

Figure 5-29. Unilateral anophthalmia. 1 = normal left eye, 2 = nose, 3 = absent right eye. Note the complex, echogenic filling of the right orbital cavity.

Associated Abnormalities

The following abnormalities are characteristically associated with anophthalmia:

- Trisomy 13
- CHARGE association
- Heterotaxy
- Lenz syndrome

Sonographic Signs

The following are the characteristic sonographic signs of anophthalmia (Figure 5-29):

- Absent anechoic eye chamber
- Echogenic filling of orbital cavity

CHIN AND NECK ABNORMALITIES

Soft tissue abnormalities of the fetal chin and neck may arise from anomalous embryologic development, such as branchial cleft cysts and thyroglossal duct cysts; from neoplastic transformation of normal structures such as teratomas or thyroid tumors; and from anomalous development of dermal layers and lymphatic channels, which can result in cystic hygromas and diffuse thickening of the nuchal soft tissue. Skeletal abnormalities of the neck include occipital or suboccipital encephalocele and cervical meningomyelocele, which are discussed in Chapter 6, "Neural Tube Defects," pages 137–143.

Micrognathia

Micrognathia describes an abnormally small mandible. It occurs as part of many syndromes and, if severe, may compromise respiration. Although charts have been developed for mandibular length, micrognathia is typically diagnosed as a subjective observation of the midline profile of the fetal face when the fetal chin is noticeably small and receding.

Associated Abnormalities

The following abnormalities[7] are characteristically associated with micrognathia:

- Achondrogenesis
- Campomelic dysplasia
- Trisomy 18 (Edwards syndrome)
- Meckel-Gruber syndrome
- Oral-facial-digital syndrome
- Treacher Collins syndrome
- Deletion syndromes

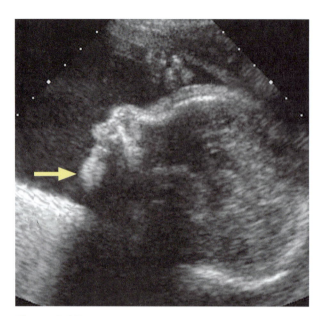

Figure 5-30. Micrognathia. Midline sagittal view of a fetus demonstrating receding chin (arrow).

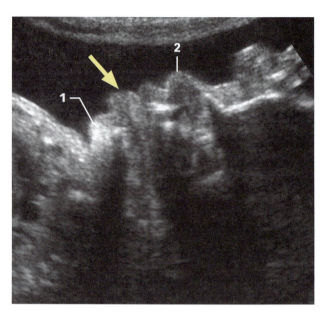

Figure 5-31. Macroglossia. Midline sagittal view of the fetal face at 18 weeks demonstrating an enlarged tongue (arrow) protruding from the mouth. 1 = chin, 2 = nose.

Sonographic Signs

Because a large portion of normal mandibular growth occurs in the third trimester, micrognathia is best diagnosed toward the latter half of pregnancy. Sonographic signs include the following:

- A true sagittal facial image demonstrates a receding chin (Figure 5-30).
- The jaw index (mandibular anteroposterior diameter divided by biparietal diameter) × 100 ≤ 23. Using a cutoff level of 23, the jaw index has 100% sensitivity and 98.1% specificity in diagnosing micrognathia, in comparison with 72.7% and 99.2%, shown by the subjective evaluation of the fetal profile. With a cutoff of 21 the jaw index yields a positive predictive value of 100%.[8]
- Polyhydramnios suggests impairment of the fetal swallowing mechanism.

Macroglossia

Macroglossia (Figure 5-31) describes an abnormally large tongue. On routine sonography of the fetal face, the tongue may be observed moving in the mouth, but if the tongue extends beyond the fetal lips repeatedly or persistently, the diagnosis of macroglossia should be considered. The most common syndrome associated with macroglossia is *Beckwith-Wiedemann syndrome*, in which omphalocele, enlargement of intra-abdominal organs, and asymmetry of the fetal limbs may also be observed. Protrusion of the tongue may also be caused by a posterior solid mass displacing it forward. The mass, such as a lymphangioma, may arise from the tongue itself or from adjacent tissue, as in the case of an epignathus (see page 104). Macroglossia is typically visualized late in pregnancy.

Associated Abnormalities

The following abnormalities are characteristically associated with macroglossia:[9]

- Beckwith-Wiedemann syndrome
- Congenital hypothyroid syndrome
- Trisomy 21
- Triploidy
- Hunter syndrome

Sonographic Signs

The following are the characteristic sonographic signs of macroglossia:

- It is best appreciated on a midline sagittal facial view as a protrusion between the upper and lower lips.
- There is the appearance of a big tongue.

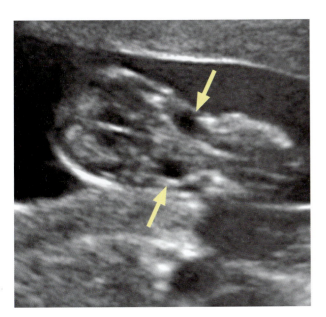

Figure 5-32. Coronal view of bilateral branchial cleft cysts (arrows) appearing as smooth-bordered, anechoic masses in both sides of the neck at 10 weeks.

- The tongue remains outside the mouth regardless of swallowing movements of the lips.
- Polyhydramnios suggests impairment of the fetal swallowing mechanism.

Neck Cysts

Branchial cleft and thyroglossal duct cysts are rarely encountered in fetal imaging studies, appearing more often as mobile, subdermal masses in children and young adults. *Branchial cleft cysts* arise from the failure of the branchial cleft to undergo normal embryologic obliteration and are located laterally in the neck between the sternocleidomastoid muscle and the pharynx. *Thyroglossal duct cysts* arise from a persistence of the thyroglossal tract and are most commonly located in the midline of the neck around the hyoid bone.

Sonographic Signs

When they do occur in the fetus, the following are the characteristic sonographic signs of neck cysts:

- Smooth-bordered, anechoic mass in neck (Figure 5-32)
- Posterior acoustic enhancement
- Displacement of normal midline anatomic structures

Neck Teratomas

Teratomas are encapsulated tumors containing tissue components derived from all three embryonic germ layers—endoderm, ectoderm, and mesoderm. Their gross pathologic appearance varies widely, from predominantly solid masses to complex heterogeneous masses containing both cystic and solid components. Some teratomas are collections of solid tissue containing bits of bone, teeth, hair, and liquefied fat. Such dramatic, gross pathologic appearances have earned the name *teratoma*, which translates literally as "monster tumor."

Most prenatally diagnosed teratomas in the neck (Figure 5-33) or in the sacrococcygeal region are of the immature variety, rendering them most likely benign. Mature teratomas, on the other hand, carry a higher probability of malignant transformation and, with that, a more ominous perinatal outcome. All teratomas, however, maintain some malignant potential.[10]

Teratomas of the neck range in size and location from small, easily resectable masses to large, airway-obstructing lesions that may lead to death—in utero, secondary to the metabolic demands that large tumors impose on the fetus, and postnatally, secondary to respiratory failure. A cervical location is rare, accounting for less than 5% of all prenatally diagnosed teratomas. However, when they do appear in the neck, they commonly arise along the anterior midline of the neck and extrude exophytically into the amniotic cavity.

Associated Abnormalities

The following abnormalities may be associated with teratomas of the neck:

- Hydrops fetalis
- Neonatal airway obstruction

Sonographic Signs

The following are the characteristic sonographic signs of teratomas of the neck:

- A complex, cystic/solid tumor is seen near the fetal neck (Figure 5-33A).
- Calcifications may be present (Figure 5-33B).
- Polyhydramnios is present in 30% of cases.

Identification of the origin of the mass is essential to determine whether a teratoma is an epignathus.

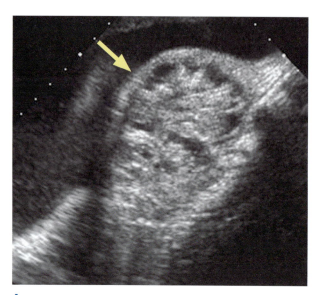 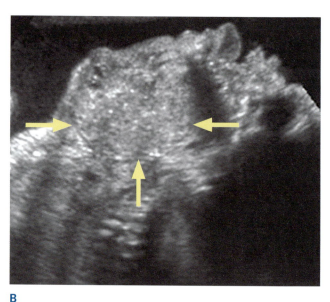

Figure 5-33. Neck teratoma. **A** Sagittal view demonstrating a complex, solid cystic tumor arising exophytically from the anterior fetal neck (arrow). **B** Sagittal view through the fetal neck demonstrating a predominantly solid mass containing focal calcifications and causing exaggerated hyperextension of the head (arrows).

Epignathus

An *epignathus* is a rare type of teratoma that arises from the oral cavity or pharynx. Most of these tumors arise from the sphenoid bone, but other sites of origin include the hard and soft palates, pharynx, tongue, and jaw. From its point of origin, an epignathus grows to fill the entire oral or nasal cavity. These masses may also invade the intracranial space. As is typical for a teratoma, the histologic composition is a combination of tissues from all three germ cell layers and may contain adipose tissue, bone, cartilage, and nerve tissue. An epignathus that fills the oral and nasal cavity obstructs swallowing and produces the polyhydramnios that is commonly present. Airway obstruction can lead to acute asphyxia immediately after birth.

Associated Abnormalities

The following abnormalities[11] are characteristically associated with epignathus:

- Cleft palate
- Facial hemangiomas
- Branchial cysts
- Hypotelorism
- Umbilical hernia
- Congenital heart defects

Sonographic Signs

The following are the characteristic sonographic signs of epignathus:

- Complex mass protruding from fetal mouth and/or neck (Figure 5-34)
- Polyhydramnios

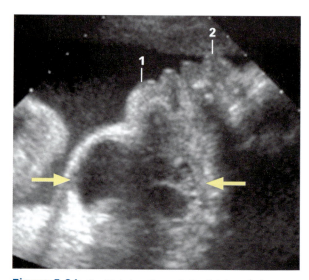

Figure 5-34. Sagittal view through the fetal neck demonstrating complex cystic/solid epignathus (arrows) arising from the oral cavity. 1 = chin, 2 = nose.

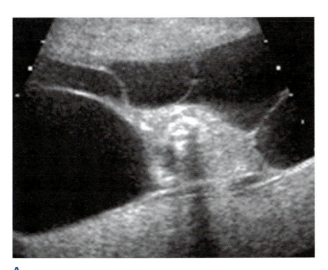 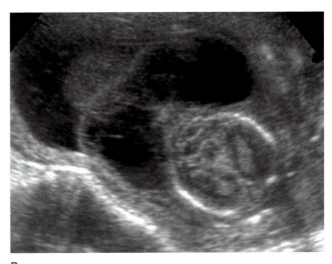

Figure 5-35. Cystic hygroma. Axial sections through **A** the neck and **B** the head demonstrating the large septated fluid collections characteristic of cystic hygroma.

Cystic Hygromas

A *cystic hygroma* is a benign developmental anomaly of lymphatic origin characterized by single or multiple cystic areas within soft tissues surrounding the neck. In the fetus, the lymphatic system drains into bilateral jugular lymphatic sacs. Atresia of the communicating lymphatic channel into the jugular vein results in lymphatic stasis and subsequent dilatation of lymph-carrying branches downstream. Overdistention of the jugular lymphatic sacs located along each side of the neck results in the collection of fluid usually partitioned by a thick fibrous band corresponding to the nuchal ligament. The thinner septa present are thought to derive from either fibrous structures of the neck or deposits of fibrin within the fluid collection. The sizes of these lesions vary greatly, from small, singular collections of fluid to enormous cysts that may be larger than the fetus itself. In cases of generalized fetal hydrops created by the fluid overload, pleural effusions, ascites, and severe skin edema are present. Cystic hygromas are frequently found in association with chromosomal aberrations, most commonly Turner syndrome.

Differential Diagnosis

Differential diagnoses of cystic hygromas include:
- Fetal hydrops fetalis
- Cervical meningomyelocele
- Teratoma
- Neural tube defects

Associated Abnormalities

The following abnormalities are characteristically associated with cystic hygromas:
- Turner syndrome
- Trisomies 13, 18, 21
- Noonan syndrome

Sonographic Signs

The following are the characteristic sonographic signs of a cystic hygroma:
- Fluid-filled structure presenting as a cystic mass contiguous with the chest wall.
- Thin-walled, multiseptated cyst usually located posterior to the fetal head/neck (Figures 5-35A and B).
- Associated with fetal ascites, fetal edema, enlarged edematous placenta, and intradermal fluid collections (cystic cutaneous lymphangiectasia).

CHAPTER 5 REVIEW QUESTIONS

1. The primordial components of the face are in place embryologically by:
    A. 4 menstrual weeks
    B. 5 menstrual weeks
    C. 6 menstrual weeks
    D. 7 menstrual weeks

2. The bony structures of the face begin to form at:
   A. 4–5 menstrual weeks
   B. 5–6 menstrual weeks
   C. 6–7 menstrual weeks
   D. 7–8 menstrual weeks

3. The hard and soft palates arise from which embryologic structure?
   A. Primary palate
   B. Secondary palate
   C. Lateral palatine processes
   D. Pharyngeal arches

4. The arrows in this image point to the:

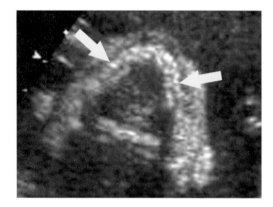

   A. Mandible
   B. Maxilla
   C. Soft palate
   D. Hard palate

5. The arrow in this image points to the:

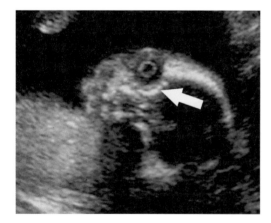

   A. Nasal septum
   B. Ethmoid bone
   C. Orbital rim
   D. Occipital bone

6. All of the following clefting abnormalities of the fetal face result from anomalous development of the primary palate EXCEPT:
   A. Simple cleft lip
   B. Complete cleft palate
   C. Premaxillary cleft lip
   D. Complete anterior cleft lip and palate

7. The most prevalent type of facial clefting is:
   A. Cleft lip and palate
   B. Cleft lip alone
   C. Cleft palate alone
   D. Median facial clefting

8. This midline sagittal sonogram through the fetal face demonstrates:

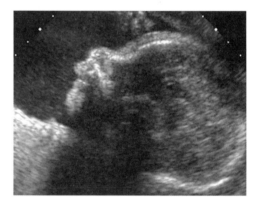

   A. Micrognathia
   B. Cleft palate
   C. Macroglossia
   D. Microglossia

9. This axial oblique image through the fetal face demonstrates:

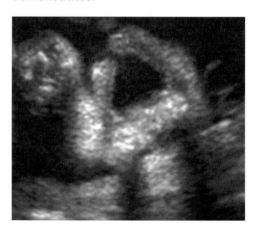

   A. Micrognathia
   B. Cleft lip

C. Cleft palate
D. Macroglossia

10. Which of the following sonographic findings is frequently associated with fetal facial clefting anomalies?
    A. Oligohydramnios
    B. Polyhydramnios
    C. Vasa previa
    D. Placenta accreta

11. A facial anomaly characterized by an increase in intraorbital distance above the 95th percentile is called:
    A. Anophthalmia
    B. Hypotelorism
    C. Hypertelorism
    D. Cyclopia

12. A facial anomaly characterized by a single midline orbit is called:
    A. Anophthalmia
    B. Hypotelorism
    C. Hypertelorism
    D. Cyclopia

13. All of the following anomalous conditions are associated with orbital hypertelorism EXCEPT:
    A. Trisomy 21
    B. Trisomy 13
    C. Turner syndrome
    D. Alobar holoprosencephaly

14. All of the following anomalous conditions are associated with cyclopia EXCEPT:
    A. Trisomy 21
    B. Trisomy 13
    C. Median facial clefting
    D. Alobar holoprosencephaly

15. The congenital absence of an eyeball within an orbit is called:
    A. Hypertelorism
    B. Hypotelorism
    C. Microphthalmia
    D. Anophthalmia

16. Sagittal and axial sections through the fetal orbits presented in this image best demonstrate:

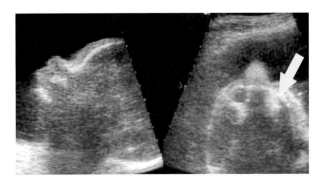

    A. Hypotelorism
    B. Hypertelorism
    C. Anophthalmia
    D. Cyclopia

17. This midline sagittal image through the fetal face best demonstrates:

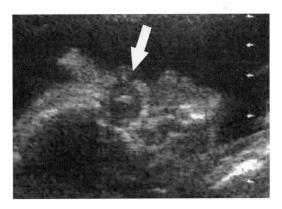

    A. Hydrocephalus
    B. Hypertelorism
    C. Anophthalmia
    D. Cyclopia

18. An abnormally small mandible is referred to as:
    A. Microglossia
    B. Micrognathia
    C. Treacher Collins syndrome
    D. Microphthalmia

19. A congenital anomaly associated with both Beckwith-Wiedemann syndrome and trisomy 21 is:
    A. Macroglossia
    B. Branchial cleft cyst
    C. Cyclopia
    D. Epignathus

20. The axial section through the fetal face presented in this image best demonstrates:

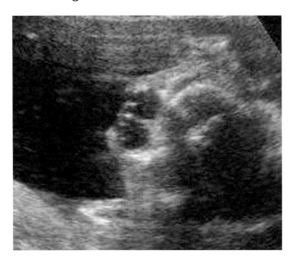

   A. Hypotelorism
   B. Hypertelorism
   C. Anophthalmia
   D. Cyclopia

21. A particular type of teratoma that arises from the oral cavity or pharynx is called a(n):
   A. Craniopharyngioma
   B. Epignathus
   C. Sacral teratoma
   D. Macroglossia

22. Teratomas contain tissue components that arise from which of the following germ cell layers?
   A. Endoderm
   B. Ectoderm
   C. Mesoderm
   D. All of the above

23. The sagittal section through the fetal neck presented in this image best demonstrates:

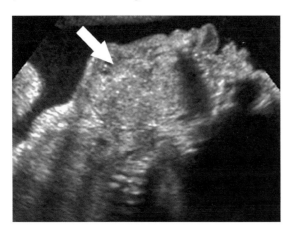

   A. Cystic hygroma
   B. Multinodular goiter
   C. Teratoma
   D. Lymphoma

24. The coronal section through the fetal neck presented in this image best demonstrates:

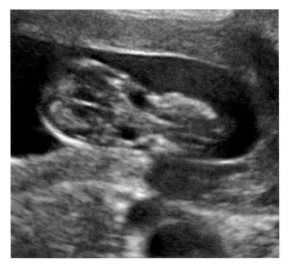

   A. Cystic hygroma
   B. Teratoma
   C. Thyroglossal duct cysts
   D. Nuchal thickening

25. Which term refers to a benign developmental anomaly of the lymphatic system that results in loculated fluid collections within the soft tissues surrounding the neck?
   A. Cystic hygroma
   B. Anasarca
   C. Hydrops fetalis
   D. Nuchal thickening

26. Cystic hygroma is most commonly found in association with which of the following abnormal congenital chromosomal conditions?
   A. Trisomy 13
   B. Trisomy 21
   C. Turner syndrome
   D. Treacher Collins syndrome

27. The axial section through the fetal head in this image demonstrates:

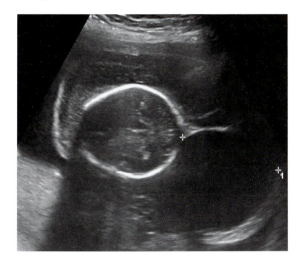

A. Cystic hygroma
B. Lymphedema
C. Hydrops fetalis
D. Teratoma

ANSWERS

See Appendix A on page 479 for answers.

REFERENCES

1. Jeanty P, Dramaix-Wilmet MS, Van Gansbeke D, et al: Fetal ocular biometry by ultrasound. Radiology 143:513–516, 1982.
2. Owens JR, Jones JW, Harris F: Epidemiology of facial clefting. Arch Dis Child 60:521–524, 1985.
3. Saraf S: Median cleft of the lip: a rare facial anomaly. Internet J Plastic Surg 2, 2013. Available at http://ispub.com/IJPS/2/2/4629.
4. Sukonpan K, Phupong V: Fetal ocular distance in normal pregnancies. J Med Assoc Thai 91:1318–1322, 2008.
5. Trout T, Budorick NE, Pretorius DH, et al: Significance of orbital measurements in the fetus. J Ultrasound Med 13:937–943, 1994.
6. Paladini D, D'Armiento M, Ardovino I, et al: Prenatal diagnosis of cerebro-oculo-facio-skeletal (COFS) syndrome. Ultrasound Obstet Gynecol 16:91–93, 2000.
7. Jones KL (ed): *Smith's Recognizable Patterns of Human Malformation*, 7th edition. Philadelphia, Saunders, 2013, pp 794–795.
8. Paladini D, Morra T, Teodoro A, et al: Objective diagnosis of micrognathia in the fetus: the jaw index. Obstet Gynecol 93:382–386, 1999.
9. Jones KL, Jones MC, del Campo Casanelles M (eds): *Smith's Recognizable Patterns of Human Malformation*, 5th edition. Philadelphia, Saunders, 1997, pp 799–800.
10. Heerema-McKenney A, Harrison MR, Bratton B, et al: Congenital teratoma: a clinicopathologic study of 22 fetal and neonatal tumors. Am J Surg Pathol 29:29–38, 2005.
11. Romero R, Pilu G, Jeanty P, et al: *Prenatal Diagnosis of Congenital Anomalies*. Norwalk, CT, Appleton & Lange, 1988, pp 106–108.

SUGGESTED READINGS

Fleischer AC, Toy E, Lee W, et al (eds): *Sonography in Obstetrics and Gynecology: Principles and Practice*, 7th edition. New York, McGraw-Hill, 2011, ch 16.

Laurenco A, Estroff J: The fetal face and neck. In Rumack CM, Wilson SR, Charboneau JW, et al (eds): *Diagnostic Ultrasound*, 4th edition. Philadelphia, Elsevier Mosby, 2011, pp 1166–1196.

Pilu G, Segata M, Perolo A: Ultrasound evaluation of the fetal face and neck. In Callen PW (ed): *Ultrasonography in Obstetrics and Gynecology*, 5th edition. Philadelphia, Elsevier Mosby, 2008, pp 392–418.

Strickland DM, Hagen-Ansert SL: The fetal face and neck. In Hagen-Ansert SL (ed): *Textbook of Diagnostic Ultrasonography*, 7th edition. St. Louis, Elsevier Mosby, 2012, pp 437–446.

CHAPTER 6

The Fetal Central Nervous System

Embryology

The Brain

The Spinal Column

Central Nervous System Abnormalities

The central nervous system comprises the brain, the spinal cord, the meninges, and the skeletal structures that contain and protect them.

EMBRYOLOGY

The central nervous system begins to develop at approximately the 5th menstrual week, with the formation of the *neural tube*—the structure that will give rise to the brain and spinal cord.

NEURULATION

The process by which the neural tube is formed is called *neurulation* (Figure 6-1) and begins 21–23 days after conception (i.e., at 35–37 menstrual days) with the formation of the neural plate and the neural folds. The *neural plate*, which is a thickening of the embryonic ectoderm and adjacent mesoderm,

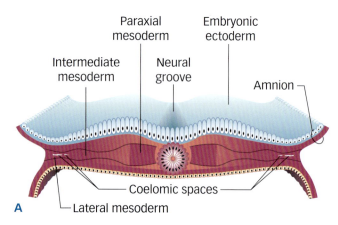
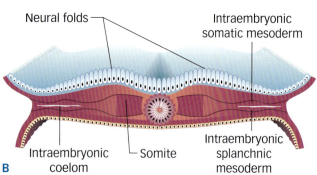
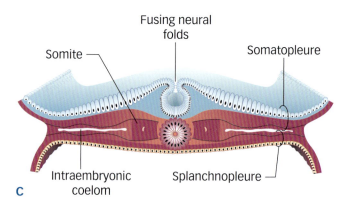

Figure 6-1. Neurulation. Development of the somites and intraembryonic coelom in transverse sections through the trilaminar embryonic disc at approximately **A** 18 conceptual (32 menstrual) days, **B** 20 conceptual (34 menstrual) days, and **C** 21 conceptual (35 menstrual) days. After Moore KL, Persaud TVN, Torchia MG: *The Developing Human: Clinically Oriented Embryology*, 9th edition. Philadelphia, Elsevier Saunders, 2013, p 64.

invaginates along its central axis to form the *neural groove*. Thickened areas adjacent to the groove, the *neural folds*, continue to rise up and grow toward the midline until they come together and fuse, creating the open-ended *neural tube*.

NEURAL TUBE

Fusion of the neural tube begins in the dorsal aspect of the mid portion of the embryo and proceeds in both cranial and caudal directions. The lumen of the neural tube, the *neural canal*, communicates freely with the amniotic cavity via openings at each end called *neuropores*. The rostral (head-end) neuropore closes at approximately conceptual day 25 (menstrual day 39), and the caudal (tail-end) neuropore (Figure 6-2) closes about two days later. When the neuropores fail to close completely, *neural tube defects* result.

INTRACRANIAL VESICLES AND VENTRICLES

After closure, the rostral neuropore evolves into three primary vesicles: the *prosencephalon* or forebrain, which ultimately gives rise to the cerebral hemispheres, lateral ventricles, and midline thalamic structures; the *mesencephalon* or midbrain, which gives rise to the cerebral peduncles, corpora quadrigemina, and cerebral aqueduct; and the *rhombencephalon* or hindbrain, which gives rise to the posterior fossa structures—pons, cerebellum, and medulla (Figure 6-3). From the prosencephalon, two secondary vesicles develop—the telencephalon and the diencephalon. From the rhombencephalon, the metencephalon and myelencephalon develop. (The mesencephalon does not divide.)

The *ventricles* take form from the residual vesicular cavities as solid brain tissue forms within each

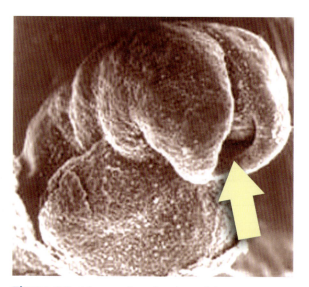

Figure 6-2. Microscopic embryology of the caudal neuropore (arrow).

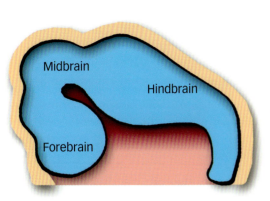
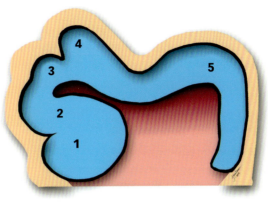

Figure 6-3. Embryonic brain vesicles. The primitive forebrain, midbrain, and hindbrain develop into the (1) telencephalon, (2) diencephalon, (3) mesencephalon, (4) metencephalon, and (5) myelencephalon.

segment of the embryonic brain. One contiguous space remains as the ventricular system of the brain and the central canal of the spinal cord. This space is initially filled with amniotic fluid and later by cerebrospinal fluid, as it is produced by the choroid plexus, which lies within the ventricular system.

THE BRAIN

The relationship between the fetal brain and the ventricles varies over gestation. Initially the ventricles are proportionately quite large when compared to normal adult intracranial anatomy, occupying most of the intracranial space. The lateral ventricles may be seen as early as 8 menstrual weeks and by 13 menstrual weeks are easily demonstrable bilaterally filled with echogenic choroid plexus (Figure 6-4A). Visualization of the rhombencephalon can occur as early as 8 menstrual weeks (Figure 6-4B).

As the gestation continues, the transverse diameter of the lateral ventricles changes little; rather, the cerebral hemispheres grow and develop around them. Between 14 and 40 menstrual weeks the atrium of the lateral ventricles measures approximately 7 mm with a standard deviation of 1 mm, creating a limit of 3 standard deviations for the normal ventricular size of 10 mm—a value that remains constant until term. During this time the paired choroid plexuses also become less prominent in the bodies and anterior horns of the lateral

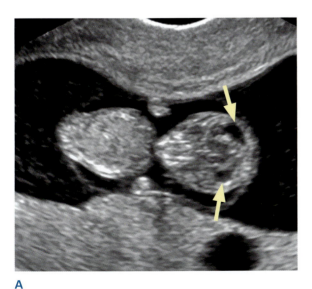
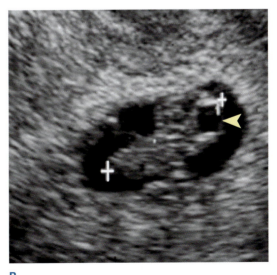

A **B**

Figure 6-4. Sonographic demonstration of normal embryonic intracranial cystic anatomy.
A Coronal section at 8 menstrual weeks demonstrating primitive lateral ventricles (arrows).
B Normal rhombencephalon at 9.5 menstrual weeks (arrowhead).

ventricles, eventually dominating the posterior aspect of these intracranial cavities. By 12 menstrual weeks the corpus callosum—the symmetric midline structure that forms the roof of the lateral ventricles—begins to develop, achieving its adult configuration by approximately 20 menstrual weeks.

In the hindbrain, the *cerebellum* begins its development at 7–8 menstrual weeks as a ridge of neural tissue lining the upper border of the primitive fourth ventricle. This ridge of tissue gives rise to the *cerebellar vermis*, which comprises the primary structural tissues that constitute the brain's functional portions. By 9–10 menstrual weeks, the superior vermis begins its formation, followed by the appearance of the inferior vermis. By 20 menstrual weeks, the hindbrain consists of paired dumbbell-shaped cerebellar hemispheres overlying the now morphologically recognizable fourth ventricle.

The fetal *calvaria* or bony skull—consisting of the frontal, occipital, and paired parietal bones—begins to ossify at about 8 menstrual weeks and should be largely intact and visible by 10–11 menstrual weeks and completely ossified by week 15.

FETAL INTRACRANIAL STRUCTURES

The anatomy of the fetal brain (Figures 6-5A and B) is different from that of an adult in several ways that are important in obstetric sonography. In the embryo, the primitive brain begins as a series of hollow, fluid-filled vesicles that twist and turn in a developmental process orchestrated by the human genetic code that finally develops into the three topographic sections of the brain: the forebrain, midbrain, and hindbrain. Identifying fluid collections in the embryonic brain up to 10 menstrual weeks is normal, whereas similar findings after 14–16 weeks would suggest the presence of some cystic intracranial abnormality. Similarly, there are normal structures seen in the fetal brain that would be considered aberrant if found in the brain of a child or an adult. The two anatomic structures that are prominent in the developing fetal brain are the cavum septi pellucidi and the choroid plexus.

Cavum Septi Pellucidi

The *cavum septi pellucidi*, or *cave of the septum pellucidum*, is an interhemispheric space containing cerebral spinal fluid (CSF) that lies between the medial walls of the frontal horns and bodies of the two lateral ventricles. It can be visualized sonographically by 18–20 menstrual weeks. The *septum pellucidum* is a thin vertical membrane that connects the corpus callosum to the columns of the *fornix of cerebrum* and separates the lateral ventricles. The space (cavum) consists of two leaves (septa pellucida), each of which is part of the ipsilateral right or left cerebral hemisphere.

The *cavum vergae* is the posterior extension of the cavum septi pellucidi, lying posterior to the columns of the fornix of cerebrum. During the sixth month of gestation, closure of this intracranial space begins

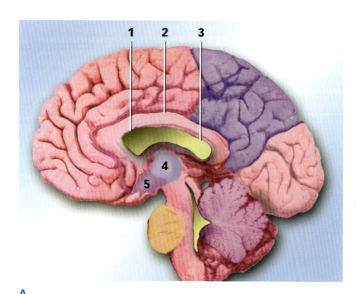

A

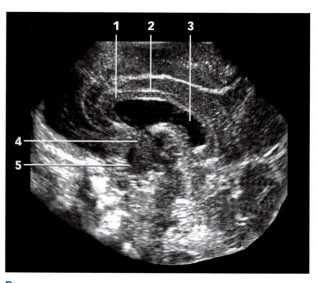

B

Figure 6-5. The cavum septi pellucidi and cavum vergae. **A** Schematic. **B** Correlative sonogram.
1 = cavum septi pellucidi, 2 = corpus callosum, 3 = cavum vergae, 4 = thalamus, 5 = hypothalamus.

posteriorly in the cavum vergae with progression anteriorly toward the cavum septi pellucidi. Complete closure does not occur until about 6 months postnatally, so visualization of the cavum septi pellucidi is always a normal finding in the fetus. Its absence is the hallmark finding in agenesis of the corpus callosum, a structure with which the cavum septi pellucidi is intimately associated (although visualization of the CSP does not rule out partial agenesis of the CC).[1]

Choroid Plexus

The *choroid plexus* (Figures 6-6A and B) is composed of a rich capillary network, inclusions of pia mater, and choroid epithelial cells. It serves as the primary source of cerebral spinal fluid. Lying along the floor of each lateral ventricle, the choroid tissue extends, via small openings called the *foramina of Monro*, onto the roof of the third ventricle. In the temporal horn of the lateral ventricle, the choroid plexus thickens to form the *glomus*, the brightly echogenic structure seen tucked within the atrium of the lateral ventricle on axial sections. The choroid plexus is confined to the body and temporal horns of the lateral ventricle. It does not extend anteriorly to the foramina of Monro, and identification of echogenic material in the forward portion of the lateral ventricle must be considered an abnormal finding.

VENTRICLES

As fluid-filled structures surrounded by solid brain parenchyma, the *ventricles* (Figure 6-7) provide an excellent series of landmarks for identifying both normal and abnormal intracranial anatomy. The two *lateral ventricles* lie within each cerebral hemisphere beneath the white fibers of the *corpus callosum*, which forms the roof of each cavity. The inferior walls of each cavity are formed by the *thalamus* medially and by the *caudate nucleus* more laterally.

The *atrium* of the lateral ventricle (Figure 6-8) is the anatomic site where the lateral, temporal, and occipital horns converge. It is easily and routinely demonstrable sonographically as an anechoic box-shaped structure in the posterior mid portion of each cerebral hemisphere, containing a section of the more obviously

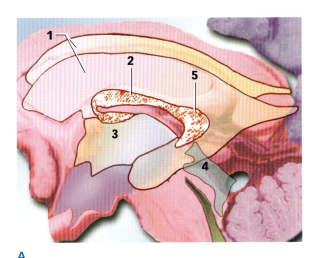

A

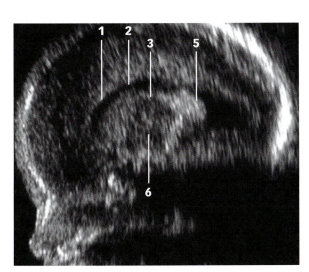

B

Figure 6-6. Choroid plexus. **A** Schematic. **B** Correlative sonographic image. 1 = lateral ventricles, 2 = choroid plexus, 3 = third ventricle, 4 = fourth ventricle (not visible in sonogram), 5 = glomus, 6 = thalamus.

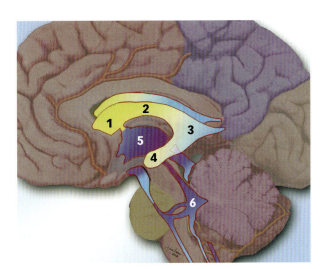

Figure 6-7. Schematic illustration of the ventricular system. 1 = frontal horn of the lateral ventricle, 2 = body of the lateral ventricle, 3 = atrium of the lateral ventricle, 4 = temporal horn of the lateral ventricle, 5 = third ventricle, 6 = fourth ventricle.

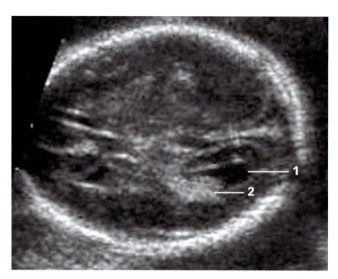

Figure 6-8. Axial sonographic section demonstrating (1) the atrium of the lateral ventricle and (2) the choroid plexus.

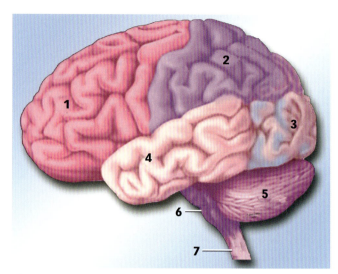

Figure 6-9. Schematic illustration of the topographic anatomy of the brain. 1 = frontal lobe, 2 = parietal lobe, 3 = occipital lobe, 4 = temporal lobe, 5 = cerebellum, 6 = brain stem, 7 = spinal cord.

echogenic choroid plexus. Measurement of the atrium in an axial plane of section along with observation of its relationship to the choroid plexus is an accurate and useful way to rule out central nervous system abnormalities that are associated with ventricular enlargement. The normal atrium measures 10 mm or less throughout gestation, and the choroid plexus should be tucked tightly between the ventricular walls. An atrial measurement greater than 10 mm, particularly when the choroid plexus appears to be "dangling" in the enlarged ventricle, is pathognomonic of ventriculomegaly.

The *third ventricle* is a symmetric midline structure whose lateral walls are formed by the inferior aspect of the thalamus and the hypothalamus; its anterior wall is formed by the *lamina terminalis* (*terminal lamina of hypothalamus*). It communicates with the lateral ventricles by means of the foramina of Monro. The *massa intermedia*, or *interthalamic adhesion*, is a column of solid thalamic tissue extending through the mid portion of the third-ventricle cavity and may serve as a useful anatomic landmark in imaging studies of both the fetal and preterm neonatal brain.

The *fourth ventricle* lies along the anterior portion of the cerebellum, behind the pons and the medulla oblongata. It communicates with the third ventricle via the slender canal called the *cerebral aqueduct* (or *aqueduct of Sylvius*). In the roof of the fourth ventricle there is an opening called the *foramen of Magendie*. In the lateral walls there are two openings called the *foramina of Luschka*. By means of these three openings, the ventricles communicate with the subarachnoid space, and the cerebrospinal fluid can circulate from one space to the other.

FOREBRAIN

Cerebral Hemispheres

The *cerebral hemispheres* constitute the largest portion of the brain and fill the entire upper portion of the intracranial cavity. Their surfaces are composed of layers of gray matter, called *cerebral cortex*, punctuated by shallow grooves called *sulci* and undulating convolutions called *gyri*. Deeper grooves, called *cerebral fissures*, serve as anatomic landmarks outlining the main topographic portions of the cerebrum: the frontal, temporal, parietal, and occipital lobes (Figure 6-9).

Lying along the midline beneath the cerebrum is the *diencephalon* (Figure 6-10), which connects each hemisphere with the midbrain and which forms the walls of much of the ventricular system. The most recognizable anatomic component of the diencephalon, sometimes referred to as the "interbrain," is the *thalamus*, which is a standard anatomic landmark in all sectional images of the brain. It is a large bilateral, ovoid structure located just above the midbrain and is the noteworthy piece of architecture supporting ventricular morphology. It forms the inferomedial walls of the lateral ventricles and surrounds most of the third ventricle. Just below the symmetric thalamic

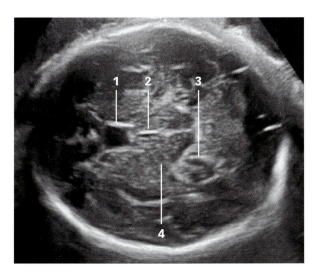

Figure 6-10. Axial sonographic section demonstrating anatomic structure in the diencephalon. 1 = cavum septi pellucidi, 2 = third ventricle, 3 = atrium of lateral ventricle, 4 = thalamus.

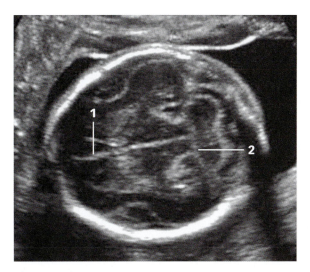

Figure 6-11. Axial sonographic section demonstrating dural structures in the fetal brain. 1 = falx cerebri, 2 = tentorium cerebelli.

lobes and perched just above the brain stem lies the *hypothalamus*, which forms the inferior portion and floor of the third ventricle.

Dural Landmarks

Covering the brain are the three meningeal layers: the pia, arachnoid, and dura mater. The *pia mater* is the thin, delicate innermost membrane surrounding the brain and spinal cord. Covering it is the *arachnoid mater*, which is attached to the inner surface of the *dura mater*. The dura is the tough, smooth, outermost covering of the brain that acts as the high-amplitude acoustic reflector seen on routine imaging sections through the fetal brain. It serves as a valuable landmark in identifying two locations in the brain: the midline *falx cerebri*, which invaginates along the intercerebral fissure, and the *tentorium cerebelli*, which forms a roof over the posterior fossa (Figure 6-11).

MIDBRAIN

The *midbrain* or *mesencephalon* (Figure 6-12) is a short, constricted portion, which connects the pons and cerebellum with the hemispheres of the cerebrum. It is directed upward and forward and consists of the corpora quadrigemina, the cerebral peduncles, and the aqueduct of Sylvius. The four solid lobes of the *corpora quadrigemina* form the dorsal borders of the *aqueduct of Sylvius*, which connects the cerebellum with the third and fourth ventricles. Inferior to it, the *cerebral peduncles* form the walls of the fourth ventricle.

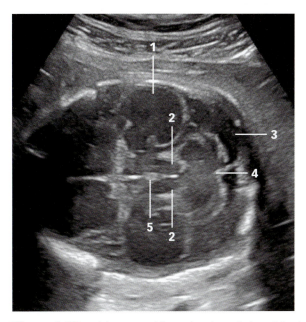

Figure 6-12. Axial sonographic section through the midbrain demonstrating normal anatomic structures. 1 = temporal lobe, 2 = cerebral peduncles, 3 = cisterna magna, 4 = cerebellum, 5 = aqueduct of Sylvius.

HINDBRAIN: POSTERIOR FOSSA STRUCTURES

The *hindbrain* (Figure 6-13), which arises from the embryonic rhombencephalon, consists of the cerebellum, pons, and medulla oblongata. The cisterna magna, located between the cerebellum and the dorsal surface of the medulla, provides a useful sonographic imaging landmark due to the presence of cerebrospinal fluid

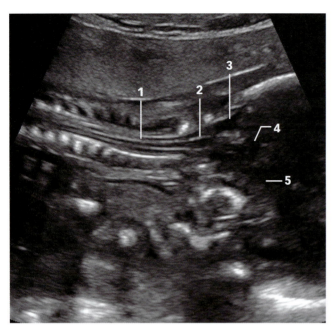

Figure 6-13. Sagittal sonographic section demonstrating normal hindbrain and cervical spine anatomy. 1 = cervical spinal cord, 2 = medulla oblongata, 3 = cisterna magna, 4 = cerebellum, 5 = pons.

contained within. All of these structures are located primarily within the posterior fossa and are sometimes referred to as the *brain stem*.

Cerebellum

The fetal *cerebellum* should be routinely imaged in an axial oblique plane of section that demonstrates the cavum septi pellucidi anteriorly and the cerebellum posteriorly. The cerebellum occupies the posteroinferior portion of the intracranial cavity. The constricted central portion is called the *vermis*, and the lateral expanded portions are called the *hemispheres*. The surface of the cerebellum consists of gray matter and is not convoluted but is traversed by numerous furrows, or *sulci*. The cerebellum is connected with the cerebrum by the *superior peduncles*, with the pons by the *middle peduncles*, and with the medulla oblongata by the *inferior peduncles*. These peduncles are bundles of fibers. Impulses from the motor centers in the cerebrum, from the semicircular canals of the inner ear, and from the muscles enter the cerebellum by way of these bundles.

Pons

The *pons* is situated in the front of the cerebellum between the midbrain and the medulla oblongata. It consists of interlaced transverse and longitudinal white fibers intermixed with gray matter. The transverse fibers are those derived from the middle peduncles of the cerebellum and serve to join its two halves. The longitudinal fibers connect the medulla with the cerebrum. Also in it are the nuclei of all or some of the fibers.

Medulla Oblongata

The *medulla oblongata* (spinal bulb) is continuous with the spinal cord, which on passing into the cranial cavity through the foramen magnum widens into a pyramid-shaped mass that extends to the lower margin of the pons. Externally, the medulla oblongata resembles the upper part of the spinal cord, but the internal structure is different.

Cisterna Magna

The *cisterna magna* (also known as the *cerebellomedullary cistern*) is the largest of the subarachnoid cisterns and should measure 10 mm or less (see Filly's rule, page 123). It is located between the cerebellum and the dorsal surface of the medulla oblongata. Cerebrospinal fluid produced in the ventricular system drains into the cisterna magna from the fourth ventricle via the median aperture (of Magendie) and the lateral apertures (of Luschka). The two other principal cisterns are the *pontine cistern*, located between the pons and the medulla oblongata, and the *interpeduncular cistern*, located between the cerebral peduncles.

BLOOD SUPPLY TO THE FETAL BRAIN

Four feed arteries supply perfusion to the brain: the two anterior internal carotid arteries and the two posterior vertebral arteries. Upon entering the intracranial cavity, each of these arteries contributes to the *circle of Willis*, an anastomotic vascular configuration located at the base of the brain (Figures 6-14A and B). Arising from both sides of the circle of Willis are the three main *cerebral arteries*: anterior, middle, and posterior. The smaller branches and arborized arterioles of the cerebral arteries provide the brain with a continuous supply of the oxygen and nutrients requisite for its constant physiologic function. When one of the feed arteries into the circle of Willis is congenitally absent or pathologically obliterated, the brain continues to receive its full perfusional requirements via collateralization through the circle. Venous drainage from the brain is through the large sinuses and into the internal jugular veins at either side of the neck.

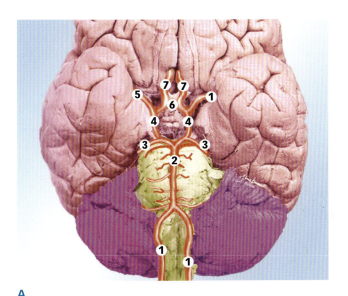 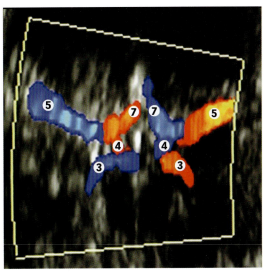

Figure 6-14. The circle of Willis. **A** Schematic showing location in brain and the vessels that define the circle: the posterior cerebral, posterior communicating, anterior cerebral, and anterior communicating arteries. **B** Correlative Doppler color flow image. 1 = vertebral artery, 2 = basilar artery, 3 = posterior cerebral artery, 4 = posterior communicating artery, 5 = internal carotid artery, 6 = anterior communicating artery, 7 = anterior cerebral artery.

Intracranial Vasculature

The *intracranial vasculature* consists of the following:

- The *anterior cerebral arteries*, each of which arises from the internal carotid artery at the inner extremity of the Sylvian fissure. Each anterior cerebral artery passes anteriorly and medially to the longitudinal fissure, where it is connected to the artery of the opposite side by the anterior communicating artery.

- The *middle cerebral arteries*, which constitute the largest branches of the right and left internal carotid arteries. The middle cerebral artery passes obliquely through the Sylvian fissure and, at the insula, divides into its terminal branches (Figure 6-15).

- The *posterior cerebral arteries*, which arise near the intersection of the posterior communicating arteries and the basilar artery, course upward, and penetrate the cerebral cortex. The cerebellum receives its arterial perfusion from various branches of the vertebral and basilar arteries.

THE SPINAL COLUMN

By 16 weeks, ossification centers in each vertebra make the spinal column easily and reliably amenable to sonographic imaging. Three brightly echogenic foci, demonstrated on axial images through each vertebral

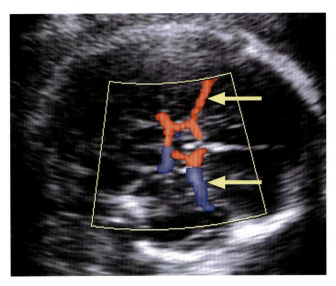

Figure 6-15. Axial color Doppler image through the base of the brain demonstrating flow in the middle cerebral arteries (arrows).

segment, represent accumulated calcium in the ossification centers: one centrally located in the vertebral body and two laterally located between the laminae and pedicles in the posterior vertebral element (Figures 6-16A–D). The spinal column consists of twenty-four articulating vertebrae in the cervical, dorsal, and lumbar regions and nine fused vertebrae in the sacrum and coccyx.

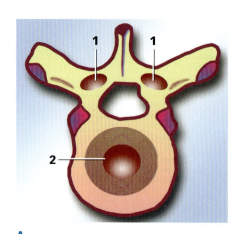

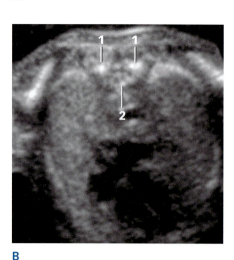

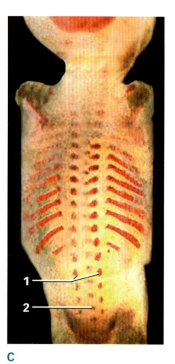

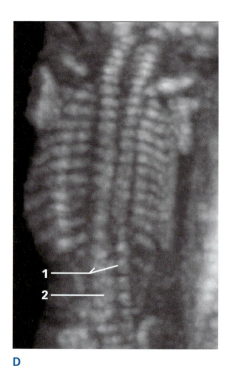

Figure 6-16. Vertebral ossification centers. **A** Schematic and **B** correlative sonogram of a vertebral ossification center. **C** Gross anatomy and **D** sonogram of the location of the vertebral ossification centers relative to the body (posterior views). 1 = ossification centers located laterally between the laminae and the pedicles, 2 = single ossification center located in the vertebral body.

In a parasagittal or coronal plane of section, the lateral ossification centers run parallel to each other and should follow the normal configuration of a spinal column. If imaging is optimal, the spinal cord itself can be visualized starting at about 14 menstrual weeks. In the longitudinal plane, the spinal cord is hypoechoic, with bright anterior and posterior margins and a bright central line (Figure 6-17). The lower tip of the spinal cord, called the *conus medullaris* (*medullary cone*), resembles a pencil point.

Real-time examination of the fetal spine is performed in at least two orthogonal planes of section throughout its length. *Transversely* (Figure 6-18), the exam is begun in the proximal cervical spine and proceeds caudally. Attention is paid to the:

- Integrity of the skin line
- Location and configuration of the ossification centers in each vertebra
- Integrity of the musculature in the back

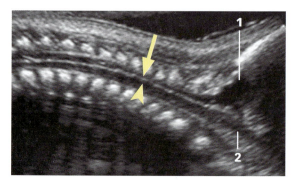

Figure 6-17. Sagittal section through the cervical and upper thoracic fetal spine demonstrating the brightly echogenic dura mater (arrow) surrounding the relatively hypoechoic spinal cord (arrowhead). 1 = cisterna magna, 2 = medulla oblongata.

Sagittally or *coronally*, the spine is examined to assess:

- Cervical and lumbosacral curvatures (Figure 6-19)
- Sacral caudal tapering
- Configuration of vertebral ossification centers (Figure 6-20)

CENTRAL NERVOUS SYSTEM ABNORMALITIES

The spectrum of congenital anomalies affecting the fetal central nervous system (CNS) is enormous and in a review text such as this can be covered only in outline. However, severe prenatal anomalies not compatible with life and those associated with poor perinatal outcomes are almost always identifiable during the course of a routine obstetric sonographic examination.

Axial images through the fetal brain obtained during the course of routine measurements of biparietal diameter and head circumference (see Chapter 4) yield a great deal of anatomic detail that, when augmented with additional targeted images, can reliably detect many serious abnormalities that portend a poor prognosis for the fetus. Most of these life-threatening abnormalities can be detected before 20 weeks' gestation. Serious abnormalities distort normal anatomic configurations and relationships, and these should catch the examiner's eye during routine biometric imaging, prompting further investigation of the entire central nervous system, from brain to *cauda equina* (the spinal roots that descend from the cord and occupy the vertebral canal below it). In addition to acquiring routine images of the specific intracranial anatomic structures, sonographic examination of the fetal head should focus attention on the integrity of the bony calvaria and overlying soft-tissue scalp echoes. In addition to the gross structural variants that define each abnormality, other sonographic findings—such as polyhydramnios and discordant biometric measurements—can direct the sonographer to a more focused look at the fetal central nervous system.

Central nervous system abnormalities can affect the brain, spinal cord, and associated musculoskeletal structures (Table 6-1). The most common and frequently encountered spinal cord anomalies—e.g., spina bifida or one of its variants—result from neural tube defects. Intracranial anomalies, on the other hand, arise from a variety of compromised developmental processes that result in a broad and diverse range of anatomic deformities. From a sonographic perspective, these abnormalities can be classified as cystic or solid in nature, which—while perhaps oversimplifying the study of intracranial anomalies—is a useful approach for sonographic imaging professionals.

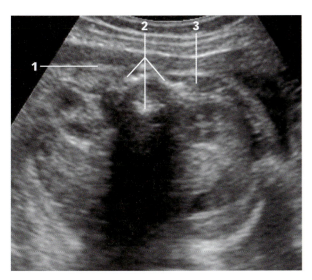

Figure 6-18. Transverse section through the fetal back demonstrating (1) an intact skin line, (2) normally configured ossification centers, and (3) intact back musculature.

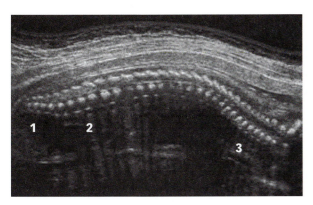

Figure 6-19. Sagittal section through the fetal spine demonstrating normal cervical and lumbosacral curves. 1 = caudal tapering, 2 = lumbosacral curve, 3 = cervical curve.

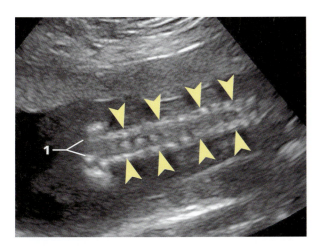

Figure 6-20. Coronal section through the thoracolumbar and sacroiliac spine demonstrating normal sacral caudal tapering (1) and parallel configuration of the lateral ossification centers in each vertebra (arrowheads).

INTRACRANIAL CYSTIC ABNORMALITIES

Cystic abnormalities found within the confines of the cranium are the result of (1) the overaccumulation of cerebrospinal fluid in otherwise normal fluid-containing anatomic structures (such as the ventricles and cisternae), (2) the accumulation of fluid in anomalously created lacunae within normally solid intracranial parenchyma, or (3) fluid-filled masses such as cysts and vascular malformations. The first task in differentiating cystic abnormalities in the head, therefore, is to determine whether the identified fluid collection conforms to normal, albeit large and exaggerated, fluid-filled anatomy or assumes a nonanatomic configuration. In the former instance, when the abnormality is found within the cerebral hemispheres, hydrocephalus is present. If the cystic collection is in the posterior fossa and conforms to the shape of the cisterna magna and/or fourth ventricle, Dandy-Walker malformation is the primary possibility. Fluid collections that present not as normal but rather as dilated anatomic structures represent another category of intracranial cystic abnormalities.

Hydrocephalus

Congenital enlargement of the ventricular system varies from mild, benign ventriculomegaly to chronic, massive hydrocephalus with concomitant compression atrophy (i.e., atrophy due to continuous pressure) of the surrounding cerebral parenchyma. On the low end of the measurement spectrum, mild cerebral ventriculomegaly as an isolated finding, with a lateral atrial dimension measuring 10–15 mm, is a condition that usually carries no significant sequelae. It may, however, be observed in a variety of conditions, including subtle forms of agenesis of the corpus callosum, and it should be carefully followed sonographically. Enlargement of the lateral ventricles to more than 15 mm is more commonly associated with obvious malformations of the central nervous system.

The terms *ventriculomegaly* and *hydrocephalus* are often used interchangeably, but there is a subtle definitional difference. *Ventriculomegaly* refers to the generic enlargement of a ventricle caused by increased intraventricular pressure resulting either from a downstream cerebrospinal fluid (CSF) flow obstruction or from passive enlargement of the ventricle as it opportunistically expands to fill a space created by adjacent atrophied cerebral parenchyma. Most commonly, these softened, ischemic areas are caused by congenital infections of the brain or periventricular infarction. As an isolated sonographic finding, mild ventriculomegaly may be seen to have resolved spontaneously on subsequent imaging studies; however, careful study of the central nervous system is warranted in all fetuses presenting with this finding. Atrial diameters exceeding 10 mm (>4 standard deviations) suggest ventriculomegaly.[2]

Hydrocephalus, on the other hand, is the dilatation of the ventricular system, almost always caused by obstruction of cerebrospinal fluid outflow through the aqueduct of Sylvius and/or the foramina of Luschka. *Communicating hydrocephalus* is a less common cause of ventricular enlargement that results from the relative overproduction of cerebrospinal fluid. In both ventriculomegaly and hydrocephalus, the ventricular system becomes dilated and stands out dramatically during sonographic examination thanks to the inherent tissue contrast created by the cystic filling of normally

Table 6-1. Summary of fetal central nervous system abnormalities.

Type of Abnormality	Anomaly
Intracranial cystic abnormalities	Hydrocephalus
	Hydranencephaly
	Holoprosencephaly
	Dandy-Walker malformation
	Vein of Galen aneurysm/malformation
	Choroid plexus cysts
Intracranial solid abnormalities	Agenesis of the corpus callosum
	Intracranial tumors
	Intracranial hemorrhage in utero
	Porencephaly (can also be cystic)
	Schizencephaly
	Intracranial calcifications
	Microencephaly
	Megalencephaly
Neural tube defects	Anencephaly
	Exencephaly (acrania)
	Cephalocele/encephalocele
	Iniencephaly
	Spina bifida

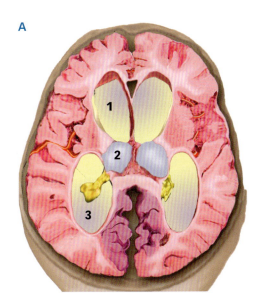 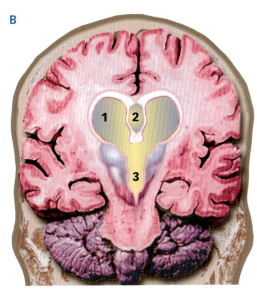

Figure 6-21. Hydrocephalus. **A** Axial oblique schematic. 1 = front horn of the lateral ventricle, 2 = thalamus, 3 = atrium of the lateral ventricle. **B** Coronal schematic. 1 = lateral ventricle, 2 = cavum septi pellucidi, 3 = third ventricle.

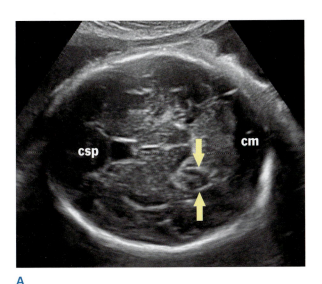 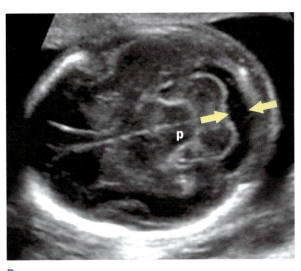

Figure 6-22. Axial sections at two different levels through the fetal head demonstrating the proper measurement locations when applying Filly's rule. **A** The atrium of the lateral ventricle (arrows) at the level of the cavum septi pellucidi (csp) and cisterna magna (cm). **B** The cisterna magna (arrows) in the posterior fossa at the level of the pons (p).

configured anatomic structures. Symmetric dilatation of the third and both lateral ventricles suggests anomalies of cerebrospinal fluid outflow such as aqueductal stenosis (Figures 6-21A and B).

The two classic sonographic signs of abnormal ventricular size are increased lateral ventricular atrial diameter (to more than 10 mm) and the presence of a "dangling choroid." The atrium of the lateral ventricle can be reliably imaged in the fetal head as soon as the brain is fully formed. As mentioned earlier in this chapter, normal values for the atrium measured in axial section at the level of the thalamus (biparietal diameter plane) are 10 mm or less. When combined with a measurement of the cisterna magna in an axial oblique section, atrial diameter is a valuable indicator of central nervous system normality. In an elegant simplification of an otherwise time-consuming and tedious sonographic trudge through the complexity of fetal neuroanatomy, Filly et al.[3] studied two reliable, easy-to-obtain measurements taken in the fetal head to determine their predictive value in identifying fetuses with normal central nervous systems. "Filly's rule" (Figures 6-22A and B) can be stated as follows: If the atrium of the lateral ventricle and the cisterna magna *both* measure 10 mm or less, there is a 95% negative predictive value for *any* central nervous system anomaly.[3]

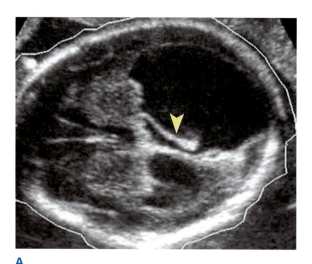 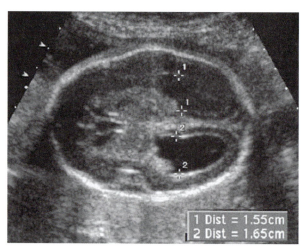

Figure 6-23. Axial sections through the fetal head demonstrating two hallmark sonographic findings for hydrocephalus. **A** Dangling choroid (arrowhead). **B** Ventriculomegaly.

Differential Diagnosis

While hydrocephalus can be differentiated from other intracranial cystic abnormalities by the identification of characteristic ventricular morphology that is dilated to some extent, it can, in some instances, be mistaken for hydranencephaly or holoprosencephaly.

Associated Abnormalities

Conditions associated with hydrocephalus include the following:

- Concomitant CNS anomalies:
  - Aqueductal stenosis
  - Chiari malformations
  - Neural tube defects
  - Dandy-Walker malformation
  - Encephalocele
  - Alobar holoprosencephaly
  - Posterior fossa cysts
  - Polymicrogyria
- Craniofacial anomalies:
  - Cleft lip/palate
  - Low-set ears
  - Bilateral optic atrophy
  - Facial bone anomalies
  - Acrocephalosyndactylia
- Syndromes:
  - Meckel-Gruber
  - Miller-Dieker
- Chromosomal anomalies:
  - Trisomy 21 (Down syndrome)
  - Triploidy

Sonographic Signs

The following are the characteristic sonographic signs of hydrocephalus:

- Normal ventricular configuration—just dilated
- Dangling choroid plexus (Figure 6-23A)
- Presence of excess fluid in lateral ventricles with an axial atrial measurement > 10 mm (Figure 6-23B)
- Observed brain echogenicity (dense texture may suggest intrauterine infection)
- Associated sonographic findings that may include polyhydramnios, abnormal fetal lie, hepatomegaly, and fetal ascites with associated infection, myelomeningocele, and other intracranial abnormalities, including Dandy-Walker malformation, encephalocele, and intracranial tumor

Hydranencephaly

Hydranencephaly (Figure 6-24A) is characterized by the near or total absence of the cerebral hemispheres in the presence of normally developed meninges and skull. The falx cerebri may be present. The midbrain, cerebellum, and basal ganglia are intact. While the exact etiology in every case cannot be known, the usual explanation for hydranencephaly is ischemic infarction of the brain along the anterior and middle cerebral artery distribution secondary to bilateral internal carotid artery occlusions. The occlusions can result from primary agenesis of normal neck vasculature or from some toxic or inflammatory intrauterine insult. The space created by the atrophic cerebral hemispheres fills with cerebrospinal fluid that completely occupies the calvarial cavity. Hydranencephaly can be differentiated from hydrocephalus in that, first, there is no cortical mantle bordering the huge intracranial fluid collection and, second, the fluid collection does not conform to the expected architecture of a ventricular system.

Differential Diagnosis

Hydranencephaly can be confidently diagnosed by the identification of fluid filling the entire cranial vault, which is absent even a thin mantle of cerebral hemispheric tissue. However, differential diagnoses include hydrocephalus and holoprosencephaly.

Associated Abnormalities

Conditions associated with hydranencephaly include the following:

- Consequential arthrogryposis
- Renal aplastic dysplasia
- Polyvalvular developmental heart defect
- Fowler syndrome
- Trisomy 13 (Patau syndrome)
- Polyhydramnios

Sonographic Signs

The following are the characteristic sonographic signs of hydranencephaly:

- Macrocephaly
- Large anechoic area in the cranial vault surrounding the midbrain and basal ganglia (Figures 6-24B and C)
- Absent cortical mantle
- Variable presence of the third ventricle
- Tentorium separating a normal posterior fossa from the anterior and middle cranial fossae
- Polyhydramnios
- Occasionally small portions of occipital lobes

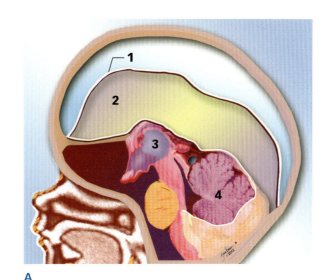

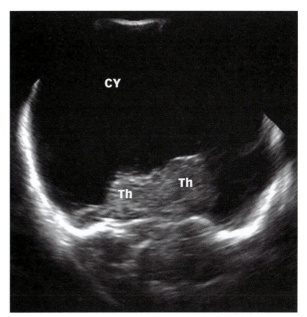

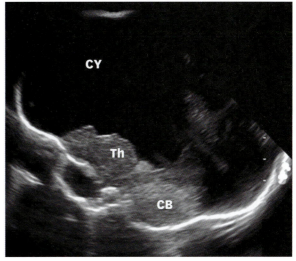

Figure 6-24. **A** Schematic illustration of hydranencephaly demonstrating absence of the cerebral hemispheres with cystic filling of the cranial vault. Normal mid- and hindbrain anatomy is present. 1 = meninges, 2 = empty intracranial cavity, 3 = midbrain, 4 = cerebellum. **B** Coronal section demonstrating cystic filling of the intracranial vault above the paired thalami. **C** Sagittal section demonstrating the intact hindbrain structures. CY = cystic filling, Th = thalamus, CB = cerebellum.

Holoprosencephaly

Holoprosencephaly (Figure 6-25) is a malformation sequence in which the forebrain (prosencephalon) fails to develop normally. The embryonic brain begins its formation around a single midline cystic cavity called the *monoventricle* (sometimes referred to as the *holoventricle*). Through a process called *forebrain diverticulation*, the symmetric cerebral hemispheres and normal ventricular system emerge from a complex series of rotations and duplications of the monoventricle that occur along the midline at the end of the 5th gestational week. Compromise of this process by chromosomal abnormalities (particularly trisomies 13 and 18) and by teratogenic insults produces a constellation of anatomic defects that are the hallmarks of holoprosencephaly. As forebrain diverticulation is closely associated with embryonic development of the face, abnormalities of the median facial structures (forehead, nose, interorbital structures, and upper lip) are frequently found in association with the intracranial defects of holoprosencephaly.

There are three types of holoprosencephaly, defined by the degree of abnormal cleavage of the prosencephalon: alobar, semilobar, and lobar. All three types are associated with severe mental retardation.

Alobar Holoprosencephaly

Alobar holoprosencephaly (Figure 6-25B) is the most severe type of holoprosencephaly, characterized by the following:

- A single horseshoe-shaped ventricle in the midline
- Absence of the lateral and third ventricles
- Absence of the midline structures: the cavum septi pellucidi, corpus callosum, interhemispheric fissure, and falx cerebri
- Associated craniofacial features: proboscis, cyclopia, mono-nostril, hypotelorism, and cebocephaly

Semilobar Holoprosencephaly

Less severe in appearance is *semilobar holoprosencephaly* (Figure 6-25C), characterized by the following:

- Partial formation of the midline interhemispheric fissure and the presence of cerebral cortex surrounding a ventricle fused in the midline
- A monoventricle with partially developed occipital and temporal horns and a more prominent cerebral mantle
- Thalami and a third ventricle that are better formed, but thalami that may be partially or completely fused
- Absence of the cavum septi pellucidi and falx cerebri anteriorly
- Agenesis or hypoplasia of the corpus callosum
- Associated craniofacial features: hypotelorism and cleft lip

Lobar Holoprosencephaly

The least severe form of holoprosencephaly is *lobar holoprosencephaly* (Figure 6-25D), characterized by the following:

- Cerebral hemispheres present with fusion of the frontal horns of the lateral ventricle
- Fused segment that communicates with the third ventricle

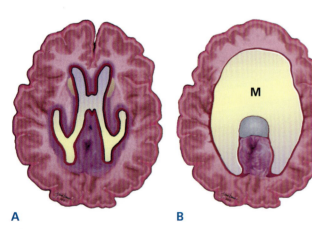
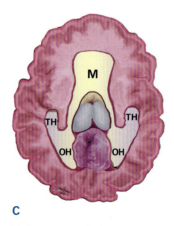
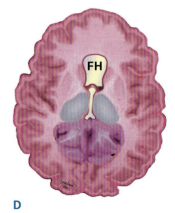

Figure 6-25. Schematic axial sectional illustration of different forms of holoprosencephaly. **A** Normal ventricles. **B** Alobar holoprosencephaly. **C** Semilobar holoprosencephaly. **D** Lobar holoprosencephaly. M = monoventricle, OH = occipital horn, TH = temporal horn, FH = fused frontal horns.

- Absence of the cavum septi pellucidi anteriorly
- Agenesis or hypoplasia of the corpus callosum
- Fully developed ventricular occipital horns

Facial Anomalies Associated with Holoprosencephaly

Holoprosencephaly presents some classic sonographic findings that result from the wide and dramatic spectrum of facial anomalies often associated with this fetal condition.

- *Proboscis* is an anterior, midline facial appendage projecting from the midline of the fetal face. It may appear at the normal topographic site of the nose, on the forehead, or between the eyes (called an *interorbital* proboscis) (Figures 6-26A and B).
- *Cyclopia* is characterized by a single palpebral fissure and a single midline orbit that may contain either a single globe or two separate globes (see Figures 6-26A–D).
- *Ethmocephaly* is a facial malformation in which there is a single palpebral fissure with a single midline orbit containing separate, closely spaced globes, with maldeveloped nasal structures and a midline proboscis extending cephalad from the orbits (Figure 6-26D).
- *Cebocephaly* is characterized by hypotelorism with a better-formed nasal bridge. There is, however, a single-nostril nose present.

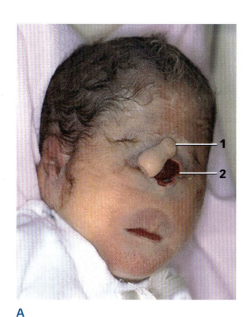
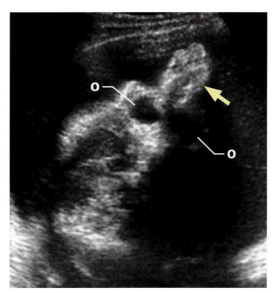
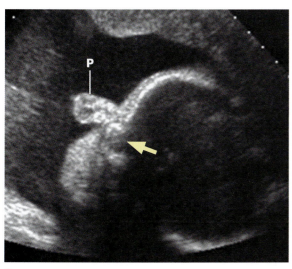
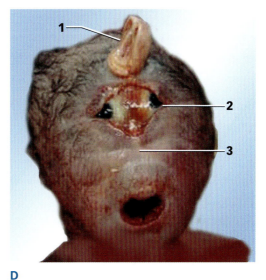

Figure 6-26. A Facial anomalies associated with holoprosencephaly include (1) proboscis and (2) cyclopia. **B** Proboscis (arrow) associated with ethmocephaly. O = orbit. **C** Cyclopia (arrow) associated with ethmocephaly. P = proboscis. **D** Gross anatomy of ethmocephay. 1 = proboscis, 2 = single palpebral fissure with (in this instance) hypotelorism of duplicate globes, 3 = malformed nasal structures.

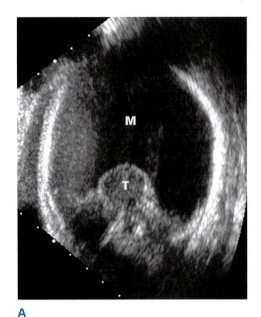

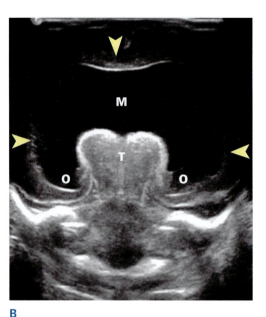

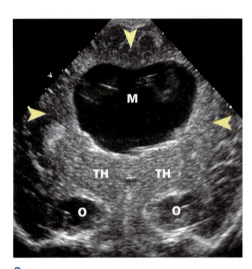

Figure 6-27. Sonographic demonstration of facial anomalies associated with holoprosencephaly. **A** Alobar anomalies, characterized by a single midline monoventricle and the absence of lateral and third ventricles. **B** Semilobar anomalies, with a more prominent cerebral mantle surrounding the monoventricle. **C** Lobar anomalies, with fusion of the frontal horns of the lateral ventricles around the monoventricle and fully developed ventricular occipital horns. M = monoventricle, T = thalamus, O = occipital horns, TH = temporal horn, arrowheads = cerebral cortex.

Holoprosencephaly associated with cyclopia, ethmocephaly, and/or cebocephaly is virtually always a lethal malformation, as the absence of normal facial respiratory apparatus precludes breathing.

Differential Diagnosis

Conditions that may be confused with holoprosencephaly include hydranencephaly and severe hydrocephalus. In both hydranencephaly and severe hydrocephalus, a well-formed falx should be present in the midline. In hydranencephaly there may be no detectable cortical tissue surrounding the large intracranial fluid collection; in severe hydrocephalus, careful examination will show a thin layer of cortical parenchyma around the grossly dilated ventricular anatomy.

Associated Abnormalities

The following abnormalities are characteristically associated with holoprosencephaly:

- Trisomy 13 (Patau syndrome)
- Trisomy 18 (Edwards syndrome)
- Congenital renal anomalies
- Congenital cardiac anomalies

Sonographic Signs

The hallmark anatomic anomalies associated with all forms of holoprosencephaly (Figure 6-27) include:

- Presence of a single midline ventricle, or *monoventricle*
- Mantle of cerebral tissue present around the monoventricle
- Associated craniofacial abnormalities

Characteristic sonographic signs of specific forms of holoprosencephaly include the following:

- *Alobar holoprosencephaly*: a single midline ventricle and the absence of lateral and third ventricles (Figure 6-27A)
- *Semilobar holoprosencephaly*: a monoventricle with partially developed occipital and temporal horns and a more prominent cerebral mantle (Figure 6-27B)
- *Lobar holoprosencephaly*: fusion of the frontal horns of the lateral ventricles around the monoventricle and fully developed ventricular occipital horns (Figure 6-27C)

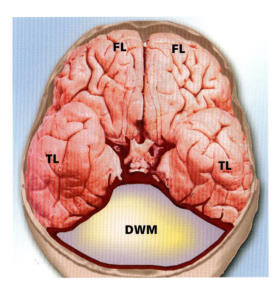

Figure 6-28. Schematic axial oblique illustration of Dandy-Walker malformation (DWM) in the posterior fossa characterized by the absence or severe dysgenesis of the cerebellar vermis with opportunistic filling of the space with cerebrospinal fluid. TL = temporal lobes, FL = frontal lobes.

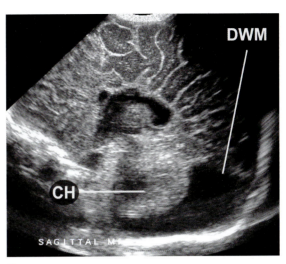

A

Figure 6-29. Sonographic findings in Dandy-Walker malformation (DWM). **A** Midline sagittal section demonstrating enlargement of the posterior fossa with opportunistic filling with cerebrospinal fluid and effacement of the cerebellar hemispheres (CH). (Figure continues . . .)

Dandy-Walker Malformation

Dandy-Walker malformation (DWM) is a cystic abnormality of the posterior fossa characterized by the absence or severe dysgenesis of the cerebellar vermis with opportunistic filling of the space with cerebrospinal fluid (Figure 6-28). While the etiology in each case is indeterminate, Dandy-Walker malformation is most often due to embryologic failure of the medullary velum (vellum medullare) to regress, combined with cerebellar cleft malformation and failure of the cerebellar commissure to develop into the vermis. The resultant obstruction of outflow from the fourth ventricle causes cystic enlargement of the posterior fossa, which in severe cases can extend upstream to affect the third and both lateral ventricles. However, Dandy-Walker malformation can be isolated to the fourth ventricle.

A *Dandy-Walker variant* is a less severe manifestation of this condition, presenting anatomically as mild dilatation of the fourth ventricle with varying degrees of cerebellar vermian dysgenesis. Because the vermis does not form inferiorly until 18 weeks, the diagnosis of Dandy-Walker variant cannot be made until later in the second trimester.

Differential Diagnosis

The differential diagnosis for Dandy-Walker malformation involves ruling out a posterior fossa arachnoid cyst. Dandy-Walker malformation can be differentiated from a posterior fossa arachnoid cyst in that an arachnoid cyst does not communicate with the fourth ventricle. Arachnoid cysts are isolated findings that are not associated with other congenital malformations.

Associated Abnormalities

The following abnormalities are characteristically associated with Dandy-Walker malformation:

- Hydrocephalus (present with Dandy-Walker malformation in about 25% of cases)
- Other abnormalities of the central nervous system: agenesis of the corpus callosum, holoprosencephaly, schizencephaly, and/or occipital encephalocele
- Cardiac anomalies
- Cleft palate
- Meckel-Gruber syndrome[4]

Sonographic Signs

The following are the characteristic sonographic signs of Dandy-Walker malformation (Figures 6-29A and B):

- Enlargement of the posterior fossa
- Cerebellar hemispheres that may be separated and flattened
- Concomitant hydrocephalus (in 25% of cases)
- Polyhydramnios
- Contiguity with the fourth ventricle (differentiates Dandy-Walker from an arachnoid cyst)

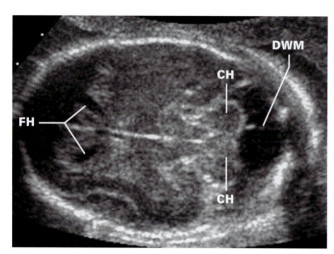

B

Figure 6-29, continued. B Axial section demonstrating an enlarged fluid-filled posterior fossa and concomitant hydrocephalus. DWM = Dandy-Walker malformation, CH = thinned cerebellar hemisphere, FH = mildly dilated lateral ventricular frontal horns.

Vein of Galen Aneurysm/Malformation

A *vein of Galen aneurysm* (VGA)—also known as a *median prosencephalic vein malformation*—is an arteriovenous malformation originating in the median prosencephalic vein in the mid portion of the fetal brain (Figure 6-30A). Anomalous anastomoses arise between the high-pressure branches of the cerebral arteries and the large, low-pressure median prosencephalic vein, a precursor of the vein of Galen, which drains the anterior and central regions of the brain into the sinuses of the posterior cerebral fossa. Concomitant outflow obstruction of the draining vein creates a dilated midline vascular mass that extends posteriorly and inferiorly into the straight sinus with drainage out via the transverse/sigmoid sinuses.

The sonographic appearance of a vein of Galen aneurysm is dramatic, with the dilated median prosencephalic vein appearing as an anechoic structure in the posterior midline that demonstrates robust arteriovenous hemodynamics with color Doppler imaging. Large systemic shunting within the fetal brain often results in a substantial steal of blood, potentially leading to cardiac failure, hydrops fetalis, and perinatal death.[5]

Differential Diagnosis

Differential diagnoses of vein of Galen malformation include arteriovenous malformation in the mid portion of the fetal brain and some rare vascular intracranial tumors.

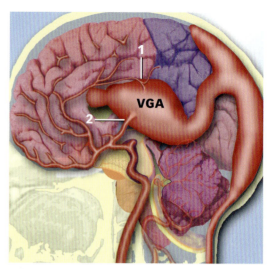

A

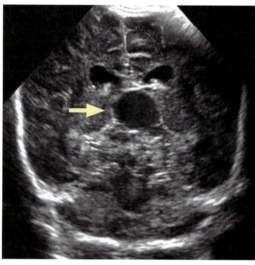

B

Figure 6-30. A Schematic illustration of a vein of Galen aneurysm (VGA) demonstrating anomalous anastomoses with the cerebral arteries. 1 = superior cerebral artery, 2 = middle cerebral artery. **B** Coronal section of VGA. (Figure continues . . .)

Associated Abnormalities

The following abnormalities are characteristically associated with vein of Galen aneurysm:

- High-output cardiac failure
- Hydrocephalus

Sonographic Signs

The following are the characteristic sonographic signs of a vein of Galen aneurysm (Figures 6-30B–D):

- Dilated cystic structure in the posterior midline
- High-amplitude, arteriovenous hemodynamic patterns with color Doppler imaging

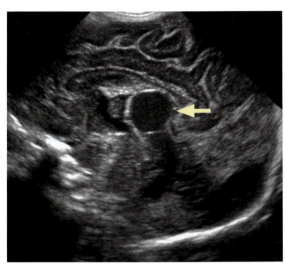

C

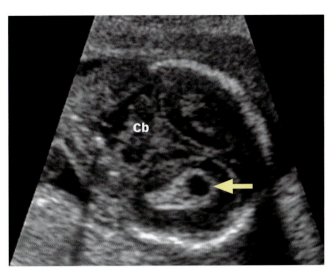

Figure 6-31. Coronal section through the posterior aspect of the fetal brain demonstrating the typical well-circumscribed, anechoic characteristics of a choroid plexus cyst. Arrow = cyst, Cb = cerebellum.

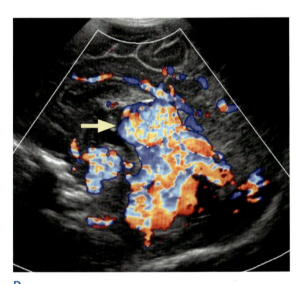

D

Figure 6-30, continued. C Sagittal section. **D** Sagittal color Doppler image demonstrating the typical arteriovenous fistula flow pattern with high-amplitude, high-velocity flow and aliasing. Arrows = VGA.

- Signs of hydrops fetalis
- Typical arteriovenous fistula (AVF) flow pattern demonstrated with color Doppler imaging

Choroid Plexus Cysts

A *choroid plexus cyst* (CP cyst) is a benign fluid collection caused by an abnormal folding in the choroid epithelium. Cerebrospinal fluid, which is produced by the choroid, becomes trapped in this pouch, creating a well-circumscribed, usually anechoic focal lesion that is observed in 1%–2% of mid-trimester fetuses. Choroid plexus cysts carry virtually no clinical significance but, because of past reports of a possible association with chromosomal aneuploidy, they elicit concern from patients and providers who have not been disabused of the myth that these benign findings predict fetal anomalies. The significance of choroid plexus cysts as a component finding in a genetic sonogram is discussed further in Chapter 11 (page 280).

Differential Diagnosis

Choroid plexus cysts have a characteristic sonographic appearance but could be confused with the rare choroid plexus xanthogranuloma, as they are so infrequently encountered during routine prenatal fetal sonography.

Associated Abnormalities

The following abnormalities are characteristically associated with choroid plexus cysts (see also Chapter 11):

- Trisomy 18
- Klinefelter syndrome
- Aicardi syndrome

Sonographic Signs

The following are the characteristic sonographic signs of choroid plexus cysts:

- Small, well-circumscribed, anechoic structures within the echogenic choroid plexus (Figure 6-31)
- May be unilateral or bilateral

INTRACRANIAL SOLID ABNORMALITIES

Solid abnormalities encountered during sonographic evaluation of the fetal brain include the absence of anatomic structures one would expect to see and the presence of structures that one should not see.

Agenesis of the Corpus Callosum

The *corpus callosum* is the midline anatomic structure of the brain, consisting of bundles of neural fibers that serve as a physical connection and method of communication between the two cerebral hemispheres. It also functions as the roof of the lateral ventricles. A teratogenic insult early (at 8–12 weeks) can result in complete *agenesis of the corpus callosum* (ACC) or in partial dysgenesis of its normal architecture. The white matter tracts that properly lie horizontally above the lateral ventricles instead are oriented vertically; they are separated and thus ascend upward (i.e., cephalad) from their normal position (Figures 6-32A and B).

Agenesis of the corpus callosum has a male predilection of about 2:1 and an association with both trisomies 13 and 18. Fetal alcohol syndrome has been implicated as an etiologic factor in cases where excessive maternal alcohol consumption has occurred during pregnancy. A host of central nervous system abnormalities usually accompany agenesis of the corpus callosum (see list below).

The spectrum of sonographic findings associated with agenesis of the corpus callosum varies widely depending on the exact configuration of anomalous anatomy present. When there is gross distortion of normal intracranial architecture secondary to concomitant pathology, routine sonographic evaluation is an extremely sensitive method for prenatal diagnosis. When the anatomic irregularities are subtle and less immediately apparent, the clinical pearl for identifying agenesis of the corpus callosum during the course of a screening sonographic examination is the absence of the cavum septi pellucidi, a landmark that should be routinely identified.

Differential Diagnosis

Agenesis of the corpus callosum can be confidently diagnosed when an interhemispheric cyst is identified along with the absence of the corpus callosum. However, if an absent corpus callosum cannot be confirmed sonographically, the cyst may also represent a normal cavum septi pellicidi, cavum vergae, cavum interpositi, or interhemispheric arachnoid cyst.

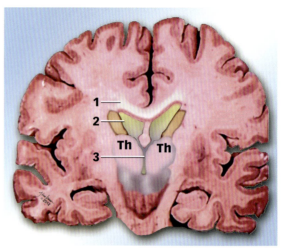

A

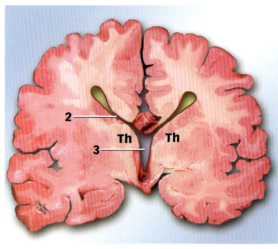

B

Figure 6-32. Comparative schematic illustration of agenesis of the corpus callosum, coronal sections. **A** Normal. **B** Absent corpus callosum with cephalad migrations of the bodies of the lateral ventricles. 1 = corpus callosum, 2 = lateral ventricle, 3 = third ventricle, Th = thalamus. (Figure continues . . .)

Associated Abnormalities

Conditions associated with agenesis of the corpus callosum include the following:

- Aneuploidy:
  - Trisomy 18 (Edwards syndrome)
  - Trisomy 13 (Patau syndrome)
  - Trisomy 8 (Warkany syndrome 2)
- Other syndromes:
  - Aicardi syndrome
  - Apert syndrome
  - Bickers-Adams-Edwards syndrome
  - Coffin-Siris syndrome

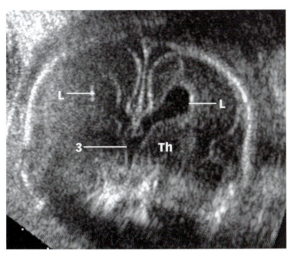

C

Figure 6-32, continued. C Coronal sonographic section in agenesis of the corpus callosum demonstrating the upward and outward migration of the bodies of the lateral ventricles. L = lateral ventricles, 3 = third ventricle, Th = thalamus.

- Fetal alcohol syndrome
- Fryns syndrome
- Gorlin syndrome
- Hydrolethalus syndrome
- Lowe syndrome
- Zellweger syndrome
• CNS anomalies:
  - Chiari II malformation
  - Dandy-Walker spectrum
  - Gray matter heterotopia
  - Holoprosencephaly
  - Hydrocephalus, particularly of the trigone and posterior horns of the lateral ventricles
  - Interhemispheric cysts
  - Intracranial lipoma
  - Polymicrogyria
  - Porencephaly

Sonographic Signs

Characteristic sonographic signs of agenesis of the corpus callosum (ACC) include the following:

- Absent cavum septi pellucidi (in complete ACC)
- Lateral ventricles displaced upward and outward (Figure 6-32C)
- Third ventricle dilated and displaced superiorly
- Posterior horn hydrocephalus

Intracranial Tumors

Intracranial tumors in the fetus are rare. Most intracranial tumors detected in utero are supratentorial, and 50% of these are teratomas. Other tumor types include glioblastomas, craniopharyngiomas, sarcomas, and oligodendrogliomas. While sonography is an extremely sensitive modality for identifying poor-prognosis brain tumors in utero, it lacks any specificity in determining the histologic nature of these large, complex masses.

Differential Diagnosis

Intracranial tumors are unique in their sonographic appearance, vascularization patterns, and the gross distortion of normal intracranial anatomic architecture that accompanies them.

Associated Abnormalities

Conditions associated with intracranial tumors include the following:

- High-output cardiac failure
- Hydrops fetalis
- Abnormal cerebral Doppler flow velocimetry

Sonographic Signs

The following are the characteristic sonographic signs of intracranial tumors:

- Large, complex, echogenic mass in the brain (Figures 6-33A and B)
- Gross distortion of normal intracranial architecture
- Hydrocephalus
- Macrocephaly
- Polyhydramnios

Intracranial Hemorrhage in Utero

Intracranial hemorrhage (ICH) in utero is rare. However, as is the case with the more commonly encountered intracranial hemorrhage in low-birthweight preterm neonates, bleeding into the fetal brain and/or ventricles occurs when significant pressure gradient changes occur secondary to cerebral hypoxic events. Common etiologic factors include severe fetal or maternal hypoxia, maternal abdominal trauma, fetal or maternal thrombocytopenia, and twin-to-twin transfusion syndrome or demise of a co-twin.[6] As the arterial compensatory mechanism kicks in to shunt more blood to the oxygen-deprived brain, increased pressure in the arterial branches supplying the choroid plexus ruptures these fragile, thin-walled vessels. Blood extravasates

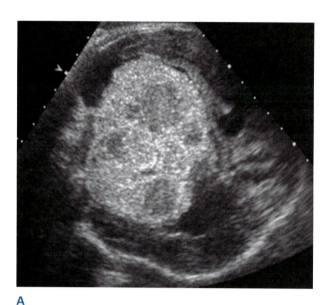
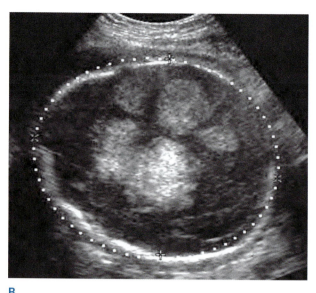

Figure 6-33. Two examples of fetal intracranial tumors demonstrating the presence of large, solid echogenic masses obliterating normal brain architecture. **A** Coronal section through a cerebral teratoma. **B** Axial section through a glioblastoma.

into the adjacent anatomy, creating an extremely variable sonographic appearance. Fresh blood and solid hematomas appear as heterogeneous, brightly echogenic areas within the ventricle or cerebral parenchyma.

Differential Diagnosis

The sonographic appearance of in utero intracranial hemorrhage is usually quite specific and can be differentiated from other cerebral pathology by its poorly marginated borders and relationship to ventricular anatomy. If, however, bleeding into the brain is well confined and localized, it could be confused with an intracranial tumor.

Sonographic Signs

The characteristic sonographic signs of intracranial hemorrhage in utero are irregularly marginated, heterogeneous echogenic areas within the cerebral parenchyma (Figure 6-34).

Porencephaly

Porencephaly (see Figure 6-34) is defined as a focal cystic area of *encephalomalacia* (softening of brain tissue) that communicates with the ventricle, subarachnoid space, or both. The term is broadly applied to any abnormal congenital or developmental cystic cavity identified in the brain; however, when found in association with intracranial hemorrhage, porencephaly specifically refers to cystic lesions created by the lysis of ischemic areas adjacent to the ventricles.

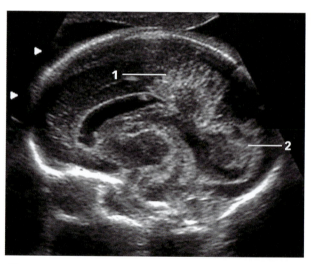

Figure 6-34. Sagittal section demonstrating an echogenic, irregularly marginated hemorrhage on the cerebral hemisphere and porencephaly extending from the occipital ventricular horn. 1 = hemorrhage, 2 = porencephaly.

Differential Diagnosis

Differential diagnoses for porencephaly include other intracranial cystic lesions, such as subarachnoid lesions or Dandy-Walker malformations.

Sonographic Signs

The characteristic sonographic sign of porencephaly is a localized fluid collection in the cerebral parenchyma communicating with the lateral ventricles or subarachnoid space.

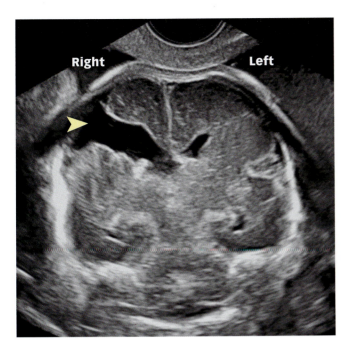

Figure 6-35. Coronal sonographic section demonstrating a unilateral cystic defect extending from brain surface to ventricular wall in a 24-week fetus with schizencephaly. Reprinted with permission from Lee W, Comstock CH, Kazmierczak, et al: Prenatal diagnostic challenges and pitfalls for schizencephaly. J Ultrasound Med 28:1379-1384, 2009.

Schizencephaly

Schizencephaly is a rare condition in which large gray-matter clefts extend through the cerebral parenchyma from the peripheral meninges to the ependymal area of the lateral ventricles.

Its etiology is believed to be related to abnormal neuronal migration during embryologic development of the brain; however, in utero vascular insults that result in encephalomalacia must also be considered.

Differential Diagnosis

The presence of a cystic intracranial defect extending from the inner surface of the calvaria deep into solid brain tissue differentiates schizencephaly from most other types of cystic intracranial anomalies. However, it may appear sonographically similar to various types of holoprosencephaly and agenesis of the corpus callosum.

Associated Abnormalities

Conditions associated with schizencephaly include the following:

- Absent cavum septi pellucidi
- Hydrocephalus

Sonographic Signs

The following are the characteristic sonographic signs of schizencephaly:

- Unilateral or bilateral cystic defect extending from brain surface to ventricular wall (Figure 6-35)
- Absence of the cavum septi pellucidi
- Hydrocephalus

Intracranial Calcifications

The presence of intracranial calcifications in the fetal brain may be an indicator of several types of pathology. Less common causes include Sturge-Weber syndrome, calcifications within a tumor, and in utero intracranial hemorrhage (of which intracranial calcifications can be a chronic indicator). The most common cause of intracranial calcifications is a congenital infection by pathogens such as toxoplasmosis and cytomegalovirus, which cross the placenta and infect the fetus (see Chapter 12).

Associated Abnormalities

Conditions associated with intracranial calcifications include the following:

- Sturge-Weber syndrome
- In utero intracranial hemorrhage

Sonographic Signs

The characteristic sonographic sign of intracranial calcification is brightly echogenic foci within the parenchyma of the fetal brain.

Microencephaly

Microencephaly is a condition characterized by an abnormally small and underdeveloped brain and skull (the latter known as *microcephaly*; see Figures 6-36A and B) with a head circumference more than 3 standard deviations below the mean for age. Microencephaly results from abnormal brain development in association with conditions such as holoprosencephaly or lissencephaly (the absence of sulci and gyri concurrently) or brain injury such as porencephaly. Microencephaly is also associated with a multitude of genetic syndromes and malformations, single-gene defects, and in utero exposure to infections, drugs, and environmental teratogens. Although diagnosis of microencephaly may be made in some cases as early as 15.5 weeks, most cases of microencephaly develop later in pregnancy. Microencephaly is associated with abnormal neurologic function and delayed mental development.

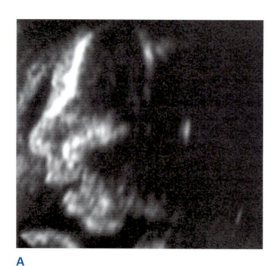 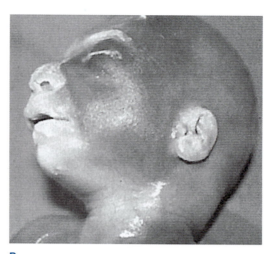

Figure 6-36. Classic facies of microcephaly. **A** Sonographic appearance. **B** Gross pathologic appearance.

Associated Abnormalities

Micreoencephaly is associated with a multitude of conditions, including the following:

- Syndromes:
  - Trisomy 13
  - Coffin-Lowry syndrome
  - Cornelia de Lange syndrome
  - Feingold syndrome
  - Holoprosencephaly
  - Miller-Dieker syndrome
  - Neu-Laxova syndrome
  - Roberts syndrome
  - Rubinstein-Taybi syndrome
  - Ruvalcaba-Myhre syndrome
  - Seckel syndrome
  - Smith-Lemli-Opitz syndrome
  - Walker-Warburg syndrome
- Other anomalies:
  - Microphthalmia
  - Hypotelorism
  - Cephaloceles
  - Porencephaly

Sonographic Signs

The following are the characteristic sonographic signs of microencephaly:

- All biometric head measurements are small relative to femur length and abdominal circumference.
- Head circumference is >3 standard deviations below mean for gestational age.
- Severe cases are differentiated from anencephaly by the presence of cerebral parenchyma within the cranial vault.

Megalencephaly

Megalencephaly is a condition characterized by an abnormally large and heavy brain exceeding the mean volume by more than twice the standard deviation. Excessive proliferation of cerebral tissue, which may be unilateral or bilateral, exerts pressure on the cranial vault, resulting in skull bossing and an enlarged head (*macrocephaly*). Genetic pathways that direct brain development (currently poorly understood) are believed to be the underyling cause. While megalencephaly may be sonographically diagnosed in utero—particularly as part of more complex fetal anomalous syndromes—it is more commonly diagnosed at birth or in early childhood development. Clinical complications associated with megalencephaly vary with the severity of abnormal neurological development and include mental retardation, autism, epilepsy, motor impairment, and/or paralysis.

Associated Abnormalities

Megalencephaly may be associated with the following syndromes:

- Achondroplasia
- Beckwith-Wiedemann syndrome
- Neurofibromatosis type 1
- Tuberous sclerosis
- Klippel-Trenaunay-Weber syndrome
- Epidermal naevus syndrome

Sonographic Signs

Although megalencephaly is more commonly diagnosed at birth and early childhood, sonographic signs suspicious for megalencephaly in utero include:

- Abnormally large head circumference measurements for dates
- HC/AC ratio above the 99th percentile

NEURAL TUBE DEFECTS

Neural tube defects comprise a spectrum of fetal anatomic abnormalities resulting from the failure of closure of the neural tube. Where along the neural axis this defect occurs determines the type of anomaly that will be manifested. If the defect occurs in the cranial portion of the embryo, anencephaly, exencephaly, encephalocele, or iniencephaly presents; if it occurs caudally in the rostral portion of the embryo, spina bifida or one of its variants will manifest itself. (See Figure 6-37.)

Relatively recent studies have implicated folic acid deficiency as a primary etiologic factor in the development of neural tube defects. The data strongly suggest that diminished folate levels (folic acid and vitamin B_{12}), which are requisite for the production and maintenance of new cells particularly in the embryologic pathway by which the neural tube is formed, impede normal neurulation, resulting in the open defects characteristic of this category of central nervous system abnormalities.[7] The major and lethal expressions of neural tube defects most commonly encountered in obstetric sonographic practice include the following:

- Anencephaly
- Exencephaly (acrania)
- Cephalocele/encephalocele
- Iniencephaly
- Spina bifida

Anencephaly

Anencephaly is the most common open neural tube defect and results from the incomplete closure of the cranial portion of the neural tube. It is a lethal fetal anomaly occurring at a rate of 1:1000 live births and carries a 4% chance of recurrence in a subsequent pregnancy.[8] It is more commonly present in female than in male fetuses. Pathologically, anencephaly is characterized by the absence of the cranial vault and cerebral hemispheres, while portions of the midbrain and the brain stem remain present. Typical facies in an anencephalic fetus include macrophthalmia (bulging eyes), macroglossia (thick tongue), and a dramatically shortened neck.

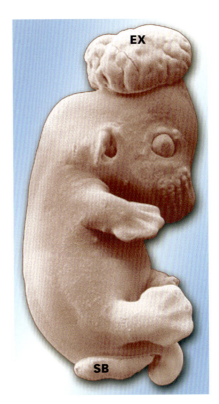

Figure 6-37. Neural tube defects induced in a mouse embryo: failure of closure of the neural tube at the cranial end, resulting in exencephaly (EX), and at the caudal end, resulting in spina bifida aperta (SB).

Polyhydramnios is commonly observed with anencephaly, presumably as a result of brain dysfunction and lack of fetal swallowing. The diagnosis of anencephaly is difficult to make before the end of the first trimester (10–11 weeks), in part because the cranium does not calcify until that time. By the beginning of the second trimester, however, sonographic findings are pathognomonic for anencephaly.

Differential Diagnosis

Several conditions characterized by the absence of all or part of the fetal cranial structures may mimic anencephaly. These include acrania, amniotic band syndrome that affects the head, and severe microcephaly.

Associated Abnormalities

The following abnormalities are characteristically associated with anencephaly:

- Spina bifida (cervical)
- Cleft lip and palate

- Clubfoot (talipes equinovarus)
- Omphalocele
- Congenital heart defects
- Hydronephrosis
- Polyhydramnios

Sonographic Signs

The following are the characteristic sonographic signs of anencephaly:

- Major portions of the cranium and intracranial structures are absent (Figure 6-38A).
- Parts of the midbrain and brain stem may be present (Figure 6-38A).
- Orbits and face present typical anencephalic facies: macrophthalmia and macroglossia (Figures 6-38B and C).
- Polyhydramnios is observed 40%–50% of the time.
- Concomitant neural tube defects are frequently identified.

Exencephaly (Acrania)

Exencephaly (*acrania*) is a rare congenital anomaly characterized by partial or complete absence of the calvaria with complete but abnormal development of brain tissue. The cerebral hemispheres are typically present but malformed and are covered by a thin membrane. The cerebellum, brain stem, and cranial nerves are present and normal.

Differential Diagnosis

Other anomalous conditions that affect the ossification and normal development of the calvarial bones may mimic acrania. These include congenital hypophosphatasia, achondrogenesis, severe osteogenesis imperfecta, and some calvarial defects secondary to amniotic band syndrome.

Associated Abnormalities

The following abnormalities are characteristically associated with acrania:

- Cleft lip and palate
- Clubfoot (talipes equinovarus)

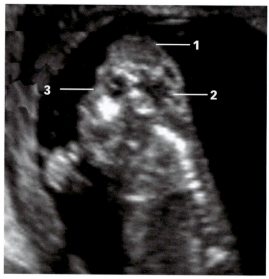

A

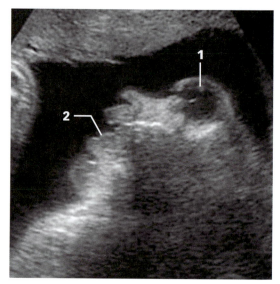

B

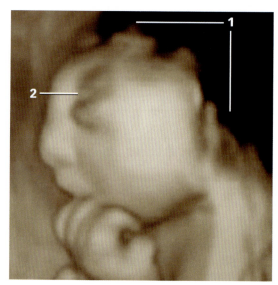

C

Figure 6-38. **A** Sagittal sonogram of a fetus with anencephaly demonstrating the absence of the cranium. 1 = absent cranium, 2 = presence of hindbrain, 3 = face. **B** Typical anencephalic facies: (1) macrophthalmia and (2) macroglossia. **C** 3D surface rendering of a fetus with anencephaly demonstrating the open defect and typical anencephalic facies. 1 = absent cranium, 2 = macrophthalmia.

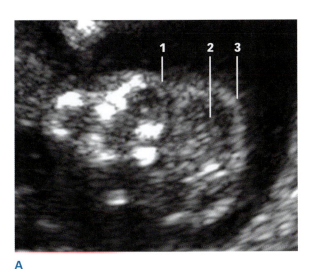
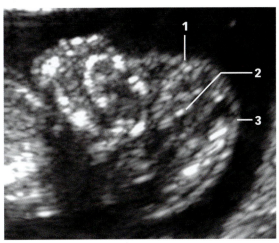

Figure 6-39. A Coronal and **B** sagittal sections demonstrating typical sonographic findings in exencephaly. 1 = absent cranial vault, 2 = cerebral hemispheres, 3 = covering membrane.

Sonographic Signs

As demonstrated in Figures 6-39A and B, the following sonographic signs are present:

- Absence of a cranial vault
- Presence of cerebral hemispheres
- Thin membrane covering cerebral hemispheres

Cephalocele/Encephalocele

Incomplete closure of the rostral end of the neural tube may also result in focal defects of the bony calvaria through which intracranial contents, specifically the meninges, can herniate. If the protruding lesion consists only of meninges, it is called a *cephalocele*; if brain tissue accompanies the herniated meninges, the lesion is called an *encephalocele* (Figure 6-40A). These defects can occur anywhere along the skull, but in the United States they are most commonly observed in the midline occipital region above the tentorium. Some cephaloceles are small and barely noticeable, whereas others are large enough to permit the entire brain to herniate through. A cranial *meningocele* differs from an encephalocele in that no brain tissue extends into the cystic sac.

Because encephaloceles are frequently associated with other syndromes and concomitant fetal anomalies, careful review of the remainder of the fetus is indicated when an encephalocele is encountered during sonographic examination. Some syndromes that include encephaloceles as a part of their presentation are Meckel-Gruber syndrome (see pages 291–292) and

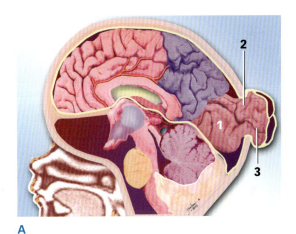

Figure 6-40. A Schematic showing an occipital encephalocele with (1) herniation of part of the occipital lobe through (2) a calvarial defect into (3) a meningeal sac. (Figure continues . . .)

amniotic band syndrome (see pages 287–288). Hydrocephalus is present in 80% of occipital lesions, spina bifida in 7%–15%.

Differential Diagnosis

Encephaloceles are confidently diagnosed sonographically by identifying the calvarial bony defect through which neural tissue herniates. A large cystic or complex mass such as a neck teratoma or cystic hygroma may in some instances mimic a large complex encephalocele. A differential diagnosis for the simpler cystic-appearing cephalocele could be a subcutaneous fluid collection associated with gross scalp edema in hydrops fetalis.

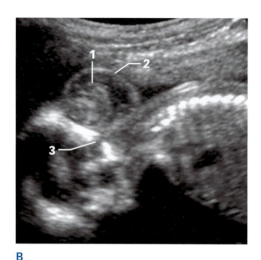
B

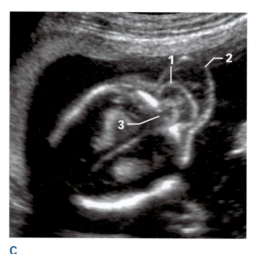
C

Figure 6-40, continued. **B** Sonographic demonstration of an occipital encephalocele in sagittal section. **C** Sonographic demonstratio n of an occipital encephalocele in axial section. The more echogenic occipital lobe (1) herniates into a meningeal sac (2) through a bony calvarial defect (3).

Associated Abnormalities

The following abnormalities are characteristically associated with encephaloceles:[9]

- Agenesis of the corpus callosum
- Orofacial clefting
- Dandy-Walker malformation
- Arnold-Chiari malformation
- Hemifacial microsomia
- Iniencephaly
- Myelomeningocele
- Hydrocephalus
- Polyhydramnios
- Spina bifida

Sonographic Signs

The following are the characteristic sonographic signs of encephalocele (Figures 6-40B and C):

- Mass extending from the calvaria; may be totally cystic (cephalocele), may be cystic with septations (meningocele), or may contain brain (encephalomeningomyelocele)
- Cranial defect (occasionally seen)
- Cranial cavity that appears small if a significant portion of brain is herniated

Iniencephaly

Iniencephaly is a rare, uniformly lethal neural tube defect of the cervical and upper thoracic regions producing anomalous features that include retroflexion of the upper spine accompanied by a short neck and trunk, defects of the thoracic cage, and anterior spina bifida. The hallmark findings of prenatal diagnosis include cervical rachischisis, occipital encephalocele, and exaggerated spinal lordosis (Figure 6-41A). The sonographic appearance of iniencephaly is that of a grossly abnormal fetus with a "stargazer" posture in which the immobile head is hyperextended with the face directed upward. The head is not observed to move independently of the fetal body.

Differential Diagnosis

The sonographic appearance of iniencephaly is so dramatically abnormal that few other anomalous conditions mimic it.

Associated Abnormalities

Other fetal anomalies are associated with iniencephaly in 84% of cases and include the following:

- Anencephaly and variants
- Myelomeningoceles
- Diaphragmatic hernia
- Pulmonary hypoplasia
- Cardiac defects

Sonographic Signs

Characteristic sonographic signs (Figure 6-41B) of iniencephaly include the following:

- Exaggerated cervicothoracic lordosis: "stargazer" posture
- Occipital bone defects including encephalocele
- Short, fused cervical vertebrae
- Polyhydramnios
- Cervical rachischisis

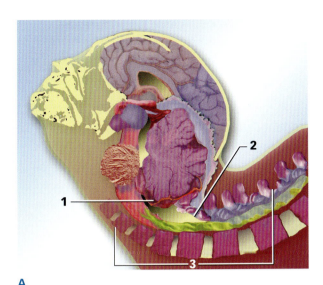
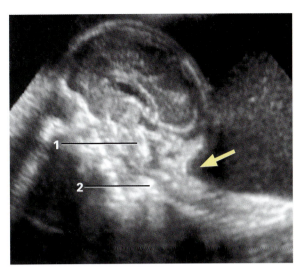

Figure 6-41. A Schematic demonstration of the characteristic pathologic findings in iniencephaly. 1 = occipital encephalocele, 2 = cervical rachischisis, 3 = exaggerated cervicothoracic lordosis. **B** Sagittal sonogram in a 20-week fetus demonstrating the hallmark findings. 1 = occipital encephalocele, 2 = cervical rachischisis, arrow = exaggerated cervicothoracic lordosis.

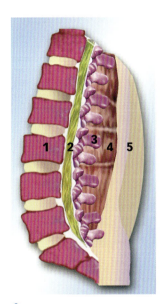
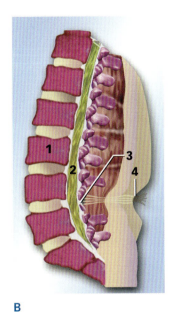

Figure 6-42. Comparative schematic illustration of spina bifida occulta demonstrating a localized defect that remains hidden by intact posterior musculature, fascia, and skin. **A** Normal spine. 1 = vertebral body, 2 = spinal cord and meninges, 3 = posterior vertebral elements, 4 = musculature, 5 = posterior fascia and skin. **B** Spina bifida occulta. 1 = vertebral body, 2 = intact spinal cord, 3 = localized defect, 4 = skin dimple/tuft.

Spina Bifida

Spina bifida, also called *spinal dysraphism*, is a neural tube defect resulting from the failure of the vertebral column to close during neurulation. The defect may occur anywhere along the spinal column but is most commonly located in the lumbosacral region. The gross pathologic appearance varies in size and content from the externally undetectable *spina bifida occulta* to the complete open splaying of the entire neural canal with accompanying severe intracranial anatomic abnormalities. Spina bifida is the most common neural tube defect affecting the spinal column, with an incidence of approximately 1:1000–2000 live births.[10] The etiology is usually multifactorial, with both genetic and environmental factors implicated as causes.

The milder form of spina bifida, *spina bifida occulta*, is characterized by a defect in the posterior bony neural arch of the spinal canal, with preservation of overlying tissue and skin (Figures 6-42A and B). Rarely demonstrable during antenatal sonography, "hidden" spina bifida is typically diagnosed postnatally as an incidental finding during imaging studies of the spine. With the exception of an occasional skin dimple or subcutaneous lipoma overlying the defect, there are no signs or symptoms of spina bifida occulta and no neurologic sequelae.

Spina bifida aperta, on the other hand, presents as a visible defect along the spine with the attendant skin, subcutaneous, bony, and neural tissue abnormalities that are hallmarks of this condition. The opening

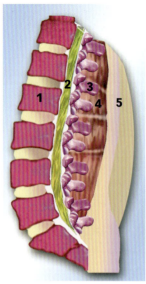
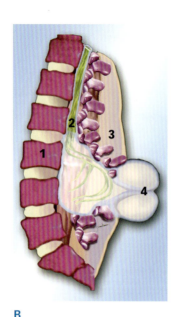

Figure 6-43. Comparative schematic illustration of spina bifida aperta demonstrating herniation of neural tissue and meninges through an open defect in the spinal column. **A** Normal spine. **B** Spina bifida aperta. 1 = vertebral body, 2 = spinal cord and meninges, 3 = posterior vertebral elements, 4 = musculature, 5 = posterior fascia and skin.

in the defective neural tube permits herniation of meninges, forming a cystic sac projecting posteriorly from the spinal canal (Figures 6-43A and B). When meninges alone are present, the herniated sac is called a *myelocele*; when neural tissue is also present, it is called a *myelomeningocele* (or *meningomyelocele*). Virtually all cases of spina bifida aperta present with myelomeningoceles of some type, although differentiation of the specific nature of the mass is moot from a sonographic and clinical perspective. The herniated sac may be small or large and may be confined to the level of a single vertebra or extend the full length of the spinal column.

Rarely, a severe form of spina bifida called *rachischisis* may be present in which the entire spinal canal is splayed open posteriorly from the neck to the sacrum. Typically, this is associated with other severe cranial anomalies, such as anencephaly or acrania. "Open" spina bifida is also associated with other intracranial anomalies such as ventriculomegaly, the "lemon sign" (frontal scalloping or indentation of the frontal bones), and the "banana sign" (obliteration of the cisterna magna around the cerebellum in the posterior fossa). Caudal torsion of the spinal cord can also pull the posterior fossa structures (cerebellum and medulla oblongata) into the upper cervical spine, creating a Chiari II malformation. Prognosis depends on severity of the lesion and is poorest in infants who have total paralysis below the lesion, kyphosis, hydrocephalus, and/or associated congenital defects.

Differential Diagnosis

The primary differential diagnosis for spina bifida aperta is a sacrococcygeal teratoma arising from the lower back. While most teratomas also have a hallmark complex cystic/solid sonographic appearance, those that are predominantly cystic may mimic a meningomyelocele.

Associated Abnormalities

The following abnormalities are characteristically associated with spina bifida:

- Trisomy 18 (Edwards syndrome)
- Trisomy 13 (Patau syndrome)
- Chiari II malformation
- Hydrocephalus
- Clubfoot (talipes equinovarus)
- Rocker bottom foot (congenital vertical talus)

Sonographic Signs

Transversely, the exam demonstrates the following sonographic signs of spina bifida (Figure 6-44A):

- Posterior ossification centers are splayed into a U or V shape.
- When a herniated sac is intact, a cystic structure can be seen extending from the back.
- The sac may appear as a small, simple cystic structure, as a cyst with septations, or as a complex cystic/solid mass.

Sagittally, the exam demonstrates these signs of spina bifida (Figures 6-44B and C):

- Discontinuity of parallel lateral ossification centers
- Herniated sac protruding posteriorly

The *intracranial view* demonstrates these signs of spina bifida:

- *Lemon sign*: overlapping of the frontal bones, creating a lemon-shaped fetal head (Figure 6-45A)
- *Banana sign*: effacement of the cisterna magna due to downward displacement of the cerebellum (Figure 6-45B), as seen with Chiari type II malformation (Figure 6-45C).

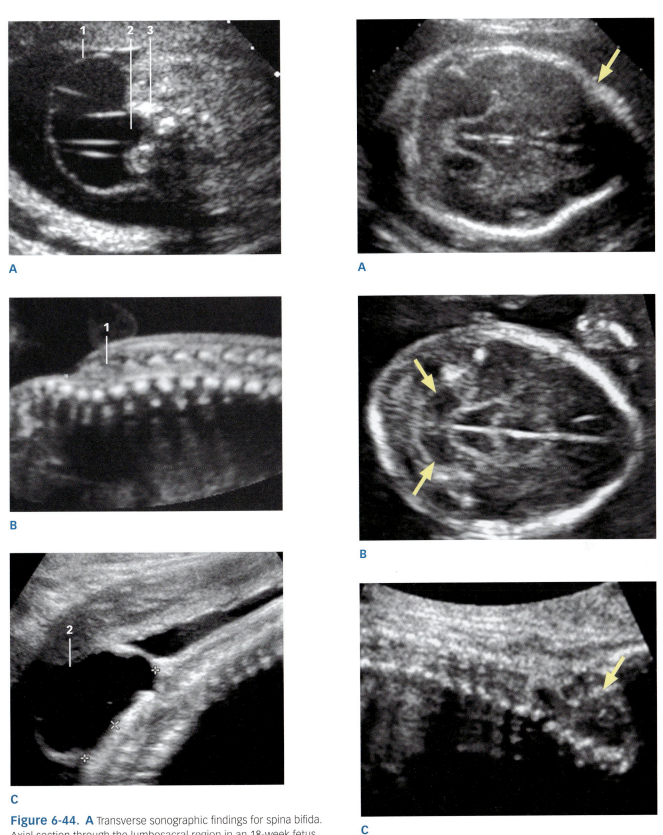

Figure 6-44. A Transverse sonographic findings for spina bifida. Axial section through the lumbosacral region in an 18-week fetus demonstrating a septated, cystic lesion arising from a defect in the posterior tissue planes. 1 = herniated sac, 2 = open defect, 3 = splaying of ossification centers. **B** and **C** Sagittal sonographic findings for spina bifida in two different fetuses at different gestational ages. 1 = discontinuity of ossification centers, 2 = herniated sac.

Figure 6-45. Intracranial sonographic findings for spina bifida. **A** Lemon sign (arrow). **B** Banana sign (arrows), visible only in axial section. **C** Chiari type II malformation (arrow).

CHAPTER 6 REVIEW QUESTIONS

1. The space lying between the frontal horns and bodies of the two lateral ventricles is the:
   A. Cavum vergae
   B. Cavum septi pellucidi
   C. Foramen of Monro
   D. Falx cerebri

2. The highly vascularized structure lying along the floor of both lateral ventricles and extending along the roof of the third ventricle is the:
   A. Cavum septi pellucidi
   B. Falx cerebri
   C. Corpus callosum
   D. Choroid plexus

3. The site where the body, posterior, and temporal horns of the lateral ventricle converge is called the:
   A. Pons
   B. Atrium
   C. Third ventricle
   D. Choroid

4. The symmetric midline intracranial structure whose lateral walls are formed by the inferior aspect of the thalamus and hypothalamus is the:
   A. Corpus callosum
   B. Third ventricle
   C. Fourth ventricle
   D. Aqueduct of Sylvius

5. The portion of dura mater that invaginates along the intercerebral fissure is called the:
   A. Falx cerebri
   B. Cavum septi pellucidi
   C. Third ventricle
   D. Aqueduct of Sylvius

6. The fluid-filled structure located between the cerebellum and the occipital bone in the posterior fossa is called the:
   A. Third ventricle
   B. Fourth ventricle
   C. Cisterna magna
   D. Interpeduncular cistern

7. The anastomotic network of arteries located at the base of the brain is the:
   A. Circle of Willis
   B. Sylvian fissure
   C. Posterior cerebral artery
   D. Vertebrobasilar circulation

8. In this image the arrow points to:

   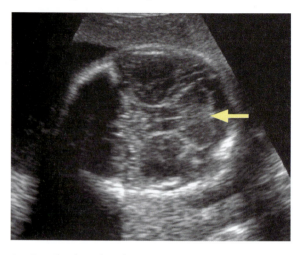

   A. Cerebral peduncles
   B. Cerebral hemispheres
   C. Cerebellar hemispheres
   D. Cisterna magna

9. In this image the arrow points to:

   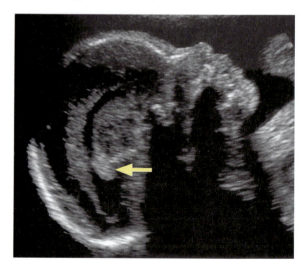

   A. Choroid plexus
   B. Cavum septi pellucidi
   C. Cerebral peduncles
   D. Thalamus

10. In this image the arrow points to:

    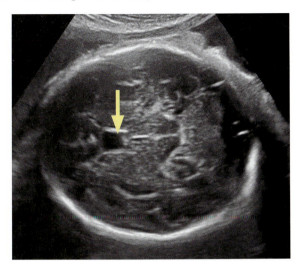

    A. Third ventricle
    B. Fourth ventricle
    C. Choroid plexus
    D. Cavum septi pellucidi

11. Ossification centers are found in the following locations within each vertebra EXCEPT:
    A. Vertebral body
    B. Spinous process
    C. Between lamina and pedicle on right side
    D. Between lamina and pedicle on left side

12. The sacral spine in this image demonstrates:

    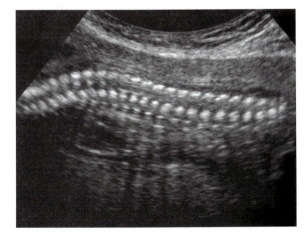

    A. Spina bifida
    B. A sacrococcygeal teratoma
    C. Splayed vertebrae
    D. A normal spine

13. Congenital enlargement of the intracranial ventricular system is called:
    A. Cystic hygroma
    B. Hydranencephaly
    C. Holoprosencephaly
    D. Ventriculomegaly

14. Hydrocephalus is best described as:
    A. Enlargement of the ventricular system with concomitant compression atrophy of adjacent cerebral parenchyma
    B. Enlargement of the ventricular system without concomitant compression atrophy of adjacent cerebral parenchyma
    C. Enlarged, single midline ventricle surrounded by a mantle of cerebral tissue
    D. Cystic dilatation of the cisterna magna with compression atrophy of the cerebellum

15. Ventriculomegaly is best described as:
    A. Enlargement of the ventricular system with concomitant compression atrophy of adjacent cerebral parenchyma
    B. Enlargement of the ventricular system without concomitant compression atrophy of adjacent cerebral parenchyma
    C. Enlarged, single midline ventricle surrounded by a mantle of cerebral tissue
    D. Cystic dilatation of the cisterna magna with compression atrophy of the cerebellum

16. This image demonstrates:

    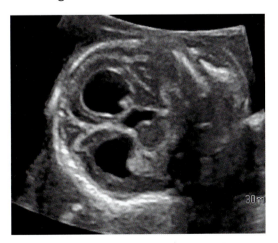

    A. Hydrocephalus
    B. Hydranencephaly
    C. Holoprosencephaly
    D. Dandy-Walker malformation

17. The near or total absence of the cerebral hemispheres is called:
    A. Holoprosencephaly
    B. Hydranencephaly
    C. Hydrocephalus
    D. Dandy-Walker anomaly malformation

18. This image demonstrates:

    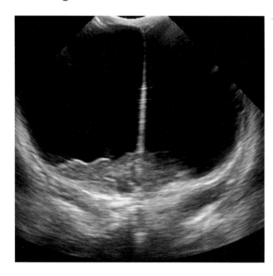

    A. Hydrocephalus
    B. Hydranencephaly
    C. Holoprosencephaly
    D. Dandy-Walker malformation

19. The abnormality of forebrain diverticulation that results in the presence of a single middle ventricle is called:
    A. Holoprosencephaly
    B. Hydranencephaly
    C. Hydrocephalus
    D. Dandy-Walker anomaly malformation

20. Bizarre facial abnormalities such as cyclopia and proboscis are usually associated with:
    A. Holoprosencephaly
    B. Hydranencephaly
    C. Hydrocephalus
    D. Median facial cleft

21. The most severe type of holoprosencephaly is:
    A. Lobar
    B. Semilobar
    C. Alobar
    D. Nonlobar

22. This image demonstrates:

    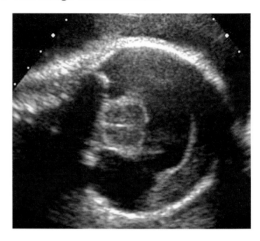

    A. Alobar holoprosencephaly
    B. Lobar holoprosencephaly
    C. Anencephaly
    D. Hydrocephalus

23. The anomaly in this image is most commonly associated with:

    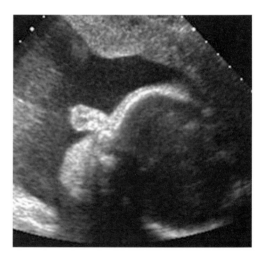

    A. Trisomy 21
    B. Trisomy 18
    C. Beckwith-Wiedemann syndrome
    D. Holoprosencephaly

24. Which of the following is a cystic abnormality of the posterior fossa that is characterized by the absence or severe dysgenesis of the cerebellar vermis with opportunistic filling of the space with cerebrospinal fluid?
    A. Hydrocephalus
    B. Hydranencephaly
    C. Subarachnoid cyst
    D. Dandy-Walker malformation

25. All of the following congenital abnormalities are associated with Dandy-Walker malformation EXCEPT:
    A. Cleft palate
    B. Cyclopia
    C. Hydrocephalus
    D. Agenesis of the corpus callosum

26. This image demonstrates:

    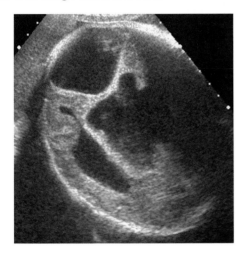

    A. Dandy-Walker malformation
    B. Alobar holoprosencephaly
    C. Lobar holoprosencephaly
    D. Hydranencephaly

27. A congenital intracranial anomaly characterized sonographically by the upward and outward displacement of both lateral ventricles is known as:
    A. Holoprosencephaly
    B. Hydranencephaly
    C. Agenesis of the corpus callosum
    D. Hydrocephalus

28. This image demonstrates:

    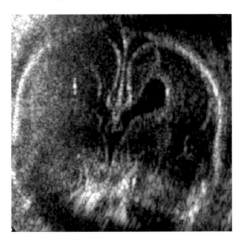

    A. Agenesis of the corpus callosum
    B. Holoprosencephaly
    C. Hydranencephaly
    D. Dandy-Walker malformation

29. All of the following are histopathologic types of intracranial tumors EXCEPT:
    A. Epignathus
    B. Glioblastoma
    C. Craniopharyngioma
    D. Sarcoma

30. An abnormally small fetal head, measuring more than 2–3 standard deviations below mean for gestational age, is called:
    A. Macrocephaly
    B. Microcephaly
    C. Anencephaly
    D. Schizencephaly

31. The fetal anatomic abnormalities resulting from the failure of the process of neurulation are referred to collectively as:
    A. Spinal dysraphism
    B. Holoprosencephaly
    C. Dandy-Walker syndrome
    D. Neural tube defects

32. All of the following congenital anatomic abnormalities are considered neural tube defects EXCEPT:
    A. Spina bifida
    B. Anencephaly
    C. Iniencephaly
    D. Holoprosencephaly

33. The most commonly occurring neural tube defect affecting the spinal column is:
    A. Encephalocele
    B. Spina bifida
    C. Iniencepaly
    D. Anencephaly

34. A fetal intracranial abnormality characterized by the absence of the cranial vault and cerebral hemispheres but with portions of the midbrain and the brain stem present is called:
    A. Holoprosencephaly
    B. Hydrocephalus

C. Dandy-Walker malformation

D. Anencephaly

35. This image demonstrates:

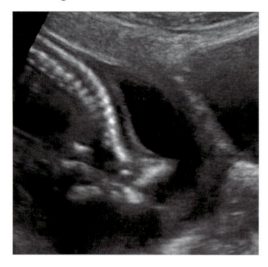

A. Spina bifida

B. Anencephaly

C. Dandy-Walker malformation

D. Cranial dysostosis

36. Protrusion of intracranial contents, such as brain and meninges, through a defect in the bony calvaria is called:

A. Encephalocele

B. Anencephaly

C. Schizencephaly

D. Holoprosencephaly

37. This image demonstrates:

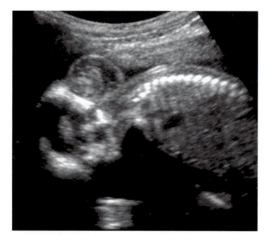

A. Neck teratoma

B. Cystic hygroma

C. Encephalocele

D. Nuchal thickening

38. The type of neural tube defect characterized sonographically by a fetus with exaggerated cervicothoracic lordosis, also called the "stargazer" posture, is:

A. Anencephaly

B. Spina bifida

C. Encephalocele

D. Iniencephaly

39. The neural tube defect characterized by an open defect along the posterior spine with protrusion of neural tissue and meninges is called:

A. Spina bifida aperta

B. Spina bifida occulta

C. Iniencephaly

D. Encephalocele

40. The arrow and cursors in this image are delineating a:

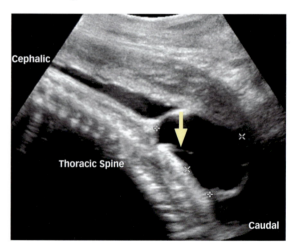

A. Cystic teratoma

B. Meningomyelocele

C. Cystic hygroma

D. Branchial cleft cyst

ANSWERS

See Appendix A on page 479 for answers.

REFERENCES

1. Winter TC, Kennedy AM, Byrne J, et al: The cavum septi pellucidi: why is it important? J Ultrasound Med 29:427–444, 2010.

2. Cardoza JD, Goldstein RB, Filly RA: Exclusion of fetal ventriculomegaly with a single measurement: the width of the lateral ventricular atrium. Radiology 169:711–714, 1988.

3. Filly RA, Cardoza JD, Goldstein RB, et al: Detection of fetal central nervous system anomalies: a practical level of effort for a routine sonogram. Radiology 172:403–408, 1989.

4. Estroff JA, Scott MR, Benacerraf BR: Dandy-Walker variant: prenatal sonographic features and clinical outcome. Radiology 185:755–758, 1992.

5. Sepulveda W, Vanderheyden T, Pather J, et al: Vein of Galen malformation: prenatal evaluation with three-dimensional power Doppler angiography. J Ultrasound Med 22:1395–1398, 2003.

6. Sherer DM, Anyaegbunam A, Onyeije C: Antepartum fetal intracranial hemorrhage: predisposing factors and prenatal sonography. Am J Perinatol 15:431–441, 1998.

7. Dunlap B, Shelke K, Salem SA, et al: Folic acid and human reproduction: ten important issues for clinicians. J Exp Clin Assist Reprod 8:2, 2011.

8. Cowchock S, Ainbender E, Prescott G, et al: The recurrence risk for neural tube defects in the United States: a collaborative study. Am J Med Genet 5:309–314, 1980.

9. Cohen MM Jr, Lemire RJ: Syndromes with cephaloceles. Teratology 25:161–172, 1982.

10. Babcock CJ, Ball RH, Feldkamp ML: Prevalence of aneuploidy and additional anatomic abnormalities in fetuses with open spina bifida: population based study in Utah. J Ultrasound Med 19:619–623, 2000.

SUGGESTED READINGS

Benacerraf BR: *Ultrasound of Fetal Syndromes*, 2nd edition. Philadelphia, Churchill Livingstone, 2008.

Fleischer AC, Toy E, Lee W, et al (eds): *Sonography in Obstetrics and Gynecology: Principles and Practice*, 7th edition. New York, McGraw-Hill, 2011, ch 15.

Henningsen CG: The fetal neural axis. In Hagen-Ansert SL (ed): *Textbook of Diagnostic Ultrasonography*, 7th edition. St. Louis, Elsevier Mosby, 2012, pp 1289–1310.

Pilu G: Ultrasound evaluation of the fetal neural axis. In Callen PW (ed): *Ultrasonography in Obstetrics and Gynecology*, 5th edition. Philadelphia, Saunders Elsevier, 2008, pp 363–391.

Sauerbrei S: The fetal spine. In Rumack CM, Wilson SR, Charboneau JW, et al (eds): *Diagnostic Ultrasound*, 4th edition. Philadelphia, Elsevier Mosby, 2011, pp 1245–1272.

Toi A, Levine D: The fetal brain. In Rumack CM, Wilson SR, Charboneau JW, et al (eds): *Diagnostic Ultrasound*, 4th edition. Philadelphia, Elsevier Mosby, 2011, pp 1197–1244.

CHAPTER 7

The Fetal Chest, Lungs, and Heart

Lung Development and Anatomy

Heart Development and Anatomy

Sonographic Anatomy

Chest Abnormalities

The thoracic cavity, commonly called the chest, encompasses the heart, lungs, great vessels, and mediastinal structures. It is bordered anterolaterally by the rib cage and sternum and posteriorly by the spine. Its inferior boundary is formed by the diaphragm, a thick bilateral muscular structure that separates it from the abdominal cavity. Sonographic examination of all these component anatomic structures is an integral part of a routine obstetric ultrasound examination beginning with the second trimester.

LUNG DEVELOPMENT AND ANATOMY

EMBRYONIC AND ALVEOLAR PERIODS

There are two periods of critical importance when monitoring for abnormalities during pulmonary development:

- The *embryonic period*, from 3 to 6 conceptual weeks (5 to 7 menstrual weeks), when the presence and integrity of normal anatomic structures in the chest is established
- The *alveolar period*, beginning at 36 conceptual (38 menstrual) weeks, which determines the maturity and proper functionality of the lungs at birth

Genetic or toxic insults that adversely affect the proper unfolding of pulmonary embryonic and developmental events will yield hallmark anatomic abnormalities. Abnormalities originating during the embryonic period result in the absence or malformation of fundamental anatomic structures, such as the trachea, bronchial tree, and alveolar bed. Abnormalities arising from later developmental defects, during the alveolar period, produce pathologic transformation of normally present pulmonary tissue, resulting in undeveloped hypoplastic lungs, cystic malformations, pleural effusion, and/or other physiologic deficiencies that deliver a neonate with acute, and often lethal, respiratory distress syndrome (RDS).

Pulmonary development begins around the end of the 5th menstrual week, when a single lung bud appears at the distal end of each primordial bronchus (embryonic period). There are four additional stages of lung development:

- *Pseudoglandular* or *embryonic* phase, conceptual weeks 7–17 (menstrual weeks 9–19): During this phase the air-conducting bronchi and terminal bronchioles form (Figure 7-1A). This includes the embryonic period described above.
- *Canalicular* phase, conceptual weeks 17–27 (menstrual weeks 19–29): During this phase lung tissue becomes vascularized and the lumina of the bronchioles and the alveolar ducts enlarge (Figure 7-1B).
- *Terminal sac* or *saccular phase*, conceptual weeks 28–36 (menstrual weeks 30–38): This phase is characterized by the appearance of primordial alveoli and a capillary bed that is sufficiently formed to permit respiratory function adequate for survival outside the uterus (Figure 7-1C).
- *Alveolar phase*, conceptual week 36 (menstrual week 38) to 2 years: During this phase the number of terminal bronchioles and alveoli increases (Figure 7-1D). The exact time of its onset overlaps with the terminal sac phase; the time of its exact onset varies among experts.

An important biochemical component of the final two stages of lung development is *pulmonary surfactant*,

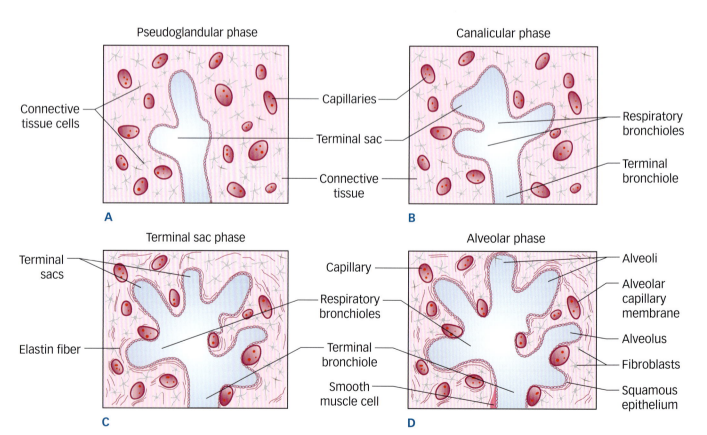

Figure 7-1. Pulmonary embryology. **A** Pseudoglandular phase, 7–17 conceptual (9–19 menstrual) weeks. **B** Canalicular phase, 17–27 conceptual (19–29 menstrual) weeks. **C** Terminal sac or saccular phase, 28–36 conceptual (30–38 menstrual) weeks. **D** Alveolar phase, beginning at 36 conceptual (38 menstrual) weeks and ending at 2 years. (Sources vary on exactly when phases begin.)

a lipoprotein produced by the alveolar cells of the lungs. Its primary physiologic function is to increase the *compliance* of the fetal lung—its ability to expand to accommodate an air volume that will permit adequate oxygen perfusion postnatally. Pulmonary surfactant also regulates the size and expansion of the alveolar bed and serves to normalize surface tension in the alveolar spaces, keeping the tiny air sacs open and available for gaseous exchange. Surfactant levels can be measured on amniotic fluid as an indicator of fetal lung maturity (see "Amniotic Fluid" below).

During the entire fetal period, four conditions are required for adequate lung development. If any of these factors is absent or significantly compromised, the lungs will not develop into the functional respiratory organs that are required to support life outside the uterus. The four conditions are:

- Adequate thoracic space
- Normal fetal breathing movements
- Fluid production in the lungs
- Adequate amniotic fluid volume

AMNIOTIC FLUID

While all four of the factors mentioned above are requisite for normal lung development, amniotic fluid plays a uniquely important role. Adequate pulmonary function at birth depends on an adequate and mature surfactant system in utero, comprising lipoproteins suspended in amniotic fluid. While in the third trimester these biochemical markers can be assessed with laboratory analysis of amniocentesis specimens, in earlier stages of pregnancy sonographic assessment of fluid volume provides valuable diagnostic and prognostic information.

Before 15–20 menstrual weeks, amniotic fluid is derived primarily from the maternal perfusion activity of the chorioamnion. However, in the mid to late second trimester and in the third trimester, it is produced primarily by fetal urine. Amniotic fluid serves several functions:

- It cushions the fetus against injury.
- It allows for free movement of the fetus.
- It is essential for fetal lung development.
- It provides a source of fetal nutrition.
- It aids in maintaining fetal temperature.

Estimating Amniotic Fluid Volume

Normally the volume of amniotic fluid surrounding the fetus gradually increases through early pregnancy until it reaches a maximum of approximately 800 ml at about 33 menstrual weeks, decreasing gradually thereafter. The increase in amniotic fluid volume during the second trimester reflects the increased urine output of the fetus. The decrease in the later part of pregnancy reflects increased fetal swallowing and decreased fetal urine output.

Many different methods have been described to estimate the amount of amniotic fluid present within the uterus. The primary methods are subjective visual assessment on sonography, the maximum vertical pocket method, and the four-quadrant amniotic fluid index (Table 7-1).

Subjective Assessment

The oldest and still one of the most accurate methods of assessing amniotic fluid volume is a subjective visual assessment of the amount of fluid present while scanning the pregnancy in real time. Early in the second trimester, the volume occupied by the fetus is about equal to the volume of amniotic fluid. The fetus does not appear confined within the uterus and is seen to move freely within the surrounding fluid. Throughout the second and third trimesters, the volume of the fetus increases relative to the volume of fluid, and in late pregnancy the amount of fluid appears small in comparison with the fetus. The disadvantage of the subjective assessment method is that it is not a metric, making it unreliable for follow-up examination.

Maximum Vertical Pocket Estimate

The *maximum vertical pocket* (MVP) method, sometimes called the *single deepest pocket* (SDP) method, is obtained by measuring the anteroposterior (AP) dimension (depth) of the largest pocket of amniotic fluid that is void of both fetal parts and umbilical cord. This metric is valid throughout the third trimester. A pocket measuring 2–8 cm is considered normal.

Four-Quadrant Amniotic Fluid Index

With the *four-quadrant amniotic fluid index* (AFI), measurements are taken in each of four uterine quadrants, and the greatest vertical (anteroposterior) measurements are summed. Except at the extreme

Table 7-1.	Amniotic fluid index (AFI) values in normal pregnancy.				
Menstrual Week	Percentile Values (cm)				
	2.5th	5th	50th	95th	97th
16	7.3	7.9	12.1	18.5	20.1
17	7.7	8.3	12.7	19.4	21.1
18	8.0	9.7	13.3	20.2	22.0
19	8.3	9.0	13.7	20.7	22.5
20	8.6	9.3	14.1	21.2	23.0
21	8.8	9.5	14.3	21.4	23.3
22	8.9	9.7	14.5	21.6	23.5
23	9.0	9.8	14.6	21.8	23.7
24	9.0	9.8	14.7	21.9	23.8
25	8.9	97	14.7	22.1	24.0
26	8.9	9.7	14.7	22.3	24.2
27	8.5	9.5	14.6	22.6	24.5
28	8.6	9.4	14.6	22.8	24.9
29	8.4	9.2	14.5	23.1	25.4
30	8.2	9.0	14.5	23.4	25.8
31	7.9	8.8	14.4	23.8	26.3
32	7.7	8.6	14.4	24.2	26.9
33	7.4	8.3	14.3	24.5	27.4
34	7.2	8.1	14.2	24.8	27.8
35	7.0	7.9	14.0	24.9	27.9
36	6.8	7.7	13.8	24.9	27.9
37	6.6	7.5	13.5	24.4	27.5
38	6.5	7.3	13.2	23.9	26.9
39	6.4	7.2	12.7	22.6	25.5
40	6.3	7.1	12.3	21.4	24.0
41	6.3	7.0	11.6	19.4	21.6
42	6.3	6.9	11.0	17.5	19.2

Source: Reprinted with permission in modified form from Moore TR, Cayle JE: The amniotic fluid index in normal human pregnancy. Am J Obstet Gynecol 162:1168, 1990.

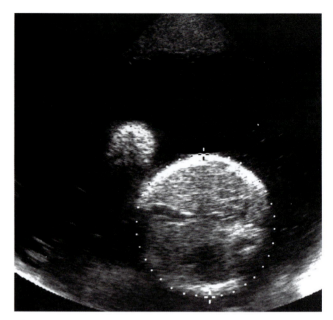

Figure 7-2. Polyhydramnios. Sector scan through the gravid uterus at 18 menstrual weeks' gestation demonstrating an excessive amount of amniotic fluid completely surrounding the fetal abdomen.

Amniotic Fluid Abnormalities

Polyhydramnios

Polyhydramnios (Figure 7-2) is commonly defined as an AFI of 20 cm or greater. It is commonly caused by conditions that result in increased urinary or respiratory fluid production or conditions that result in decreased fetal swallowing. Common causes of polyhydramnios include:

- Idiopathic causes, which may be related to:
  - Fetal swallowing abnormalities
  - Fetal renal insufficiency
  - Gastrointestinal tract absorption abnormalities
- Fetal anomalies:
  - Fetal neural tube defects
  - Fetal gastrointestinal obstructive anomalies
  - Fetal hydrops
  - Trisomy 18 (Edwards syndrome)
  - Cystic hygromas
- Placental abnormalities
- Intrauterine infection
- Maternal diabetes mellitus
- Twin-to-twin transfusion syndrome

percentiles, a progressive increase in the AFI is noted until approximately 28 menstrual weeks (Table 7-1). After that, the AFI slowly decreases.

- After 30 menstrual weeks, the normal AFI generally falls between 10 and 20 cm at the 50th percentile (AFI varies at higher and lower percentiles).
- An AFI ≤ 5 cm is consistent with oligohydramnios.
- An AFI ≥ 20 cm is consistent with polyhydramnios.[1,2]

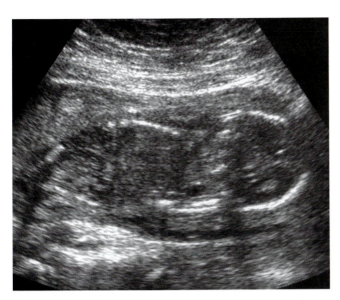

Figure 7-3. Severe oligohydramnios. This scan through the long axis at 24 menstrual weeks' gestation demonstrates a severely growth-restricted fetus with no evidence of amniotic fluid in the uterine cavity. (The complete absence of amniotic fluid is anhydramnios.)

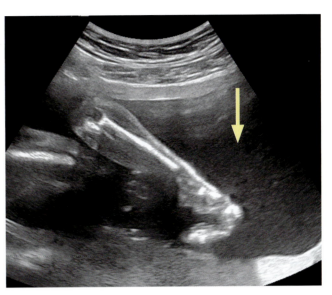

Figure 7-4. Echogenic amniotic fluid (arrow) in a normal fetus at 22 menstrual weeks' gestation.

Oligohydramnios

A number of different definitions of *oligohydramnios* have been proposed, including total amniotic fluid volume less than 300–500 ml, a maximum vertical pocket less than 2 cm, or an amniotic fluid index less than 5 cm (Figure 7-3).[1,2] In the third trimester oligohydramnios carries with it a perinatal mortality rate 40–50 times greater than that of normal pregnancies. *Anhydramnios* is the complete absence of amniotic fluid.

Common causes of oligohydramnios are many and include:

- Pregnancy-related causes:
  - Premature rupture of membranes
  - Post-term pregnancy
  - Intrauterine infection
  - Placental insufficiency or abruption
- Fetal genitourinary anomalies:
  - Renal atresia
  - Bilateral renal anomalies
  - Bladder outlet obstruction
  - Posterior urethral valves
- Fetal chromosomal abnormalities
- Intrauterine growth restriction (IUGR)
- Pharmaceutical causes
- Idiopathic causes

Echogenic Amniotic Fluid

Normal amniotic fluid is anechoic during the first trimester. Presence of diffuse low-level echoes within the fluid, frequently seen swirling as the fetus or mother moves, may represent vernix (desquamated fetal epithelial cells), blood, or meconium. Before 15 menstrual weeks this appearance is most commonly created by blood; after that, vernix. After 15 weeks, in the second and third trimesters, amniotic fluid becomes more echogenic as desquamation of fetal epithelial cells increases (Figure 7-4). Markedly hyperechoic fluid is rare but may represent intra-amniotic hemorrhage, particularly in a patient with a coagulation disorder.

Fetal Pulmonic Maturity Studies

Maturity of the fetal lungs is an important clinical consideration when managing a patient in preterm labor or who may need surgical intervention prior to term. The standard method of establishing fetal lung maturity is through the use of biochemical tests, which measure substances in the amniotic fluid that are produced by the fetal lung. The following laboratory tests can be performed on fluid obtained by amniocentesis:

- *Lecithin/sphingomyelin ratio* (L/S ratio) is the most accurate measure of fetal lung maturity. A ratio greater than 2:1 indicates that postnatal respiratory distress syndrome (RDS) will be unlikely.

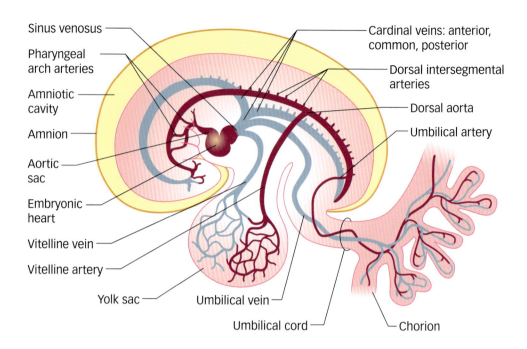

Figure 7-5. The human cardiovascular system at 6 menstrual (4 conceptual) weeks. Reprinted with permission from Moore KL, Persaud TVN, Torchia MG: *The Developing Human: Clinically Oriented Embryology*, 9th edition. Philadelphia, Elsevier Saunders, 2013, p 291. (Re-rendered for this publication.)

- *Phosphatidylglycerol* (PG) appears at about the time of lung maturity (35 menstrual weeks). If phosphatidylglycerol is identified in amniotic fluid, it is unlikely that the fetus will develop respiratory distress after delivery.
- *Surfactant-protein A* (SP-A) measures the level of a protein synthesized primarily in the alveoli of the lung and excreted into amniotic fluid. Diminished levels are associated with neonatal respiratory distress.

HEART DEVELOPMENT AND ANATOMY

EMBRYOLOGY

The cardiovascular system begins its nonstop supporting role in the life of a human organism when the primitive circulatory system, powered by a single-chambered tube, begins to beat at 22 days after conception. By the beginning of the 6th menstrual week, the bulbous, hollow cardiovascular channel has already established vascular communication with the maternal circulation in the chorion and with the main embryonic circulation via the cardinal veins and intersegmental arteries (Figure 7-5).

The drumstick-shaped *truncus arteriosus*, sitting craniad to the bilobed *bulbus cordis*, partitions into the great arteries—the *aorta* and the *pulmonary trunk*—by the end of the 7th menstrual week (Figure 7-6). Ridges of tissue arise along the walls of the bulbus cordis and, over several days, spiral into the *aorticopulmonary septum*, which partitions the aorta and pulmonary trunk. Interference with this embryonic partitioning mechanism will result in a congenital conotruncal cardiovascular anomaly, as described on pages 176–180.

Partitioning of the primordial heart begins around the middle of the 6th and is complete by the end of the 7th menstrual week (Figure 7-7). The membranous *septum primum* grows from the roof of the single atrial chamber toward the centrally located *endocardial cushions* (plugs of cardiac mesenchymal tissue). The septum secundum also grows adjacent to the septum primum and together they form the embryonic atrial septum. This septum partitions the right and left atria, leaving a gap that will ultimately become the *foramen ovale*. In the single lower chamber, the primordial *interventricular septum* arising from the apex grows upward to separate right and left ventricles, leaving an *interventricular foramen* that permits cross-circulation until the end of the 9th menstrual week.

In the central portion of the primordial heart, endocardial cushions grow outward and upward, fusing with the septum primum descending from above and with the interventricular septum arising from below to form the complex, valve-containing atrioventricular partitions.

Embryologic development of the fetal heart can be summarized as follows:

- *Cardiovascular tube formation*, menstrual weeks 4.1–4.6: A linear tube forms and begins beating as soon as it is formed.

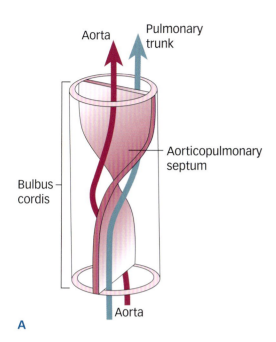

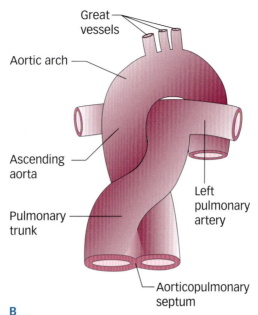

Figure 7-6. Embryologic origin of **A** the truncus arteriosus, which develops into **B** the great vessels. Ridges of tissue arise along the walls of the bulbus cordis and, over several days, spiral into the *aorticopulmonary septum*, which partitions the aorta and pulmonary trunk. Reprinted with permission from Moore KL, Persaud TVN, Torchia MG: *The Developing Human: Clinically Oriented Embryology*, 9th edition. Philadelphia, Elsevier Saunders, 2013, p 311. (Re-rendered for this publication.)

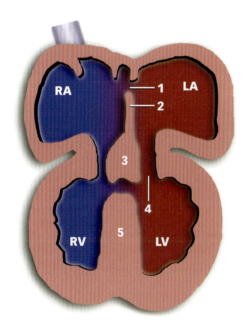

Figure 7-7. Chamber partitioning. Endocardial cushions grow outward and upward, fusing with the septum primum descending from above and with the interventricular septum arising from below to form the complex, valve-containing atrioventricular partitions. 1 = foramen ovale, 2 = septum primum, 3 = endocardial cushions, 4 = interventricular foramen, 5 = interventricular septum, RA = right atrium, LA = left atrium, RV = right ventricle, LV = left ventricle.

- *Looping*, menstrual weeks 5–6: The linear tube bends into asymmetric right and left sides; distinct chambers begin to form.
- *Atrial septation*, menstrual weeks 6.8–9: The atria separate (septate) by the septum primum and septum secundum; endocardial cushions form.
- *Outflow tract* separation, menstrual weeks 7–10: The single outflow tract, or truncus arteriosus, begins to develop into the aorta and pulmonary artery.
- *Ventricular septation*, menstrual weeks 7.4–8.6: The two ventricular chambers are formed by the growth of the interventricular septum. Embryologic development of the heart is complete by approximately 9 menstrual weeks.

FETAL HEART ANATOMY AND CARDIOVASCULAR CIRCULATION

By 11 menstrual weeks' gestation, the primitive embryonic heart has evolved into a four-chambered pump that receives blood through a venous inflow system, ejects blood via an arterial outflow system, and regulates flow within its chambers with a series of valves and temporary communication channels that seal off after birth.

As in postnatal cardiac circulation, blood enters both sides of the heart by way of large venous structures that empty into the atria. On the right side, the *superior* and *inferior venae cavae* empty into the *right atrium*. Blood is pumped past the *tricuspid valve* into the *right ventricle* during diastole and out into the lungs across the *pulmonic valve* via the *pulmonary arteries* during systole. After circuiting through the pulmonary microvasculature, blood returns to the *left atrium* via the *pulmonary vein*. Crossing the *mitral valve* during systole, blood fills the *left ventricle* and is pumped across the *aortic valve* into the systemic circulation during systole.

Fetal cardiovascular circulation (Figure 7-8), however, begins at the placenta. As the gaseous physiologic exchange performed in prenatal lungs is carried out by the placenta, fetal cardiovascular circulation shunts a large volume of blood away from the nonfunction-ing lungs and directly into the systemic circulation. Oxygenated blood from the fetal side of placental circulation travels through the single *umbilical vein*, which pierces the fetal abdominal wall, courses upward to the undersurface of the liver, and is directed through and around the liver via the *ductus venosus* and *portal sinus*. The portal sinus directs blood into the

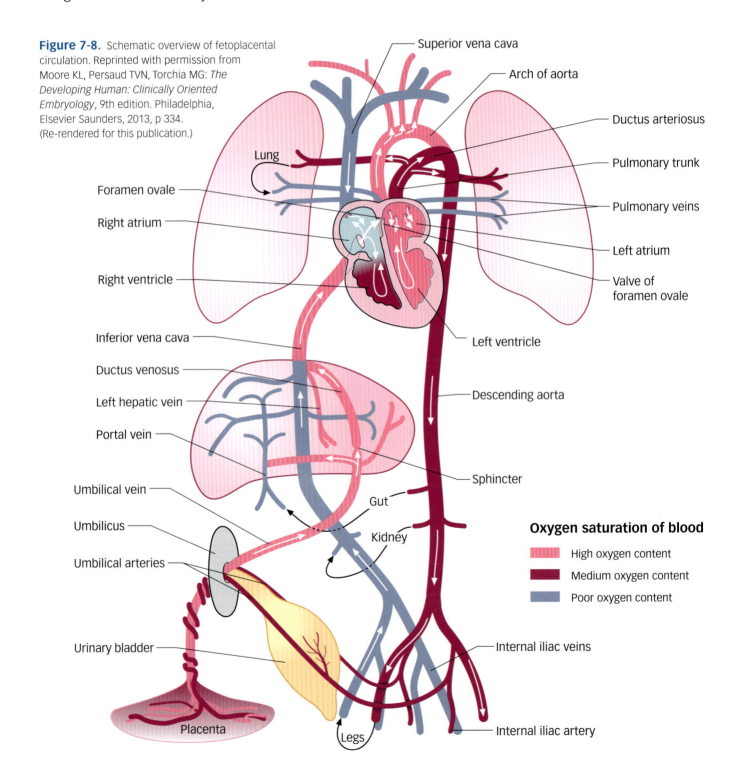

Figure 7-8. Schematic overview of fetoplacental circulation. Reprinted with permission from Moore KL, Persaud TVN, Torchia MG: *The Developing Human: Clinically Oriented Embryology*, 9th edition. Philadelphia, Elsevier Saunders, 2013, p 334. (Re-rendered for this publication.)

liver, where it enters the hepatic microcirculation and ultimately empties into the inferior vena cava via the three hepatic veins. Blood circuiting through the ductus venosus, however, bypasses the liver and empties directly into the inferior vena cava.

Several anatomic features of the right side of the fetal heart shunt blood away from the pulmonary and directly into the systemic circulation. In the right atrium, the *eustachian valve* and the *crista dividens* channel blood toward the *foramen ovale*, which redirects it to the left atrium, away from the right. This is the first shunting of blood away from the lungs. Of the blood volume that does enter the right ventricle, most of it is directed to the systemic circulation via the *ductus arteriosus*—a communication between the *main pulmonary artery* and the *aortic arch*. This is the second shunting of blood away from the lungs. During a normal transition from fetal to neonatal cardiovascular circulation, both the foramen ovale and the ductus arteriosus close and seal within the first 24 hours after birth. Blood flow through the fetal heart is proportioned as follows:

- 40% right atrial blood → foramen ovale → left atrium → systemic
- 60% right atrial blood → right ventricle; of this 60%, right ventricular output is as follows:
  - 92% → main pulmonary artery → ductus arteriosus → systemic
  - 8% → right ventricular blood → pulmonary artery → lungs

SONOGRAPHIC ANATOMY

Sonographic visualization of the major anatomic structures of the fetal chest can usually be carried out by 16 menstrual weeks. A complete sonographic evaluation of the fetal chest includes the following:

- Assessment of the integrity and symmetry of bony elements of the thorax
- Assessment of chest size in relationship to the fetus in general and the fetal abdomen in particular
- Assessment of the lungs
- Identification of the presence and integrity of the diaphragm
- Assessment of the great vessels
- Evaluation of the fetal heart

BONY THORAX

Axial and coronal sections demonstrate integrity of the thorax, fetal breathing movements, and overall size and shape of these structures (Figures 7-9A and B). During the second and third trimesters, bony elements of the thorax that should be visualized during a real-time anatomic survey include the following:

- Clavicles
- Ribs
- Scapulae
- Vertebral bodies

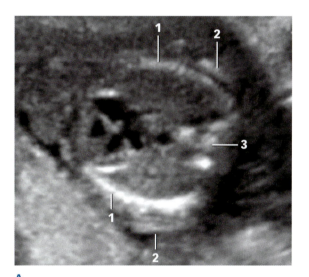

A

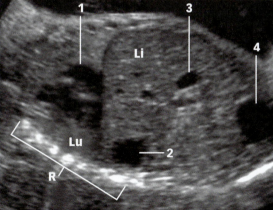

B

Figure 7-9. Sonographic demonstration of the essential elements of the bony thorax. **A** Axial section through the chest of a fetus at 16 menstrual weeks. 1 = ribs, 2 = scapulae, 3 = vertebra. **B** Coronal section through a different fetus (also 16 weeks) demonstrating the normal thoracoabdominal contour. 1 = heart, 2 = stomach, 3 = gallbladder, 4 = urinary bladder, Li = liver, Lu = lung, R = ribs.

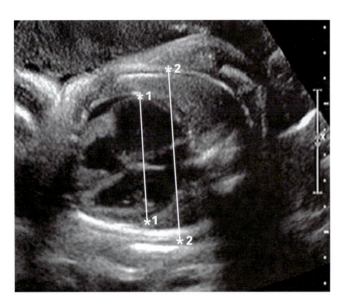

Figure 7-10. Axial section through a fetal chest in which the heart occupies more than one-third of the thoracic space, demonstrating cardiomegaly. 1 = transcardiac diameter, 2 = transthoracic diameter.

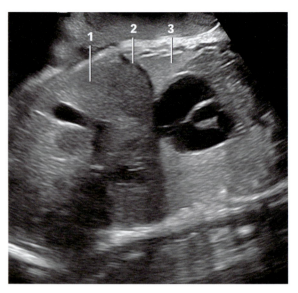

Figure 7-11. Coronal section through a fetus at 20 menstrual weeks demonstrating the normal comparative variation of pulmonary and hepatic echogenicity. 1 = liver, 2 = diaphragm, 3 = lung.

CHEST SIZE

The circumference of the fetal chest is an indirect indicator of the normality of its contents, specifically the size of the heart and lungs. An axial section obtained just above the level of the diaphragm should demonstrate the heart occupying approximately one-third of the thoracic cavity, with the lungs filling the remaining space. Deviations from this relationship raise the concern that abnormalities may be present in the lungs, such as pulmonary hypoplasia, or in the heart, such as cardiomegaly (Figure 7-10).

LUNGS

The fetal lungs appear as solid, homogeneously echogenic structures, filling the thoracic space between the centrally positioned heart and the peripherally encompassing rib cage. Pulmonary parenchyma is normally slightly more echogenic than adjacent abdominal parenchymal viscera, such as the parenchyma of the spleen and liver. A coronal section (Figure 7-11) demonstrates the relationship of pulmonary parenchyma separated from the abdominal viscera by the hypoechoic, curvilinear hemidiaphragms.

The lungs are visualized from the late first trimester onward and early on are defined by adjacent structures: the ribs superolaterally and the heart medially. In the normal chest, the fetal heart should occupy approximately one-third of the thoracic volume on transverse images. Typically, the right lung is slightly larger than the left because of the left-sided cardiac apex. Normally, the right atrium and a portion of the left atrium lie to the right of midline. In the sagittal plane, the diaphragm can be visualized, with adjacent stomach, spleen, and liver below the diaphragm.

The echogenicity of the lungs should be homogeneous and of medium level. The lung and liver are initially equal in echogenicity, but as pregnancy progresses the lung becomes slightly more echogenic than the liver.

DIAPHRAGM

The fetal *diaphragm* is the muscular structure that forms the inferior border of the thoracic cavity. By the beginning of the second trimester, the diaphragm is best demonstrated sonographically in a coronal plane of section (see Figure 7-11) as a curvilinear, hypoechoic crescent partitioning the thoracic and abdominal cavities. It is a useful landmark in assessing the integrity and correct location of the thoracoabdominal viscera, an important consideration when assessing for diaphragmatic hernia.

GREAT VESSELS

The *great vessels* of the fetal thorax include the *superior vena cava*, the *ascending and descending thoracic aorta*, the *pulmonary artery*, and the *ductus arteriosus* (coursing from the pulmonary artery to the descending

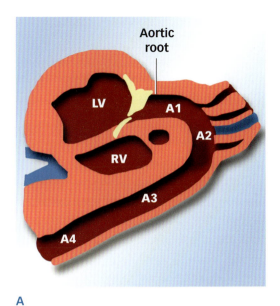
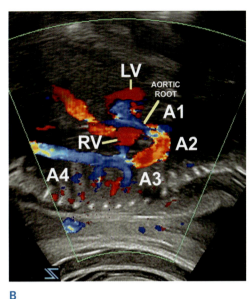

Figure 7-12. Sagittal section through the aortic arch demonstrating its main thoracic segments. **A** Schematic. **B** Sonogram. A1 = ascending aorta, A2 = aortic arch, A3 = descending aorta, A4 = thoracic aorta, LV = left ventricle, RV = right ventricle. (The blue vessel in the schematic is the internal jugular vein, not visible in the accompanying sonogram.)

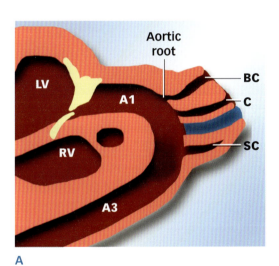
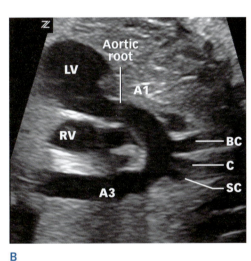

Figure 7-13. Sagittal close-up section through the aortic arch demonstrating the major vessels arising from it. **A** Schematic. **B** Sonogram. LV = left ventricle, RV = right ventricle, A1 = ascending aorta, A3 = descending aorta, BC = brachiocephalic artery, C = left common carotid artery, SC = left subclavian artery. (The blue vessel in the schematic is the internal jugular vein, not visible in the accompanying sonogram.)

thoracic aorta). These vessels can be visualized as early as 14 menstrual weeks in an axial view through the upper mediastinum. At the same gestational age, a sagittal plane can demonstrate the segments of the aortic arch (Figures 7-12A and B) and the vessels arising from it (Figures 7-13A and B)—including the *brachiocephalic* (also called the *innominate*), *left common carotid*, and *left subclavian arteries*. The *common carotid arteries* and *jugular veins* are also commonly seen in the neck of an older fetus.

Concomitant with fetal lung development is the development of associated pulmonary vasculature. The *pulmonary arteries* arise from six different developmental configurations of embryonic aortic arches. These primitive vascular structures, which develop at different times during early gestation, give rise to the fetal aortic arch and all of its branches and to pulmonary arterial vasculature. The *pulmonary veins* develop as an outgrowth of the dorsal atrial wall.

HEART

The fetal heart can be most clearly imaged if the fetus is in a supine position within the uterus. If the fetus is lying on its side, the heart can still be imaged fairly well through the ribs. If the fetus is lying in the spine-up position, however, imaging cardiac structures is much more difficult. To define the cardiac position and situs, the sonographer must determine the position of the fetus in the uterus (i.e., the fetal lie; see Chapter 12, pages 330–331) and must establish fetal laterality independent of the position of fetal internal organs. A complete cardiac evaluation includes examining the fetal heart in its entirety—its chambers, valves, and connections to the great vessels.

Three main cardiac segments are assessed during the course of a routine sonographic examination of the fetal heart:

- The *visceroatrial situs*, which is important in localization and lateralization of the atrium
- The *ventricular loop*, which is important in diagnosing the relation of the ventricles to each atrium
- The *truncus arteriosus*, which is important for determining the relation between the great arteries and the ventricles

The four valves of the heart that can be routinely visualized sonographically are the following:

- *Tricuspid valve*: located between the right atrium and the right ventricle
- *Pulmonic valve*: located between the right ventricle and the pulmonary artery
- *Mitral (bicuspid) valve*: located between the left atrium and the left ventricle
- *Aortic valve*: located between the left ventricle and the aorta

Four-Chamber View

The *four-chamber view* (Figure 7-14A) is the single most important view of the fetal heart and should be obtained during the course of every routine sonographic examination of a fetus. A large proportion of cardiovascular anatomic abnormalities can be detected on this single image. While additional views are often necessary to evaluate and diagnose a particular abnormality completely, variations seen in the four-chamber view can direct the examiner to the additional echocardiographic information that should be obtained.

The four cardiac chambers can be identified by their unique sonographic characteristics:

- The *right atrium* may be identified when scanning in different anatomic planes and noting the hepatic veins, inferior vena cava, and superior vena cava draining into that structure. The flap of the foramen ovale is noted opening from the right atrium into the left atrium.
- The *left atrium* is posterior in location in comparison to the right atrium, with the foramen ovale opening into this chamber. The position of the spine is noted, with the left atrium lying close to the vertebral column.
- The *right ventricle* is retrosternal in location, with the tricuspid valve lower in position within the right ventricle than the mitral valve is within the left ventricle. There is also a large echogenic structure lying within the apex of the right ventricle, the *muscular moderator band*. The right ventricle lies retrosternal in location.
- The *left ventricle* can be identified by the presence of papillary muscles within the chamber. Echogenic foci may be identified within the left ventricle. These are thought to be attachments of the papillary muscles and are not abnormal. The mitral valve is in a higher location within the left ventricle than the tricuspid is within the right ventricle. The apex of the heart and the interventricular septum are just cephalad to the

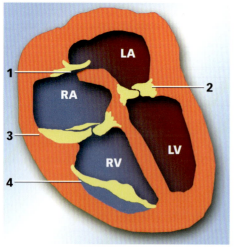

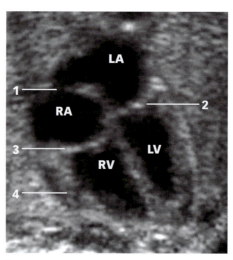

Figure 7-14. Four-chamber view of the fetal heart demonstrating the major anatomic landmarks. **A** Schematic. **B** Sonogram. LV = left ventricle, RV = right ventricle, LA = left atrium, RA = right atrium, 1 = foramen ovale, 2 = mitral valve, 3 = tricuspid valve, 4 = moderator band.

fetal stomach. The left ventricle is smooth-walled. Chordae tendineae may sometimes be imaged extending from the ventricular wall to the edges of the atrioventricular valves.

Anatomic Structures Visualized in the Four-Chamber View

The following are visualized in a normal four-chamber view (Figure 7-14B):

- The heart is seen located within the left side of the chest.
- The heart should occupy about one-third of the fetal thorax.
- The apex of the heart points approximately 45° to the left of the anterior chest wall.
- The ventricles are approximately the same size (although the right is larger than the left later in pregnancy).
- The flap of the foramen ovale opens into the left atrium.
- Prominent moderator bands are present in the apex of the right ventricle.
- Valves separate both atria from the ventricles.

Conditions Visualized in the Four-Chamber View

The following conditions are some of the more common and sonographically recognizable in the four-chamber view:

- Atrioventricular canal defect
- Single ventricle
- Ebstein's anomaly
- Hypertrophied or dilated ventricles
- Ventricular hypoplasia
- Tricuspid or mitral valve atresia
- Cardiomyopathy
- Ventricular septal defect
- Atrial septal defect
- Endocardial cushion defect
- Aortic/pulmonary stenosis
- Arrhythmias
- Masses

Left Ventricular Outflow Tract View

The relation of the aorta to the left ventricle is best evaluated using the left ventricular long-axis view of the fetal heart, which is most commonly called the left ventricular outflow tract (LVOT) view. This LVOT view (Figure 7-15A) is obtained by rotating the transducer from the four-chamber view into a plane angled from the fetal stomach toward the right shoulder of the fetus. The LVOT view is helpful in evaluating the anatomic relationship between the ascending aorta and the left ventricle.

Anatomic Structures Visualized in the LVOT View

The following are visualized with the long-axis view of the fetal heart (Figure 7-15B):

- Aortic and left ventricular continuity
- Left atrium
- Aortic root
- Ventricular septum

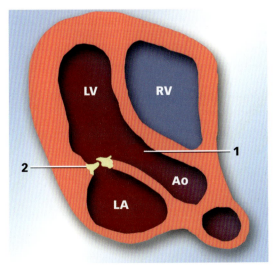

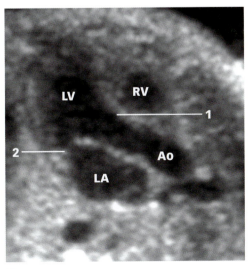

Figure 7-15. Long-axis view of the fetal heart demonstrating the left ventricular outflow tract (LVOT) and the major anatomic landmarks. **A** Schematic. **B** Sonogram. LV = left ventricle, RV = right ventricle, LA = left atrium, Ao = aorta, 1 = aortic root, 2 = mitral valve.

A   B

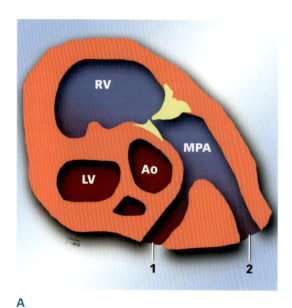
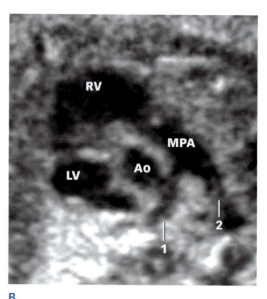

Figure 7-16. Right ventricular outflow tract (RVOT) view of the fetal heart. **A** Schematic. **B** Sonogram. RV = right ventricle, LV = left ventricle, Ao = aorta, MPA = main pulmonary artery, 1 = left pulmonary artery, 2 = right pulmonary artery.

Right Ventricular Outflow Tract View

The *pulmonary outflow tract* or *right ventricular outflow tract* (RVOT) view (Figure 7-16A) demonstrates the main pulmonary artery exiting the right ventricle and crossing over the ascending aorta. This crisscross relation is the result of normal rotation of the great vessels early in cardiogenesis. If the pulmonary artery and aorta are parallel rather than forming this crisscross, there is a rotational abnormality of the great vessels, most commonly transposition of the great vessels.

Anatomic Structures Visualized in the RVOT View

The following are visualized with the right ventricular outflow tract view (Figure 7-16B):

- Pulmonary artery in long axis arising anteriorly in an axial section through the ascending aorta
- Pulmonic valve separating the right ventricle from the main pulmonary artery
- Right ventricle

Conditions Visualized in Outflow Tract Views

The following are some of the more common ventricular loop and truncus abnormalities demonstrable sonographically with both the left and right ventricular outflow tract views:

- Transposition of the great vessels
- Tetralogy of Fallot
- Double-outlet right ventricle
- Pulmonary stenosis

Apical Five-Chamber View

An apical five-chamber view (Figure 7-17A) is obtained cephalad to the routine four-chamber view in the same transverse plane. It is a useful adjunct to the four-chamber view in assessing the integrity of the cardiac chambers and septa and left ventricular outflow tract. It demonstrates the mitral valve, interventricular septum anterior to the mitral valve, anterior wall of the ventricular septum as it joins the anterior wall of the aortic outflow tract, and right and left atrial chambers. Short-axis views may also be obtained at the level of the ventricular chambers.

Anatomic Structures Visualized in the Apical Five-Chamber View

The following are visualized with the apical five-chamber view of the fetal heart (Figure 7-17B):

- Both ventricles and the interventricular septum
- Both atria and the interatrial septum
- Aortic root and left ventricular outflow tract

Conditions Visualized in the Apical Five-Chamber View

The following are some of the more common cardiac abnormalities demonstrable sonographically with the apical five-chamber view:

- Anomalies demonstrable on a four-chamber view, most of which can be identified on the five-chamber view as well (see pages 162–163)
- Transposition of the great vessels

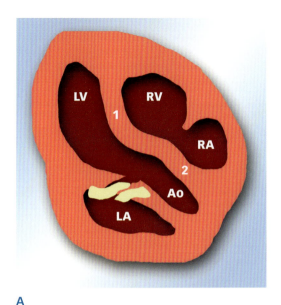
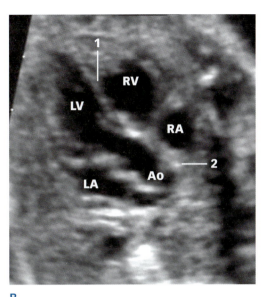

Figure 7-17. Apical five-chamber view of the fetal heart demonstrating major anatomic landmarks. **A** Schematic. **B** Sonogram. LV = left ven-tricle, RV = right ventricle, LA = left atrium, RA = right atrium, Ao = aorta, 1 = interventricular septum, 2 = interatrial septum.

Fetal Echocardiography

Fetal echocardiography is a comprehensive ultrasound evaluation of the prenatal heart that, when indicated, is typically performed between 18 and 22 menstrual weeks of gestation. While most routine screening sonograms carried out during the second trimester include imaging of the overall size, shape, and configuration of the cardiac chambers, outflow tracts, and great vessels, fetal echocardiography is a more specialized dynamic study. It is typically performed by sonographers and physicians specifically trained to do so.

In addition to the standard views obtained during a screening sonogram, still images and real-time clips of the inflow tracts, cardiac valves, myocardium, great vessels, and their connections to respective chambers are acquired. Using B-mode, color Doppler imaging, pulsed Doppler interrogation, and M-mode tracing, the examiner conducts cardiac biometry and assessment of cardiac function. (See the AIUM practice guidelines in Appendix C on the performance of fetal echocardiography.)

Indications for Fetal Echocardiography

Echocardiographic studies are not included in the course of routine sonographic examination. Indications for fetal echocardiography include the following:[3,4,5]

- Situs inversus
- Asplenia
- Dextrocardia
- Enlarged heart
- Sustained cardiac arrhythmia
- Increased nuchal translucency diameter in pregnancy
- Fetus that is small for gestational age
- Extracardiac abnormalities
- Two-vessel umbilical cord
- Osteogenesis imperfecta
- Other abnormal findings in the fetal heart

CHEST ABNORMALITIES

Anomalies affecting the fetal chest can be divided into two categories: those affecting the thoracic cavity and lungs and those affecting the heart and great vessels (Table 7-2). Thoracic and pulmonary abnormalities are typically significant enough to be detected during the course of a routine obstetric sonographic examination of fetal anatomy. Cardiovascular anomalies, on the other hand—particularly subtle ones—require a complete fetal echocardiographic examination by an individual trained in performing a detailed assessment of the heart and great vessels.

THORACIC AND PULMONARY ABNORMALITIES

The primary thoracic and pulmonary abnormalities demonstrable during a complete obstetric sonogram include almost all that are incompatible with life and several that may change the management of the

Table 7-2. Summary of fetal thoracic abnormalities.

Type of Abnormality	Anomaly
Thoracic and pulmonary	Pulmonary hypoplasia
	Pleural effusion
	Pulmonary sequestration
	Congenital diaphragmatic hernia (CDH)
	Cystic adenomatoid malformation of the lung (CAML)
	Tracheal atresia
	Chest masses
Heart and great vessels	Septal defects
	Conotruncal anomalies
	Single ventricle anomalies
	Disproportionate ventricular size
	Positional abnormalities
	Cardiac wall abnormalities
	Heart rate/rhythm abnormalities

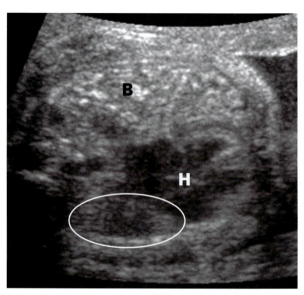

Figure 7-18. Pulmonary hypoplasia in a diaphragmatic hernia. Axial section through the fetal thorax. H = heart, B = bowel, circled = hypoplastic lung.

pregnancy. These anomalies include pulmonary hypoplasia, pulmonary sequestration, diaphragmatic hernia, cystic adenomatoid malformation of the lung, tracheal atresia, and chest masses. Pleural effusion, which is frequently an indicator of concomitant structural anomalies or physiologic complications, is also detectable during the routine examination of the fetal chest as described above.

Pulmonary Hypoplasia

Pulmonary hypoplasia is a condition characterized by deficient or incomplete development of the lungs. Typically the trachea and bronchial apparatuses are present but the alveolar beds are incompletely formed and atrophic. Pulmonary hypoplasia is most commonly a sequela to an inadequacy of one or more of the four conditions necessary for normal lung development outlined on page 153, but it may also be caused by genetic factors and other extra- and intrathoracic fetal anatomic abnormalities. In general, a fetus that has a thoracic circumference smaller than the 5th percentile is likely to experience respiratory distress, which can be lethal. If the chest is (by subjective criteria) visibly small compared with the abdomen and if there is a sharp change in diameter of the anterior/posterior dimension from the chest to the abdomen, the possibility of pulmonary hypoplasia should be considered.

Associated Abnormalities

The following conditions reduce the thoracic cavity space necessary for normal lung expansion and growth and commonly result in pulmonary hypoplasia:

- Diaphragmatic hernia (Figure 7-18)
- Sequestration of the lung
- Agenesis of the diaphragm
- Intrathoracic masses
- Thanatophoric lung (Figure 7-19)

Sonographic Signs

The following are the characteristic sonographic signs of pulmonary hypoplasia:

- Reduced chest-to-head ratio (<1 is associated with a poor outcome).
- Reduced thoracic circumference.
- Oligohydramnios is a frequently associated finding.

Pleural Effusion

Pleural effusion, also called *hydrothorax*, is a collection of fluid in the pleural cavity. Its causes are many and its pathophysiology is varied. In the fetus, it is a nonspecific finding that may represent a *chylothorax*, a primary type of pleural effusion caused by lymphatic leakage or a

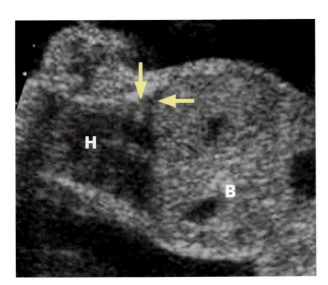
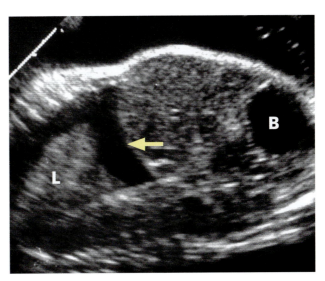

Figure 7-19. Pulmonary hypoplasia in thanatophoric dysplasia. Coronal section through the fetal chest and abdomen. H = heart, B = hyperechogenic bowel, arrows = hypoplastic lung.

Figure 7-20. Pleural effusion in hydrops fetalis. Sagittal section through the fetal chest and abdomen demonstrating fluid surrounding the lung. L = lung, B = bladder, arrow = pleural fluid.

secondary effusion related to various causes of hydrops fetalis (fetal hydrops). While fetal hydrops, with its myriad etiologies, is the most common cause of pleural effusion in the fetus, other causes include the following:

- Congenital cardiac anomalies
- Congenital lung anomalies:
  - Airway malformations
  - Bronchopulmonary sequestration
  - Diaphragmatic hernia
- Chromosomal abnormalities:
  - Trisomy 21 (Down syndrome)
  - Trisomy 18 (Edwards syndrome)
  - Turner syndrome

Sonographic Signs

The following are the characteristic sonographic signs of pleural effusion:

- Anechoic fluid surrounding the lung and conforming to the shape of the pleural cavity (Figure 7-20).
- May be unilateral or bilateral.

Pulmonary Sequestration

Pulmonary sequestration is an anomalous condition characterized by an accessory fragment of lung that has no connection to the tracheobronchial tree and that maintains its own, separate arterial circulation. There are two distinct types of sequestration based on the relationship that the aberrant bit of lung has to the pleura and its venous drainage.

Intralobar sequestration is the most common type, accounting for almost 85% of cases.[6] Venous drainage typically occurs via the pulmonary veins but there may be drainage into the hemiazygos system, portal vein, or inferior vena cava. The sequestered segment is closely connected to adjacent normal lung and there is no separate pleura associated with it.

Extralobar sequestration is less common, with venous drainage through the systemic veins into the right atrium. The sequestered segment of lung is separated from adjacent lung and is surrounded by its own individual pleura. It is supplied by an arterial branch arising directly from the aorta, not from the pulmonary artery. Color and spectral Doppler are extremely helpful in establishing a diagnosis of extralobar sequestration by identifying a separate vessel arising from the aorta and supplying the echogenic mass of tissue.

Rarely, "pulmonary" sequestrations are found in the abdomen rather than the chest; approximately 10%–15% of extralobar sequestrations are found below the diaphragm and appear as brightly echogenic masses within the abdomen.

Associated Abnormalities

The following abnormalities are characteristically associated with pulmonary sequestration:

- Congenital diaphragmatic hernia
- Diaphragmatic eventration
- Congenital heart disease

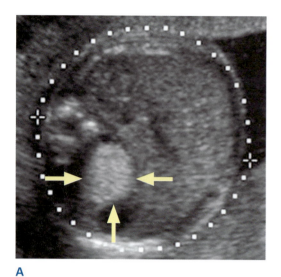

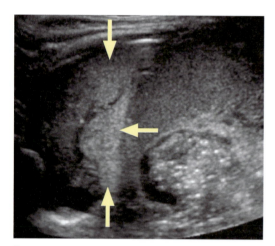

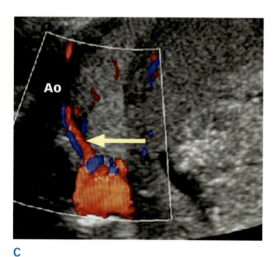

Figure 7-21. Sonographic findings for pulmonary sequestration. **A** Axial section through the fetal thorax demonstrates a well-marginated, hyperechoic solid mass (arrows) in the lower lobe of the left lung. **B** Coronal section through the chest and upper abdomen demonstrates an echogenic sequestered lobe in the right lung (arrows). **C** Color Doppler imaging in the same fetus shows the feed vessel (arrow) originating from the thoracic aorta (Ao).

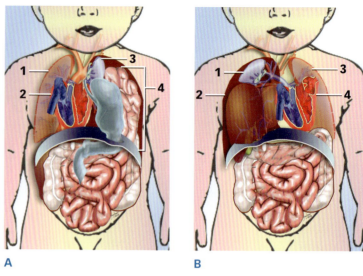

Figure 7-22. Schematic demonstration of the two common types of diaphragmatic hernia. **A** Posterior, left-sided (Bochdalek) type. 1 = right lung, 2 = displaced heart, 3 = hypoplastic left lung, 4 = herniated viscera. **B** Anterior, right-sided (Morgagni) type. 1 = hypoplastic right lung, 2 = liver, 3 = left lung, 4 = displaced heart.

Sonographic Signs

The following are the characteristic sonographic signs of pulmonary sequestration:

- Well-defined, solid echogenic mass adjacent to a normal-appearing lung (Figures 7-21A and B)
- Identification of a feed vessel originating from the aorta with color Doppler imaging (Figure 7-21C)
- Possible sonographic signs of hydrops (may or may not be present)

Congenital Diaphragmatic Hernia

Congenital diaphragmatic hernia (CDH) is a result of incomplete fusion of the diaphragmatic structures at 6–10 menstrual weeks. The diaphragmatic defect may be either right- or left-sided, but left-sided diaphragmatic hernias are more commonly observed during ultrasound examination because of herniation of stomach, intestines, and spleen into the chest in left-sided hernia. Left-sided hernias are usually of the posterolateral (Bochdalek) variety (Figure 7-22A) and account for approximately 95% of all prenatal diaphragmatic hernias. Right-sided diaphragmatic defects are typically obstructed by the liver, although if the defect is large enough, the liver, gallbladder, and part of the gut may herniate into the thoracic cavity. Right-sided hernias are usually of the anterior (Morgagni) variety (Figure 7-22B) and are rare, accounting for approximately 2% of all congenital diaphragmatic hernias.

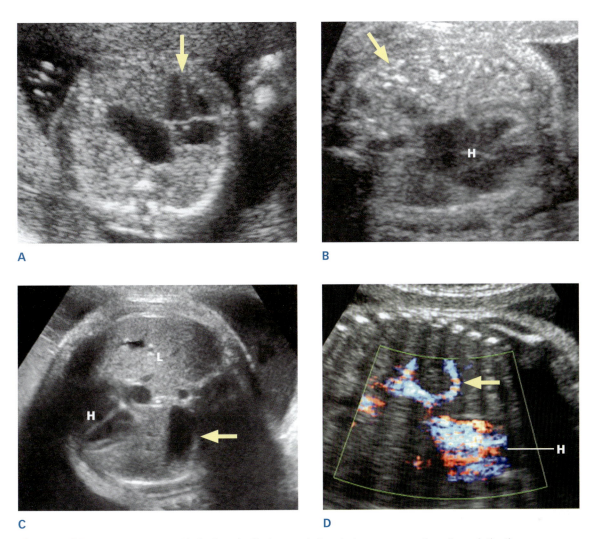

Figure 7-23. Hallmark sonographic findings in diaphragmatic hernia, transverse sections through the thorax. **A** Cardiomediastinal shift (arrow). **B** Bowel loops (arrow) at the same level of the heart (H). **C** Stomach (arrow) in the thorax; H = heart, L = liver. **D** Color Doppler image of an hepatic vein (arrow) in the thorax; H = heart.

Associated Abnormalities

The following abnormalities are characteristically associated with diaphragmatic hernia:

- Pulmonary hypoplasia
- Pulmonary sequestration
- Trisomies 13, 18, and 21
- Turner syndrome
- Neural tube defects
- Congenital cardiac anomalies

Sonographically, the most notable intrathoracic abnormality in congenital diaphragmatic hernia is displacement of the fetal heart toward the right chest wall. Typically, the cardiac apex will be angled to the left. More careful examination usually suggests either bowel or stomach in the left hemithorax. A diaphragmatic hernia can be differentiated from an intrathoracic mass by failure to visualize the diaphragm on the affected side. Typically in patients who have pulmonary sequestration or cystic adenomatoid malformation, the diaphragm will be visible below the lesion.

Sonographic Signs

The following are the characteristic sonographic signs of diaphragmatic hernia:

- Cardiomediastinal shift to the nonherniated side of the chest (Figure 7-23A)
- Stomach/bowel loops at the same level as the heart (Figures 7-23B and C)
- Hepatic veins and liver in the thorax (Figure 7-23D)
- Absent bowel loops in the abdomen
- Polyhydramnios

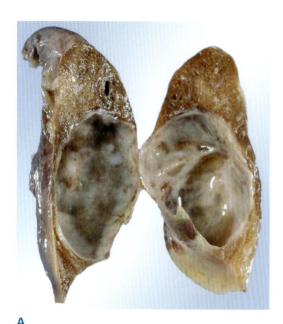
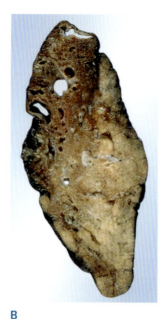

Figure 7-24. Gross pathologic specimens of cystic adenomatoid malformation of the lung (CAML). **A** Type I: large, macrocystic lesion. **B** Type II: multiple small cysts. **C** Type III: in this example, noncystic lesions that have produced a mediastinal shift.

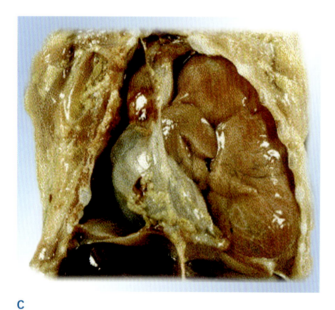

Cystic Adenomatoid Malformation of the Lung

Also called *congenital pulmonary airway malformation* (CPAM), *cystic adenomatoid malformation of the lung* (CAML) is an abnormality of lung development in which normal lung is replaced by nonfunctioning cystic tissue. It is usually unilateral and involves an entire lobe of the affected lung. The prognosis for neonates born with CAML varies widely and is dependent primarily on the extent of lung replacement with anomalous tissue. Mediastinal shift by a cystic adenomatoid malformation mass is associated with an increased likelihood of fetal demise. It is well established that many cystic adenomatoid malformation lesions become relatively smaller when compared with total lung volume as the pregnancy progresses.

Three categories of cystic adenomatoid malformation of the lung exist and are based on the size of the cysts present in the lung:

- *Type I*: macrocystic, consisting of large cysts of variable sizes, usually 2–10 cm; this is the most common type, accounting for 70% of cases (Figure 7-24A).
- *Type II*: multiple small cysts (<1.2 cm); this is a less common type, accounting for 15%–20% of cases (Figure 7-24B).
- *Type III*: microcystic (<0.5 cm) or noncystic lesions producing a mediastinal shift; this type accounts for less than 10% of cases (Figure 7-24C).

Associated Abnormalities

The following abnormalities are characteristically associated with cystic adenomatoid malformation of the lung:

- Pulmonary sequestration
- Renal agenesis

Sonographic Signs

The following are the characteristic sonographic signs of cystic adenomatoid malformation of the lung:

- *Type I*: nonvascular cystic masses in the fetal lung (Figure 7-25A)
- *Type II*: homogeneously echogenic lobe(s) (Figure 7-25B)
- *Type III*: mediastinal shift with lateral displacement of the heart (Figure 7-25C)

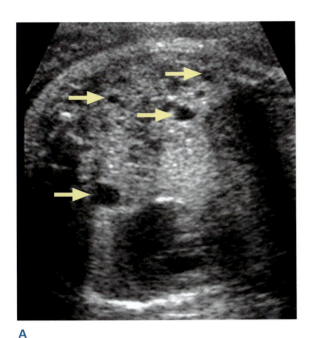
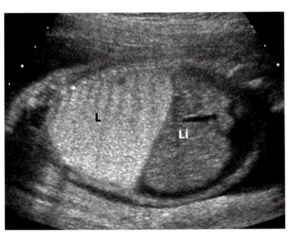
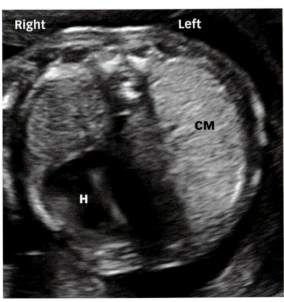

Figure 7-25. Hallmark sonographic findings in cystic adenomatoid malformation of the lung (CAML). **A** Type I: nonvascular cystic lesions in the lung (arrows). **B** Type II: homogeneously echogenic lung lobe. L = lung, Li = liver. **C** Type III: mediastinal shift with heart (H) displaced to the right by cystic mass (CM) in the left hemithorax.

Tracheal Atresia

Tracheal atresia is a rare pulmonary anomaly in which the trachea fails to form or is obliterated by external compression of the airway structures. It is a uniformly lethal condition. The level of tracheal obstruction is typically at the larynx.

Associated Abnormalities

The following abnormalities are characteristically associated with tracheal atresia:

- Renal anomalies
- Central nervous system malformations
- Tracheoesophageal atresia

Sonographic Signs

The following are the characteristic sonographic signs of tracheal atresia:

- Bilateral diffusely echogenic lungs
- Fluid-filled trachea (Figure 7-26)
- Enlarged lungs adjacent to a relatively small, compressed heart
- Reduced cardiothoracic circumference ratio
- Polyhydramnios

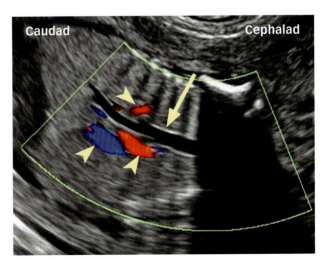

Figure 7-26. Coronal section through the fetal chest in a fetus with tracheal atresia demonstrating a fluid-filled trachea (arrow) coursing between the pulmonary vasculature (arrowheads).

Table 7-3.	Sonographic appearance of chest masses.
Appearance	Mass
Cystic	CAML type I
	Bronchogenic cyst
	Congenital diaphragmatic hernia
	Enteric cyst
	Mediastinal meningocele
	Esophageal duplication cyst
Cystic and solid	CAML type II
	Enteric cyst
	Teratoma (pericardial)
	Congenital diaphragmatic hernia
	Mixed CAML type II and sequestration
	Pulmonary sequestration
	Thoracic neuroblastoma
Solid	CAML type III
	Pulmonary sequestration
	Congenital diaphragmatic hernia

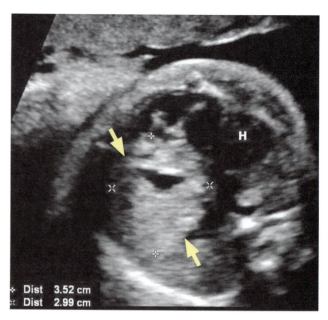

Figure 7-27. Sonographic findings in a fetus with a chest mass. Transverse section demonstrates a complex mass (arrows) in the thoracic cavity with a laterally displaced heart (H).

Chest Masses

Unilateral fetal chest masses are summarized in Table 7-3. Mediastinal masses—including teratomas, enteric cysts, and thymic masses—are rare, but because they dramatically distort the normal sonographic appearance of the fetal chest they are easily detected. However, pathologic differentiation is impossible with prenatal ultrasound.

Associated Abnormalities

The following abnormalities are characteristically associated with fetal chest masses:
- Pulmonary hypoplasia
- Congenital heart disease
- Tracheal atresia

Sonographic Signs

The following are the characteristic sonographic signs of fetal chest masses:
- Presence of a sonographically complex mass in the thoracic cavity (Figure 7-27)
- Displaced mediastinal structures
- Pleural effusions

HEART AND GREAT VESSEL ABNORMALITIES

Cardiovascular abnormalities are among the most common congenital defects. The incidence of congenital heart disease is estimated to be approximately 1 in 100 live births.[7, 8, 9, 10] Like the range of central nervous system anomalies assessed in sonographic studies, the spectrum of cardiovascular defects subject to ultrasound examination spans a breadth that is beyond the scope of a sonography review text. However, major abnormalities that are incompatible with postnatal life or that portend significant clinical sequelae are identifiable during the course of a routine obstetric sonogram.

Anomalous conditions that can be detected during a routine sonographic survey of the fetal anatomy are presented here. If cardiac abnormalities are detected on an initial obstetric examination, or if there is strong suspicion on the basis of clinical data that there is a cardiovascular problem, a complete fetal echocardiographic study should be performed as a separate procedure by those with expertise in the field.

As a means of review for sonographic practitioners, the universe of cardiac anomalies is distilled into categories consistent with how the condition may appear during the course of a routine obstetric ultrasound examination (Table 7-4): septal defects, conotruncal anomalies,

Table 7-4.	Categories of congenital cardiac abnormalities.
Category	Defect
Septal defects (VSD)	Ventricular septal defect
	Atrial septal defect (ASD)
	Atrioventricular septal defect (AVSD)
Conotruncal anomalies	Tetralogy of Fallot
	Transposition of the great arteries
	Persistent truncus arteriosus
	Double-outlet right ventricle
Single ventricle anomalies	Hypoplastic heart syndromes
	Tricuspid atresia
	Double-inlet left ventricle
Disproportionate ventricular size	Ebstein's anomaly
	Coarctation of the aorta
Positional abnormalities	Situs abnormalities
	Ectopia cordis
Cardiac wall abnormalities	Cardiomyopathy
	Cardiac tumors
	Fetal pericardial effusion
Heart rate/rhythm abnormalities	Fetal supraventricular tachycardia
	Atrial flutter
	Premature ventricular contractions
	Premature atrial contractions
	Atrioventricular block

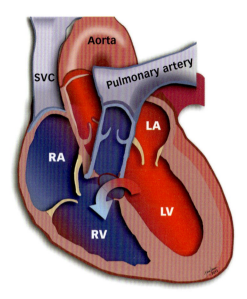

Figure 7-28. Ventricular septal defect. **A** Schematic showing a ventricular septal defect (curved arrow): an abnormal communication between the right and left ventricles though a defect in the interventricular septum, which allows shunting of blood from the left to right ventricle (curved arrow). SVC = superior vena cava, RA = right atrium, LA = left atrium, RV = right ventricle, LV = left ventricle. (Figure continues . . .)

single ventricle anomalies, disproportionate ventricles, positional abnormalities, cardiac wall abnormalities, and abnormalities of fetal heart rate and rhythm.

Septal Defects

Septal defects are structural abnormalities of the inside of the heart that allow anomalous circulatory communication between the chambers. They are some of the most common congenital cardiac abnormalities. They arise from failure of the embryologic processes that seal off cross-chamber foramina that are normal prior to 7 menstrual weeks. The persistent defects can appear between the atria, the ventricles, or a combination of the two and include the following:

- Ventricular septal defects
- Atrial septal defects
- Atrioventricular septal defects

Ventricular Septal Defects

A *ventricular septal defect* (VSD) is an abnormal communication between the right and left ventricles through a defect in the interventricular septum (Figure 7-28A). It is the most common congenital cardiac anomaly, occurring in about 1 in 400 live births.[11] A ventricular septal defect may be an isolated defect but may also be seen in association with many other cardiac anomalies.

Associated Abnormalities

The following abnormalities are characteristically associated with ventricular septal defects:

- Tetralogy of Fallot
- Truncus arteriosus
- Double-outlet right ventricle
- Aortic coarctation
- Tricuspid atresia

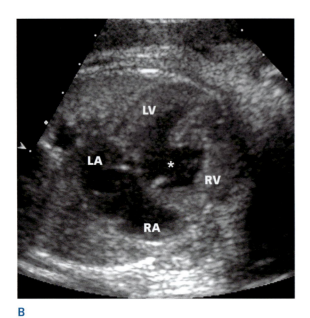 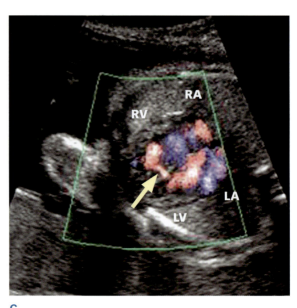

Figure 7-28, continued. B Axial image of a ventricular septal defect (*asterisked) in a 22-week fetus. **C** Color Doppler demonstration of a ventricular septal defect (arrow). RV = right ventricle, LV = left ventricle, RA = right atrium, LA = left atrium.

Sonographic Signs

The following are the characteristic sonographic signs of ventricular septal defects:

- Visualization of a defect in the interventricular septum (Figure 7-28B)
- Shunting of blood between ventricles seen with color Doppler imaging (Figure 7-28C)

Atrial Septal Defects

An *atrial septal defect* (ASD) is an abnormal communication between the right and left atria (Figure 7-29A). It is the second most common type of congenital heart anomaly after ventricular septal defects. In the fetus, there is a normal communication between the atria via the foramen ovale, making the prenatal diagnosis of an atrial septal defect a diagnostic challenge. There are three major types of atrial septal defects:[12]

- *Secundum ASD*: Usually an isolated anomaly that accounts for 60%–90% of all atrial septal defects. An ostium secundum atrial septal defect involves the fossa ovalis and is mid-septal in location. This type of atrial septal defect is a true deficiency of the interatrial septum and is distinct from the frequently identified patent foramen ovale. The shape of the defect ranges from circular to oval. Less often, strands of tissue cross the defect, creating a fenestrated appearance that suggests multiple defects.

- *Primum ASD*: Associated with other cardiac anomalies, this atrial septal defect accounts for 5%–20% of all atrial septal defects. An ostium primum atrial septal defect involves atrial and ventricular septa. Primum defects do not always involve the ventricular septum. If both the atrial and the ventricular septa are involved, the defect is called an *atrioventricular canal* or *atrioventricular septal defect* (see pages 175–176).

- *Sinus venosus*: Associated with anomalous right pulmonary venous return (5%), the third form of atrial septal defect involves defects of the sinus venosus type, which are high in the interatrial septum near the junction with the superior vena cava.

Associated Abnormalities

Atrial septal defects tend to be isolated anatomic anomalies; however, they may be associated with the following conditions:

- Down syndrome
- Holt-Oram syndrome
- Ellis–van Creveld syndrome
- Mitral valve prolapse
- Lutembacher syndrome
- Total anomalous pulmonary venous return

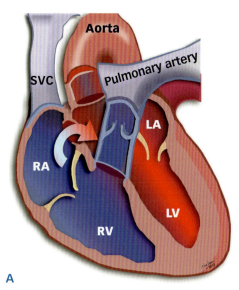
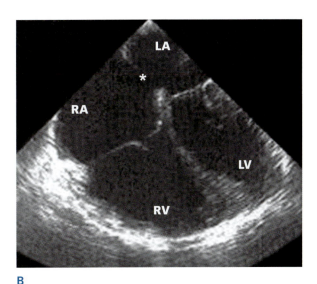

Figure 7-29. Atrial septal defect. **A** Schematic showing the abnormal communication between the right and left atria, which allows shunting of blood from the right to left (curved arrow). **B** Four-chamber visualization of a large defect (*asterisked) in the interatrial septum. RV = right ventricle, LV = left ventricle, RA = right atrium, LA = left atrium, SVC = superior vena cava.

Sonographic Signs

The following are the characteristic sonographic signs of atrial septal defects:

- Difficult diagnosis secondary to a normal foramen ovale
- Visualization of a large defect in the interatrial septum (Figure 7-29B)
- Enlarged pulmonary vasculature
- Left atrium of normal size; other chambers that may be enlarged

Atrioventricular Septal Defects

An *atrioventricular septal defect* (AVSD), also called an *endocardial cushion defect* and an *atrioventricular canal*, is a combination of cardiac anomalies affecting the atrial and ventricular septa and one or both of the tricuspid and mitral valves (Figure 7-30A). A complete atrioventricular septal defect consists of both atrial and ventricular septal defects with a common atrioventricular valve and presents with a deformity caused by narrowing of the left ventricular outflow tract. An incomplete atrioventricular septal defect consists of an atrial septal defect with separate mitral and tricuspid valve orifices. Both types arise from incomplete closure of the embryonic endocardial cushions.

Associated Abnormalities

The following abnormalities are characteristically associated with atrioventricular septal defects:

- Trisomy 21 (50% of fetuses)[13]
- Trisomy 18 (25% of fetuses)[13]
- Holt-Oram syndrome
- Ellis–van Creveld syndrome
- Total anomalous pulmonary return

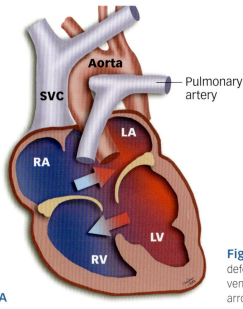

Figure 7-30. Atrioventricular septal defect. **A** Schematic demonstrating defects in both atrial and ventricular septa. RV = right ventricle, LV = left ventricle, RA = right atrium, LA = left atrium, SVC = superior vena cava, arrows = mixing of right and left heart blood. (Figure continues . . .)

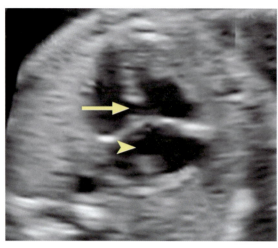

B

Figure 7-30, continued. B Four-chamber view demonstrating septal defects. Arrow = ventricular septal defect, arrowhead = atrial septal defect.

Sonographic Signs

The following are the characteristic sonographic signs of atrioventricular septal defects:

- Large defect along the cardiac midline (Figure 7-30B)
- Common valve cusps meeting at the same level during systole
- Valve cusps opening toward the atrioventricular septal defect during diastole

Conotruncal Anomalies

Conotruncal anomalies are malformations of the cardiac outflow tracts and the great arteries arising from the heart. They result from the failure of the growth, partitioning, and rotation of the primitive ductus arteriosus and its connections to the two ventricles. While there are numerous variants to be found, the four most common presentations encountered in routine sonography practice include the following:

- Tetralogy of Fallot
- Transposition of the great arteries
- Persistent truncus arteriosus
- Double-outlet right ventricle

Tetralogy of Fallot

Tetralogy of Fallot is a relatively common cardiac anomaly that accounts for approximately 10% of all congenital heart disease.[14] It is characterized by four features—hence the term "tetralogy" (Figure 7-31A):

- Overriding aorta with the aortic valve connected to both right and left ventricles.
- Ventricular septal defect, usually in the superior aspect of the septum.
- Right ventricular outflow obstruction caused by stenosis of the proximal-most part of the pulmonary artery (infundibulum) near the pulmonic valve.
- Right ventricular hypertrophy caused by the chronic pressure increase associated with outflow stenosis. This is a variable finding, not always seen in the fetus; it is more commonly identified in the neonate or child with tetralogy of Fallot.

Associated Abnormalities

The following abnormalities are characteristically associated with tetralogy of Fallot:

- Pulmonary hypoplasia
- Patent ductus arteriosus
- Atrial septal defect
- Prune belly syndrome
- Transposition of the great vessels

Sonographic Signs

The following are the characteristic sonographic signs of tetralogy of Fallot:

- Y-shaped overriding aorta with outflow from both ventricles (Figure 7-31B)

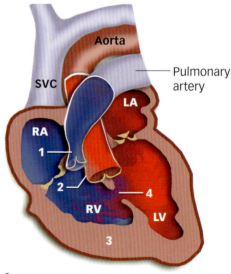

A

Figure 7-31. Tetralogy of Fallot. **A** Schematic demonstrating the four main pathologic features: 1 = pulmonary artery stenosis, 2 = overriding aorta, 3 = right ventricular hypertrophy, 4 = ventricular septal defect. RV = right ventricle, LV = left ventricle, RA = right atrium, LA = left atrium, SVC = superior vena cava. (Figure continues . . .)

- Ventricular septal defect (Figure 7-31C)
- Right ventricular outflow abnormalities (Figure 7-31D)
- Hydrops fetalis
- Polyhydramnios

Transposition of the Great Arteries

In *transposition of the great arteries* (TGA), also called *transposition of the great vessels*, the aorta arises from the right ventricle and the pulmonary trunk arises from the left ventricle (Figure 7-32A). There are two types of transposition of the great vessels: complete, or dextro-transposition (D-TGA), and congenitally corrected transposition, or levo-transposition (L-TGA). D-TGA is the most common type, accounting for approximately 80% of cases. It is characterized by a normal size relationship between the atria and the ventricles with or without a ventricular septal defect and pulmonary stenosis. Postnatally, complete transposition is a lethal condition; corrected transposition is not. Preexisting maternal diabetes mellitus is a risk factor for the fetus with transposition of the great arteries.

Associated Abnormalities

The following congenital cardiac abnormalities are characteristically associated with transposition of the great arteries:

- Ventricular septal defect
- Patent ductus arteriosus

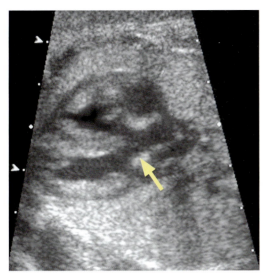

B

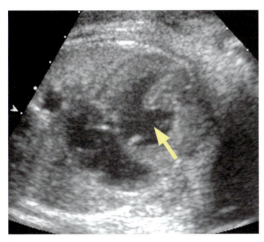

C

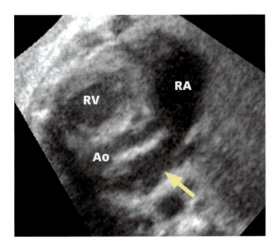

D

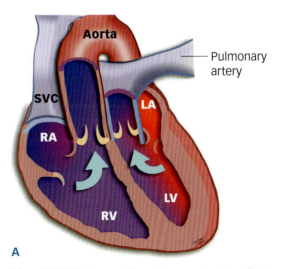

A

Figure 7-31, continued. **B** Y-shaped overriding aorta (arrow). **C** Ventricular septal defect (arrow). **D** Right ventricular outflow obstruction. RV = right ventricle, RA = dilated right atrium, Ao = aorta, arrow = dilated pulmonary artery.

Figure 7-32. Transposition of the great arteries. **A** Schematic demonstrating aberrant takeoff of the aorta from the right ventricle and the pulmonary artery from the left ventricle. RV = right ventricle, LV = left ventricle, RA = hypoplastic right atrium, LA = hypoplastic left atrium, SVC = superior vena cava, curved arrows = direction of blood flow. (Figure continues . . .)

Figure 7-32, continued. B Main pulmonary artery (arrow) arising from the left ventricle, in transposition of the great arteries. **C** Aorta (arrow) arising from the right ventricle. **D** Doppler color imaging highlights the "parallel channel" sign as both outflow channels course anomalously out of the heart. RV = right ventricle, LV = left ventricle, MPA = main pulmonary artery, AA = aortic arch.

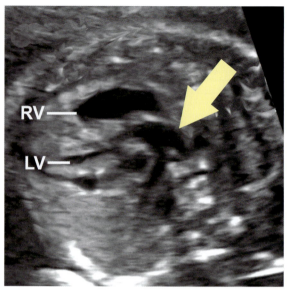

B

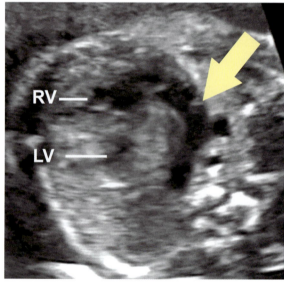

C

- Patent foramen ovale in neonates
- Atrial septal defect

Sonographic Signs

The following are the characteristic sonographic signs of transposition of the great arteries:

- Pulmonary artery arising from the left ventricle (Figure 7-32B)
- Aorta arising from the right ventricle (Figure 7-32C)
- "Parallel channel" sign—aorta and pulmonary artery coursing side by side (Figure 7-32D)

Persistent Truncus Arteriosus

The *truncus arteriosus* is the single tubular embryonic conduit arising cranially from the primitive heart, or bulbus cordis (Figure 7-6A). In normal cardiac development the truncus has partitioned into two separate conduits, the ascending aorta and the pulmonary trunk, by the end of the 5th conceptual week. Failure of this normal embryonic partitioning results in a cardiovascular abnormality called *persistent truncus arteriosus* (PTA), or more commonly just *truncus arteriosus* (TA) or *common arterial trunk*. Persistent truncus arteriosus is characterized pathologically by a single great artery arising from the two ventricles and a concomitant large ventricular septal defect (Figure 7-33A). An abnormal truncal valve may be present, consisting of 2–4 cusps of the anomalously developed aortic and pulmonic valves.

Associated Abnormalities

The following abnormalities are characteristically associated with persistent truncus arteriosus:

- Ventricular septal defect
- Right-sided aortic arch

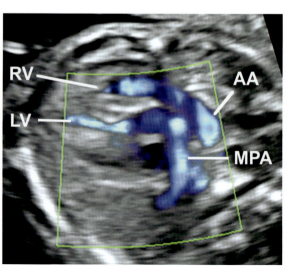

D

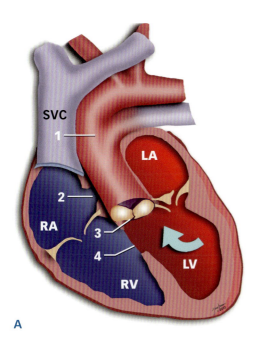

Figure 7-33. Persistent truncus arteriosus. **A** Schematic demonstrating a single artery arising from the truncal root. 1 = truncus arteriosus, 2 = atrial septal defect, 3 = truncal valve, 4 = ventricular septal defect, RV = right ventricle, LV = left ventricle, RA = hypoplastic right atrium, LA = hypoplastic left atrium, SVC = superior vena cava, curved arrow = direction of blood flow. **B** LVOT view showing a single great artery arising from the truncal root (arrow). RV = right ventricle, LV = left ventricle, LA = left atrium, 1 = ventricular septal defect, 2 = abnormal truncal valve. **C** Aorta and main pulmonary artery arise from a common arterial trunk. LSA = left subclavian artery, LPA = left pulmonary artery, RPA = right pulmonary artery.

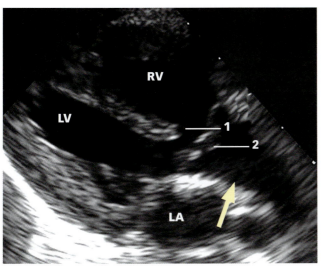

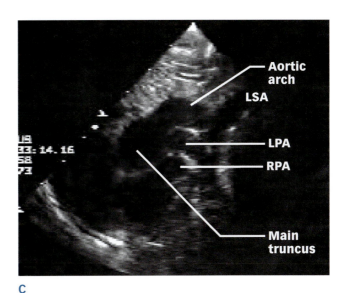

Sonographic Signs

The following are the characteristic sonographic signs of persistent truncus arteriosus:

- Single great artery arising from the truncal root (Figure 7-33B)
- Abnormal truncal valve
- Aorta and main pulmonary artery arising from a common arterial trunk (Figure 7-33C)
- Ventricular septal defect

Double-Outlet Right Ventricle

In *double-outlet right ventricle* (DORV), both the aorta and the pulmonary artery arise from the right ventricle (Figure 7-34A). It is rarely an isolated finding; rather it is typically one morphologic component in other complex congenital cardiac anomalies. A ventricular septal defect is virtually always present. Double-outlet right ventricle is demonstrated sonographically in the fetus by visualizing at least 50% of the luminal diameter of both great arteries taking off from the right ventricle.

Associated Abnormalities

The following abnormalities are characteristically associated with double-outlet right ventricle:

- Trisomy 18 (Edwards syndrome)
- Trisomy 13 (Patau syndrome)
- Pulmonary stenosis

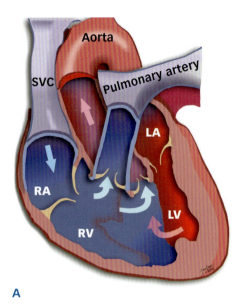 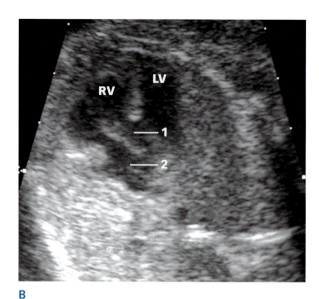

Figure 7-34. Double-outlet right ventricle. **A** Schematic showing both the aorta and the pulmonary artery arising from the right ventricle. RV = right ventricle; LV = left ventricle; RA = right atrium; LA = left atrium; SVC = superior vena cava; blue arrows = double outlet, aorta, and pulmonary artery; pink arrows = aortic outflow. **B** Linear alignment of the aorta and pulmonary trunk. RV = right ventricle, LV = left ventricle, 1 = aorta, 2 = pulmonary trunk.

- Coarctation of the aorta
- Anomalous pulmonary venous return
- Tracheoesophageal fistula

Sonographic Signs

The following are the characteristic sonographic signs of double-outlet right ventricle:

- Linear alignment of the aorta and pulmonary trunk (Figure 7-34B)
- Ventricular septal defect
- Shared origin of the aortic root and pulmonary trunk

Single Ventricle Anomalies

Single ventricle anomaly is a generic term that refers to any fetal congenital cardiac anomaly characterized by the presence of only one functionally adequate ventricle. These anomalies include the following:

- Hypoplastic heart syndromes
- Tricuspid atresia
- Double-outlet right ventricle (see pages 179–180)
- Double-inlet left ventricle (see page 182)

Hypoplastic Heart Syndromes

Hypoplastic left heart syndrome (HLHS) is a cardiac anomaly characterized by the incomplete development of structures comprising the left side of the heart, including the ventricle, atrium, mitral valve, aortic valve, and aorta (Figure 7-35A). It is the most common cause of postnatal congestive cardiac failure and is lethal in the presence of a closed foramen ovale.

Hypoplastic right ventricle—the anomaly characterized by the incomplete development of the structures on the right side of the heart—is less common than its left-sided counterpart but also poses a risk for serious postnatal sequelae. The inability of the right ventricle to accommodate an adequate volume of blood to pump into the lungs for oxygenation results in poor outcomes for the neonate.

Associated Abnormalities

The following abnormalities are characteristically associated with hypoplastic heart syndromes:

- Hypoplastic left heart syndrome:
  - Coarctation of the aorta
  - Aortic atresia/hypoplasia
  - Mitral atresia
- Hypoplastic right ventricle:
  - Tricuspid atresia
  - Pulmonary atresia

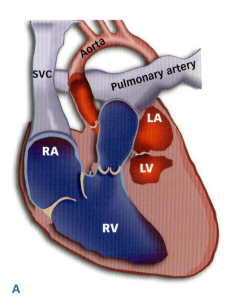
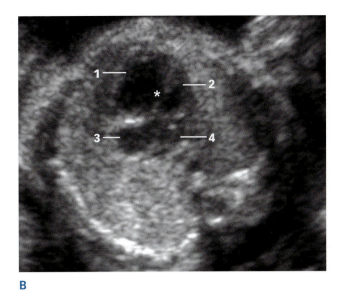

Figure 7-35. Hypoplastic left heart syndrome. **A** Schematic showing hypoplastic chambers of the left heart. RA = right atrium, RV = right ventricle, LV = hypoplastic left ventricle, LA = hypoplastic left atrium, SVC = superior vena cava. **B** Four-chamber demonstration of small, thick-walled left atrium and ventricle. 1 = right ventricle, 2 = left ventricle, 3 = right atrium, 4 = left atrium, asterisk (*) = presence of an associated ventricular septal defect.

Sonographic Signs

The following are the characteristic sonographic signs of hypoplastic heart syndromes:

- Small, thick-walled cardiac chambers seen in the four-chamber view (Figure 7-35B)
- Concentric ventricular thickening
- Small ascending aorta (left-sided)
- Hypoplastic pulmonary artery
- Malformation of the atrioventricular valve on the affected side

Tricuspid Atresia

Tricuspid atresia is a congenital cardiac anomaly in which the tricuspid valve and right ventricular inlet fail to form properly, if at all. As a result, there is no direct communication between the right atrium and the right ventricle, compromising outflow of blood into the pulmonary artery (Figure 7-36A). In the fetus, venous blood returning to the right atrium can cross the foramen ovale into the left heart, where the increased volume and pressure can cause volume overload. Some blood does reach the lungs via the ductus arteriosus, but regression of this normal fetal circulatory vessel postnatally presents the risk of serious sequelae. When a concomitant ventricular septal defect is present, shunting of blood from the left to the right ventricle helps maintain systemic oxygenation.

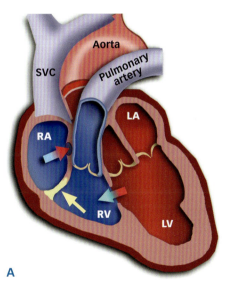

Figure 7-36. Tricuspid atresia. **A** Schematic showing atresia of the tricuspid valve (yellow arrow) with concomitant atrial septal defect (arrow in the RA) and ventricular septal defect (arrow entering the RV). RV = small right ventricle, LV = large left ventricle, RA = right atrium, LA = left atrium, SVC = superior vena cava. (Figure continues . . .)

Associated Abnormalities

The following abnormalities are characteristically associated with tricuspid atresia:[7,8,9,10]

- Atrial septal defect
- Ventricular septal defect (Figure 7-36B)
- Right-sided aortic arch

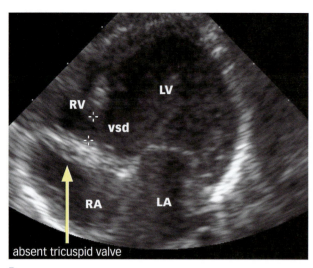

Figure 7-36, continued. B Four-chamber view demonstrating a hypoplastic right ventricle (RV) and absent tricuspid valve (arrow) in a fetus with tricuspid atresia. RA = right atrium, LV = left ventricle, vsd = ventricular septal defect. Reprinted from Gibson CM, Shafer K, Singh P, et al (eds): Tricuspid atresia echocardiography. © WikiDoc, available at http://www.wikidoc.org/index.php/Tricuspid_atresia_echocardiography.

- Enlarged left ventricle
- Atrial and/or ventricular septal defects

Double-Inlet Left Ventricle

Double-inlet left ventricle is another type of conotruncal congenital defect affecting both the cardiac chambers and the valves. Both the left and right atria feed directly into the left ventricle, the right ventricle being hypoplastic or completely absent (Figure 7-37A).

Associated Abnormalities

The following abnormalities are characteristically associated with double-inlet left ventricle:

- Coarctation of the aorta
- Pulmonary atresia
- Pulmonic valve stenosis

- Transposition of the great vessels
- Pulmonary atresia/stenosis

Sonographic Signs

The following are the characteristic sonographic signs of tricuspid atresia (Figure 7-36B):

- Absent tricuspid valve
- Hypoplastic right ventricle
- Hypoplastic pulmonary artery
- Absent or diminished blood flow into the pulmonary artery with color Doppler
- Enlarged right atrium

Sonographic Signs

The following are the characteristic sonographic signs of double-inlet left ventricle (Figures 7-37B–D):

- Single ventricular chamber on a four-chamber view
- Two atria with valves present on a four-chamber view

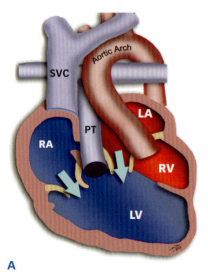
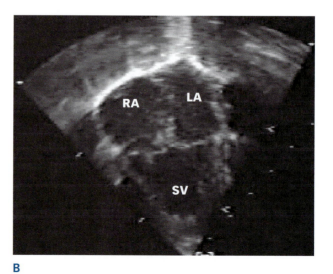

Figure 7-37. Double-inlet left ventricle. **A** Schematic showing both atria (arrows) feeding into the left ventricle. **B** Apical four-chamber view in systole. Note the double-inlet left ventricle. RV = reversed hypoplastic right ventricle (sometimes completely absent), LV = reversed left ventricle, RA = right atrium, LA = left atrium, SVC = superior vena cava, PT = pulmonary trunk, SV = single ventricle. (Figure continues . . .)

Disproportionate Ventricular Size

Several congenital cardiac anomalies are characterized by the presence of disproportionate ventricular size. While this finding may be apparent on a four-chamber view, a complete fetal echocardiographic workup is required to fully delineate the constellation of findings associated with each specific condition.

Ebstein's Anomaly

Ebstein's anomaly is a rare congenital cardiac anomaly in which the tricuspid valve is displaced inferiorly in the right ventricle (Figure 7-38A). The valve leaflets are incompletely separated and may be adherent to the chordae tendineae, which anchor them to the ventricular wall. Tricuspid regurgitation is common and may be severe enough to cause right ventricular overload and compromise of the outflow tract. Concomitant abnormalities include pulmonary stenosis and atrial septal defects.[15]

Associated Abnormalities

The following abnormalities are characteristically associated with Ebstein's anomaly:

- Trisomy 13 (Patau syndrome)
- Trisomy 18 (Edwards syndrome)
- Turner syndrome
- Pulmonary atresia/stenosis

Sonographic Signs

The following are the characteristic sonographic signs of Ebstein's anomaly:

- Enlarged right atrium
- Inferior displacement of the tricuspid valve (Figure 7-38B)
- Tricuspid regurgitation (Figure 7-38C)
- Pericardial effusion if cardiac function is severely compromised

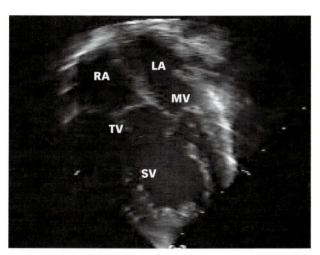

C

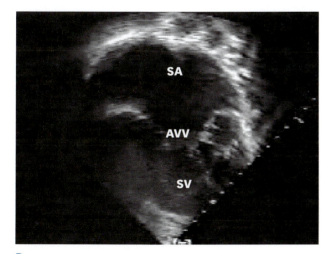

D

Figure 7-37, continued. C Slightly different view in systole, also demonstrating a double-inlet left ventricle. **D** Apical four-chamber view in diastole demonstrating a complete atrioventricular canal with a single ventricle. RA = right atrium, LA = left atrium, TV = tricuspid valve, MV = mitral valve, SV = single ventricle, SA = single atrium, AVV = atrial ventricular valve.

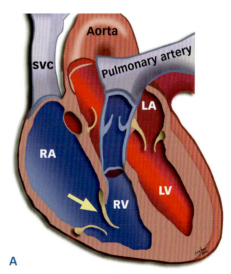

A

Figure 7-38. Ebstein's anomaly. **A** Schematic showing the inferiorly displaced tricuspid valve (arrow). SVC = superior vena cava, RA = right atrium, RV = right ventricle, LV = left ventricle, LA = left atrium. (Figure continues . . .)

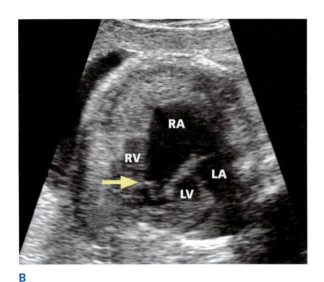
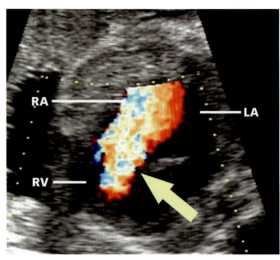

B
C

Figure 7-38, continued. B Four-chamber view demonstrating low-set tricuspid valve (arrow). RV = right ventricle, RA = right atrium, LV = left ventricle, LA = left atrium, SVC = superior vena cava. **C** Four-chamber view with color Doppler demonstrating tricuspid regurgitation (arrow). RA = right atrium, LA = left atrium, RV = right ventricle.

Coarctation of the Aorta

Coarctation of the aorta describes a narrowing of the aortic lumen (Figure 7-39A). This hemodynamically significant stenosis reduces the volume of blood flow into the aortic arch, resulting in arch hypoplasia. A hallmark sonographic finding described in neonates with coarctation of the aorta is the *contraductal shelf*, which may represent residual fibrotic tissue derived from the ductus arteriosus.

There are infantile and adult types of coarctation, the infantile form obviously being the one detectable with prenatal sonography. Infantile coarctation is characterized by diffuse narrowing of the aorta proximal to the ductus arteriosus.

Associated Abnormalities

The following abnormalities are characteristically associated with coarctation of the aorta:

- Ventricular septal defects
- Mitral valve anomalies
- Single ventricle
- Transposition of the great vessels
- Double-inlet left ventricle
- Tetralogy of Fallot
- Hypoplastic left heart syndrome
- Neonatal patent ductus arteriosus

Sonographic Signs

The following are the characteristic sonographic signs of coarctation of the aorta:

- Narrowed aortic arch (Figure 7-39B).
- Contraductal shelf (Figure 7-39C).
- Ventricular disproportion (Figure 7-39D).
- Doppler may demonstrate elevated velocities distal to the stenotic area.

Positional Abnormalities

As nicely demonstrated in a routine four-chamber view, the fetal heart sits in the center of an intact thoracic cavity with its apex directed approximately 45° to the left. It is bordered on both sides by homogeneously echogenic lung. Deviations from this normal anatomic configuration raise the specter of congenital positional abnormalities, such as:

- Diaphragmatic hernia (see pages 168–169)
- Situs abnormalities
- Ectopia cordis

Situs Abnormalities

Situs abnormalities are variations in the laterality of thoracic and abdominal organs. As this finding may be a harbinger of other complex congenital anomalies, care should be taken during routine examination of the chest to correctly assign laterality based on the sonographer's determination of external landmarks

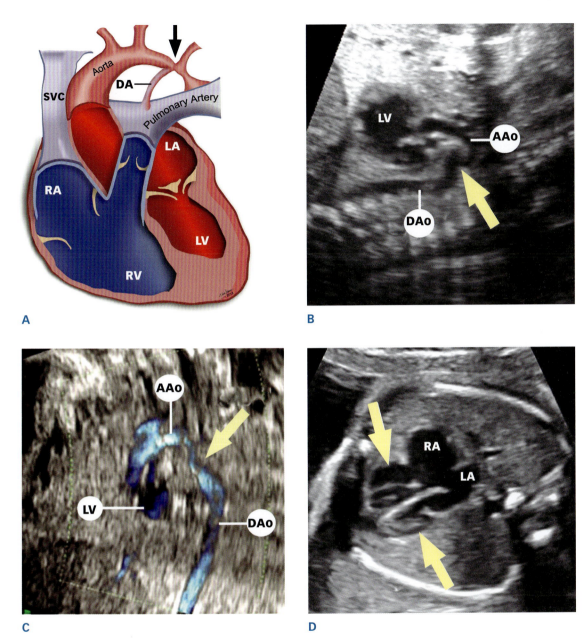

Figure 7-39. Infantile-type coarctation of the aorta. **A** Schematic showing characteristic diffuse narrowing (arrow) proximal to the ductus arteriosus (DA); note the enlarged right ventricle and small left ventricle. SVC = superior vena cava, RA = right atrium, LA = left etrium, RV = right ventricle, LV = left ventricle. **B** Sagittal section demonstrating the coarcted segment (arrow). **C** Sagittal color Doppler image demonstrating the contraductal shelf (arrow). **D** Ventricular disproportion (arrows). LV = left ventricle, RA = right atrium, LA = left atrium, AAo = aortic arch, DAo = descending aorta.

(fetal lie, etc.), not depend on the heart's relationship to adjacent internal anatomic landmarks.

There are two primary situs abnormalities:

- *Situs inversus* is a rare anomaly characterized by the complete reversal of normal right-left laterality of organs in the chest and abdomen.
- *Situs ambiguus* (commonly also spelled as *situs ambiguous*)—also known as *heterotaxy syndrome*—is characterized by the incomplete right-left mirroring of intrathoracic content. Paired thoracic and abdominal organs, such as the lungs and kidneys, appear as partial mirror images of each other instead of having the unique characteristics normally present right and left. There are typically many complex anatomic abnormalities associated with heterotaxy syndrome.

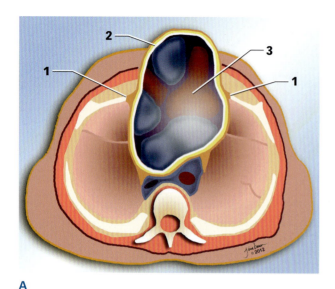
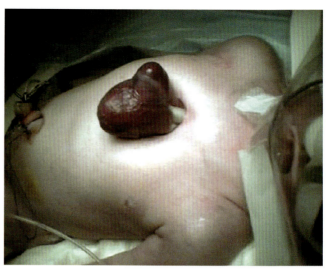

Figure 7-40. Ectopia cordis. **A** Schematic axial section demonstrating the heart herniated through a sternal defect. 1 = sternal defect, 2 = pericardium, 3 = herniated heart. **B** Gross pathology of ectopia cordis in a neonate. (Figure continues . . .)

Associated Abnormalities

The following abnormalities are characteristically associated with situs abnormalities:[16]

- Intestinal malrotation
- Cardiac defects:
  - Dextrocardia syndrome
  - Transposition of the great vessels
- Biliary atresia
- Total anomalous pulmonary return
- Polysplenia

Sonographic Signs

The following are the characteristic sonographic signs of situs abnormalities:

- Reversal of laterality of landmark anatomic structures, i.e., heart on the right, liver and stomach on the left
- Frequent congenital cardiac abnormalities

Ectopia Cordis

Ectopia cordis is a rare congenital malformation in which part or all of the heart is located outside of the thoracic cavity (Figures 7-40A and B). Failure of the lateral embryonic mesoderm to migrate and fuse in the midline leaves a defect along the anterior body wall, usually in the thoracic region, through which the heart can herniate. Other ectopic locations of ectopia cordis are along the thoracoabdominal, abdominal, or cervical surface of the fetus.

Associated Abnormalities

Ectopia cordis may occur as an isolated defect or in conjunction with other anterior body wall herniation abnormalities, including the following:

- Omphalocele
- Congenital diaphragmatic hernia
- Congenital heart disease
- Pentalogy of Cantrell

Sonographic Signs

The following are the characteristic sonographic signs of ectopia cordis:

- Identification of the heart outside the thoracic cavity (Figures 7-40C and D)
- Small thorax

Cardiac Wall Abnormalities

Focal or diffuse distortion of the normal, symmetric appearance of the cardiac walls suggests the presence of a congenital anomaly. Conditions involving the aberrant appearance of the cardiac wall include the following:

- Cardiomyopathy
- Cardiac tumors
- Fetal pericardial effusions

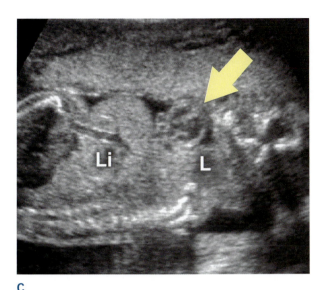
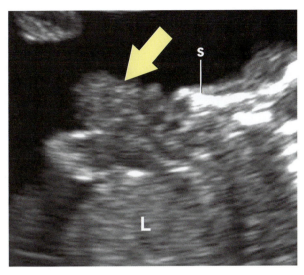

Figure 7-40, continued. C Sagittal scan through the fetus demonstrating a herniated heart (arrow). **D** Transverse scan through the anterior thorax showing a herniated heart (arrow). Li = liver, L = lung, S = sternum.

Cardiomyopathy

Cardiomyopathy (CMP) is an abnormality of myocardial function that ultimately leads to heart failure. Its cause can be extrinsic, where the primary pathology originates outside the heart muscle itself (as in ischemic cardiomyopathy), or it can be an intrinsic weakness of the myocardium caused by genetic or idiopathic etiologies. In the fetus, cardiomyopathy presents sonographically as an abnormally large heart with either dilated chambers (dilated cardiomyopathy) or thick ventricular septum and walls (hypertrophic cardiomyopathy).

To an experienced obstetric sonographer, *cardiomegaly* is apparent as a subjective finding wherein the heart is too big for the chest. A quantitative method that measures the relative size of the heart and thoracic cage and is a useful tool in the assessment of fetal cardiac and thoracic wall anomalies is the *fetal cardiothoracic (C/T) circumference ratio*: the ratio of the cardiac circumference to the thoracic circumference. As a rule of thumb, the C/T ratio should be less than 0.5 throughout gestation.

Atrioventricular valve (mitral or tricuspid) regurgitation is present in about 60% of fetuses with cardiomyopathy.[17] M-mode of the short- or long-axis left ventricle in either type of cardiomyopathy is helpful to determine chamber size, to measure left ventricular wall and septum thickness, and to evaluate cardiac function.

Associated Abnormalities

The following abnormalities are characteristically associated with cardiomyopathy:

- Congenital infection
- Endocardial fibroelastosis
- Twin-to-twin transfusion syndrome
- Maternal diabetes
- Barth syndrome
- Noonan syndrome

Sonographic Signs

The following are the characteristic sonographic signs of cardiomyopathy:

- Cardiomegaly
- Dilated cardiac chambers (Figure 7-41A)
- Thickened ventricular septum and myocardium (Figures 7-41A and B)
- Atrioventricular valve regurgitation (Figure 7-41C)

Cardiac Tumors

On rare occasions an echogenic mass may be seen within the fetal heart. Among cardiac tumors, rhabdomyoma is the most common. Less common cardiac tumors include teratomas, fibromas, hemangiomas, and myxomas. None of these can be histologically differentiated with ultrasound.

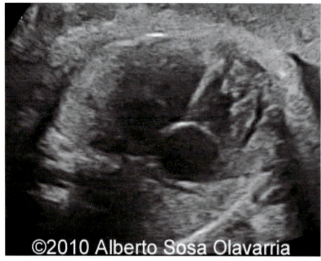

A

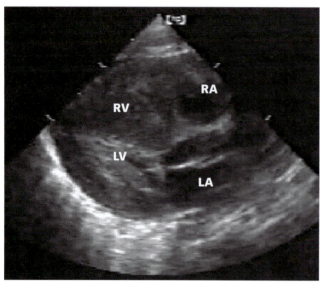

B

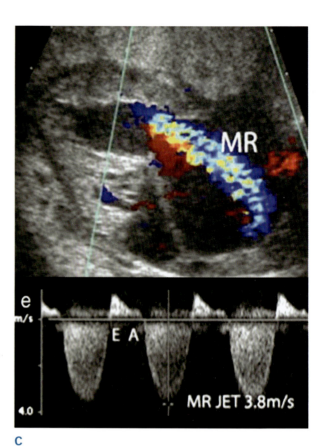

C

Figure 7-41. Cardiomyopathy. **A** Four-chamber view demonstrating a thickened myocardium with dilated cardiac chambers. © Alberto Sosa Olavarria; reprinted with permission from TheFetus.net. **B** Hypertrophic cardiac walls. RA = right atrium, RV = right ventricle, LA = left atrium, LV = left ventricle **C** Atrioventricular valve regurgitation demonstrated in a color and spectral Doppler display of a high-velocity mitral valve regurgitation jet. MR = mitral regurgitation.

Associated Abnormalities

The following abnormalities are characteristically associated with cardiac tumors:

- Pericardial effusion
- Pleural effusion
- Hydrops fetalis
- Pulmonary hypoplasia

Sonographic Signs

The following are the characteristic sonographic signs of cardiac tumors:

- Echogenic masses within the fetal heart (Figure 7-42A)
- Solid or complex appearance
- Distortion of normal cardiac morphology
- Displacement of the heart from its normal position in the chest (Figure 7-42B)

Fetal Pericardial Effusion

Fetal pericardial effusion (FPE) is an accumulation of fluid in the pericardial sac. A small rim of fluid outlining the myocardium is a normal finding if it measures less than 2 mm. A larger fluid collection warrants a careful sonographic examination of the fetal cardiovascular system and correlation with clinical findings to assess risks for hydrops fetalis. Fetal pericardial effusion is one of the earliest indicators of impending hydrops. In the absence of other sonographic abnormalities, an isolated fetal pericardial fluid collection up to 7 mm in thickness is not thought to be associated with an adverse outcome.[18]

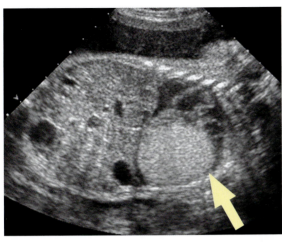

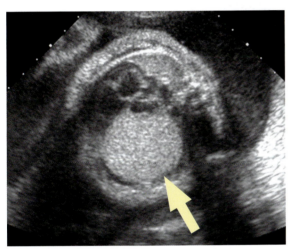

Figure 7-42. Cardiac tumors (arrows). **A** Coronal section demonstrating a cardiac tumor (rhabdomyoma). **B** Axial section through the thorax of the same fetus. Note lateral displacement of the fetal heart from its normal position.

Associated Abnormalities

The following abnormalities are characteristically associated with fetal pericardial effusion:

- Hydrops fetalis
- Cardiac anomalies
- Cardiac tumors
- Trisomy 21 (Down syndrome)

Sonographic Signs

The following is the characteristic sonographic sign of fetal pericardial effusion (Figure 7-43):

- Anechoic fluid collection conforming to the pericardial sac
- Hypoplastic lungs due to fluid compression

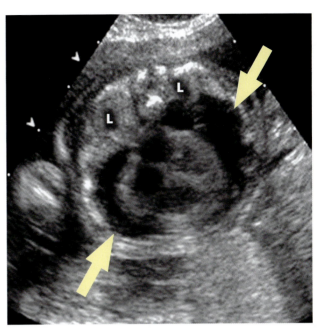

Figure 7-43. An axial section through the fetal chest demonstrates large bilateral pericardial effusions (arrows) compressing the lungs (L) of this 28-week growth-restricted fetus.

Abnormalities of Fetal Heart Rate and Rhythm

In the second and third trimesters, the fetal heart rate may vary. An average heart rate in the fetus is 100–180 beats per minute. Variations in heart rate and rhythm are commonly encountered during routine obstetric ultrasound examination and are rarely of any significance. However, persistent elevation (tachyarrhythmia) or reduction (bradyarrhythmia) of heart rate may predispose the fetus to heart failure and its fluid-overload sequela, hydrops fetalis. M-mode and spectral Doppler are both methods of quantifying and documenting abnormalities of fetal cardiac rate and rhythm. The five main abnormalities of cardiac rate and rhythm encountered in utero are discussed below.

Fetal Supraventricular Tachycardia

Fetal supraventricular tachycardia is the most common cardiac tachyarrhythmia identified (accounting for 60%–90% of cases)[19] and is characterized by a heart rate of >180 beats per minute (bpm). It is often associated with other intra- or extracardiac anomalies. If it persists after birth and is not associated with fetal hydrops or other anatomic or physiologic abnormalities, it can usually be successfully treated pharmacologically.

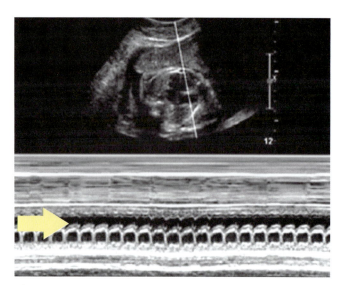

Figure 7-44. Supraventricular tachycardia. M-mode demonstration of a subjectively rapid heart rate (arrow).

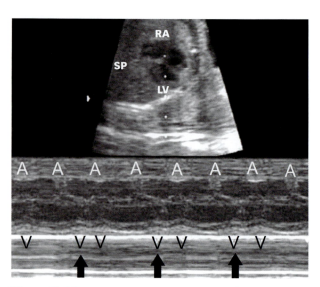

Figure 7-46. Premature ventricular contractions (arrows). M-mode demonstration of excess ventricular contractions (V) in relation to atrial contractions (A).

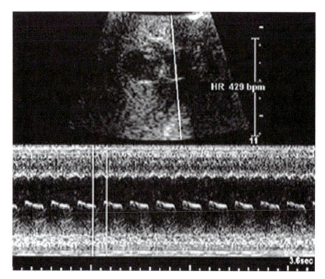

Figure 7-45. Atrial flutter. M-mode demonstration of rapid atrial contractions greater than 300 beats per minute.

Sonographic Signs

The following are the characteristic sonographic signs seen with fetal supraventricular tachycardia:

- Real-time demonstration of a subjectively rapid heart rate (Figure 7-44)
- M-mode demonstration of heart rate > 180 bpm

Atrial Flutter

Atrial flutter, another form of tachyarrhythmia, is characterized by an atrial contraction rate of 300–600 bpm with a variable, but increased, ventricular contraction rate (Figure 7-45). While atrial flutter may be an isolated finding, it can be associated with Ebstein's anomaly and pulmonary stenosis. If it persists throughout gestation, hydrops fetalis becomes a serious concern.

Sonographic Signs

The following are the characteristic sonographic signs seen with atrial flutter:

- Real-time demonstration of subjectively rapid atrial contractions with normal to increased ventricular contraction rate.
- M-mode demonstration of an atrial contraction rate > 300 bpm

Premature Ventricular Contractions

Premature ventricular contractions (PVCs) (Figure 7-46) are ectopic ventricular contractions usually punctuated by compensatory pauses as the heart's electrical system "reboots." PVCs can be associated with concomitant cardiac pathology such as myocarditis, cardiac tumors, long QT syndrome, electrolyte imbalances, and complete atrioventricular block. Most isolated sonographically identified PVCs resolve spontaneously prior to birth or within 6 weeks after birth.

Sonographic Signs

The characteristic sonographic sign seen with premature ventricular contractions is a real-time demonstration of early contraction of the ventricle without a preceding atrial contraction.

Premature Atrial Contractions

Premature atrial contractions (PACs) (Figure 7-47) are ectopic atrial contractions also punctuated by

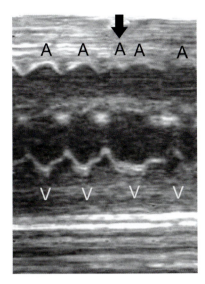

Figure 7-47. Premature atrial contraction (arrow). M-mode demonstration of atrial contractions (A) before passive ventricular filling (V).

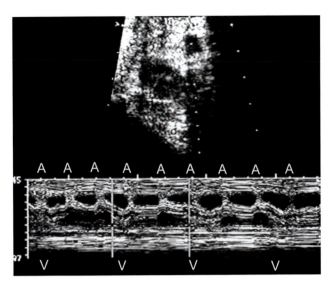

Figure 7-48. Atrioventricular block. M-mode demonstration of atrial contraction (A) rhythm independent of ventricular contraction (V) rhythm.

compensatory pauses. They are rarely associated with other congenital cardiac anomalies and are usually self-limiting, do not compromise cardiac function, and resolve spontaneously either in utero or shortly after birth.

Sonographic Signs

The characteristic sonographic sign seen with premature atrial contractions is early atrial contraction before passive ventricular filling.

Atrioventricular Block

Atrioventricular block (AV block) is a bradyarrhythmia caused by abnormalities in cardiac conduction. This condition is characterized by an atrial contractile rhythm independent of ventricular contractile rhythm. While dissociated atrial and ventricular contractions can be an isolated and serendipitous observation during routine sonographic examination, persistent congenital complete AV block (CAVB) is also associated with concomitant cardiac anomalies, accompanied by the risk of developing hydrops fetalis, in 35%–53% of cases.[20]

Sonographic Signs

The following are the characteristic sonographic signs seen with atrioventricular block:

- Real-time demonstration of atrial contraction rhythm independent of ventricular contraction rhythm (Figure 7-48)
- M-mode demonstration of a ventricular contraction rate < 70 bpm

CHAPTER 7 REVIEW QUESTIONS

1. All of the following cardiac segments are assessed during the course of a routine sonographic examination of the fetal heart EXCEPT:
   A. Visceroatrial situs
   B. Ventricular loop
   C. Truncus arteriosus
   D. Abdominal visceral situs

2. Which of the following would be an indication for fetal echocardiography?
   A. Dextrocardia
   B. Two-vessel umbilical cord
   C. Increased diameter of nuchal lucency
   D. All of the above

3. Approximately what percentage of fetal blood flows across the foramen ovale into the left atrium?
   A. 20%
   B. 30%
   C. 40%
   D. 60%

4. All of the following fetal cardiac anomalies can be detected on a four-chamber view EXCEPT:
   A. Transposition of the great vessels
   B. Single ventricle

C. Ebstein's anomaly

D. Ventricular hypoplasia

5. All of the following anatomic structures can be identified on the left ventricular outflow tract (LVOT) view EXCEPT:
   A. Left atrium
   B. Aortic root
   C. Pulmonary artery
   D. Ventricular septum

6. What is the name for the condition characterized by deficient or incomplete development of the fetal lungs?
   A. Diaphragmatic hernia
   B. Pulmonary sequestration
   C. Pulmonary hypoplasia
   D. Congenital cystic adenomatoid malformation

7. A congenital abnormality of lung development characterized by the replacement of normal tissue with nonfunctioning cystic tissue is called:
   A. Diaphragmatic hernia
   B. Pulmonary sequestration
   C. Pulmonary hypoplasia
   D. Cystic adenomatoid malformation

8. The most common congenital cardiac anomaly, occurring in about 1 in 400 births, is:
   A. Tetralogy of Fallot
   B. Ventricular septal defect
   C. Atrial septal defect
   D. Aortic coarctation

9. All of the following anatomic defects are associated with tetralogy of Fallot EXCEPT:
   A. Transposition of the great vessels
   B. Overriding aorta
   C. Ventricular septal defect
   D. Tricuspid atresia

10. The congenital cardiac anomaly characterized by the aorta arising from the right ventricle and the pulmonary trunk arising from the left ventricle is called:
    A. Tetralogy of Fallot
    B. Conotruncal abnormality
    C. Persistent truncus arteriosus
    D. Transposition of the great vessels

11. A congenital cardiac anomaly characterized by the incomplete development of structures comprising the left side of the heart is called:
    A. Tetralogy of Fallot
    B. Conotruncal abnormality
    C. Persistent truncus arteriosus
    D. Hypoplastic left heart syndrome

12. The congenital narrowing of the aortic lumen is called:
    A. Coarctation of the aorta
    B. Tetralogy of Fallot
    C. Ebstein's anomaly
    D. Aortic stenosis

13. The rare congenital chest anomaly in which all or part of the heart is located outside of the thoracic cavity is called:
    A. Ebstein's anomaly
    B. Ectopia cordis
    C. Diaphragmatic hernia
    D. Omphalocele

14. Ebstein's anomaly is characterized primarily by:
    A. Tricuspid valve displaced inferiorly in the right ventricle
    B. Mitral valve displaced inferiorly in the left ventricle
    C. Overriding aorta
    D. All or part of heart located outside the thoracic cavity

15. The primary anatomic abnormality associated with persistent truncus arteriosus is:
    A. Aorta arising from the right ventricle
    B. Pulmonary artery arising from the left ventricle
    C. Pulmonary hypoplasia
    D. Single great artery arising from truncal root

16. An atrioventricular septal defect is also called:
    A. Endocardial cushion defect
    B. Conotruncal abnormality
    C. Situs inversus
    D. Truncus arteriosus

17. An anomalous condition characterized by an accessory fragment of lung that has no connection to the tracheobronchial tree and that maintains its own, separate arterial circulation is:
    A. Cystic adenomatoid malformation
    B. Diaphragmatic hernia
    C. Pulmonary sequestration
    D. Diaphragmatic eventration

18. Fetal pleural effusion is also called:
    A. Hydrothorax
    B. Pyothorax
    C. Hydrops fetalis
    D. Pulmonary hypoplasia

19. In this image the structure identified as #1 is the:

    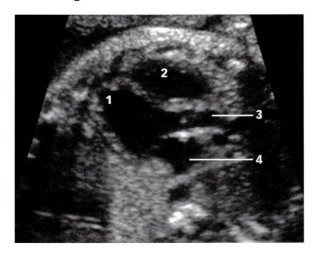

    A. Right ventricle
    B. Left ventricle
    C. Right atrium
    D. Left atrium

20. In the image accompanying question 19 the structure identified as #2 is the:
    A. Right ventricle
    B. Left ventricle
    C. Right atrium
    D. Left atrium

21. In the image accompanying question 19 the structure identified as #3 is the:
    A. Pulmonary artery
    B. Pulmonary vein
    C. Inferior vena cava
    D. Aortic root

22. In the image accompanying question 19 the structure identified as #4 is the:
    A. Right atrium
    B. Left atrium
    C. Pulmonary artery
    D. Superior vena cava

23. The anomaly demonstrated in this image is:

    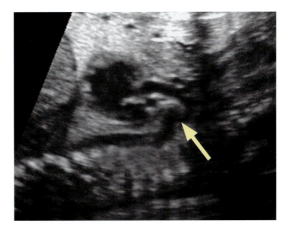

    A. Aortic coarctation
    B. Transposition of great vessels
    C. Patent ductus arteriosus
    D. Pulmonary stenosis

24. The arrow in this image points to:

    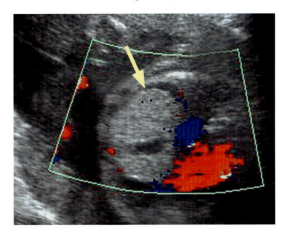

    A. Pulmonary sequestration
    B. Pericardial tumor
    C. Cystic adenomatoid malformation of the lung
    D. Pleural effusion

25. The anomaly demonstrated in this image is:

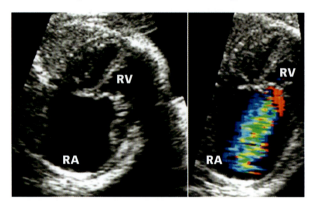

A. Mitral atresia
B. Pulmonary stenosis
C. Patent foramen ovale
D. Patent ductus arteriosus

26. This image demonstrates:

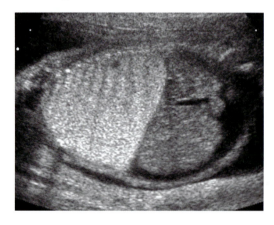

A. Normal lung/liver echogenicity
B. Pulmonary sequestration
C. Cystic adenomatoid malformation of the lung
D. Cystic fibrosis

27. This image demonstrates:

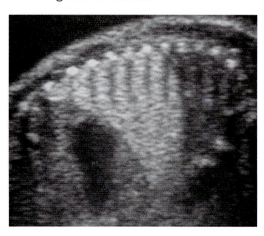

A. Diaphragmatic hernia
B. Pulmonary sequestration
C. Cystic adenomatoid malformation of the lung
D. Cystic fibrosis

28. This image best demonstrates:

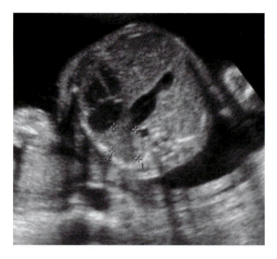

A. Diaphragmatic hernia
B. Duodenal atresia
C. Ectopia cordis
D. Cystic adenomatoid malformation

ANSWERS

See Appendix A on page 480 for answers.

REFERENCES

1. Ghidini A, Schillrò M, Locatelli AL: Amniotic fluid volume: when and how to take action. Contemporary Ob/Gyn: Expert Advice for Today's Ob/Gyn. Available at http://contemporaryobgyn.modernmedicine.com/contemporary-obgyn/content/tags/amniotic-fluid-volume/amniotic-fluid-volume-when-and-how-take-action?page=full.

2. Magann EF, Chauhan SP, Barrilleaux PS, et al: Amniotic fluid index and single deepest pocket: weak indicators of abnormal volumes. Obstet Gynecol 96(5 Pt 1):737–740.

3. Moss AJ, Adams FH, Emmanouilides GC: *Moss and Adams' Heart Disease in Infants, Children, and Adolescents: Including the Fetus and Young Adult*, 5th edition. Baltimore, Lippincott, Williams and Wilkins, 1995, p 555.

4. Benacerraf BR, Barss VA, Laboda A: A sonographic sign for the detection in the second trimester of the fetus with Down's syndrome. Am J Obstet Gynecol 151:1078–1079, 1985.

5. Lee W: Performance of the basic fetal cardiac ultrasound examination [published erratum appears in J Ultrasound Med 17:796, 1998]. J Ultrasound Med 17:601–607, 1998.

6. Berrocal T, Madrid C, Novo S, et al: Congenital anomalies of the tracheobronchial tree, lung, and mediastinum: embryology, radiology, and pathology. RadioGraphics 24:1–17, 2004.

7. Ianniruberto A: Management of fetal cardiac structural abnormalities. Fetal Ther 1:89–91, 1986.

8. Hoffman JI: Incidence of congenital heart disease. II. Prenatal incidence. Pediatr Cardiol 16:155–165, 1995.

9. Hoffman JI, Christianson R: Congenital heart disease in a cohort of 19,502 births with long-term follow-up. Am J Cardiol 42:641–647, 1978.

10. Hoffman JI: Incidence of congenital heart disease. I. Postnatal incidence. Pediatr Cardiol 16:103–113, 1995.

11. Goo HW, Park IS, Ko JK, et al: CT of congenital heart disease: normal anatomy and typical pathologic conditions. RadioGraphics 23:147–165, 2003.

12. Dinsmore RE, Wismer GL, Guyer D, et al: Magnetic resonance imaging of the interatrial septum and atrial septal defects. Am J Roentgenol 145:697–703, 1985.

13. Langford K, Sharland G, Simpson J: Relative risk of abnormal karyotype in fetuses found to have an atrioventricular septal defect (ASVD) on fetal echocardiography. Prenat Diagn 25:137–139, 2005.

14. Entezami M, Albig M, Gasiorek-Wiens A, et al: *Ultrasound Diagnosis of Fetal Anomalies*. New York, Thieme, 2003, p 93.

15. Watson H: Natural history of Ebstein's anomaly of tricuspid valve in childhood and adolescence: an international co-operative study of 505 cases. Br Heart J 36:417–427, 1974.

16. Applegate KE, Goske MJ, Pierce G, et al: Situs revisited: imaging of the heterotaxy syndrome. RadioGraphics 19:837–852, 1999.

17. Pedra SR, Smallhorn JF, Ryan G, et al: Fetal cardiomyopathies: pathogenetic mechanisms, hemodynamic findings, and clinical outcome. Circulation 106:585–591, 2002.

18. Di Salvo DN, Brown DL, Doubilet PM, et al: Clinical significance of isolated fetal pericardial effusion. J Ultrasound Med 13:291–293, 1994.

19. Hornberger LK, Sahn DJ: Rhythm abnormalities of the fetus. Heart 93:1294–1300, 2007.

20. Schmidt KG, Ulmer HE, Silverman NH, et al: Perinatal outcome of fetal complete atrioventricular block: a multicenter experience. J Am Coll Cardiol 17:1360–1366, 1991.

SUGGESTED READINGS

Callen PW: Amniotic fluid volume: its role in fetal health and disease. In Callen PW (ed): *Ultrasonography in Obstetrics and Gynecology*, 5th edition. Philadelphia, Saunders Elsevier, 2008, pp 758–779.

Drose JA: *Fetal Echocardiography*, 2nd edition. St. Louis, Saunders Elsevier, 2010.

Fleischer AC, Toy E, Lee W, et al (eds): *Sonography in Obstetrics and Gynecology: Principles and Practice*, 7th edition. New York, McGraw-Hill, 2011, ch 6.

Hagen-Ansert SL: The fetal thorax. In Hagen-Ansert SL (ed): *Textbook of Diagnostic Ultrasonography*, 7th edition. St. Louis, Elsevier Mosby, 2012, pp 1311–1322.

Joo S-J, Jaeggi E: Ultrasound evaluation of the fetal heart. In Callen PW (ed): *Ultrasonography in Obstetrics and Gynecology*, 5th edition. Philadelphia, Saunders Elsevier, 2008, pp 511–586.

Moss AJ, Adams FH, Emmanouilides GC: *Moss and Adams' Heart Disease in Infants, Children, and Adolescents: Including the Fetus and Young Adult*, 8th edition. Baltimore, Lippincott, Williams and Wilkins, 2013.

Stamm ER, Drose JA: The fetal heart. In Rumack CM, Wilson SR, Charboneau JW, et al (eds): *Diagnostic Ultrasound*, 4th edition. Philadelphia, Elsevier Mosby, 2011, pp 1294–1326.

CHAPTER 8

The Fetal Skeleton

Skeletal Anatomy

Skeletal Abnormalities

SKELETAL ANATOMY

The presence of calcium in the ossified portion of each fetal bone provides the acoustic impedance differential that produces the high-amplitude echoes characteristic of skeletal structures. While the nonossified, cartilaginous portions of skeletal structures can be visualized sonographically, the ossified components of each bone stand out in distinct contrast to adjacent soft tissue structures.

AXIAL SKELETON

The *axial skeleton* consists of the cranium, facial bones, pelvis, and spine.

- *Skull*: Cranium, frontal, temporal, occipital, and facial bones (Figure 8-1). The sphenoid bone and petrous ridges are seen at the base of skull separating the cranial fossae (Figure 8-2).
- *Facial bones*: Orbits, maxilla, mandible, and bony nasal septum (see Figure 8-1).
- *Pelvis*: Iliac ossification centers, seen from the early second trimester; ischial ossification centers are seen at about 20 menstrual weeks (Figure 8-3).
- *Spine*: Composed of three ossification centers, two posterior and one anterior. The spine can be seen with great clarity especially after 22 weeks. Sagittal images offer the best method of evaluation (Figures 8-4A and B).

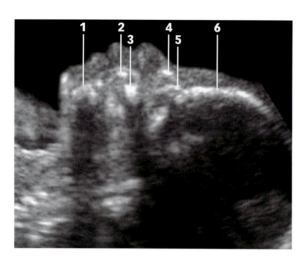

Figure 8-1. Sagittal section through the fetal face demonstrating normal skeletal anatomy of the frontal and facial bones. 1 = mandible, 2 = tooth bud, 3 = maxilla, 4 = nasal bone, 5 = orbital rim, 6 = frontal bone.

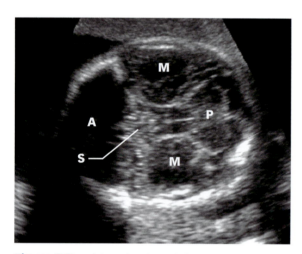

Figure 8-2. Axial section through the base of the fetal skull demonstrating cranial fossae. M = middle cranial fossa, A = anterior cranial fossa, P = posterior cranial fossa, S = sphenoid bone.

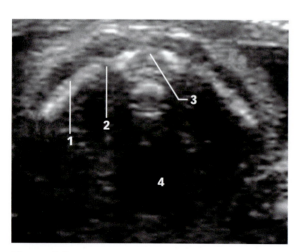

Figure 8-3. Fetal pelvis in transverse section. 1 = iliac ossification center, 2 = sacroiliac joint, 3 = sacrum, 4 = urinary bladder.

APPENDICULAR SKELETON

The *appendicular skeleton* consists of the bones of the appendages—the upper and lower extremities—most of which are well visualized by early to mid second trimester. The ossified portion of the long bones, particularly the proximal femora and humeri (Figures 8-5A and B), are easily seen and should be imaged during the course of a routine obstetric ultrasound examination. In the late third trimester, ossification centers begin to appear in the epiphyses (an *epiphysis* is the rounded end of a long bone located at its joint with an adjacent bone). These easily identified sonographic landmarks are indicators of fetal maturity. (See also Chapter 4, "Epiphyseal Appearance," pages 79–80.)

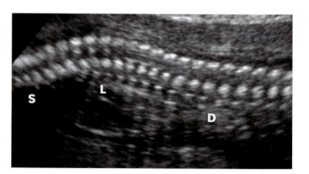

A

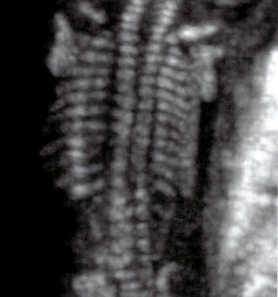

B

Figure 8-4. Ossification centers in the fetal spine. **A** Sagittal 2D section demonstrating sacral (S), lumbar (L), and dorsal (D) spine. **B** 3D coronal rendering through the entire fetal spine at 14 menstrual weeks.

Upper Extremity

In the upper extremity, the scapulae and clavicles can be seen by 7 menstrual weeks. The radius and ulna are routinely demonstrable by the mid second trimester and typically end distally at the same level. (Figure 8-6A). The fingers of the hand may be easier to visualize than the toes of the foot, because fingers are longer than toes. The metacarpals are well ossified by 16 menstrual weeks; the carpal bones remain cartilaginous throughout pregnancy and cannot be visualized sonographically, although the metacarpals can (Figure 8-6B). Although the fetal hand is frequently clenched in a fist-like position, which can hinder visualization, careful and persistent scanning will reveal all four fingers and the thumb in the normal fetus by the mid second trimester (Figure 8-6C).

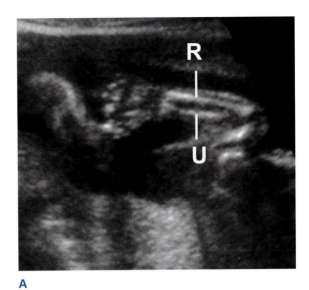

A

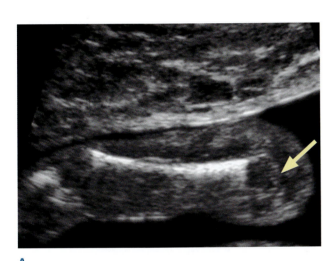

A

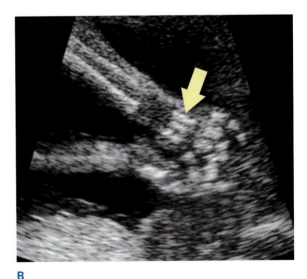

B

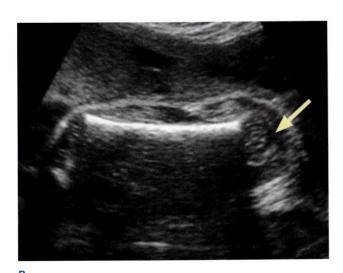

B

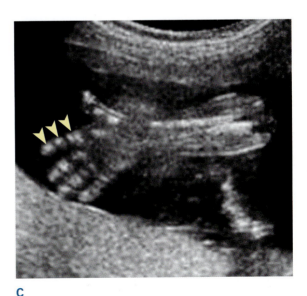

C

Figure 8-5. Proximal long bones easily demonstrable sonographically by the mid second trimester include **A** the femur and **B** the humerus; arrows = nonossified heads of these long bones.

Figure 8-6. **A** Distal long bones of the upper extremity: radius (R) and ulna (U). **B** Ossified metacarpal bones (arrow). **C** Fetal hand demonstrating proximal, mid, and distal phalanges (arrowheads).

Lower Extremity

In the lower extremity, the tibia, fibula, and ankle mortise are seen in the mid second trimester ending at about the same level proximally, with the fibula being slightly longer distally (Figure 8-7A). Fetal metatarsals can be identified by 16 menstrual weeks, and the toes, while smaller than fingers, can usually be imaged around the same age (Figures 8-7B and C). While the other tarsal bones do not begin the ossification process until after birth, the partially ossified calcaneus appears between the fifth and sixth months (Figure 8-7D).

As in the upper extremity, ossification centers begin appearing in the long bones of the lower extremity in the late third trimester—first in the distal femoral epiphysis and later in the proximal tibial epiphysis. In normal female fetuses, the distal femoral epiphysis ossifies at about 32 menstrual weeks and the proximal tibial epiphysis ossifies at about 35 weeks. In males, the ossification of these epiphyses occurs about 2 weeks later. The patella can also be visualized, but this bone does not ossify until after birth.

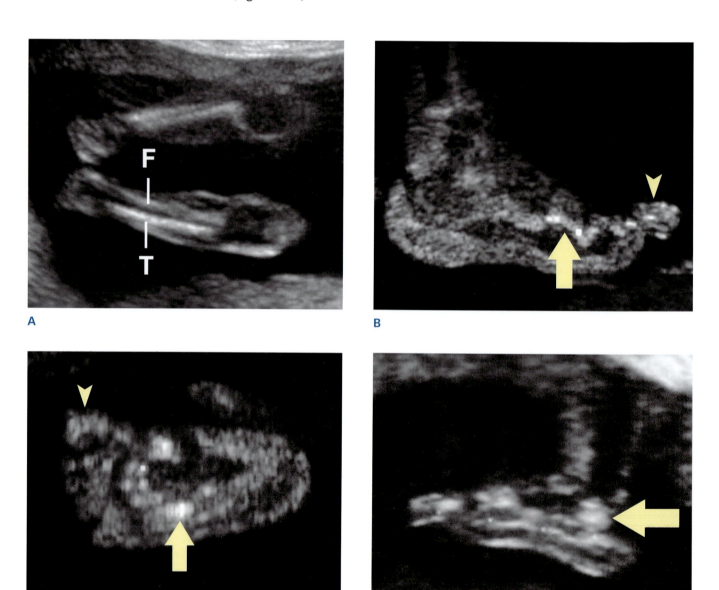

Figure 8-7. A Distal long bones of the lower extremity: tibia (T) and fibula (F). **B** Lateral and **C** plantar views of a fetal foot at 16 menstrual weeks demonstrating the metatarsals (arrows) and toes (arrowheads). **D** Partially ossified calcaneus (arrow) at 20 weeks.

SKELETAL ABNORMALITIES

The spectrum of fetal skeletal abnormalities is vast—from minor defects associated with the malformation of a single bone to systemic disorders that are lethal as early as 24 menstrual weeks' gestation. While it is improbable that single, minor bony defects will be detected during the course of a routine obstetric sonographic examination, skeletal abnormalities that are incompatible with life or that are associated with poor perinatal outcomes present such dramatic imaging findings that they can reliably be detected prenatally. Such lethal anomalies not only alter the normal appearance of the bony skeleton but also result in somatic variations that make them readily apparent. There are many ways to classify skeletal anomalies and syndromes. The schema followed in this chapter is outlined in Table 8-1.

DEFINITION OF TERMS

Since most lethal skeletal dysplasias are associated with shortening of the limbs, command of the medical terminology that describes the type and extent of limb shortening is an integral part of the sonographic examination (Figure 8-8). The following terms are key:

- *Rhizomelia*: shortening of the proximal segment of an extremity (such as the humerus or the femur) (Figure 8-8B)

Table 8-1. Summary of prenatally detectable skeletal anomalies.

Type of Abnormality	Anomaly
Osteochondrodysplasias	Defects of growth of tubular bones
	Disorganized development of cartilage and fibrous skeleton
	Abnormalities of density of cortex
Idiopathic osteolyses	Osteogenesis imperfecta
	Hypophosphatasia
Dysostoses	With cranial and facial involvement
	With predominant axial involvement
	With predominant involvement of extremities

- *Mesomelia*: shortening of the distal segment of an extremity (such as the radius/ulna or the tibula/fibula) (Figure 8-8C)
- *Micromelia*: shortening of both proximal and distal segments of an extremity (Figure 8-8D)
- *Amelia*: absence of an extremity

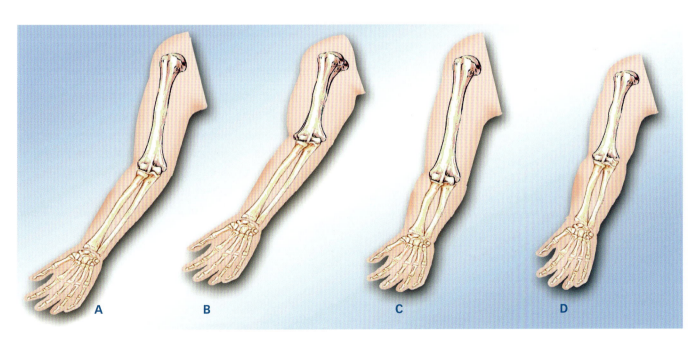

Figure 8-8. Schematic demonstration of the types of limb-shortening anomalies associated with skeletal dysplasias. **A** Normal. **B** Rhizomelia. **C** Mesomelia. **D** Severe micromelia. (Figure continues . . .)

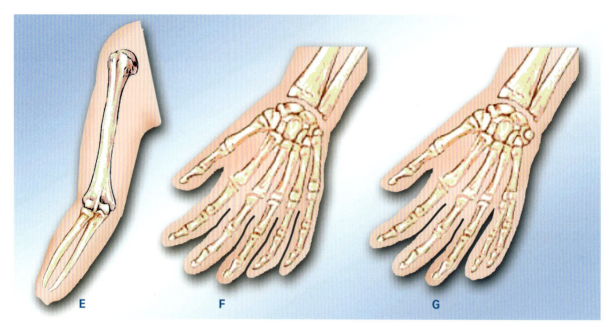

Figure 8-8, continued. E Meromelia. **F** Polydactyly. **G** Syndactyly.

- *Meromelia*: partial absence of a limb (Figure 8-8E)
- *Polydactyly*: presence of more than five digits on a single hand or foot (fingers or toes) (Figure 8-8F)
- *Syndactyly*: soft tissue or bony fusion of digits (fingers or toes) (Figure 8-8G)

SONOGRAPHIC CONSIDERATIONS

In addition to the routine sonographic examination of the fetus, the following must be assessed more carefully if a short-limb skeletal dysplasia is suspected:

- *Long bones*: All the long bones—including both femora, tibiae, fibulae, humeri, radiae, and ulnae—should be imaged and the lengths measured. Also, the morphology of the long bones and the sonographic reflectivity of the long bones should be evaluated.
- *Fetal skull*: The shape and density of the skull should be evaluated. If the skull appears to be underossified, compressing the skull with the transducer (see Figures 8-14K and L, page 211) may indicate whether the skull is abnormally flexible.
- *Fetal ribs and chest*: If a fetal skeletal dysplasia is suspected, fetal chest circumference should be obtained at the level of the fetal heart, and the length and character of the ribs should be observed. Irregular or fractured ribs should be noted. The fetal scapula should be specifically imaged in transverse and longitudinal planes.
- *Fetal spine*: The fetal spine should be imaged with particular attention to the ossified vertebral bodies.
- *Fetal hands and feet*: The fetal hands and feet should be carefully examined to evaluate the length of the fingers and toes, to check for polydactyly or syndactyly, and to check for positioning abnormalities such as clubfeet or rocker bottom feet.
- *Fetal face*: During the late second and early third trimesters, there may be clues in the appearance of the fetal face that will help differentiate among skeletal dysplasias.

OSTEOCHONDRODYSPLASIAS

Osteochondrodysplasias—also called *skeletal dysplasias* or *short-limb dysplasias*—are a group of skeletal anomalies resulting from abnormalities of bony formation. There are several ways to categorize the broad spectrum of specific manifestations that skeletal dysplasias present. From a sonographic imaging perspective, it is useful to separate them into two general categories:

- Long bones that are notably shortened before 20 menstrual weeks
- Long bones that are notably shortened later in the pregnancy

Skeletal dysplasias in which limbs are notably short before 20 weeks are usually lethal at birth. In the much larger group of skeletal dysplasias occurring after 20 weeks, fetal limb lengths are more mildly shortened; in this group, the limbs will not demonstrate significant shortening until the end of the second trimester. Only a few of these conditions can be specifically identified in utero.

Achondrogenesis

Achondrogenesis is a rare, lethal form of short-limb dysplasia in which there is virtually no ossification of the vertebral bodies; however, the posterior elements of the spine may demonstrate the presence of normal calcification. There are two types:

Type I, also known as *Parenti-Fraccaro achondrogenesis*, is characterized by:

- Absent vertebral ossification centers
- Incomplete ossification of the skull
- Rib fractures
- Extremely short and stubby arms
- Head that is not enlarged compared to the trunk

Type II, also known as *Langer-Saldino achondrogenesis*, is characterized by:

- Head that is large compared to the body
- Prominent skin folds over a short neck
- Small chest
- Distended abdomen and possible fetal hydrops
- Very short limbs held away from the body

Associated Abnormalities

In addition to the plethora of anatomic abnormalities listed above, the following abnormalities are characteristically associated with achondrogenesis:

- Intrauterine growth restriction (IUGR)
- Cleft soft palate
- Cystic hygroma
- Hydrops fetalis

Sonographic Signs

The following are the characteristic sonographic signs of achondrogenesis:

- Lack of vertebral ossification (Figures 8-9A and B)
- Small chest (Figures 8-9A and B)
- Large head with slightly decreased ossification of the cranium, or caput membranaceum (Figures 8-9C and D)
- Severely shortened limbs, usually involving all limbs (Figures 8-9E and F)

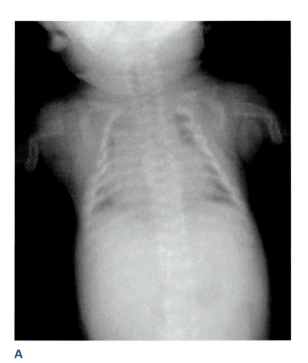
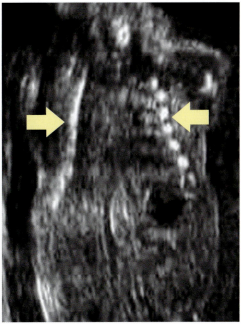

A **B**

Figure 8-9. Achondrogenesis. **A** Postnatal radiograph demonstrating diminished ossification in vertebrae and ribs. **B** Prenatal sonogram demonstrating small chest (arrows). (Figure continues . . .)

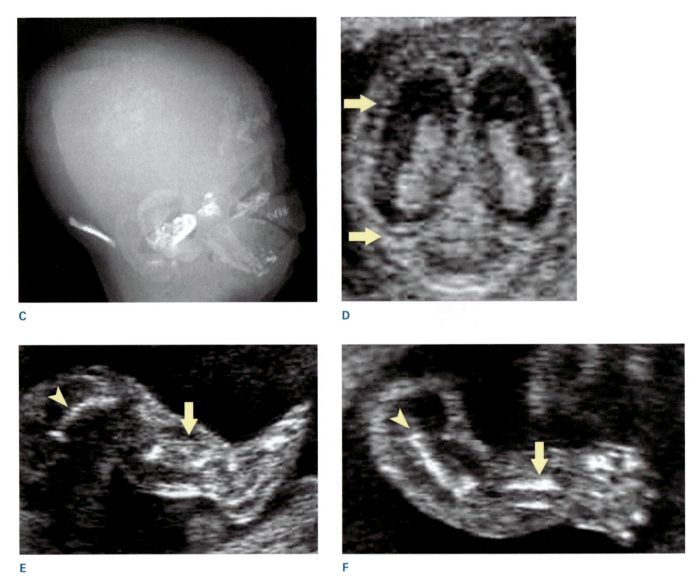

Figure 8-9, continued. C Postnatal radiograph demonstrating caput membranaceum. **D** Prenatal sonogram demonstrating caput membranaceum; arrows = diminished ossification of the cranial bones. **E** Micromelia of the lower extremity and **F** micromelia of the upper extremity; arrows = shortened distal segments, arrowheads = shortened proximal segments.

Achondroplasia

Achondroplasia is a genetic disorder that affects normal growth and development of the skeletal system. It is the most common cause of short-limb dwarfism, occurring in approximately 1 in 25,000–50,000 births. It may be transmitted as either a heterozygous or a homozygous trait.

Heterozygous achondroplasia is the nonlethal type and is characterized by mild rhizomelic shortening of the limbs and drop-off of femur length after 20 menstrual weeks. Heterozygous achondroplasia may be difficult to diagnose prenatally unless one of the parents has achondroplasia. *Homozygous dominant achondroplasia* is the lethal, short-limb type and occurs in fetuses in which both parents have achondroplasia. In 80% of homozygous cases, a spontaneous genetic mutation is the cause. In some cases, the trait is carried as autosomal dominant.

Associated Abnormalities

Other abnormalities and anatomic anomalies associated with both types of achondroplasia include the following:

- Macrocephaly
- Low nasal bridge with prominent forehead
- Mid-facial hypoplasia

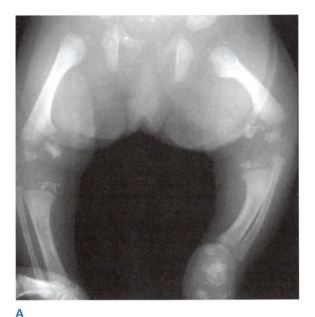 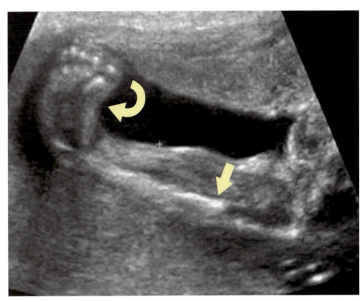

Figure 8-10. Heterozygous achondroplasia—rhizomelia. **A** Postnatal radiograph. **B** Prenatal sonogram; straight arrow = femur, curved arrow = concomitant talipes equinovarus (clubfoot).

- Small cuboidal vertebral bodies
- Short, tubular bones
- Trident hand
- Hydrocephalus
- Spinal cord compression

Sonographic Signs

The following are the characteristic sonographic signs of achondroplasia:

- Rhizomelia (Figures 8-10A and B)
- Frontal bossing of the skull
- Abnormal femur length measurements:
  ▸ Homozygous: femur length below the 5th percentile by the second trimester
  ▸ Heterozygous: normal femur length prior to 20 menstrual weeks
  ▸ Femur lengths below the 99% prediction interval by 27 weeks

Thanatophoric Dysplasia

Thanatophoric dysplasia is the most common short-limb skeletal dysplasia, with a reported incidence of 1 in 25,000 births.[1] It is a lethal skeletal dysplasia characterized by extreme rhizomelia, bowed long bones, a hypoplastic thorax with normal trunk length, and a relatively large head. The fetal long-bone lengths may be normal until 12–13 weeks. The vertebral bodies are typically flattened (a condition called *platyspondyly*). It is the extremely narrowed chest and pulmonary hypoplasia that give rise to postnatal respiratory distress, which is the typical cause of death.

Thanatophoric dysplasia is associated with numerous anatomic abnormalities, including cloverleaf skull (kleeblattschädel), horseshoe kidney, atrial septal defects, and imperforate anus. Cloverleaf skull results from premature closure of coronal and lambdoidal sutures and is pathognomonic for this condition.

Associated Abnormalities

The following abnormalities are characteristically associated with thanatophoric dysplasia:

- Macrocephaly
- Hydrocephalus
- Patent ductus arteriosus
- Atrial septal defect
- Horseshoe kidney
- Hydronephrosis
- Imperforate anus

Sonographic Signs

The following are the characteristic sonographic signs of thanatophoric dysplasia:

- Markedly shortened and densely ossified bowed long bones

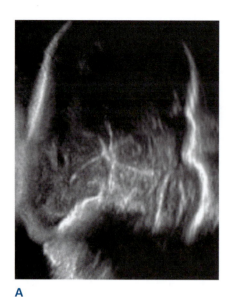
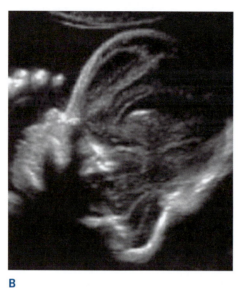
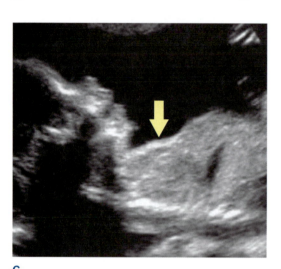
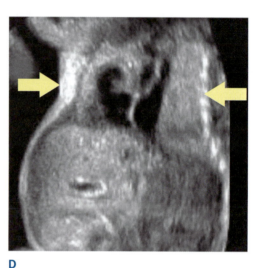

Figure 8-11. Thanatophoric dysplasia. **A** Coronal section demonstrating cloverleaf skull. **B** Cloverleaf skull in sagittal section. **C** Bell-shaped chest (hypoplastic thorax) in sagittal section; arrow = diminished thoracic volume. **D** Bell-shaped chest in coronal section; arrows = diminished thoracic volume. (Figure continues . . .)

- Cloverleaf and relatively large skull (Figures 8-11A and B)
- Hypoplastic thorax (bell-shaped chest) (Figures 8-11C and D)
- Trident hand deformity (Figures 8-11E and F)
- Polyhydramnios (71% of cases)
- Flattened vertebral bodies

Short Rib–Polydactyly Syndrome

Short rib–polydactyly syndrome (SRPS) is a lethal osteochondrodysplasia characterized by short limbs (micromelia), an excessive number of digits (polydactyly), and an extremely narrowed thorax. Typically the trunk is short with horizontal ribs that reach only to the posterior axillary line. There are two types—type I (Saldino-Noonan) and type II (Majewski)—which manifest differences in concomitant craniofacial, cardiac, and long-bone anomalies. However, both result in lethal postnatal respiratory insufficiency secondary to severe pulmonary hypoplasia. Commonalities also include a wide range of genitourinary and cloacal abnormalities.[2] An association with choroid plexus cysts has also been reported.[3]

Associated Abnormalities

The following abnormalities are characteristically associated with short rib–polydactyly syndrome:

- Cardiac defects:
  - Double-outlet right ventricle
  - Endocardial cushion defect
  - Hypoplastic right heart
- Polycystic kidneys
- Imperforate anus

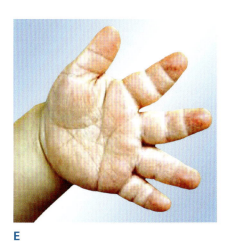
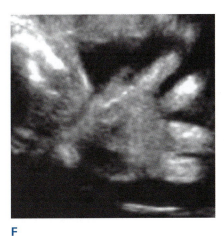

Figure 8-11, continued. E Postnatal gross pathologic appearance of trident hand deformity. **F** Sonographic appearance of trident hand deformity.

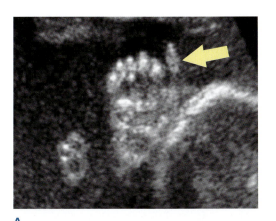
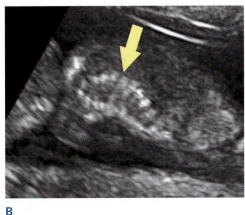
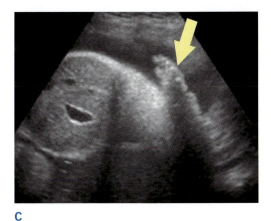
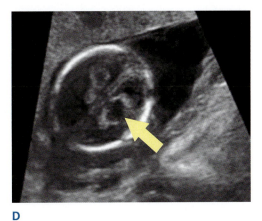

Figure 8-12. Short rib–polydactyly syndrome. **A** Polydactyly; arrow = extra digit. **B** Narrowed thorax with short ribs (arrow). **C** Extreme micromelia (arrow), upper extremity. **D** Choroid plexus cysts (arrow).

Sonographic Signs

The following are the characteristic sonographic signs of short rib–polydactyly syndrome:

- Polydactyly (Figure 8-12A)
- Narrowed thorax (Figure 8-12B)
- Striking micromelia (Figure 8-12C)
- Choroid plexus cysts (Figure 8-12D)

Campomelic Dysplasia

Campomelic dysplasia is a rare osteochondrodysplasia reported to occur in 1 in 100,000–200,000 births. It is alternatively referred to as *campomelia*, from the French word meaning "bent limb." The limb shortening is variable, but specific features—such as a sharp midfemoral bend on each side—may suggest the diagnosis. Bowing of the distal tibia and/or a short fibula may occur as well. Clubfeet are common. The prognosis for this condition is variable, but there is a high mortality rate during early postnatal life. Demise is associated with a wide range of concomitant anomalies found in campomelic dysplasia.

Associated Abnormalities

The following abnormalities are characteristically associated with campomelic dysplasia:[4]

- Hydrocephalus
- Genitourinary and gonadal dysgenesis
- Micrognathia
- Hydronephrosis
- Cardiovascular anomalies:
  - Patent ductus arteriosus
  - Ventricular septal defects
  - Coarctation of the aorta
- Inner ear anomalies resulting in hearing loss
- Polyhydramnios

Sonographic Signs

The following are the characteristic sonographic signs of campomelic dysplasia:

- Severe bowing of long bones, especially in the lower extremity (Figures 8-13A, B, and C)
- Narrowed thorax (Figure 8-13D)
- Hypoplastic scapulae (Figure 8-13E)
- Associated hydronephrosis or hydrocephalus

Asphyxiating Thoracic Dystrophy

Asphyxiating thoracic dystrophy, also called *Jeune thoracic dystrophy* or *Jeune syndrome*, is a short-limb skeletal dysplasia sometimes classified as a type of short rib–polydactyly syndrome. It is characterized by a severely narrowed thorax, renal cystic dysplasia, polydactyly, and biliary dysgenesis. It is not uniformly lethal; however, the long-term prognosis for those who survive the neonatal period is poor, with renal failure,

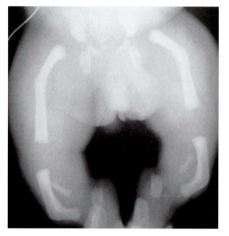
A

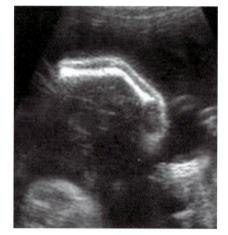
B

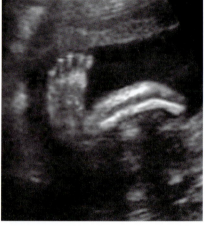
C

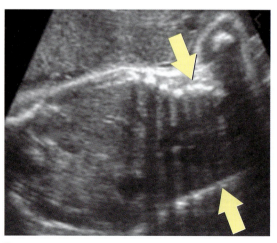
D

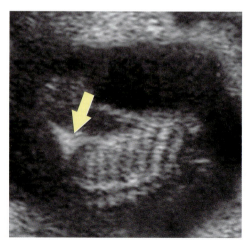
E

Figure 8-13. Campomelic dysplasia. **A** Limb bowing, postnatal radiograph. **B** Bowed femur, longitudinal sonographic appearance. **C** Bowed tibia with clubfoot, lateral sonographic view. **D** Narrowed thorax; arrows = short ribs and diminished thoracic volume. **E** Hypoplastic scapula (arrow).

hepatic dysfunction, and chronic pulmonary problems all contributing to the demise of the individual.

Associated Abnormalities

The following abnormalities are characteristically associated with asphyxiating thoracic dystrophy:

- Polydactyly
- Lacunar skull
- Situs inversus
- Pancreatic cysts

Sonographic Signs

The following are the characteristic sonographic signs of asphyxiating thoracic dystrophy:

- Shortened long bones
- Narrowed thorax
- Cystic dysplastic kidneys
- Polydactyly

Metatropic Dysplasia

Another rare condition that is diagnosable in utero is *metatropic dysplasia*. This condition is characterized by a small thorax, severe thoracic kyphoscoliosis, and short limbs with flaring enlargement of the metaphyseal ends of the bones. As a result there is usually restricted mobility of the knee and hip joints. Macrocephaly with ventriculomegaly may be present.

Associated Abnormalities

The following abnormalities are characteristically associated with metatropic dypalsia:

- Macrocephaly
- Ventriculomegaly
- Spinal cord compression

Sonographic Signs

The following are the characteristic sonographic signs of metatropic dysplasia:

- Shortened long bones
- Narrowed thorax

Chondroectodermal Dysplasia

Also called *Ellis–van Creveld syndrome*, *chondroectodermal dysplasia* is a type of osteochondrodysplasia characterized by disproportionate and irregularly shortened extremities, polydactyly, and a narrowed thorax. It is associated about half the time with an atrial septal defect, often with a single atrium.

Associated Abnormalities

The following abnormalities may be associated with chondroectodermal dysplasia:

- Mental retardation
- Dandy-Walker malformation
- Cryptorchidism
- Talipes equinovarus
- Renal agenesis

Sonographic Signs

The following are the characteristic sonographic signs of chondroectodermal dysplasia:

- Shortened long bones
- Narrow thorax
- Polydactyly

Rhizomelic Chondrodysplasia Punctata

Rhizomelic chondrodysplasia punctata is an autosomal recessive type of osteochondrodysplasia, the dominant feature of which is proximal limb shortening. There is typically symmetric shortening of both femora and humeri, a low nasal bridge, congenital cataracts, respiratory problems, and significant delays in growth and mental development. Most of these individuals die before reaching two years of age.

Associated Abnormalities

The following abnormalities may be associated with rhizomelic chondrodysplasia punctata:

- Microcephaly
- Multiple joint contractures

Sonographic Signs

The following are the characteristic sonographic signs of rhizomelic chondrodysplasia punctata:

- Symmetric shortening of the proximal long bones (humerus/femur)
- Low nasal bridge

IDIOPATHIC OSTEOLYSES

The idiopathic osteolyses are rare autosomal dominant bone disorders characterized by abnormal bone remodeling in which the normal ossification process fails. The two types most commonly encountered prenatally are osteogenesis imperfecta and hypophosphatasia.

Osteogenesis Imperfecta

Osteogenesis imperfecta (OI) is a disorder of production, secretion, or function of type I collagen, which serves as the matrix upon which bone is built. There are eight types, ranging from mild manifestation of clinical features to severe, lethal forms that are deemed incompatible with life when detected in utero. The overriding characteristic of osteogenesis imperfecta is hypomineralization of bone, resulting in abnormal fragility of skeletal structures. In utero fractures result in long-bone shortening. Neonates with osteogenesis imperfecta are at risk for delivery trauma leading to intracranial hemorrhage and stillbirth. There is no known treatment.

Associated Abnormalities

The following abnormalities are characteristically associated with osteogenesis imperfecta:

- Intrauterine growth restriction (IUGR)
- Macrocephaly
- Umbilical hernia

Hypophosphatasia

Similar in manifestation to osteogenesis imperfecta, *hypophosphatasia* is a metabolic disorder that results in demineralization of bony structures. Rather than being a disorder of collagen production, however, it is a deficiency of serum alkaline phosphatase that produces the clinical and anatomic abnormalities associated with this condition.

There are several subtypes of hypophosphatasia; it is the perinatal subtype that is uniformly lethal and that is detectable in utero. The hallmark sonographic findings are similar to those found in osteogenesis imperfecta: The fetal long bones are markedly shortened with deep cupping of the metaphyses, the ribs may be short and fragmented, and the skull may be markedly underossified. The spine may have groups of three ossified vertebral bodies followed by three unossified and then another three ossified in an alternating pattern.

Associated Abnormalities

The following abnormalities are characteristically associated with hypophosphatasia:

- Polyhydramnios
- Intrauterine growth restriction (IUGR)

Sonographic Signs

The sonographic signs of the various forms of idiopathic osteolysis are essentially the same and include:

- Presence of long-bone fractures or excessive callus formation (Figures 8-14A, B, and C)
- Rib cage deformity with fractures (Figures 8-14D and E)
- Drastically shortened long-bone length with bowing (Figures 8-14F, G, and H)
- Hypomineralized skeletal structures (Figure 8-14I)
- Enhanced spatial resolution of intracranial anatomy and increased posterior acoustic enhancement due to hypomineralized skull bones (Figure 8-14J)
- Decreased calvarial ossification, permitting deformity when compressed with a transducer or by accompanying oligohydramnios (Figures 8-14K and L)

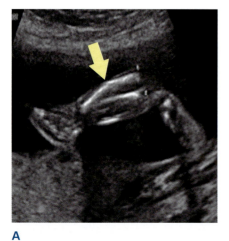
A

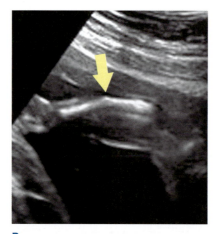
B

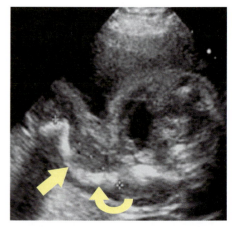
C

Figure 8-14. Osteogenesis imperfecta. Long bone fractures (arrows) of **A** the tibia, **B** the radius, and **C** the femur; curved arrow = callus formation. (Figure continues . . .)

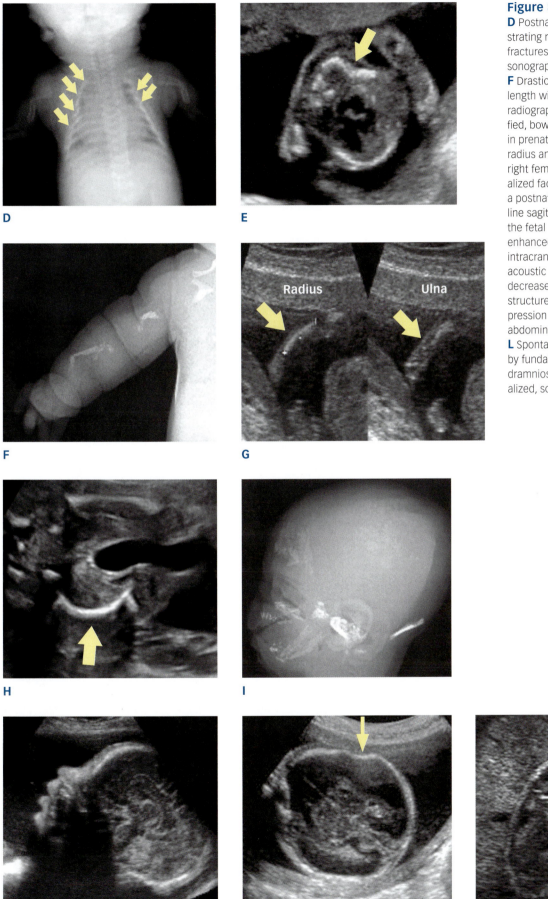

Figure 8-14, continued.
D Postnatal radiograph demonstrating multiple bilateral rib fractures (arrows). **E** Prenatal sonographic correlation (arrow). **F** Drastically shortened long-bone length with bowing in postnatal radiograph. **G** Shortened, deossified, bowed long bones (arrows) in prenatal sonogram showing radius and ulna. **H** Bowing of the right femur (arrow). **I** Hypomineralized facial bones and calvaria in a postnatal radiograph. **J** Midline sagittal section through the fetal head demonstrating enhanced spatial resolution of intracranial anatomy and absent acoustic shadowing resulting from decreased ossification of skeletal structures. **K** Focal cranial compression deformity from transabdominal transducer pressure. **L** Spontaneous cranial deformity by fundal placenta and oligohydramnios resulting from demineralized, soft cranial bones.

DYSOSTOSES

A *dysostosis* is an isolated bony malformation that may occur alone or in conjunction with various syndromes. It results from the defective ossification of fetal cartilage.

Radial Ray Anomaly

A *radial ray anomaly* is the partial to complete absence of the radius, usually associated with abnormalities of the bones in the wrist and thumb. There is a large spectrum of specific appearances: The radius may be shortened, curved, or absent, often with the hand in medial rotation.

Associated Abnormalities

A radial array anomaly is a component of many syndromes, including the following:

- Trisomy 18 (Edwards syndrome)
- Amniotic band syndrome
- Holt-Oram syndrome
- VACTERL association (vertebral defects, anal atresia, cardiac defects, tracheoesophageal fistula, renal anomalies, and limb abnormalities)
- In utero teratogen exposure, especially to thalidomide and valproic acid

Sonographic Signs

The following are the characteristic sonographic signs of radial ray anomaly[5] (Figures 8-15A and B):

- Absent or hypoplastic radius
- Sharp medial rotation of the hand
- Absent thumb in some cases

Talipes Equinovarus

Talipes equinovarus, better known as *clubfoot*, is the most common skeletal anomaly detected during routine obstetric sonographic examination. It is estimated to occur in 0.5%–5% of live births.[6] Clubfoot can occur as an isolated anomaly or in association with a broad spectrum of other anatomic abnormalities and syndromes. The etiology can be genetic, environmental, or associated with uterine constraint resulting from oligohydramnios, amniotic band syndrome, and/or uterine tumors. There are scores of associated anomalous conditions and they include chromosomal and other syndromes, genitourinary and spinal anomalies, and connective tissue disorders. Sonographic detection is based on knowledge of the relative orientation of the foot and lower extremity long bones. When the tibia and fibula are imaged in a lateral view, the foot should also appear in a lateral view; in talipes, with the lower leg in a lateral view, the foot will appear in an anteroposterior (AP) view. The pathologic changes in the foot include inversion of the foot, with flexion of the sole and deviation of the navicular bone closer to the medial aspect of the calcaneus (Figures 8-16A, B, and C).

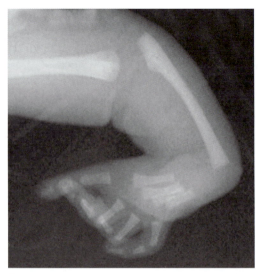

A

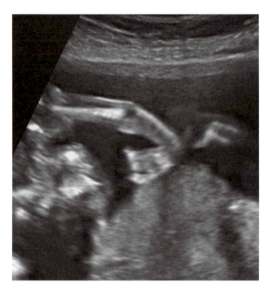

B

Figure 8-15. Radial ray anomaly. **A** Postnatal radiograph. **B** Prenatal sonographic appearance.

Associated Abnormalities

Although clubfoot can be associated with numerous anomalous conditions and syndromes, the following

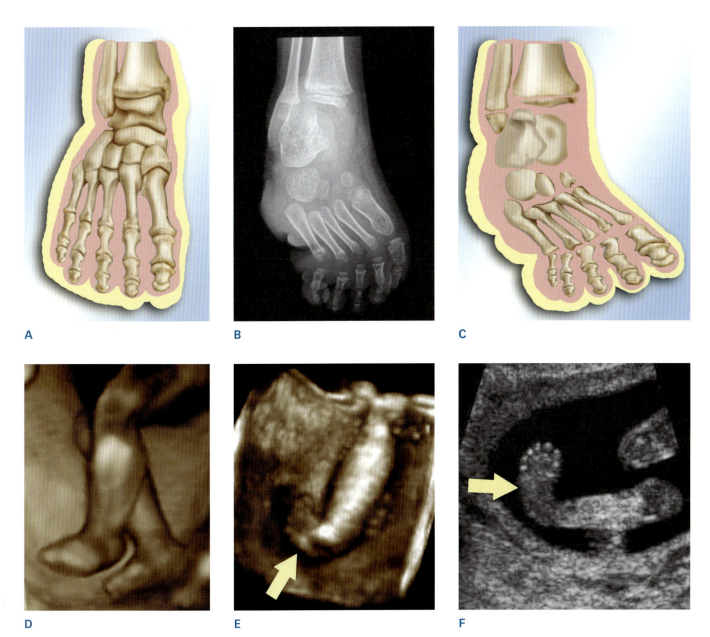

Figure 8-16. Talipes equinovarus (clubfoot). **A** Schematic of normal foot anatomy. **B** Radiograph of clubfoot. **C** Schematic of clubfoot anatomy. **D** 3D surface rendering of a normal foot. **E** 3D surface rendering of a clubfoot (arrow); note medial deviation of the foot and flexion of the sole. **F** Standard 2D imaging of a clubfoot (arrow).

abnormalities are characteristically associated with talipes equinovarus and are among the more commonly encountered:

- Meckel-Gruber syndrome
- Triploidy syndrome
- Ehlers-Danlos syndrome
- Ellis–van Creveld syndrome
- Noonan syndrome
- Trisomy 13 (Patau syndrome)
- Trisomy 18 (Edwards syndrome)

Sonographic Signs

The following are the characteristic sonographic signs of talipes equinovarus (Figures 8-16A–F):

- Foot deviated from the normal position
- Inversion of the foot and flexion of the sole

Rocker Bottom Foot

In a rocker bottom foot, there is dorsal and lateral dislocation of the talonavicular joint and a prominent calcaneus mimicking the appearance of the rocker of a rocking chair. The presence of a rocker bottom foot in an antenatal ultrasound scan is sometimes classified as a soft sign of aneuploidic anomalies.

Associated Abnormalities

The following abnormalities may be associated with rocker bottom foot:

- Trisomy 13 (Patau syndrome)
- Trisomy 18 (Edwards syndrome)
- 18q deletion syndrome
- Spina bifida

Sonographic Signs and Diagnostic Criteria

The characteristic sonographic sign of rocker bottom foot is visualization of a convex, rounded sole of the foot (Figures 8-17A and B).

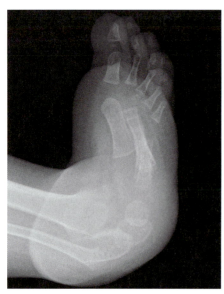

A

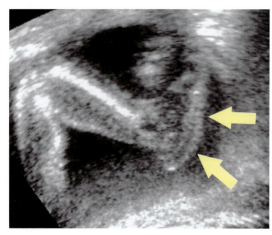

B

Figure 8-17. Rocker bottom foot. **A** Radiographic and **B** sonographic demonstrations of a convex, rounded sole (arrows).

CHAPTER 8 REVIEW QUESTIONS

1. The axial skeleton consists of all of these bony structures EXCEPT:
   A. Long bones
   B. Cranium
   C. Facial bones
   D. Pelvis

2. This image best demonstrates:

   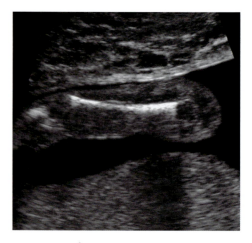

   A. Normal ossified metaphysis
   B. Normal ossified epiphysis
   C. Femoral bowing
   D. Micromelia

3. Congenital limb shortening that affects both proximal and distal segments of an extremity is called:
   A. Rhizomelia
   B. Mesomelia
   C. Micromelia
   D. Amelia

4. Congenital limb shortening that affects only the proximal segment of an extremity is called:
   A. Rhizomelia
   B. Mesomelia
   C. Micromelia
   D. Amelia

5. The presence of more than five digits on a single hand or foot is called:
   A. Syndactyly
   B. Mesomelia
   C. Polydactyly
   D. Exodactyly

6. Congenital skeletal syndromes characterized by abnormal shortening of the long bones resulting from abnormalities of bony formation are called:
   A. Achondrogenesis
   B. Osteochondrodysplasia
   C. Osteogenesis imperfecta
   D. Hypophosphatasia

7. Abnormal congenital hypomineralization of fetal bony structure is called:
   A. Achondrogenesis
   B. Osteochondrodysplasia
   C. Osteogenesis imperfecta
   D. Campomelic dysplasia

8. The hallmark sonographic finding in a fetus affected by campomelic dysplasia is:
   A. Bell-shaped chest
   B. Severe demineralization of the long bones
   C. Absent vertebral ossification
   D. Severe bowing of the long bones

9. All of the following congenital skeletal abnormalities are types of osteochondrodysplasia EXCEPT:
   A. Hypophosphatasia
   B. Asphyxiating thoracic dystrophy
   C. Metatropic dysplasia
   D. Chondroectodermal dysplasia

10. The idiopathic osteolyses are a group of congenital skeletal abnormalities characterized primarily by:
    A. Severe micromelia
    B. Hypomineralization of bone
    C. Polydactyly
    D. Bell-shaped thorax

11. Congenital clubfoot is also known as:
    A. Noonan syndrome
    B. Radial ray anomaly
    C. Pectus excavatum
    D. Talipes equinovarus

12. Dorsal and lateral dislocation of the talonavicular joint with a prominent calcaneus is called:
    A. Talipes equinovarus
    B. Clubfoot
    C. Rocker bottom foot
    D. Syndactyly

13. An isolated bony malformation that may occur alone or in conjunction with various syndromes is called:
    A. Dysostosis
    B. Osteochondrodysplasia
    C. Achondroplasia
    D. Achondrogenesis

14. The congenital skeletal abnormality characterized primarily by absent ossification of the vertebral bodies is:
    A. Achondrogenesis
    B. Thanatophoric dysplasia
    C. Achondroplasia
    D. Diastrophic dysplasia

15. A cloverleaf skull and a bell-shaped chest are two hallmark sonographic findings in which type of fetal skeletal abnormality?
    A. Short rib–polydactyly syndrome
    B. Campomelic dysplasia
    C. Chondrodysplasia punctata
    D. Thanatophoric dysplasia

16. This image best demonstrates:

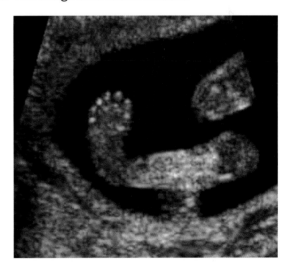

   A. Talipes equinovarus
   B. Rocker bottom foot
   C. Amniotic band syndrome
   D. Radial ray anomaly

17. This image best demonstrates:

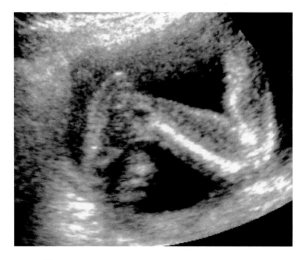

   A. Talipes equinovarus
   B. Rocker bottom foot
   C. Amniotic band syndrome
   D. Radial ray anomaly

18. The nonlethal skeletal dysplasia characterized by mild rhizomelic shortening of the limbs and drop-off of femur length after 20 menstrual weeks is:
   A. Achondrogenesis
   B. Achondroplasia
   C. Thanatophoric dysplasia
   D. Campomelic dysplasia

19. Parenti-Fraccaro and Langer-Saldino are two types of:
   A. Achondroplasia
   B. Idiopathic osteolysis
   C. Achondrogenesis
   D. Dysostosis

20. Syndactly is defined as:
   A. Presence of extra digits on a single hand or foot
   B. Partial absence of a limb
   C. Absence of an extremity
   D. Soft tissue or bony fusion of digits

21. The lethal type of short-limb dysplasia characterized by severe rhizomelic shortening of the limbs, limb bowing, lordotic spine, and a bulky head is:
   A. Homozygous dominant achondroplasia
   B. Heterozygous achondroplasia
   C. Short rib–polydactyly syndrome
   D. Osteogenesis imperfecta

22. Campomelic dysplasia is characterized by all of the following sonographic findings EXCEPT:
   A. Hydrocephalus
   B. Micrognathia
   C. Narrowed thorax
   D. Cloverleaf skull

23. One of the congenital metabolic disorders that results in demineralization of fetal bone is:
   A. Hypophosphatasia
   B. Radial ray anomaly
   C. Talipes equinovarus
   D. Meckel-Gruber syndrome

24. This image of the femur best demonstrates:

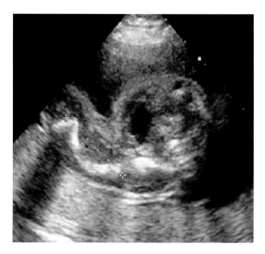

   A. Radial ray anomaly
   B. Homozygous achondroplasia
   C. Heterozygous achondroplasia
   D. Osteogenesis imperfecta

25. The anatomic abnormality demonstrated in this image is a hallmark sonographic finding in:

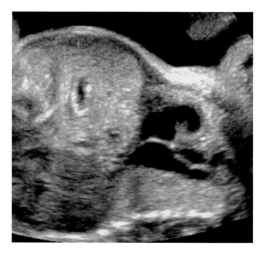

A. Osteogenesis imperfecta
B. Thanatophoric dysplasia
C. Campomelic dysplasia
D. Heterozygous achondroplasia

ANSWERS

See Appendix A on page 480 for answers.

REFERENCES

1. Miller E, Blaser S, Shannon P, et al: Brain and bone abnormalities of thanatophoric dwarfism. Am J Roentgenol 192:48–51, 2009.

2. Jones KL (ed): *Smith's Recognizable Patterns of Human Malformation*, 5th edition. Philadelphia, Saunders, 1997, pp 334–336.

3. Chen CP, Chang TY, Chen CY, et al: Short rib–polydactyly syndrome type II (Majewski): prenatal diagnosis, perinatal imaging findings and molecular analysis of the NEK1 gene. Taiwan J Obstet Gynecol 51:100–105, 2012.

4. Gilbert-Barnes E: Pathological case of the month. Arch Pediatr Adolesc Med 154:748, 2000.

5. Ryu JK, Cho JY, Choi JS: Prenatal sonographic diagnosis of focal musculoskeletal anomalies. Korean J Radiol 4:243–251, 2003.

6. Bromley B, Benacerraf B: Abnormalities of the hands and feet in the fetus: sonographic findings. Am J Roentgen 165:1239–1243, 1995.

SUGGESTED READINGS

Fleischer AC, Toy E, Lee W, et al (eds): *Sonography in Obstetrics and Gynecology: Principles and Practice*, 7th edition. New York, McGraw-Hill, 2011, ch 19.

Glanc P, Chitayat D, Unger S: The fetal musculoskeletal system. In Rumack CM, Wilson SR, Charboneau JW, et al (eds): *Diagnostic Ultrasound*, 4th edition. Philadelphia, Elsevier Mosby, 2011, pp 1389–1423.

Goncalves LF, Kusanovic JP, Gotsch F, et al: The fetal musculoskeletal system. In Callen PW (ed): *Ultrasonography in Obstetrics and Gynecology*, 5th edition. Philadelphia, Saunders Elsevier, 2008, pp 419–492.

Henningsen CG: The fetal skeleton. In Hagen-Ansert SL (ed): *Textbook of Diagnostic Ultrasonography*, 7th edition. St. Louis, Elsevier Mosby, 2012, pp 1380–1394.

CHAPTER 9
The Fetal Abdomen and Pelvis

Embryology

Abdominal and Pelvic Anatomy

Abdominal and Pelvic Abnormalities

The fetal abdomen and related anatomic structures typically are examined in serial transverse planes of section. Morphologically, the abdomen has a smooth, rounded contour covered externally by a contiguous layer of soft tissue and skin. The inner aspect of the abdominal wall consists of a thin (1–3 mm) hypoechoic zone of muscle, which should not be confused with ascites (Figure 9-1).

EMBRYOLOGY

The primordial gut (Figure 9-2) forms during the 6th menstrual week as the lateral folds arising from the central portion of the embryonic mesoderm incorporate part of the yolk sac into the interior of the embryo. This hollow tube extends the length of the embryo from the primordial mouth (*stomodeum*) to the anal pit (*proctodeum*). Simultaneously, the tissues surrounding the yolk sac and the allantois fuse to form the umbilical cord.

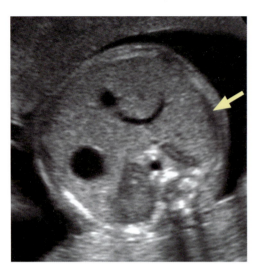

Figure 9-1. Abdominal soft tissue contour. Arrow = hypoechoic muscular layer.

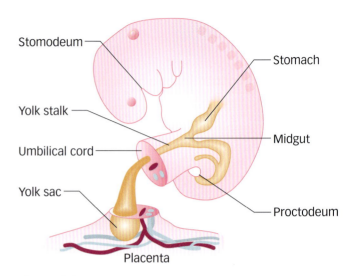

Figure 9-2. The primordial gut.

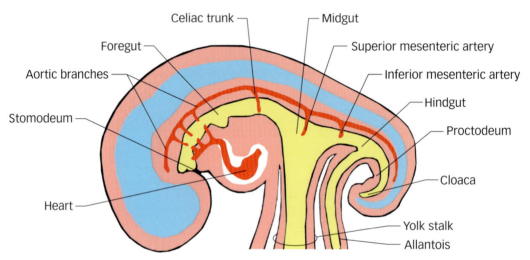

Figure 9-3. The embryonic gut.

The primitive gastrointestinal (GI) tract consists of three parts (Figure 9-3):

- *Foregut*: The foregut gives rise to the esophagus, stomach, liver, biliary tract, pancreas, and part of the duodenum. The arterial supply is via the celiac artery.
- *Midgut*: The midgut consists of the distal duodenum, jejunum, ileum, cecum, appendix, ascending colon, and proximal transverse colon. The arterial supply is via the superior mesenteric artery.
- *Hindgut*: The hindgut consists of the distal transverse colon, descending colon, sigmoid colon, rectum, upper anal canal, and urogenital sinus. The arterial supply is via the inferior mesenteric artery.

The anterior abdominal wall forms as a part of a complex process early in the embryonic period. At the beginning of the 8th menstrual week, the gastrointestinal tract begins to elongate, and as it does its size exceeds the volume that can be contained within the developing peritoneal cavity.

A portion of the intestinal tract herniates into the base of the cord in a process referred to as *midgut* or *physiologic herniation*. After undergoing further development and a series of rotational maneuvers, the hernia is reduced as the bowel returns to the peritoneal cavity by about the 12th menstrual week (Figures 9-4A and B). Identification of the point where the bowel herniates into the base of the umbilical cord is a normal sonographic finding in the first trimester (Figures 9-4C and D). In about 20% of fetuses, a small, persistent bulge at the base of the umbilical cord may be identified until the

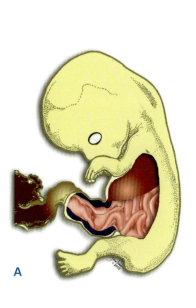
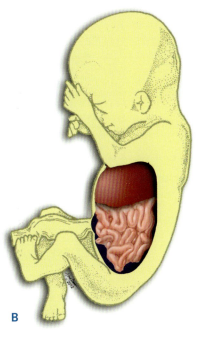
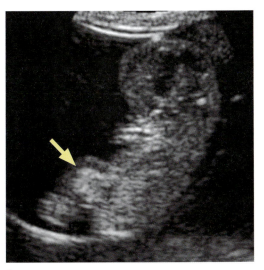
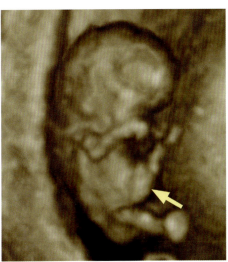

Figure 9-4. Schematics of physiologic herniation. **A** Physiologic herniation at 9 menstrual weeks. **B** Hernia reduction after bowel has returned to the peritoneal cavity by 12 weeks. **C** Sonographic appearance (sagittal section) of physiologic herniation (arrow) at 9 weeks. **D** 3D surface rendering of physiologic herniation (arrow) at 9 weeks. Figures 9-4A and B reprinted with permission from Cyr DR, Mack LA, Schoenecker SA, et al: Bowel migration in normal fetus: US detection. Radiology 161:119-121, 1986.

12th menstrual week.[1] Diagnosis of omphalocele, therefore, cannot reliably be made until after the reduction of the midgut herniation is completed—although herniation present after menstrual week 12 merits further study. (See "Omphalocele," pages 226–227.)

ABDOMINAL AND PELVIC ANATOMY

LIVER

The fetal *liver* is the predominantly visible structure within the fetal cavity due to its large size in comparison with adult human anatomy (Figure 9-5). It occupies most of the upper abdomen in the fetus. Its anatomic landmarks provide useful criteria in obstetric sonography, and knowledge of its vascular anatomy is essential to the practice of obstetric sonography. The left lobe can be seen filling most of the left upper quadrant anterior to the spleen and fluid-filled stomach.

UMBILICAL CORD AND VESSELS

The *umbilical cord* inserts on the inferior portion of the anterior abdominal wall just above the level of the urinary bladder.

The *umbilical vein*, coursing in from the umbilical cord, demarcates the left lobe of the liver from the medial margin of the right lobe, which occupies the entire right upper quadrant (Figure 9-5). This large vein

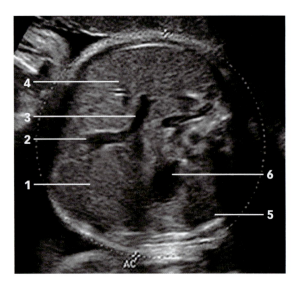

Figure 9-5. Sonographic appearance of the normal fetal liver at 20 menstrual weeks. 1 = left lobe, 2 = umbilical vein, 3 = right portal vein, 4 = right lobe, 5 = stomach, 6 = spleen.

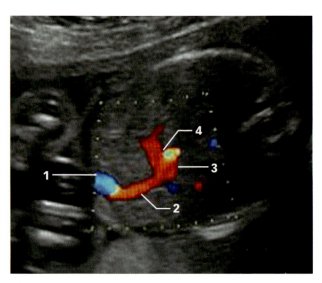

Figure 9-6. Color Doppler demonstration of blood flow into the fetal abdomen via the umbilical vein. 1 = umbilical vein, 2 = portal sinus, 3 = extrahepatic portal vein, 4 = portal vein bifurcation.

courses upward and into the liver, bringing oxygenated and nutrient-rich blood from the placenta to the fetal circulatory system. As it enters the *porta hepatis*, the end of the umbilical vein joins the extrahepatic portal vein. The confluence of the umbilical vein with the portal vein is called the *portal sinus* and is an important landmark in determining the correct level of section for abdominal circumference measurements. Following delivery, the portal sinus becomes the left branch of the portal vein[2] (Figure 9-6).

As it reaches the undersurface of the liver, the umbilical vein gives rise to the *ductus venosus*, which penetrates the liver and empties into the inferior vena cava and the portal sinus (Figure 9-7). The *hepatic veins* join the inferior vena cava at their confluence with it, just beneath the diaphragm, and drain into the right atrium (Figure 9-8).

The smaller paired *umbilical arteries* course downward from the fetal aorta, pass laterally along each side of

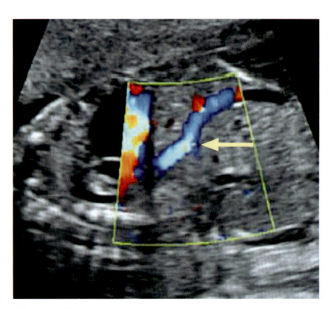

Figure 9-7. Longitudinal color Doppler demonstration of the ductus venosus (arrow) coursing through the liver and emptying into the inferior vena cava.

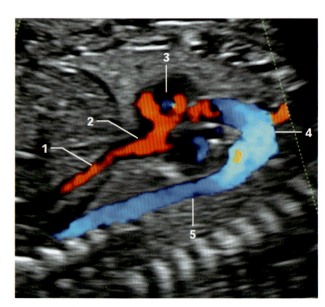

Figure 9-8. Color Doppler imaging demonstrating the left hepatic vein emptying into the hepatic confluence and inferior vena cava. 1 = left hepatic vein, 2 = inferior vena cava, 3 = right atrium, 4 = aortic arch, 5 = descending aorta.

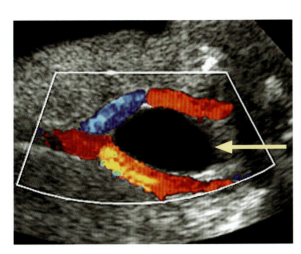

Figure 9-9. Color Doppler demonstration of the paired umbilical arteries coursing cephalad along the lateral aspects of the fetal bladder (arrow).

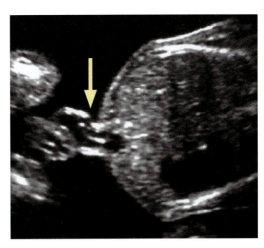

Figure 9-10. Cord insertion (arrow) on the anterior abdominal wall.

the bladder, and exit the abdominal cavity at the base of the cord. They can be reliably seen with color Doppler imaging by the second trimester (Figure 9-9).

The site of the *cord insertion* on the fetal abdomen is routinely imaged during the course of an obstetric ultrasound examination to search for and help classify any anterior abdominal wall herniation defects that may be present (Figure 9-10).

Umbilical artery Doppler is a noninvasive technique that is useful in obtaining information about the hemodynamic resistance of the placenta, a physiologic indicator of fetal growth and developmental deficits. Spectral Doppler signals are obtained in the mid portion of the cord near its insertion on the placental surface. Normal hemodynamic patterns in the umbilical arteries begin with relatively high resistance in early gestation, and resistance decreases as the pregnancy progresses (Figure 9-11). A reversal of this pattern, where resistance increases as gestation progresses, is universally indicative of real or potential fetal compromise.

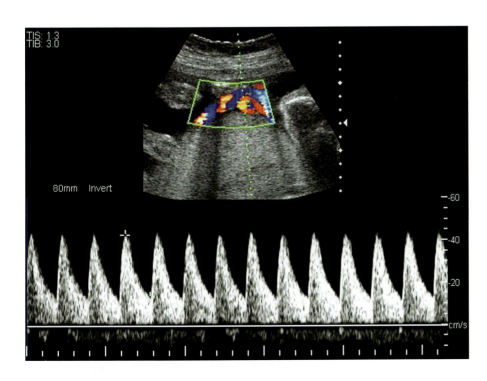

Figure 9-11. Normal umbilical cord Doppler in a 30-week fetus. Hemodynamic patterns in the umbilical arteries begin with relatively high resistance in early gestation; resistance decreases as the pregnancy progresses, as the filled spectral window demonstrates.

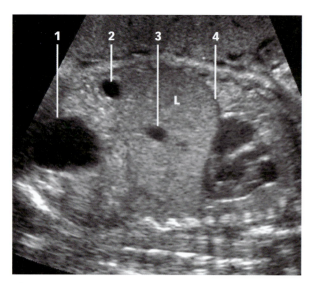

Figure 9-12. The fetal gallbladder is a fluid-filled structure located on the undersurface of the liver. 1 = fetal urinary bladder, 2 = gallbladder, 3 = portal vein, 4 = diaphragm, L = liver.

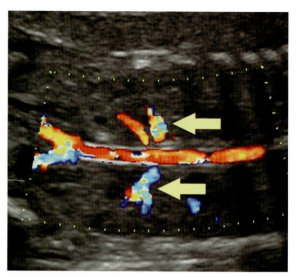

Figure 9-13. Color Doppler demonstration of the abdominal aorta terminating in the umbilical arteries of the pelvis. Both renal arteries are seen (arrows). Note duplication of the renal arteries in the upside of this fetus, a normal variant.

GALLBLADDER

The *gallbladder* is a fluid-filled structure located on the undersurface of the liver, separating the right lobe from the medial left lobe of the liver (Figure 9-12). The gallbladder is physiologically inactive in utero and can be seen in 84% of fetuses.[3] The absence of its appearance on sonographic examination raises the possibility of biliary atresia. The gallbladder can be differentiated from the umbilical vein by its teardrop shape, its off-midline location, and its position within the abdominal cavity with no exterior extension. It is one of only three intra-abdominal anatomic structures that are normally filled with simple fluid, the other two being the urinary bladder and the stomach. Any other prominent fluid-filled structure in the abdominal or pelvic cavity should be viewed with suspicion and investigated further.

AORTA

The *aorta* and its branching *renal arteries* can be seen in the fetal retroperitoneum terminating in the umbilical arteries of the pelvis (Figure 9-13). In fetuses with abnormal masses found in the renal fossae, color Doppler imaging can be useful in differentiating renal from adrenal origins.[4]

STOMACH

The *stomach* is seen as an ovoid/spherical fluid collection in the left upper quadrant of the abdomen. Coronal imaging can demonstrate the fundus, body, and pylo-

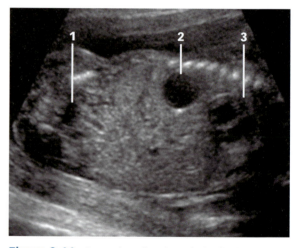

Figure 9-14. Coronal section through the fetal abdomen demonstrating the anatomic relationship between the fetal bladder (1), stomach (2), and heart (3).

rus. The muscular layer is very thin in normal fetuses and may be thickened in cases of hypertrophic pyloric stenosis. A single coronal image can demonstrate the stomach, bladder, and heart when all these organs are in their proper locations (Figure 9-14).

SMALL AND LARGE BOWEL

The fetal *small bowel* occupies a relatively smaller portion of the abdominal cavity than it does in adult human anatomy. While the stomach is normally filled with amniotic fluid and identifiable sonographically, bowel loops are collapsed and specific segments

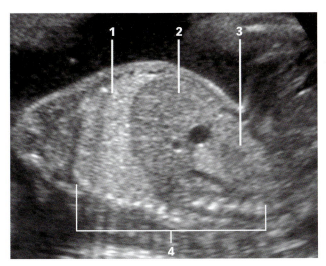

Figure 9-15. Sagittal section through the fetal abdomen demonstrating the normal fetal bowel echogenicity relative to that of the lung, liver, and posterior skeletal structures (vertebrae). 1 = lung, 2 = liver, 3 = bowel, 4 = vertebrae.

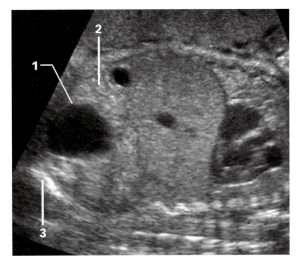

A

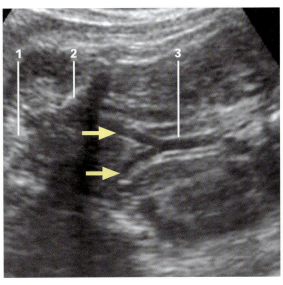

B

Figure 9-16. Normal fetal pelvic anatomy. **A** Coronal section. 1 = urinary bladder, 2 = small bowel, 3 = iliac wing. **B** Axial oblique section. 1 = symphysis pubis, 2 = iliac wing, 3 = aorta, arrows = internal iliac arteries.

cannot be identified unless there is sufficient fluid content to provide sonographic contrast. Normally the small intestine demonstrates a mixed echogenic/cystic appearance that is less echogenic than skeletal structures (Figure 9-15). Peristalsis should be seen by the late second trimester. Meconium (a mixture of bile and swallowed vernix, desquamated epithelium, and fetal hairs) becomes packed in the large bowel and may appear as highly echogenic areas within the bowel.

The fetal *large bowel* (colon) is usually visible by about 22 menstrual weeks and becomes more prominent as it fills with meconium. The colon is relatively hypoechoic and should not be mistaken for dilated small bowel. The colon lies near the kidneys, and when a kidney is absent, the colon will often occupy the renal fossa.

DIAPHRAGM AND PELVIC STRUCTURES

The *diaphragm* is the muscular dome that separates the abdominal from the thoracic cavity. It appears as a hypoechoic band between the echogenic lungs above it and echogenic liver below it (see Figure 9-12). It serves as a useful anatomic landmark during examination of the thoracoabdominal contents in the course of an obstetric sonogram and is particularly useful in identifying herniation defects.

The structures usually visible in the fetal pelvis include the iliac bones, sacrum, symphysis pubis, urinary bladder, rectum, small bowel, and pelvic vessels (Figures 9-16A and B). The rectum normally lies directly posterior to the bladder and is similar in echogenicity to the bladder. If the bladder is empty or small, the colon may be confused with the bladder.

ABDOMINAL AND PELVIC ABNORMALITIES

Prenatally detectable congenital abdominal abnormalities can be grouped into several categories: herniation defects resulting from aberrant embryologic development of the anterior abdominal wall; developmental

Table 9-1.	Fetal abdominal and pelvic anomalies.
Type of Abnormality	**Anomaly**
Herniation abnormalities	Omphalocele
	Gastroschisis
	Limb–body wall complex
	Cloacal exstrophy
Internal abdominal abnormalities	Gastrointestinal atresia
	Small bowel obstruction
	Imperforate anus
	Meconium peritonitis
	Echogenic fetal bowel
Liver abnormalities	Hepatomegaly
	Loss of hepatic parenchymal homogeneity
	Solid hepatic masses
	Cystic hepatic masses
	Hepatic calcifications
Gallbladder abnormalities	Fetal gallstones
Splenic abnormalities	Splenomegaly
	Splenic cysts
Pelvic masses	Ovarian cysts
	Sacral teratomas

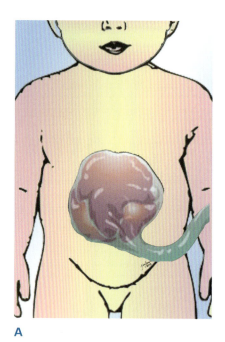

Figure 9-17. Omphalocele. **A** Schematic representation of the extrusion of abdominal contents into the base of the umbilical cord. (Figure continues . . .)

anomalies of the tubular gastrointestinal tract; abnormalities affecting the solid organs such as liver and spleen; and, finally, pelvic masses. (See Table 9-1.)

HERNIATION ABNORMALITIES

Several anterior abdominal wall herniation abnormalities are demonstrable during routine prenatal sonographic examination. Early diagnosis of these conditions gives managing clinicians time to prepare for a potentially complicated delivery and to have the neonatal team on hand to receive the neonate.

Omphalocele

An *omphalocele* is a midline defect of the abdominal wall with extrusion of gut into the base of the umbilical cord (Figure 9-17A). As noted above under "Embryology" (pages 220–221), a small, persistent bulge at the base of the umbilical cord may be identified until the 12th menstrual week in approximately 20% of fetuses. Therefore it is not feasible to diagnose omphalocele until after the reduction of the midgut herniation is completed at around that time.

While intestinal herniation is most common, other abdominal viscera may be present, depending on the size of the defect. Unlike a gastroschisis, an omphalocele is covered by a membrane consisting of parietal peritoneum and amnion.

The incidence of omphalocele is similar to that of gastroschisis, approximately 2.5 per 10,000 live births; however, there is a higher incidence of concomitant anomalies with omphalocele primarily because of an association between omphalocele and chromosomal abnormalities. The underlying pathogenic mechanism is a failure of the intestines to return to the abdomen during the second stage of intestinal rotation. However, omphalocele may also result from defective closure of midline musculature, in which case there may be total eventration of all the abdominal viscera. Rupture of the sac during vaginal delivery causes sepsis; therefore, prenatal diagnosis is essential.

Absent other significant congenital abnormalities, an isolated omphalocele can be treated in the neonate with surprisingly good outcomes. However, about 50% of fetuses with an omphalocele also have other abnormalities that can increase postnatal morbidity and mortality to between 80% and 100%.

Figure 9-17, continued. B Axial section through the fetal abdomen demonstrating a large, complex mass arising from the anterior abdomen. A = fetal abdomen in cross section. **C** Membranous sac seen containing the herniated abdominal contents. M = membrane, Li = liver, PV = portal vein segment, St = stomach. **D** Omphalocele with herniated liver. Li = liver, PV = portal vein segment, CI = cord insertion, St = stomach.

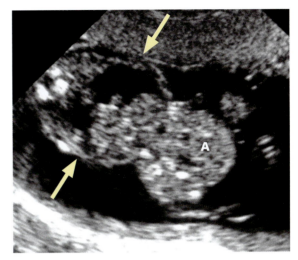

B

Associated Abnormalities

The following abnormalities may be associated with omphalocele:

- Trisomies 13, 18, and 21
- Beckwith-Wiedemann syndrome
- Pentalogy of Cantrell
- Turner syndrome
- Klinefelter syndrome
- Cloacal exstrophy
- Cardiac anomalies:
  - Transposition of the great vessels
  - Atrial and ventricular septal defects
  - Tetralogy of Fallot
  - Pulmonary artery stenosis
  - Double-outlet right ventricle
  - Coarctation of the aorta

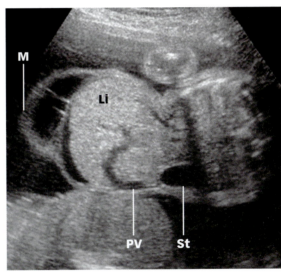

C

Sonographic Signs

The following are the characteristic sonographic signs of omphalocele:

- Complex mass extending from the anterior abdomen contiguous with the umbilical cord (Figure 9-17B).
- Membranous sac covering herniated organs (Figure 9-17C).
- Mass may contain fluid-filled bowel loops, mesentery, omentum, liver, pancreas, spleen, and/or liver (Figure 9-17D).
- Smaller-than-expected abdominal circumference.
- Polyhydramnios.

Gastroschisis

Gastroschisis is an anterior abdominal wall anomaly characterized by a small defect adjacent to the cord insertion through which abdominal viscera herniates. It has also been called *paraomphalocele, laparoschisis,* and *abdominoschisis.* The exact etiology of gastroschisis

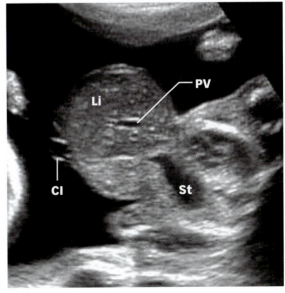

D

Figure 9-18. Gastroschisis. **A** Schematic representation of the extrusion of small bowel through an anterior abdominal wall defect not covered by a membrane and adjacent to the umbilical cord insertion. **B** Axial section through the anterior abdominal wall demonstrating an echogenic mass of bowel (B) extruding into the amniotic cavity. The herniated bowel is adjacent to the cord insertion. UV = umbilical vein. **C** Color Doppler demonstration of flow through the umbilical vein at the cord insertion (CI), which is adjacent to the herniated bowel (B).

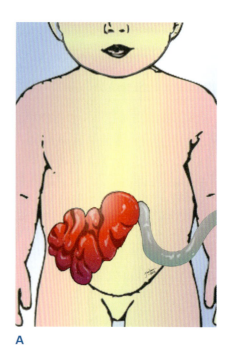

A

is uncertain; the predominant theory suggests that compromise of the vascular supply to the rectus abdominis muscle and anterior abdominal fascia results in a defect secondary to ischemic necrosis.[5]

In most cases of gastroschisis, only the small bowel is herniated (Figure 9-18A); however, in rare cases the stomach and other organs, including the liver, may herniate. Typically the herniated bowel is nonrotated and there is no covering membrane. The abdominal wall defect almost always lies to the fetal right of the umbilical cord insertion.

Gastroschisis is most commonly an isolated anomaly; when other abnormalities are present they are typically confined to the bowel. With aggressive neonatal management, survival is typically 90% or greater in neonates delivered with a gastroschisis. If there is associated bowel wall thickening or bowel distention, or if other organs are herniated, the prognosis is less favorable.

Associated Abnormalities

The following abnormalities may be associated with gastroschisis:

- Intestinal malrotation
- Intestinal atresia
- Intestinal stenosis
- Intrauterine growth restriction (IUGR)

Sonographic Signs

The following are the characteristic sonographic signs of gastroschisis:

- Thick-walled free-floating loops of bowel seen extruding into the amniotic cavity[6] (Figure 9-18B)
- Cord insertion identified adjacent (lateral) to the herniation defect (Figure 9-18C)
- No membranous sac covering the hernia
- Smaller-than-expected abdominal circumference

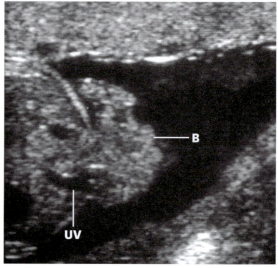

B

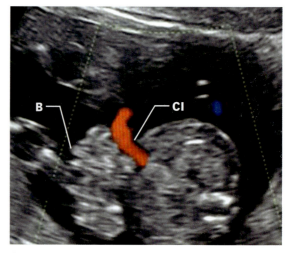

C

Sonographic Considerations

Anterior abdominal wall defects typically present a dramatically abnormal sonographic appearance. The challenge in arriving at a correct prenatal sonographic diagnosis, therefore, lies not in detecting abdominal viscera situated outside the smaller-than-expected abdominal cavity but in differentiating the two major types of herniation defect, i.e., omphalocele and gastroschisis. The following schema provides a systematic approach to identifying the correct anomaly:

- *The relationship of the abdominal wall defect to the umbilical cord*: Omphalocele occurs in the midline at the base of the cord insertion; gastroschisis is located lateral to the cord insertion, with a propensity to occur on the right side.
- *The presence or absence of a membrane covering the herniated structures*: Omphalocele is covered by a membrane; gastroschisis is not.
- *The organs herniated*: In omphalocele, liver, pancreas, and other solid abdominal organs may herniate in addition to bowel; in gastroschisis, usually only small bowel herniates. Of course, any variation may be possible.
- *Other anomalies present in the fetus*: Omphalocele is associated with other fetal anomalies; gastroschisis is rarely associated with other fetal anomalies.

Diagnostic Pitfalls

Incorrect diagnoses may result from incorrect interpretation of the following:

- Small bowel herniation into the umbilical cord between 8 and 12 menstrual weeks is a normal part of embryologic development.
- External mechanical compression of the anterior abdominal wall, i.e., in oligohydramnios, may lead to a suspicion of an abdominal wall defect or may mask a small herniation.
- Cord masses, including omphalomesenteric duct cysts or allantoic cysts, may resemble an omphalocele.

Limb–Body Wall Complex

Limb–body wall complex (LBWC), also called *body stalk anomaly*, is a uniformly lethal constellation of disruptive anatomic abnormalities involving the anterior abdominal wall of the fetus. The primary defect is a typically left-sided abdominoschisis, absent umbilical

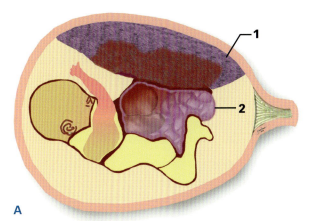

A

Figure 9-19. Limb–body wall complex (body stalk anomaly). **A** Schematic representation of the exteriorization of abdominal contents attached directly to the placental surface. 1 = placenta, 2 = exteriorized viscera. (Figure continues . . .)

cord, and exteriorization of the abdominal viscera, which are attached directly to the placental surface (Figure 9-19A). The pathogenetic mechanism may be related to early rupture of the amniotic membrane, an early ischemic insult to the abdominal wall from vascular abnormalities, or disruption of the normal embryologic formation of the anterior body folds. In addition to these complex abdominal and thoracic visceral abnormalities, myriad other congenital anomalies are associated with limb–body wall complex.

Associated Abnormalities

The following abnormalities may be associated with limb–body wall complex:

- Neural tube defects
- Facial clefts
- Encephalocele
- Exencephaly
- Caudal regression syndrome
- Limb anomalies:
  - Clubfoot (talipes equinovarus)
  - Oligodactyly, brachydactyly, syndactyly
  - Arthrogryposis
  - Absent limbs (amelia)

Sonographic Signs

The sonographic appearance of limb–body wall complex is grossly and dramatically abnormal and immediately apparent. The deformed fetus appears tethered to the placenta and free fetal movement is absent.

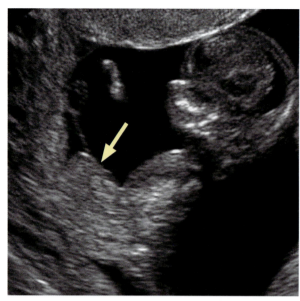

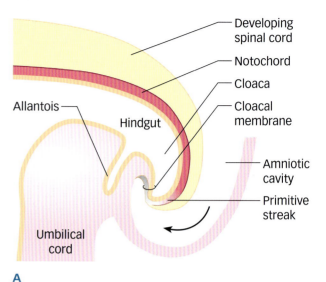

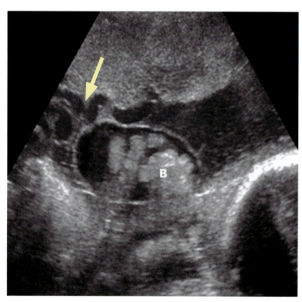

Figure 9-19, continued. B Sagittal section through a fetus at 14 weeks demonstrating the appearance of the fetus tethered (arrow) to the placenta. **C** Short umbilical cord (arrow) attaching the herniated bowel–containing mass to the placental surface. B = bowel.

There is no free-floating cord observed. Delineation of specific visceral abnormalities is difficult if not impossible because of exteriorization and compression of anatomic structures. The limbs may be difficult to locate if scoliosis is severe. While the spectrum of concomitant congenital anomalies is broad, pathognomonic sonographic findings include the following:

- Fetus appears tethered to placenta (Figure 9-19B)
- Short umbilical cord (Figure 9-19C)

Figure 9-20. Cloacal exstrophy. **A** Schematic demonstrating normal embryology of the cloaca. (Figure continues . . .)

- Herniation of the liver and abdominal viscera
- No membrane present
- No free-floating umbilical cord identified in the amniotic cavity

Cloacal Exstrophy

Cloacal exstrophy is a rare association of anomalies arising from the abnormal embryologic development of the cloaca. The *cloaca*, an early embryologic structure forming the terminal end of the hindgut (Figure 9-20A), undergoes a series of developmental changes and usually evolves into a normal rectum and urinary bladder. Disruption of this process results in extensive abnormalities of the lower abdominal wall. The triad of congenital anomalies associated with cloacal exstrophy includes a lower abdominal wall defect, exstrophy of the bladder, and omphalocele. If other anatomic abnormalities are present, such as imperforate anus and spinal defects, the condition is called *OEIS complex* (omphalocele, exstrophy, imperforate anus, and spinal defects).

Associated Abnormalities

The following abnormalities may be associated with cloacal exstrophy:

- Multicystic dysplastic kidney
- Hydronephrosis
- Undescended testicles
- Cleft clitoris
- Epispadias

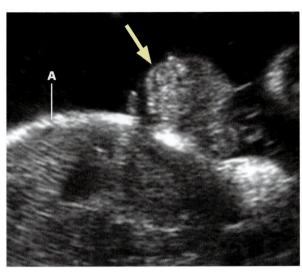

B

Figure 9-20, continued. B Axial section through the lower anterior abdominal wall (A) demonstrates an everted bladder (arrow).

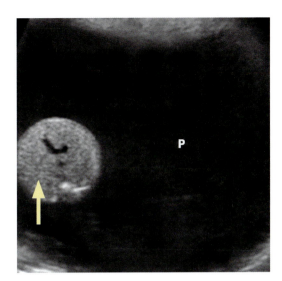

Figure 9-21. Esophageal atresia. Polyhydramnios (P) and failure to demonstrate fluid in the fetal stomach (arrow).

Sonographic Signs

The following are the characteristic sonographic signs of cloacal exstrophy:

- Bladder not identified over 30 minutes of scanning but normal amniotic fluid volume present
- Bladder exstrophy demonstrated by a soft tissue mass protruding from the lower anterior abdominal wall (Figure 9-20B)
- Microphallus in the male fetus

INTERNAL ABDOMINAL ABNORMALITIES

Gastrointestinal Atresia

Gastrointestinal atresia is a generic term applied to a narrowing of the hollow lumen of the gut at any level from the esophagus to the anus. As the passage of swallowed amniotic fluid is impeded by an atretic segment, fluid accumulates in bowel upstream from (proximal to) the site of obstruction. In some cases, the sonographic identification of which segments of bowel are dilated can provide a clue to the level of the atresia; however, this proves technically difficult and clinically moot if the atresia is distal to the first portion of the small bowel.

Esophageal Atresia

Esophageal atresia refers to interruption of the esophageal lumen, typically in the chest. It arises at about 4 weeks' gestation from the failure of the embryonic foregut to divide properly into the trachea anteriorly and the esophagus posteriorly. In 90% of cases of esophageal atresia, there is a concomitant *tracheoesophageal fistula* present, which is characterized by a pathologic communication between these two hollow tubular structures as they descend through the thorax. Associated anatomic abnormalities are common.

Associated Abnormalities

The following abnormalities may be associated with esophageal atresia:

- VACTERL association (vertebral defects, anal atresia, cardiac defects, tracheoesophageal fistula, renal anomalies, and limb abnormalities)
- CHARGE association (coloboma of the eye, heart defects, atresia of the nasal choanae, retardation of growth and/or development, genital and/or urinary abnormalities, and ear abnormalities and deafness)
- Other levels of intestinal atresia
- Pyloric stenosis
- Trisomy 18 or 21

Sonographic Signs

The following are the characteristic sonographic signs of esophageal atresia:

- Failure to demonstrate a stomach on serial sonograms (Figure 9-21)
- Polyhydramnios (Figure 9-21)
- Intrauterine growth restriction (40% of cases)[7]

Duodenal Atresia

Duodenal atresia is an interruption of the gastrointestinal tract in descending and inferior portions of the duodenum. The pathogenetic mechanism may be related to a failure of recanalization of the solid intestinal tube in early embryonic life or to external compression of the duodenum by choledochal cysts, an annular pancreas, or other upper abdominal masses that chronically obliterate the lumen.

Associated Abnormalities

The following abnormalities may be associated with duodenal atresia:

- Trisomy 21 (Down syndrome)
- Congenital heart disease
- VACTERL association
- Other intestinal atresias
- Annular pancreas

Sonographic Signs

The classic sonographic hallmark of duodenal atresia is the "double bubble" sign. Typically, on a cross section through the fetal abdomen, the first "bubble" corresponds to the stomach and the second to the postpyloric and prestenotic dilated duodenal loop. Accordingly, the following are the characteristic sonographic signs of duodenal atresia:

- Double bubble sign (Figure 9-22A)
- Identification of a focal atretic segment (Figure 9-22B)
- Polyhydramnios

Small Bowel Obstruction

Small bowel obstructions may occur at any level in the jejunum or ileum. The most common pathogenetic mechanisms are intestinal atresia, volvulus secondary to intestinal malrotation, and ischemic vascular insult to a portion of the bowel. While the subjective observation of multiple, dilated, fluid-filled loops of bowel in the peritoneal cavity during the third trimester is often adequate for the diagnosis of prenatal intestinal obstruction, several quantitative schemata have been published to assist in an earlier diagnosis. As a rule of thumb, if the inner diameter of a loop of small bowel in the mid abdomen measures greater than 7 mm during the second trimester, intestinal atresia should be considered.[8] Other sonographic observations that suggest the presence of bowel obstruction include

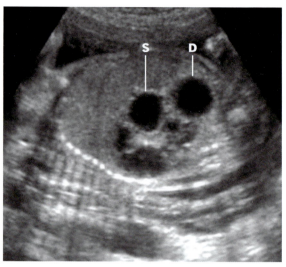

A

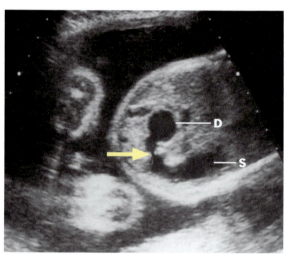

B

Figure 9-22. Duodenal atresia. **A** Sagittal section through a 14-week fetus demonstrating the "double bubble" sign. S = stomach, D = duodenum. **B** Axial oblique section demonstrating a focal atretic segment (arrow). D = duodenum, S = stomach.

hyperperistalsis, gross distention of the fetal abdomen, intra-abdominal calcifications, and polyhydramnios. While in utero bowel obstructions may occur in the colon, they are uncommon occurrences and are not usually demonstrable sonographically.

Sonographic Signs

The following are the characteristic sonographic signs of small bowel obstruction:

- Multiple dilated fluid-filled bowel loops (Figure 9-23A)
- Small bowel inner diameter of >7 mm (Figure 9-23B)
- Abdominal distention (AC measurements greater than expected for dates)

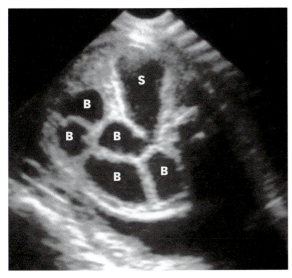

A

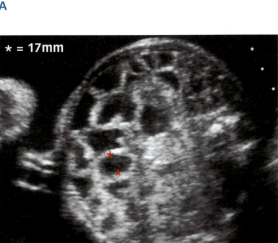

B

Figure 9-23. Small bowel obstruction. **A** Axial section through the fetal abdomen demonstrating multiple dilated, fluid-filled bowel loops (B) and dilated stomach (S). **B** Small bowel; inner diameter (calipers) measures 17 mm (>7 mm = obstruction).

Imperforate Anus

Imperforate anus is the obliteration of the anal opening. The appearance of the anomaly ranges from simple membranous separation of the anal introitus from the exterior (anal atresia) to complete absence of the entire anal mechanism (anorectal atresia). Prenatal diagnosis of congenital anorectal malformations is very difficult—first because routine visualization of the "anal echogenic spot" during prenatal sonographic examination is difficult in many cases (Figure 9-24A), and second because the presence of large, dilated loops of bowel, characteristic of other types of gastrointestinal atresia, is not a common finding associated with anal atresia.

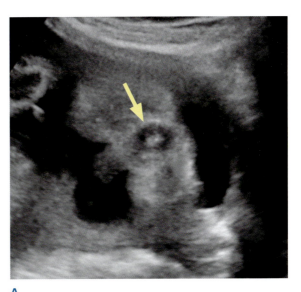

A

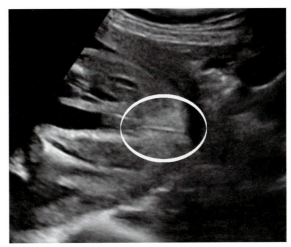

B

Figure 9-24. Imperforate anus. **A** Normal anal echogenic spot (arrow). **B** Absent perineal echogenic spot (circled).

Associated Abnormalities

The following abnormalities may be associated with imperforate anus:

- VACTERL association
- Trisomy 21
- Caudal regression syndrome
- Esophageal atresia

Sonographic Signs

The following are the characteristic sonographic signs of imperforate anus:

- Absent perineal "echogenic spot"[9] (Figure 9-24B)
- Dilated colon
- Meconium peritonitis

Meconium Peritonitis

Meconium peritonitis is an inflammatory reaction to the spillage of sterile, but irritating, fetal meconium (stool) into the peritoneal cavity. Increased intraintestinal pressure, as is typically present with all types of gastrointestinal atresia, can cause the bowel to perforate, or, in fetuses with cystic fibrosis, the abnormally viscous and sticky meconium can obstruct the bowel (*meconium ileus*), resulting in perforation. In either case, meconium seeps into the peritoneal cavity, causing a secondary inflammatory response (*meconium peritonitis*) that produces the pathophysiologic changes noted during sonographic examination: ascites, calcification, and cyst/pseudocyst formation. The perforation site seals itself off and the bowel is intact at birth; then the intraperitoneal meconium calcifies, sometimes within twenty-four hours.

Associated Abnormalities

The following abnormalities may be associated with meconium peritonitis:

- Cystic fibrosis
- Intestinal atresia
- Polyhydramnios

Sonographic Signs

The following are the characteristic sonographic signs of meconium peritonitis:

- Echogenic bowel
- Fetal ascites (Figure 9-25A)
- Intraperitoneal calcifications (Figures 9-25B and C)
- Meconium pseudocysts (Figure 9-25D)
- Polyhydramnios

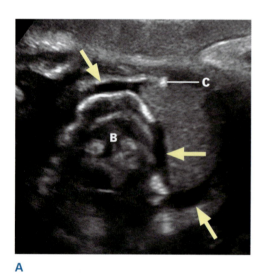
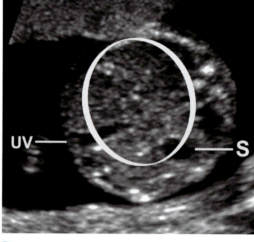

Figure 9-25. Meconium peritonitis. **A** Axial section through the abdomen of a hydropic fetus with meconium peritonitis demonstrating echogenic bowel (B), ascites (arrows), and a focal calcification (C). **B** Axial section through the fetal abdomen demonstrates diffuse, echogenic intraperitoneal calcifications (circled). UV = umbilical vein, S = fetal stomach. **C** Magnified view of multiple calcifications, appearing as hyperechogenic spots. **D** Coronal section through the abdomen of a growth-restricted fetus with meconium peritonitis and a pseudocyst (P). L = liver, T = thorax.

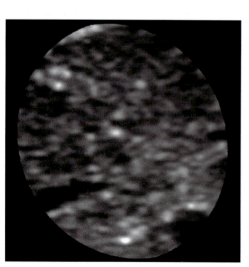
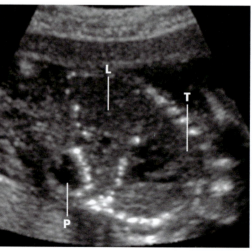

Echogenic Fetal Bowel

Echogenic fetal bowel (EFB) is the prenatal observation of an abnormal increase in the acoustic brightness of the fetal small bowel. Echogenic fetal bowel is an isolated finding in up to 70% of cases, but, because there is a small but definite association between echogenic fetal bowel and trisomy as well as several other clinically significant congenital sequelae, its observation should trigger a careful investigation of all fetal organ systems. As a rule of thumb, fetal bowel should be less echogenic than the adjacent skeletal structures, particularly the iliac bone.

Associated Abnormalities

The following abnormalities may be associated with echogenic fetal bowel:

- Trisomies 13, 18, and 21
- Meconium ileus
- Cystic fibrosis
- Intrauterine cytomegalovirus infection
- Intrauterine growth restriction (IUGR)

Sonographic Signs

The characteristic sign of echogenic fetal bowel is bowel echogenicity greater than or equal to that of the iliac bone (Figure 9-26).

LIVER ABNORMALITIES

Abnormalities of the fetal liver that are reliably demonstrable prenatally can be categorized along three sonographic parameters: size, parenchymal heterogeneity, and solidity/cysticity.

Hepatomegaly

Hepatomegaly, or enlargement of the fetal liver, may occur in association with a number of conditions, including Rh isoimmunization, congenital infection, and some syndromes (particularly Beckwith-Wiedemann and Zellweger syndromes) that result in the liver filling the epigastrium and right upper quandrant.

Sonographic Signs

The characteristic sonographic sign of hepatomegaly is an enlarged liver occupying the right and left upper quadrants (Figure 9-27).

Loss of Hepatic Parenchymal Homogeneity

The normal sonographic appearance of the fetal liver is that of a moderately echogenic, homogeneous solid structure. Its internal architecture is punctuated by numerous multisized and circuitous vascular conduits coursing in all directions. These represent the four vascular networks resident in the liver: hepatic arteries, hepatic veins, portal veins, and biliary vascular

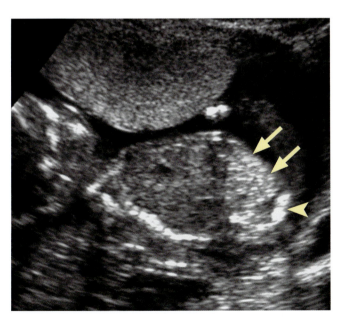

Figure 9-26. Echogenicity of fetal bowel (arrows) is greater than or equal to that of adjacent iliac bone (arrowhead).

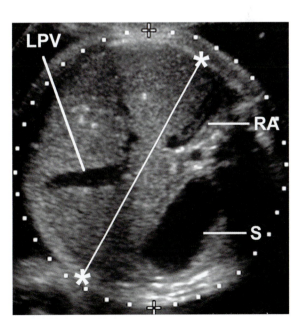

Figure 9-27. Hepatomegaly in cytomegalovirus infection. Axial section demonstrating an enlarged liver (calipers). S = stomach, LPV = left branch of portal vein, RA = right adrenal gland.

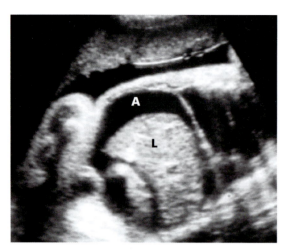

Figure 9-28. Coronal section demonstrating loss of parenchymal homogeneity and resolution loss in a fetus with hepatitis. A = ascites, L = echogenic, heterogeneous liver.

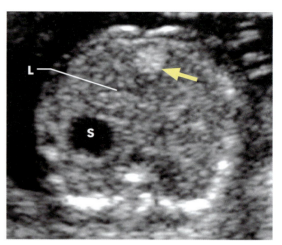

A

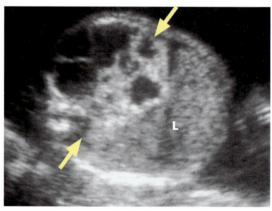

B

Figure 9-29. Solid hepatic masses. **A** Hemangioma (arrow) in a fetal liver. S = stomach, L = liver. **B** Mesenchymal hamartoma with cystic components (arrows) in a fetal liver. L = liver. (Figure continues . . .)

structures. Loss of parenchymal homogeneity (Figure 9-28) is an abnormal sonographic finding and is suggestive of several types of pathology.

Associated Abnormalities

The following abnormalities may be associated with loss of parenchymal homogeneity:

- Hepatitis
- Ischemic insults
- Portal and hepatic venous thromboembolism
- Infections:
  - Cytomegalovirus (CMV)
  - Herpes simplex
  - Varicella zoster
  - Toxoplasmosis

Sonographic Signs

Loss of parenchymal homogeneity is itself a sign that alerts sonographers to the potential presence of one or more of the pathologies listed above. Specifically, it is characterized by the appearance of increased coarseness (resolution loss) in the parenchymal echo pattern.

Solid Hepatic Masses

Solid masses in the liver are always an ominous sonographic finding. As the liver is embryologically derived from both mesenchymal and endodermal tissues, it can develop a wide variety of both benign and malignant neoplasms. Collectively, liver masses represent approximately 5% of all congenital tumors.[10]

The lesions most commonly seen in the perinatal period include the following:

- Hemangioma (benign vascular tumor) (Figure 9-29A)
- Mesenchymal hamartoma (Figure 9-29B)
- Hepatoblastoma (Figure 9-29C)
- Metastases (particularly those from neuroblastoma and leukemia)

Sonographic Signs

The following are the characteristic sonographic signs of solid masses in the liver:

- Focal, echogenic, or complex mass located in the liver.
- Doppler demonstrates arterial blood supply to the mass, with either high- or low-resistance flow patterns (Figures 9-29D and E).

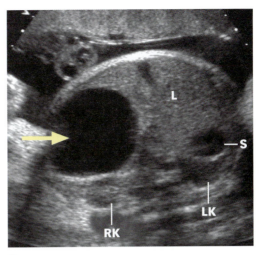

A

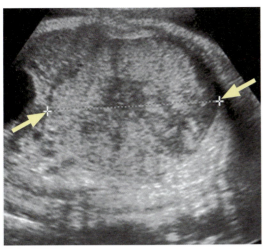

C

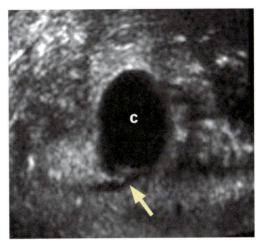

B

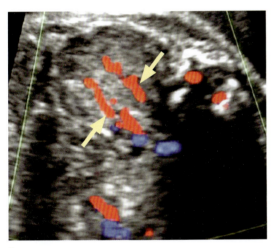

D

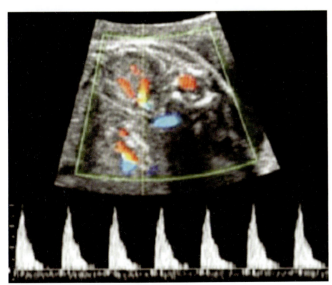

E

Figure 9-29, continued. C Hepatoblastoma (arrows). **D** Color Doppler demonstrates primary arterial blood supply to a mass (arrows). **E** Duplex imaging in which the spectral Doppler waveform demonstrates a high-resistance waveform in a different mass.

Figure 9-30. Cystic hepatic masses. **A** Axial section demonstrating a simple hepatic cyst (arrow). L = liver, S = stomach, RK = right kidney, LK = left kidney. **B** Choledochal cyst (C) in the fetal liver seen arising from the biliary ductal connection (arrow).

Cystic Hepatic Masses

Cystic masses in the liver (Figure 9-30A) are uncommon findings that are usually of little clinical significance. Most are biliary in origin, and hepatic cysts can range in size from small, submillimeter intraparenchymal inclusions to large masses that displace and distort adjacent anatomic structures. The first criterion in the correct sonographic identification of a hepatic cystic mass is the ability to clearly and distinctly differentiate it from the gallbladder.[11] A *choledochal cyst*, a rare disorder of biliary tract development, will demonstrate dilated bile ducts entering the cyst (Figure 9-30B). A choledochal cyst is a sporadic occurrence and no specific associations have been reported.

Sonographic Signs

The following are the characteristic sonographic signs of cystic masses in the liver:

- Well-circumscribed, anechoic mass within the liver (Figure 9-30A)
- Separate from the gallbladder (Figure 9-30B)
- Posterior acoustic enhancement

Hepatic Calcifications

Hepatic calcifications (calcifications in the fetal liver) are a relatively common finding, identified at 1 of every 1750 second trimester ultrasound examinations.[11] The site, size, and distribution of the lesions are major factors in determining further management. The presence of an associated liver, abdominal, or retroperitoneal mass and the association with ascites are important considerations. If the liver calcifications are single, no other fetal morphologic abnormalities are detected, and screening tests for infectious diseases are negative, then the prognosis is promising. In such cases, follow-up sonography typically shows stability or regression of the finding, and no further workup is required.

Calcifications in the liver occur in a wide range of patterns with variable distribution. They can be single or multiple, small or large. Diffuse intraparenchymal calcium deposition creates echogenic foci that may or may not cast posterior acoustic shadows. Large, single punctate echogenic lesions on the surface of the liver usually represent peritoneal calcifications, the most common source of which is meconium peritonitis. Isolated subcapsular calcifications also can be due to emboli from the portal or hepatic vein.

Infections Associated with Hepatic Calcifications

The following infections can be associated with hepatic calcifications:

- Cytomegalovirus
- Toxoplasmosis
- Rubella
- Syphilis
- Herpes simplex

Sonographic Signs

The following are the variable characteristic sonographic signs of hepatic calcifications:

- *Diffuse*: small, multiple echogenic foci within the liver parenchyma that may or may not cast acoustic shadows (Figure 9-31A)

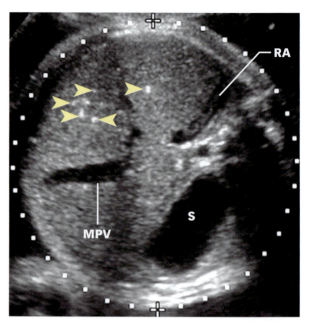

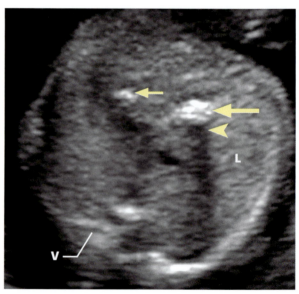

Figure 9-31. Hepatic calcifications. **A** Diffuse intraparenchymal calcium deposition creating echogenic foci that may or (as here) may not cast a posterior acoustic shadow. S = stomach, RA = right adrenal gland, MPV = main portal vein. **B** Large, single punctate echogenic lesions on the surface of the liver, which do cast acoustic shadows. Arrows = calcifications, arrowhead = acoustic shadow, L = liver, V = vertebra. (Figure continues . . .)

- *Focal*: large, focal calcifications within the liver parenchyma that do cast acoustic shadows (Figure 9-31B)
- *Extrahepatic*: small, multiple echogenic foci scattered over the peritoneal layer of the liver that may or may not cast acoustic shadows (Figure 9-31C)

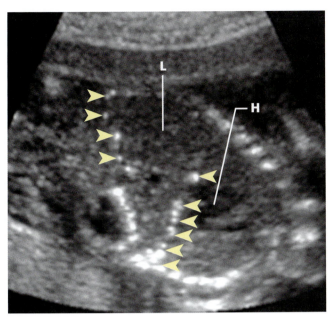

C

Figure 9-31, continued. C Peritoneal hepatic calcifications (arrowheads), most commonly attributable to meconium peritonitis, as seen here. H = heart, L = liver.

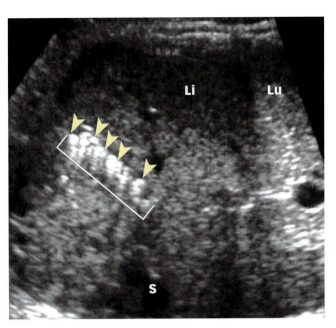

Figure 9-32. Coronal section through the fetal abdomen demonstrating multiple echogenic foci in the gallbladder with posterior ring-down artifact (bracket). Li = liver, Lu = lung, S = stomach, arrowheads = gallstones.

GALLBLADDER ABNORMALITIES

The fetal gallbladder is visualized in 82%–100% of all second and third trimester sonographic examinations.[12] In fetuses after 28 weeks, it is not uncommon to observe echogenic material in the lumen of the gallbladder, sometimes containing echogenic foci that cast posterior acoustic shadows. In the adult, these B-mode sonographic findings are hallmarks for biliary sludge and gallstones, which are often accompanied by a sick patient.

What these findings represent in the fetus, however, is less clear. Despite many scholarly attempts to assign predictive or associative value of fetal "gallstones" to a plethora of congenital abnormalities and postnatal complications, it remains impossible to do so. In general, echogenic filling of the fetal gallbladder is an incidental finding in the third trimester that does not warrant further follow-up.

Sonographic Signs

The following are the characteristic sonographic signs for assessing the fetal gallbladder:

- Echogenic filling of the fetal gallbladder
- Echogenic foci that cast posterior acoustic shadows or ring-down artifact (Figure 9-32)

SPLENIC ABNORMALITIES

Congenital splenic abnormalities are few and rare. There are two primary types:

- *Splenomegaly* may be observed in fetuses exposed to in utero infections, such as cytomegalovirus.
- Congenital *splenic cysts* are rare. There are two histologic types:
  - *Primary cysts*, which arise from cellular layers. Primary cysts may also have a neoplastic origin in dermoids, epidermoids, hemangiomas, or lymphangiomas that infarct, necrose, and liquefy.
  - *Pseudocysts*, which are an accumulation of physiologic detritus from an associated pathologic process. Pseudocysts appear in association with post-traumatic, inflammatory, or necrotic events and exude serous fluid, blood, and inflammatory byproducts.

Sonographic Signs

The following are the characteristic sonographic signs for assessing the fetal spleen (Figures 9-33A and B):

- Well-circumscribed, anechoic lesion in the splenic parenchyma
- Posterior acoustic enhancement

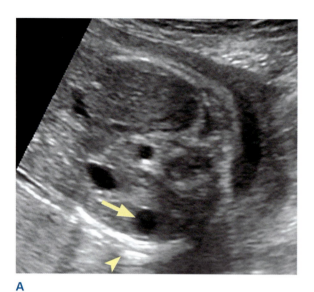
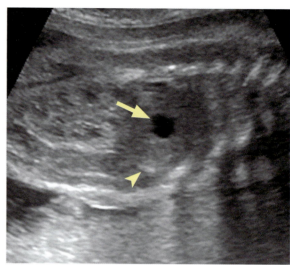

Figure 9-33. Splenic cyst (arrows). **A** Axial and **B** sagittal sections through the upper abdomen of the same fetus, demonstrating a well-circumscribed anechoic structure (arrows) with the posterior acoustic enhancement (arrowheads) that is typical of a simple cyst.

PELVIC MASSES

Ovarian Cysts

Stimulation of fetal ovaries by maternal hormones may cause functional cysts in the fetus. These lesions may be small and undetected or large enough to fill the entire fetal pelvis. Unilateral occurrence is more frequent than bilateral, and most of these cysts resolve spontaneously during the early neonatal period.

Sonographic Signs and Tips

The following are the characteristic sonographic signs of fetal ovarian cysts:

- Simple cystic mass is found in the fetal pelvis separate from the gastrointestinal tract, kidney, ureter, and bladder (Figure 9-34).
- Female gender is identified.
- It may be difficult to distinguish ovarian from urachal or mesenteric cysts.

Sacral Teratomas

When they arise in a sacral area, *teratomas*—congenital germ cell tumors derived from all three embryonic tissue layers—are generally neoplastically benign but can grow to such an enormous size that they threaten the viability of the fetus. As a rule, mature types of teratomas present sonographically as more cystic, immature types as more solid; however, there is poor correlation between sonographic appearance and malignant potential. These tumors frequently are

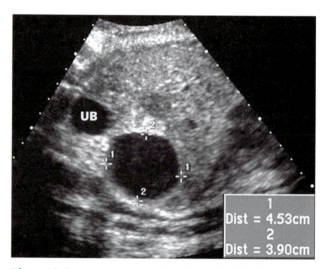

Figure 9-34. Cursors measuring a large physiologic ovarian cyst in a term fetus. UB = urinary bladder.

hypervascularized masses of solid, cystic, and calcific components. Arteriovenous shunting through the complex vascular network within the mass can lead to high-output cardiac failure, hydrops fetalis, and fetal demise. Sacral teratomas are the most common tumor of the neonate.[13] Fetal sacral teratomas are described by locus of origin:

- *Presacral teratomas* arise from the anterior aspect of the sacrum and grow into the fetal pelvis.
- *Sacrococcygeal teratomas* arise from the posterior sacrococcygeal area and project exophytically from the fetal sacrum into the amniotic cavity.

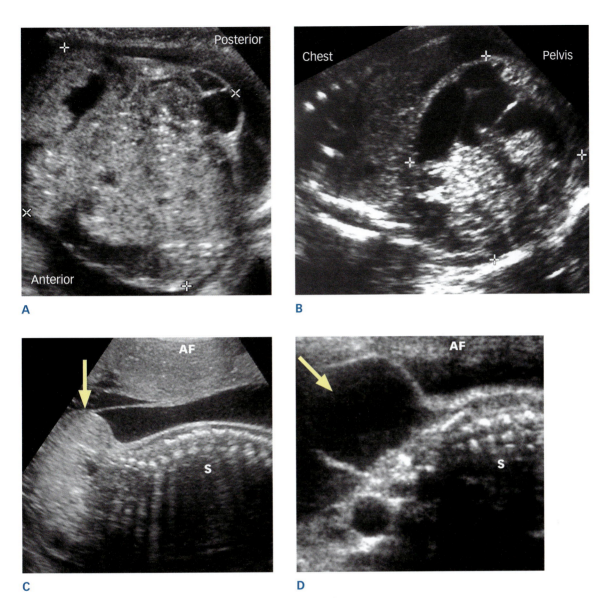

Figure 9-35. A Axial section demonstrating a large, predominantly solid presacral teratoma projecting into the abdominopelvic cavity. **B** Coronal section in a different fetus showing a mixed cystic and solid mass filling the abdomen. (Cursors are measuring the tumor in both A and B.) **C** Sagittal section through the posterior aspect of a fetus with a solid sacrococcygeal teratoma projecting exophytically from the lower back. **D** A cystic sacrococcygeal teratoma. AF = amniotic fluid, S = spine.

Associated Abnormalities

The following abnormalities may be associated with sacral teratomas:

- Myelomeningocele
- Vertebral anomalies
- Hydrops fetalis
- Ureteral obstruction
- Gastrointestinal obstruction
- Tumor rupture
- Dystocia

Sonographic Signs

The following are the characteristic sonographic signs of a sacral teratoma:

- Complex, large mass is seen in the fetal pelvis or arising from the fetal rump.
- May contain cystic, solid, and calcific components.
- Presacral tumors project into the fetal abdomen (Figures 9-35A and B).
- Sacrococcygeal tumors project exophytically off the fetus into the amniotic fluid (Figures 9-35C and D).

CHAPTER 9 REVIEW QUESTIONS

1. In this image the arrow points to:

   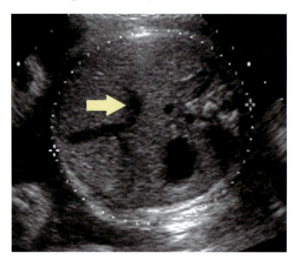

   A. Hepatic vein
   B. Right portal vein
   C. Ductus venosus
   D. Umbilical vein

2. In this image color Doppler demonstrates blood flow in the:

   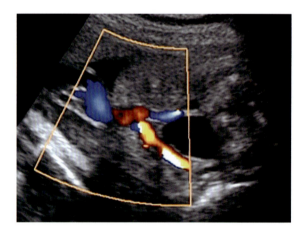

   A. Hepatic veins
   B. Umbilical veins
   C. Umbilical arteries
   D. Ductus venosus

3. In this image the arrow points to:

   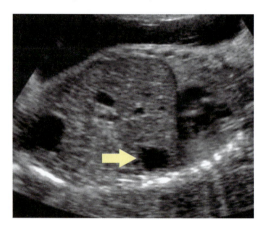

   A. Gallbladder
   B. Stomach
   C. Renal cyst
   D. Ovarian cyst

4. Which of the following statements about fetal bowel echogenicity is true?
   A. It is more echogenic than bone and less echogenic than liver.
   B. It is less echogenic than bone and more echogenic than liver.
   C. It is more echogenic than liver and less echogenic than spleen.
   D. It is more echogenic than spleen and isoechoic with liver.

5. The congenital defect characterized by a midline defect in the abdominal wall through which intra-abdominal content herniates into the base of the umbilical cord is:
   A. Omphalocele
   B. Gastroschisis
   C. Umbilical hernia
   D. Rachischisis

6. The congenital defect characterized by a defect in the abdominal wall lateral to the cord insertion through which intra-abdominal content herniates into the amniotic cavity is:
   A. Omphalocele
   B. Gastroschisis
   C. Umbilical hernia
   D. Rachischisis

7. Which of the following congenital abdominal wall defects is associated with Beckwith-Wiedemann syndrome?
   A. Omphalocele
   B. Gastroschisis
   C. Umbilical hernia
   D. Rachischisis

8. A uniformly lethal congenital abdominal wall defect characterized by absent umbilical cord and exteriorization of abdominal contents that attach directly to the placental surface is called:
   A. Gastroschisis
   B. Cloacal exstrophy
   C. Abdominoschisis
   D. Limb–body wall complex

9. The narrowing of the hollow lumen of a segment of gut is called:
   A. Cloacal exstrophy
   B. Gastrointestinal atresia
   C. Gastrointestinal ischemia
   D. Caudal regression

10. The classic sonographic sign associated with duodenal atresia is:
    A. Short umbilical cord
    B. Double bubble
    C. Echogenic bowel
    D. Tip of the iceberg

11. All of the following sonographic findings are associated with meconium peritonitis EXCEPT:
    A. Ascites
    B. Intraperitoneal calcifications
    C. Polyhydramnios
    D. Hepatosplenomegaly

12. All of the following sonographic findings are associated with congenital small bowel obstruction EXCEPT:
    A. Abdominal circumference measurements less than expected for dates
    B. Abdominal circumference measurements greater than expected for dates
    C. Multiple fluid-filled bowel loops
    D. Small bowel lumen diameter >7 mm

13. Echogenic fetal bowel is associated with all of the following conditions EXCEPT:
    A. Trisomy 13
    B. Cytomegalovirus infection
    C. Cystic fibrosis
    D. Duodenal atresia

14. Exposure to all EXCEPT which of the following infectious agents is associated with fetal hepatic calcifications?
    A. Cytomegalovirus
    B. Toxoplasmosis
    C. Gonorrhea
    D. Syphilis

15. Imperforate anus is associated with all of the following congenital abnormalities EXCEPT:
    A. VACTERL association
    B. Trisomy 21
    C. External sacrococcygeal teratoma
    D. Caudal regression syndrome

16. This image best demonstrates:

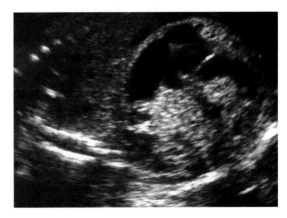

    A. Spina bifida
    B. Limb–body wall complex
    C. Sacrococcygeal teratoma
    D. Presacral teratoma

17. This image best demonstrates:

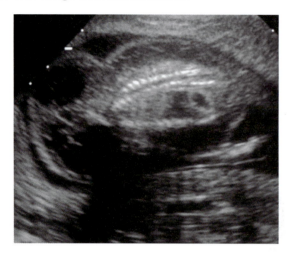

   A. Spina bifida
   B. Limb–body wall complex
   C. Sacrococcygeal teratoma
   D. Presacral teratoma

18. This image best demonstrates:

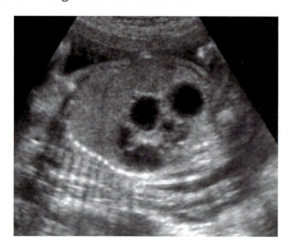

   A. Duodenal atresia
   B. Hepatic cysts
   C. Ovarian cysts
   D. Meconium peritonitis

19. This image demonstrates:

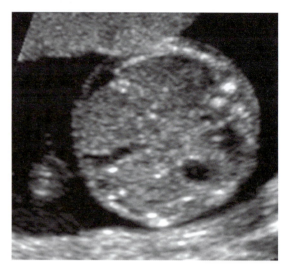

   A. Normal fetal abdomen
   B. Bilateral renal agenesis
   C. Hepatosplenic calcifications
   D. Echogenic bowel

20. The sonographic findings seen in this image are most consistent with:

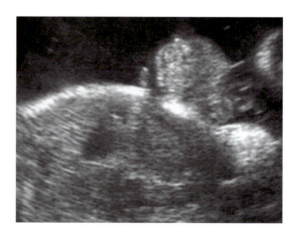

   A. Bladder exstrophy
   B. Diaphragmatic hernia
   C. Omphalocele
   D. Sacrococcygeal teratoma

ANSWERS

See Appendix A on page 481 for answers.

REFERENCES

1. Green JJ, Hobbins JC: Abdominal ultrasound examination of the first-trimester fetus. Am J Obstet Gynecol 159:165–175, 1988.

2. Czubalski A, Aleksandrowicz R: Connection types between portal vein and portal sinus during foetal life. Folia Morphol (Warsz) 59:97–98, 2000.

3. Wei J, Haller J, Rachlin S, et al: Sonographic evaluation of the fetal gallbladder in utero: incidence of visualization and morphology. J Diag Med Sonography 9:291–296, 1993.

4. Baun J, Garcia K: Prenatal diagnosis of neuroblastoma: color Doppler imaging may increase accuracy. J Diag Med Sonography 20:134–137, 2004.

5. Hoyme HE, Higginbottom MC, Jones KL: The vascular pathogenesis of gastroschisis: intrauterine interruption of the omphalomesenteric artery. J Pediatr 98:228–231, 1981.

6. Font GE, Solari M: Prenatal diagnosis of bowel obstruction initially manifested as isolated hyperechoic bowel. J Ultrasound Med 17:721–723, 1998.

7. Hill LM: Ultrasound of fetal gastrointestinal tract. In Callen PW: *Ultrasonography in Obstetrics and Gynecology*, 4th edition. Philadelphia, Saunders Elsevier, 2000, p 458.

8. Parulekar SG: Sonography of normal fetal bowel. J Ultrasound Med 10:211–220, 1991.

9. Vijayaraghavan SB, Prema AS, Suganyadevi P: Sonographic depiction of the fetal anus and its utility in the diagnosis of anorectal malformations. J Ultrasound Med 30:37-45, 2011.

10. Isaacs H Jr: Liver tumors. In *Tumors of the Fetus and Newborn*. Philadelphia, Saunders, 1997, pp 278–297.

11. Agarwal R: Sonographic assessment of fetal abdominal cystic lesions: a pictorial essay. Fetal Med 9:169–182, 1999.

12. Chan L, Rao BK, Jiang Y, et al: Fetal gallbladder growth and development during gestation. J Ultrasound Med 14:421–425, 1995.

13. Roman AS, Monteagudo A, Timor-Tritsch I, et al: First-trimester diagnosis of sacrococcygeal teratoma: the role of three-dimensional ultrasound. Ultrasound Obstet Gynecol 23:612–614, 2004.

SUGGESTED READINGS

Abbott JF: The fetal abdominal wall and gastrointestinal tract. In Rumack CM, Wilson SR, Charboneau JW (eds): *Diagnostic Ultrasound*, 4th edition. Philadelphia, Elsevier Mosby, 2011, pp 1327–1352.

Bronshtein M, Blazer S, Zimmer EZ: The gastrointestinal tract and abdominal wall. In Callen PW (ed): *Ultrasonography in Obstetrics and Gynecology*, 5th edition. Philadelphia, Saunders Elsevier, 2008, pp 587–639.

Fleischer AC, Toy E, Lee W, et al (eds): *Sonography in Obstetrics and Gynecology: Principles and Practice*, 7th edition. New York, McGraw-Hill, 2011, chs 2, 17.

Hagen-Ansert SL: The fetal abdomen. In Hagen-Ansert SL (ed): *Textbook of Diagnostic Ultrasonography*, 7th edition. St. Louis, Elsevier Mosby, 2012, pp 1336–1349.

Hagen-Ansert SL, Spradley D: The fetal anterior abdominal wall. In Hagen-Ansert SL (ed): *Textbook of Diagnostic Ultrasonography*, 7th edition. St. Louis, Elsevier Mosby, 2012, pp 1323–1335.

CHAPTER 10

The Fetal Genitourinary Tract

Embryology

Genitourinary Anatomy

Genitourinary Abnormalities

The fetal genitourinary system comprises the anatomic structures of both the urinary and genital systems. The *urinary system* consists of the kidneys, ureters, urinary bladder, and urethra; the *genital system* includes the gonads, the internal and external organs of reproduction, and their anatomic scaffolding. While each system follows its own set of genetic instructions for proper development, there is a close association and synergy between the two.

EMBRYOLOGY

The genital and urinary systems are intimately related from the standpoint of embryologic development; anomalous development of one system portends anomalies in the other. The gender of a conceptus is determined at fertilization and is dependent on the sex chromosome provided by the sperm cell. A normal ovum always contains an X chromosome. If the fertilizing male gamete contributes another X chromosome, the progeny will be female; if it contributes a Y chromosome, the progeny will be male. The genital tract arises from the intermediate mesoderm and initially manifests as wolffian (mesonephric) and müllerian ducts, embryonic structures that will evolve into the permanent male and female reproductive organs (Figures 10-1A–D).

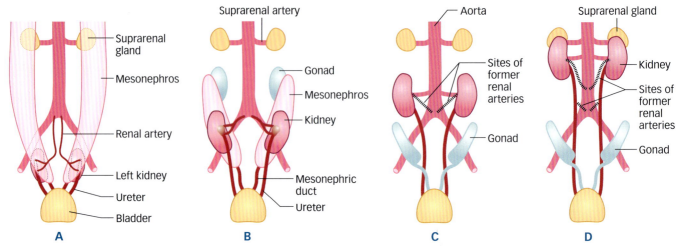

Figure 10-1. Renal embryology. These ventral views of the embryonic (A and B) and fetal (C and D) abdominopelvic region demonstrate how the kidneys rotate medially and "ascend" into the abdomen from the pelvis. **A** Menstrual week 8 and **B** menstrual week 9: Note the size regression of the mesonephroi. **C** Menstrual week 10 and **D** menstrual week 11: Note that as the kidneys ascend, they are supplied by arteries at successively higher levels and the hilum of the kidney (where the vessels and nerves enter) is eventually directed anteromedially. Reprinted with permission from Moore KL, Persaud TVN, Torchia MG: *The Developing Human: Clinically Oriented Embryology*, 9th edition. Philadelphia, Elsevier Saunders, 2013, p 253. (Re-rendered for this publication.)

The urogenital precursors arise from bits of the intermediate mesoderm that are interiorized and encapsulated during the horizontal folding of the embryo at about the beginning of the 6th menstrual week. The fetal kidneys begin to develop at the beginning of the 6th menstrual week as nonfunctional buds of tissue (*pronephroi*) near the tail end (*cloaca*) of the embryo. Within a few days, the buds have degenerated, leaving behind a primitive set of ducts around which primitive, functioning kidneys (*mesonephroi*) will grow. These well-developed excretory organs serve the embryo until the permanent kidneys (*metanephroi*) begin to function toward the end of the first trimester, around the 9th menstrual week. The metanephroi initially reside low in the pelvis in front of the sacrum. As the embryo grows, they ascend into the mid portion of retroperitoneal space, where they remain throughout life. The fetal genitourinary system is fully formed by the 9th menstrual week.

GENITOURINARY ANATOMY

KIDNEYS

Fetal kidneys can be identified as early as 12–14 menstrual weeks as two relatively hypoechoic structures adjacent to the spine as seen in transverse sections; however, they are best examined later in gestation, at 17–21 weeks. By the end of the second trimester, *renal pyramids* (conical masses that form the renal medulla) may be visible. Echopenic (hypoechoic) renal pyramids are distributed evenly throughout the renal parenchyma. Renal sinus fat is more echogenic than surrounding parenchymal tissue and can be seen in the hilum of the kidney. The *renal capsule*—the thin echogenic rim surrounding the renal parenchyma—is a useful landmark when evaluating the contour of the kidney (Figures 10-2A and B).

In many fetuses, the renal pelvis may contain a small amount of fluid (Figure 10-3), which is a normal finding and is not indicative of obstructive uropathy unless other diagnostic criteria are met. A rule of thumb for normal renal size is an anteroposterior (AP) diameter of about 1 mm per week of gestation. Color or power Doppler imaging of the renal vessels may help confirm the presence of the kidneys if gray-scale imaging is equivocal. In the normal fetus, the ureters are rarely visible.

BLADDER

The fetal bladder can be definitively identified by 16–20 weeks (frequently before that), and its sonographic demonstration is an important indicator of active renal function. The iliac wings and pelvic vascular structures are important anatomic landmarks in demonstration of the fetal bladder.

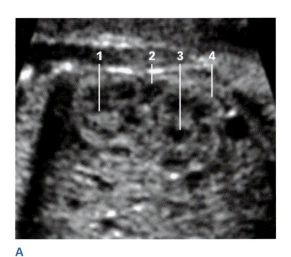
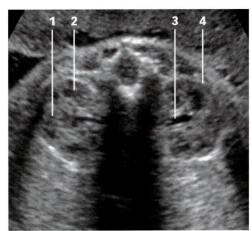

Figure 10-2. Fetal kidney. **A** Sagittal and **B** axial sections demonstrating the normal sonographic appearance of the fetal kidney at 18 weeks. 1 = renal sinus fat, 2 = renal pyramid, 3 = renal pelvis, 4 = renal capsule.

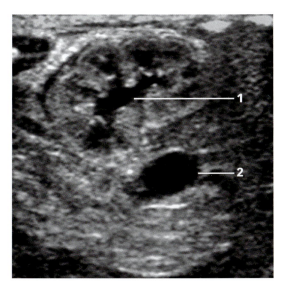

Figure 10-3. Axial oblique section through the fetal lower abdomen showing a normal amount of fluid in the fetal renal pelvis. 1 = renal pelvic fluid, 2 = urinary bladder.

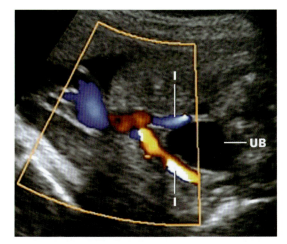

Figure 10-4. Axial oblique section through the fetal pelvis with color Doppler demonstrating the paired iliac vessels (I) as they course around the fetal urinary bladder (UB).

Sitting in the midline, the normal fetal bladder can be seen as an anechoic structure in the anterior pelvis. The iliac vessels, which run posterolateral to the bladder, can be reliably imaged with color Doppler imaging (Figure 10-4). The urinary bladder is a dynamic structure that empties and fills in cycles of 30–45 minutes. The fetus *micturates* (urinates) into the amniotic cavity and is thereby responsible for virtually all of the amniotic fluid as gestation advances. The apparent absence of the bladder during the early minutes of an obstetric ultrasound exam does not necessarily indicate abnormality. A recheck after 20–30 minutes frequently demonstrates the bladder after it has filled with urine.

ADRENAL GLANDS

The adrenal glands are not functionally a part of the genitourinary system, but since they reside in the renal fossae they are included in the anatomic examination of the fetal kidneys. The glands are relatively large in the fetus compared to those of the normal adult human anatomy. About 90% of the gland is composed of cortex, which quickly involutes after birth.

The adrenals can be seen sonographically as oval masses of echopenic tissue lying superior to the kidney on the sagittal or coronal plane of section (Figure 10-5A). Transversely (axially), the gland appears as a long, thin, echogenic line of medulla surrounded by the thicker sonolucent rim of cortex (Figure 10-5B). The adrenal gland should be smaller than the normal kidney. In fetuses with renal agenesis, the adrenals frequently opportunistically hypertrophy into the empty renal fossae.

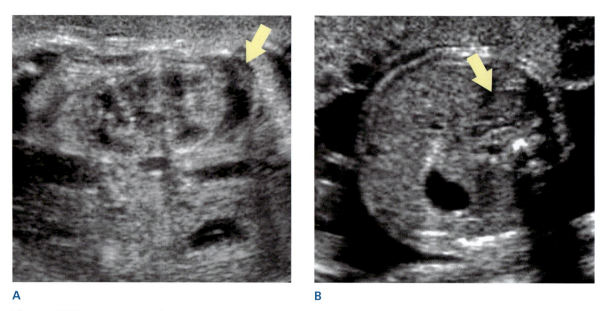

Figure 10-5. Adrenal gland. **A** Coronal section through the renal fossa showing an oval mass of echopenic tissue (arrow) lying superior to the kidney. **B** Axial section demonstrating a long, thin echogenic line of medulla (arrow) surrounded by the thicker sonolucent rim of cortex.

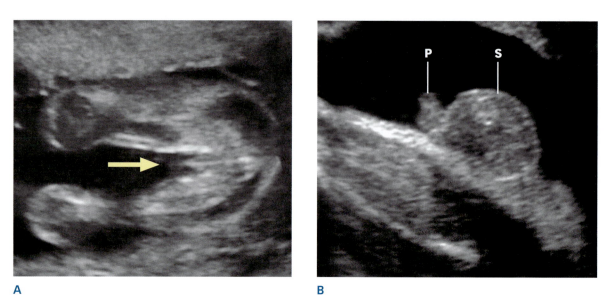

Figure 10-6. A Sonographic demonstration of fetal external genitalia in the second trimester. Arrow = labia majora. **B** Sonographic demonstration of fetal male genitalia in the second trimester. P = penis, S = scrotum.

GENITALIA

Fetal gender can be determined sonographically in virtually all normal pregnancies. The pitfalls of the early days of sonography have been obviated by enhanced imaging resolution and color Doppler imaging. With submillimeter imaging resolution, external genitalia can be identified and differentiated as early as 12 menstrual weeks. By 18–20 menstrual weeks, the external genitalia can be reliably determined during the course of a routine sonographic examination of the fetus. The external female genitalia demonstrable with ultrasound are primarily the labia majora, which appear as three parallel linear echoes aligned along the midline of the perineum (Figure 10-6A). In some male fetuses, the penis and scrotum can be seen as early as 11 menstrual weeks; in all normal male fetuses external genitalia should be seen by 16 weeks (Figure 10-6B). Confusion cast by the presence of the umbilical cord between the legs can be dispelled with the use of color Doppler imaging. Another potential pitfall in the correct detection of fetal genitalia is the misidentification (in early gestation, around 14–16 weeks) of normally edematous labia as a scrotum.

GENITOURINARY ABNORMALITIES

Abnormalities of the genitourinary tract can be divided into two broad categories: those affecting the excretory anatomy and physiology and those affecting reproductive components (see Table 10-1). Most anomalies of the excretory anatomy and physiology are easily demonstrable during routine prenatal examination of the fetus. In addition to the gross morphologic changes that may affect the kidneys, ureter, and/or bladder, impaired renal function frequently results in oligohydramnios—always a telltale sign that something is amiss with a pregnancy. These conditions are discussed at length below. Anomalies of the reproductive components of genitourinary system, on the other hand, are rarely diagnosed in utero; rather, they present at birth or later in life, particularly when the female reproductive system becomes hormonally and functionally active. Therefore these anomalies are not usually the subject of fetal ultrasound studies and are not discussed here.

Table 10-1. Summary of fetal genitourinary abnormalities.

Type of Abnormality	Anomaly
Excretory components	Renal agenesis
	Renal ectopia
	Renal cystic disease (including Potter-related)
	Obstructive uropathies
	Genitourinary neoplasms
Reproductive components	Genital agenesis or dysmorphia
	Ambiguous genitalia
	True hermaphroditism
	Wolffian and müllerian duct abnormalities

RENAL AGENESIS

Renal agenesis (RA) is a condition characterized by the absence of one or both kidneys. Its etiology is currently unknown but is thought to be multifactorial. Embryologically, renal agenesis results from failure of the metanephroi to develop as described above. Both unilateral and bilateral forms of renal agenesis are associated with Potter sequence (see "Renal Cystic Disease," pages 253–258).

Unilateral Renal Agenesis

Unilateral renal agenesis is three to four times more common than bilateral renal agenesis. It is found at autopsy in approximately 1 in 1000 individuals.[1] Most of these individuals live into middle or late life without knowing that they are absent one kidney. As long as the kidney in situ provides adequate renal function, there is no reason to suspect unilateral renal agenesis.

Associated Abnormalities

The following abnormalities may be associated with unilateral renal agenesis:

- Trisomy 21 (Down syndrome)
- Turner syndrome
- Potter sequence
- Müllerian duct anomalies
- Congenital heart disease
- Obstructive uropathies:[2]
  - Vesicoureteral reflux
  - Ureterovesical junction (UVJ) obstruction
  - Ureteropelvic junction (UPJ) obstruction
- VACTERL association (vertebral defects, anal atresia, cardiac defects, tracheoesophageal fistula, renal anomalies, and limb abnormalities)
- Sirenomelia (mermaid syndrome)

Sonographic Signs

The following are the characteristic sonographic signs of unilateral renal agenesis:

- Absent kidney (Figure 10-7A)
- Compensatory hypertrophy of the contralateral kidney (Figure 10-7B)
- Opportunistic hypertrophy of the ipsilateral adrenal gland
- Normal filling of the urinary bladder
- Normal amount of amniotic fluid

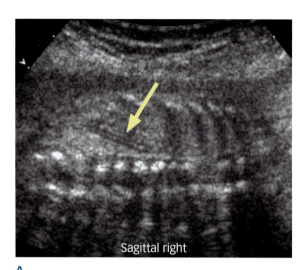 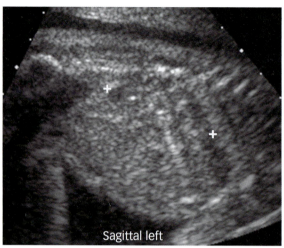

Figure 10-7. Unilateral renal agenesis. Sagittal sections through both renal fossae. **A** Absent right kidney with the characteristic long, thin appearance of the adrenal gland in the renal fossa (arrow). **B** Compensatory hypertrophy of the contralateral left kidney (cursors).

Bilateral Renal Agenesis

Bilateral renal agenesis (BRA) is a uniformly lethal anomaly characterized by the congenital absence of both kidneys. There is no urine production at any time during the gestation and therefore amniotic fluid volume is dramatically diminished, depriving the fetal lungs of the necessary lipids, proteins, and glycoproteins found in the surfactants that are essential for normal lung development. Without amniotic fluid, the lungs fail to develop and mature, and following delivery the neonate dies quickly from severe pulmonary hypoplasia.

Bilateral renal agenesis can occur as an isolated phenomenon or as part of a syndrome. It has an incidence of approximately 1 in 4000 births. One causative mechanism is posited to be a disruption of the normal embryologic sequence from pronephros to metanephros. Another is the failure of the ureteral buds to grow as a sequela to early vascular insult. Both etiologies produce true (Potter-type) bilateral renal agenesis, in which neither kidneys nor ureters are present.

Associated Abnormalities

The following abnormalities may be associated with bilateral renal agenesis:

- Potter sequence
- Genital malformations
- Sirenomelia (mermaid syndrome)
- Cardiac anomalies (full range)
- Central nervous system anomalies:
  - Hydrocephalus
  - Microcephaly
  - Meningocele
  - Holoprosencephaly
  - Iniencephaly
- Gastrointestinal malformations:
  - Duodenal atresia
  - Imperforate anus
  - Tracheoesophageal fistula
  - Omphalocele

Sonographic Signs

The following are the characteristic sonographic signs of bilateral renal agenesis:

- Empty renal fossae bilaterally (Figure 10-8)
- Oligohydramnios
- Long, thin "lying-down" adrenal glands (Figure 10-7A)
- Absent renal arteries (color Doppler)
- Absent urinary bladder
- Compression deformities secondary to extreme oligohydramnios

RENAL ECTOPIA

Renal ectopia is the presence of a kidney outside of its usual location in the retroperitoneal renal fossae. The most common types are abdominal, lumbar, pelvic,

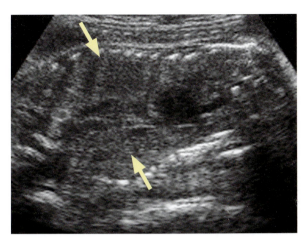

Figure 10-8. Bilateral renal agenesis. Coronal section through the fetal retroperitoneum showing empty renal fossae bilaterally (arrows), accompanied by oligohydramnios.

thoracic, and cross-fused ectopic kidneys. Abnormal location results from the stalling of the ascent of the kidney from the pelvis into the abdomen. *Cross-fused renal ectopia* is an anomaly whereby the kidneys are fused and lie along one side of the midline. There is a 2:1 male-to-female ratio with this type of embryologic maldevelopment. It is rarely detected in utero; however, after 24 weeks the adjunctive use of color Doppler imaging is helpful in confirming the presence of blood flow into renal parenchyma on one side of the abdomen and the absence of blood flow into the empty contralateral renal fossa.[3]

Associated Abnormalities

The following abnormalities may be associated with renal ectopia:

- Multicystic dysplastic kidney
- Ureterocele
- Patent urachus
- Vesicoureteric reflux
- Vaginal agenesis
- Hypospadias
- Ureteropelvic junction obstruction
- Vertebral column abnormalities

Sonographic Signs

Renal ectopia is rarely detected in utero; however, soft sonographic signs associated with this anomaly include:

- Long, thin "lying-down" adrenal glands (Figure 10-7A)
- Vesicoureteral reflux
- Contralateral renal dysplasia

RENAL CYSTIC DISEASE

Potter Sequence

Potter sequence is a constellation of abnormal facies, intrauterine growth restriction, and limb anomalies demonstrated postnatally and resulting from chronic mechanical compression of the fetus in a severely oligohydramniotic sac. The cause is severe and chronic absence of amniotic fluid, most commonly resulting from the anuria associated with severely compromised or absent renal function. While this scenario is most commonly associated with bilateral renal agenesis or severe prenatal renal cystic disease, it can also occur when severe, long-standing oligohydramnios results from a chronic leakage of fluid following a premature rupture of membranes (PROM) during the second trimester, or from a twin-to-twin transfusion. Chronic absence of amniotic fluid in a severely oligohydramniotic sac induces structural and developmental abnormalities in the severely compressed fetus.

With Potter sequence the fetus assumes a typical appearance referred to traditionally as *Potter syndrome* but more recently as *Potter sequence*. It consists of a constellation of the following postnatal findings:

- Pulmonary hypoplasia—severe and incompatible with life
- Abnormal facies (Potter facies):
  - Low-set ears
  - Flattened nose
  - Wrinkled skin
  - Micrognathia
- Intrauterine growth restriction (IUGR)
- Limb abnormalities, e.g., talipes equinovarus (clubfoot), contractures

Potter sequence is associated with several types of renal cystic disease, described as Potter types I through IV. This classification schema is used to describe the pathologic and prognostic characteristics of a broad realm of congenital kidney disease. Table 10-2 provides a summary of renal cystic disease by Potter type.

Potter Type I—Autosomal Recessive Polycystic Kidney Disease

Autosomal recessive polycystic kidney disease (ARPKD), better known as *infantile polycystic kidney disease* (IPKD), is an autosomal recessive condition characterized by the replacement of normal renal parenchyma with microcystic disease tissue in the distal convoluted tubules and collecting ducts, along with fibrotic infiltration of the renal interstices. The kidneys are bilaterally enlarged and sponge-like in texture (Figure 10-9A). Compression of functional excretory tissue by fibrocystic encroachment reduces renal function in proportion to the severity of the disease.

Morbidity and mortality, in turn, increase as renal function diminishes. The degree of renal impairment is variable; in the most severe cases, findings may be observed as early as 16 menstrual weeks, and there may be oligohydramnios throughout most of the pregnancy. In milder cases, however, the findings may not be detectable until after 24 weeks or even after birth. Fetuses with 90% or more of both kidneys affected die within the first postnatal week.[4] All fetuses affected with autosomal recessive polycystic kidney disease have some component of liver disease, and biliary duplication cysts may be visible within the liver late in pregnancy.

The primary sonographic finding in infantile polycystic kidney disease is that of markedly enlarged, echogenic kidneys bilaterally. The minute dimensions of the individual cysts preclude individual sonographic resolution; large, demonstrable anechoic lesions are not a hallmark finding with infantile polycystic kidney disease. Rather, the net effect of the thousands of specular reflectors along the back wall of each cyst is acoustic amplification that renders the kidney uniformly echogenic.

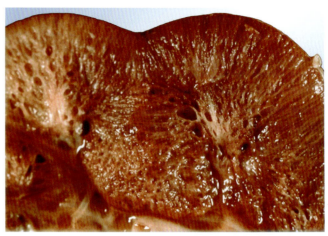

A

Figure 10-9. Potter type I, infantile polycystic kidney disease (IPKD). **A** Gross pathology. Note microcystic disease with fibrotic infiltration of the interstices. (Figure continues . . .)

Table 10-2. Potter classification of renal cystic disease.

	Type I	Type II	Type III	Type IV
Nomenclature	Autosomal recessive polycystic kidney disease (infantile polycystic kidney disease)	Multicystic renal dysplasia (multicystic dysplastic kidney disease)	Autosomal dominant polycystic kidney disease (adult polycystic kidney disease)	Obstructive cystic renal dysplasia
Location	Bilateral	Bilateral or unilateral	Bilateral	Dependent on etiology of hydronephrosis
Sonographic appearance	Enlarged kidneys, echogenic	Noncommunicating cysts of variable size	Rare in utero; enlarged and echogenic	Hydronephrosis with cortical cysts
Amniotic fluid	Frequent oligohydramnios	Normal to diminished	Normal	Varies with etiology
Prognosis	Poor	Good	Adult onset	Varies with etiology
Risk in subsequent pregnancies	25%	<5%	50%	Varies with etiology

Source: Data from Porto M, McGahan JP: The fetal abdomen and pelvis. In McGahan JP, Porto M (eds): *Diagnostic Obstetrical Ultrasound*. Philadelphia, Lippincott, 1994, p 442.

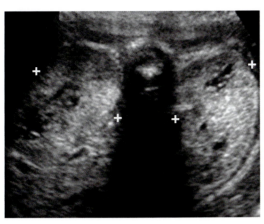
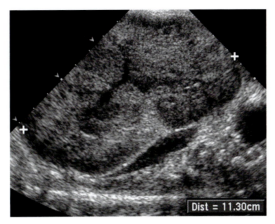

B

C

Figure 10-9, continued. **B** Sonographic findings. **C** Postnatal demonstration of gross pathology. Cursors measure enlarged, echogenic kidneys.

Associated Abnormalities

Enlarged kidneys are associated with:

- Beckwith-Wiedemann syndrome
- Meckel-Gruber syndrome
- Trisomy 13 (Patau syndrome)
- Glomerulocystic disease
- Congenital hypernephroid nephromegaly

Sonographic Signs

The following are the characteristic sonographic signs of autosomal recessive polycystic kidney disease:

- Large and homogeneously hyperechoic kidneys (Figures 10-9B and C)
- Increased kidney-to-abdominal-circumference ratio
- Loss of corticomedullary differentiation
- Kidneys that may appear normal in early pregnancy (14–16 menstrual weeks)
- Presence or absence of fetal urinary bladder
- Oligohydramnios in cases of impaired renal function

Potter Type II—Multicystic Renal Dysplasia

Multicystic renal dysplasia (MRD), also called *multicystic dysplastic kidney disease* (MCKD), arises as a result of early ureteral obstruction. Urine backs up into the renal collecting tubules, causing areas of dilatation that chronically develop into cysts (Figure 10-10A). The affected kidney, or segment, has no functional excretory tissue present; the cysts vary considerably in size and may reach up to 6 cm in diameter. Multicystic renal dysplasia is usually a sporadic congenital anomaly, although a rare autosomal dominant form does exist.

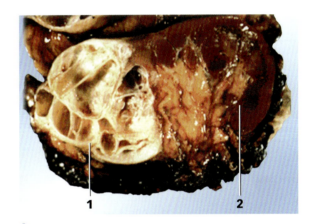

A

Figure 10-10. Potter type II, multicystic renal dysplasia (MRD). **A** Gross pathology. 1 = cystic dysplastic tissue, 2 = normal renal parenchyma. (Figure continues . . .)

The outcome in infants born with multicystic renal dysplasia is related to the severity of the disease. Multicystic renal dysplasia can affect both kidneys, a single kidney, or a segment of a single kidney. As the presence of normal parenchyma and its functionality are critical to the production of amniotic fluid, fetuses with adequate renal mass and a patent urinary outflow tract many times do quite well. About 60% of cases of multicystic renal dysplasia resolve spontaneously as the cysts involute over the first decade of life.[5] Fetuses with inadequate renal mass and/or outflow-obstructing lesions will spend several months in an oligohydramniotic environment, subjecting them to the chronic pathophysiologic insult of the Potter sequence. Pulmonary hypoplasia is the ultimate mechanism of postnatal demise.

Associated Abnormalities

The following abnormalities may be associated with multicystic renal dysplasia:

- Vesicoureteric reflux
- Ureteropelvic junction obstruction
- Ureterocele
- Meckel-Gruber syndrome
- Zellweger syndrome

Sonographic Signs

The following are the characteristic sonographic signs of multicystic renal dysplasia:

- Multiple noncommunicating cysts (Figures 10-10B and C)
- Lobulated renal contour
- Echogenic renal parenchyma
- Urinary bladder that may be present or absent
- Oligohydramnios in cases where renal function is impaired

Potter Type III—Autosomal Dominant Polycystic Kidney Disease

Autosomal dominant polycystic kidney disease (ADPKD), also called *adult polycystic kidney disease* (APKD), is rarely manifested prenatally, instead making its first appearance in adulthood as the etiology for unexpected chronic renal failure and end-stage renal disease (ESRD). By 30 years of age, about 70% of individuals with autosomal dominant polycystic kidney disease will demonstrate cysts on ultrasound.[6] About half will progress to end-stage renal disease that requires hemodialysis and/or renal transplant by 60 years of age.

Autosomal dominant polycystic kidney disease can be demonstrated in utero in a fetus with a severe form of the disease, but diagnosis is typically made later in life. ADPKD affects the kidneys bilaterally, with many variably sized cysts replacing progressively more renal parenchyma as the disease advances. There is usually hemorrhage into the cysts and fibrotic encroachment on elements of the collecting system (Figure 10-11). Frequently there is a concomitant polycystic involvement of the liver and, occasionally, the pancreas.

Sonographic Signs

Because ADPKD/Potter III does not manifest prenatally, there are no fetal sonographic signs associated with it.

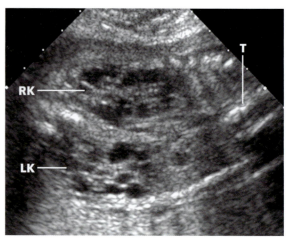

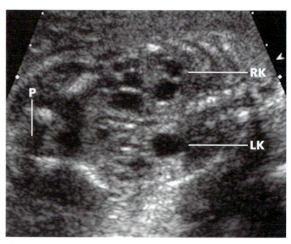

Figure 10-10, continued. B Sonographic findings in coronal section through the fetal abdomen demonstrating multiple noncommunicating cysts replacing normal renal parenchyma. **C** Sonographic findings in oblique section through the fetal abdomen demonstrating multiple noncommunicating cysts replacing normal renal parenchyma. RK = right kidney, LK = left kidney, T = fetal thorax, P = fetal pelvis.

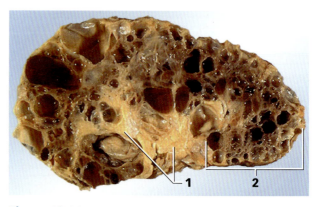

Figure 10-11. Gross pathology of Potter type III, adult dominant polycystic kidney disease (ADPKD). 1 = fibrotic tissue, 2 = cystic tissue (throughout).

Potter Type IV—Obstructive Cystic Renal Dysplasia

Obstructive cystic renal dysplasia (OCRD) is characterized by the appearance of dysplastic cysts in the kidneys secondary to chronic obstruction of urinary outflow (Figure 10-12A). Early disruption of any portion of the excretory path causes urine to back up into the renal collecting system, resulting in hydronephrosis with subsequent formation of dysplastic cysts scattered throughout the renal parenchyma. Obstructive cystic renal dysplasia may be confined to the medullary or cortical portions of the kidney and may totally or partially affect one or both kidneys. As with other types of congenital renal dysplasia, outcomes are dependent on the functioning renal mass present. Potter type IV can occur as an isolated congenital condition but is found in association with concomitant abnormalities about half the time.[7]

Associated Abnormalities

The following abnormalities may be associated with obstructive cystic renal dysplasia:

- Posterior urethral valves
- Duplex collecting system
- Ureterovesical obstruction
- VACTERL association
- Congenital heart disease
- Central nervous system abnormalities
- Gastrointestinal abnormalities

Sonographic Signs

The following are the characteristic sonographic signs of obstructive cystic renal dysplasia (Figures 10-12B and C):

- Scattered, noncommunicating cysts
- Echogenic renal cortex

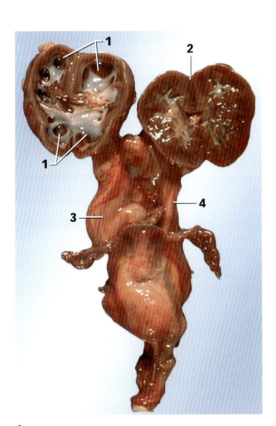
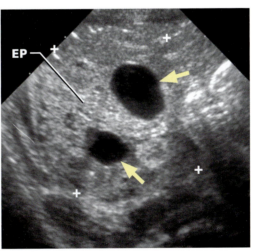
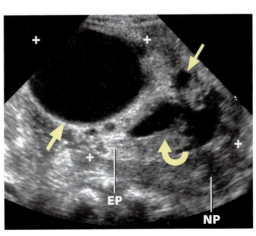

Figure 10-12. Potter type IV, obstructive cystic renal dysplasia (OCRD). **A** Gross pathology. 1 = cystic dysplasia, 2 = normal contralateral kidney, 3 = obstructed ureter, 4 = normal contralateral ureter. **B** Axial and **C** sagittal sections showing scattered, noncommunicating cysts and echogenic renal parenchyma. Cursors = kidney borders, straight arrows = cystic dysplastic tissue, curved arrow = obstructive uropathy, EP = echogenic parenchyma, NP = normal renal parenchyma.

- Evidence of obstructive uropathy on affected side:
  - Dilated renal pelvis
  - Dilated collecting system
  - Dilated ureter
  - Bladder that may or may not be dilated, depending on the location of the obstructive lesion

OBSTRUCTIVE UROPATHIES

Obstructive uropathy is a generic term for any congenital or acquired process that results in disruption of the normal outflow of the urinary tract. The obstruction may be unilateral or bilateral, temporary or permanent, and may occur at any level along the excretory system. Unilateral or spontaneously resolving obstructions are rarely associated with subsequent clinical sequelae.

Chronic pressure against the encompassing solid tissue by urine-engorged collecting structures causes permanent damage to both the kidneys and the fluid tracts. Outcomes depend on the extent and severity of the obstructive uropathy; severe, chronic, bilateral disease can compromise renal development and function to the extent that demise occurs in utero.

Obstructive uropathies are generally categorized based on the level of obstruction:

- Kidney:
  - Hydronephrosis
- Ureter:
  - Ureteropelvic junction (UPJ) obstruction
  - Ectopic ureterocele
  - Congenital primary megaureter
  - Duplicated collecting system
- Urethra:
  - Bladder outlet obstruction
  - Posterior urethral valves
  - Urethral atresia/stenosis
  - Prune belly syndrome

Hydronephrosis

Hydronephrosis is the dilatation of the renal collecting system (a subjectively milder form of dilatation is called *fetal pyelectasis*) (Figure 10-13A). A not uncommon finding during routine prenatal sonographic screening, it is discovered in 1%–3% of all pregnancies and its significance varies with the extent and chronicity of the dilatation. High-resolution ultrasound imaging can routinely demonstrate a small, normal amount of fluid in the fetal renal pelvis. However, as a rule of thumb, when the anteroposterior diameter (APD) of the renal pelvis in cross section measures less than 6 mm before 20 menstrual weeks' gestation and more than 7 mm after 20 weeks, hydronephrosis is present. See Table 10-3.[8]

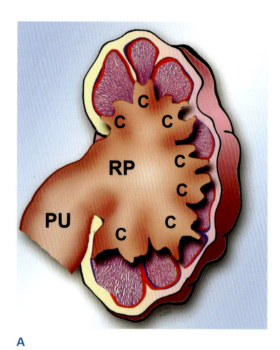

A

Figure 10-13. Hydronephrosis. **A** Schematic. PU = dilated proximal ureter, RP = dilated renal pelvis, C = caliectasis. (Figure continues . . .)

Table 10-3.	Fetal renal pelvic measurements of anteroposterior diameter (APD).	
Status	**Renal Pelvic APD (mm)**	
	Second Trimester (13–27 Weeks)	Third Trimester (28–40 Weeks)
Normal	<4 mm	<7 mm
Mild hydronephrosis	4–6 mm	7–9 mm
Moderate hydronephrosis	7–10 mm	10–15 mm
Severe hydronephrosis	>10 mm	>15 mm
Persistent hydronephrosis	>10 mm	>15 mm

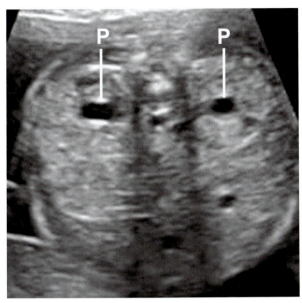

Figure 10-13, continued. B Axial section through both kidneys showing cystic dilatation of both renal pelves in a 20-week fetus. P = bilateral dilated renal pelves. **C** Caliectasis (arrows) communicating with the renal pelvis in a 16-week fetus. P = renal pelvis. **D** Thinning of the renal cortex (arrow) in a 32-week fetus. P = dilated renal pelvis, C = dilated calyces.

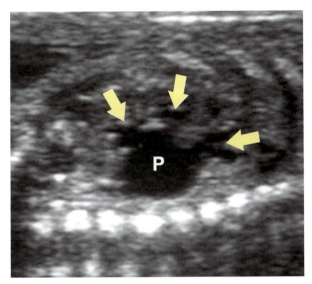

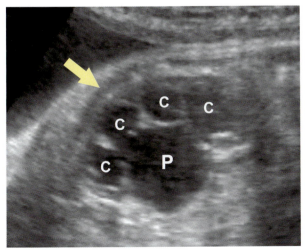

Sonographic Signs

The following sonographic signs are characteristic of hydronephrosis:

- Cystic dilatation of the renal pelvis (Figure 10-13B)
- Communication with *caliectasis* (dilated calyces) (Figure 10-13C)
- Possible presence of dilated proximal ureter
- Thinning of the renal cortex (Figure 10-13D)

Ureteropelvic Junction Obstruction

Ureteropelvic junction (UPJ) *obstruction*, also called *pelviureteric junction* (PUJ) *obstruction*, results from the failure of complete canalization of the renal pelvis and proximal ureter in the embryo at about 10–12 menstrual weeks' gestation. External compression on the ureteropelvic junction by bands of fibrous tissue, kinks, and aberrant blood vessels can also obstruct normal outflow. Unable to flow freely into the ureter, urine dams up behind the obstruction and dilates the collecting system. The condition is relatively common, occurring at a rate of approximately 1 in 1000–2000 newborns, and is most frequently unilateral and on the left side.

Sonographic Signs

The following are the characteristic sonographic signs of ureteropelvic junction obstruction (Figures 10-14A and B):

- Cystic dilatation of the renal pelvis
- Caliectasis
- Thinning of the renal cortex
- Enlarged kidney

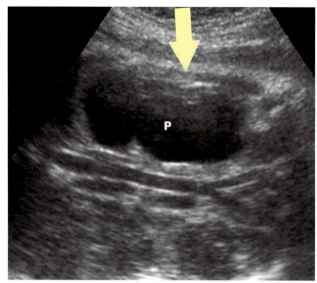

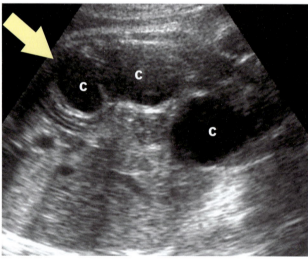

B

Figure 10-14. Ureteropelvic junction obstruction. **A** Coronal section through the retroperitoneum in a 28-week fetus demonstrating cystic dilatation of the renal pelvis. **B** Caliectasis. P = renal pelvis, C = dilated calyces, arrows = thinning of the renal cortex.

Ectopic Ureterocele

A *ureterocele* is the cystic dilatation of the distal-most portion of the ureter, just as it approaches the trigone of the bladder. A *simple ureterocele* is one that occurs at a normal location of the vesicoureteral junction (VUJ); an *ectopic ureterocele*, accounting for about 75% of all fetal ureteroceles, results from an abnormal location of the vesicoureteral junction insertion into the bladder. Weakening of the bladder wall at the insertion site allows the distal ureter to herniate into the bladder (Figure 10-15A). Regardless of etiology, chronic imped-

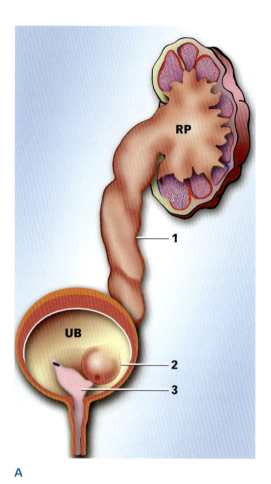

A

Figure 10-15. Ecoptic ureterocele. **A** Schematic representation of a ureterocele projecting into the lumen of the urinary bladder (UB) just above the trigone with concomitant hydroureter and hydronephrotic dilatation of the renal pelvis (RP). 1 = hydroureter, 2 = ureterocele, 3 = trigone. (Figure continues . . .)

ance of outflow into the bladder will cause the collecting system to dilate upstream from the vesicoureteral junction, putting the fetus at risk for the complications of obstructive uropathy as discussed above.

Sonographic Signs

The following are the characteristic sonographic signs of ectopic ureterocele:

- Large, tortuous, fluid-filled ureter filling the abdomen (Figure 10-15B)
- Cystic structure projecting into the bladder (Figure 10-15C)
- Ipsilateral hydronephrosis

Congenital Primary Megaureter

Congenital primary megaureter refers to the chronic dilatation of a ureter related to abnormalities of the ureter per se, rather than distal obstructive pathology.

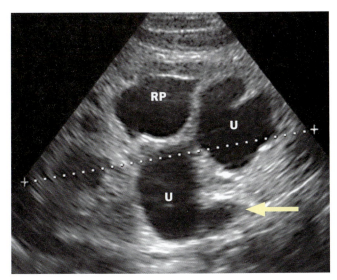
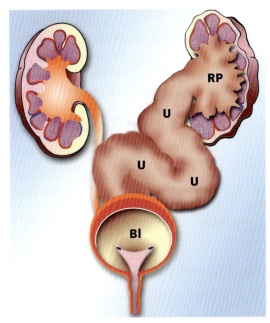
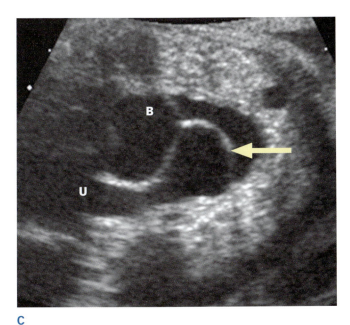
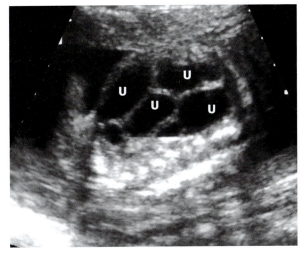

Figure 10-15, continued. B Dilated renal pelvis (RP) and a large, dilated, and tortuous ureter (U) filling the abdomen. Arrow = distal ureter. **C** Ectopic ureterocele herniating (arrow) into the bladder. U = distal ureter, B = urinary bladder.

Figure 10-16. Congenital megaureter. **A** Schematic representation of a chronically dilated ureter (U) and dilatation of the renal pelvis (RP). Bl = urinary bladder. **B** Sagittal section through the fetal abdomen demonstrating a large, tortuous ureter with dilated ureteric folds (U) filling the fetal abdomen.

It may result from reflux at the ureterovesical junction secondary to abnormalities of structure or function at the ureteral insertion site, or it may be a physiologic obstruction by an adynamic distal ureteral segment. Most etiologies are indeterminate. Pathologically, the ureter is grossly enlarged, with dilated, tortuous loops occupying most of the fetal abdomen, altering the normal architectural relationships among the visceral organs (Figure 10-16A).

Sonographic Signs

The following are the characteristic sonographic signs of congenital megaureter:

- Large, tortuous ureter with dilated ureteric folds filling the fetal abdomen (Figure 10-16B)
- Tapering of the dilated distal ureter (adynamic obstructive type)
- Dilated distal ureter at ureterovesical junction
- Normal bladder filling and emptying

Renal Duplications

Duplication of the renal collecting system can result in a *duplex* (or *bifid*) *collecting system* (Figure 10-17A). The ureters are either partially or completely duplicated, unilaterally or bilaterally, as a result of incomplete fusion of the upper- and lower-pole segments of the excretory apparatus during early renal development. The ureteral segment that arises from the upper pole is often obstructed by marked dilatation of the upper-pole portion of the collecting system. In some cases this may appear to resemble a cyst in the upper pole. The lower-pole ureteral segment is usually not obstructed but may permit reflux.

Associated Abnormalities

The following abnormalities may be associated with renal duplications:

- Ectopic ureterocele
- Vesicoureteral reflux
- Hydronephrosis

Sonographic Signs

The following are the characteristic sonographic signs of renal duplications:

- Cystic dilatation of the upper-pole collecting system (Figure 10-17B)
- Ipsilateral ureteral dilatation down to the bladder
- Presence of ureterocele (common)
- Nondilated lower-pole collecting system

Bladder Outlet Obstruction

Bladder outlet obstruction is the generic term for blockage of the urinary tract at the urethral level. In the male fetus, obstruction is most commonly caused by posterior urethral valves; in the female, by urethral atresia or congenital cloacal abnormalities. Urine accumulates in the bladder proximal to the obstruction and, as the pressure increases over time, typically causes reflux into both renal collecting systems, resulting in bilateral hydroureter and hydronephrosis.

Sonographic Signs

The sonographic appearance of bladder outlet obstruction is similar across etiologies: The hallmark finding on sonography is a massively distended urinary bladder, usually but not always accompanied by bilateral hydroureter and hydronephrosis.

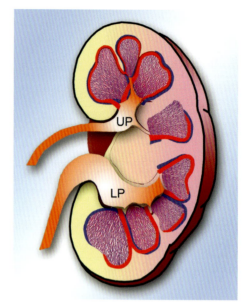

A

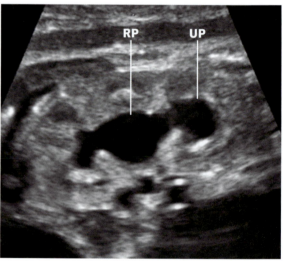

B

Figure 10-17. Renal duplication. **A** Schematic illustration of a bifid collecting system with upper-pole (UP) and lower-pole (LP) segments. **B** Cystic dilatation of the upper-pole collecting system (UP) in a fetus with renal duplication. RP = renal pelvis.

Posterior Urethral Valves

The most common cause of obstructive uropathy in male fetuses is *posterior urethral valves* (PUV), membranous remnants of the mesonephric duct projecting into the urethral lumen.[9] There are three pathologic types of PUV; all are characterized by the physical impedance of urinary outflow at the level of the prostatic urethra. In the most common manifestation of PUV, there is a hypertrophic ridge of muscle tissue at

Urethral Atresia

Urethral atresia or *agenesis* is the congenital absence of the urethra. When it occurs as an isolated anomaly, the urinary bladder will become grossly distended and appear indistinct from other types of bladder outlet obstruction. However, in instances where the urinary bladder is also congenitally absent, there may be dilatation of the upper excretory tract. In both cases, severe chronic oligohydramnios is present and, unless fetal intervention ensues, the condition is not compatible with life.[10]

Sonographic Signs

The characteristic sonographic signs of bladder outlet obstruction, including both urethral atresia and posterior urethral valves, are the following:

- Massive distention and hypertrophy of the urinary bladder
- Keyhole sign from bladder distention and dilated prostatic urethra (Figure 10-18B)
- Hydroureter and/or hydronephrosis (90% of cases)[11]
- Oligohydramnios

Prune Belly Syndrome

Prune belly syndrome (PBS), also known as *Eagle-Barrett syndrome*, is a rare, congenital obstructive uropathy associated with severe oligohydramnios, a megacystic bladder, and visible deformity of the anterior abdominal wall. It derives its name from the wizened, wrinkled skin that covers the anterior abdomen, resembling the surface of a prune (Figure 10-19A). More than 95% of cases of prune belly syndrome are found in male fetuses.[12] As with most prenatal complications involving severe oligohydramnios, it is primarily pulmonary hypoplasia that creates the associated postnatal morbidity and mortality of affected fetuses.

The constellation of pathologic findings associated with prune belly syndrome includes:

- Anterior abdominal wall atrophy
- Genitourinary anomalies:
  - Megacystis
  - Megaureter
  - Dilated prostatic urethra
- Undescended testes

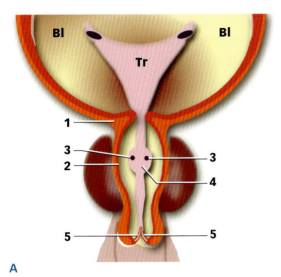

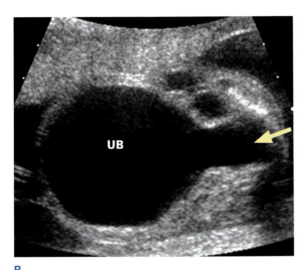

Figure 10-18. Posterior urethral valves. **A** Schematic illustration of posterior urethral valves obstructing bladder outflow. Bl = bladder, Tr = trigone, 1 = hypertrophic ridge, 2 = prostatic urethra, 3 = ejaculatory ducts, 4 = verumontanum, 5 = posterior urethral valves. **B** Coronal section through the fetal pelvis at 32 weeks demonstrating a classic keyhole sign from distention of the bladder (UB) and dilated prostatic urethra (arrow).

the bladder neck, encompassing the proximal urethral sphincter and valve-like membranes, which obstruct bladder outflow at the level of the *verumontanum* (the elevated ridge of tissue in the wall of the prostatic urethra where the seminal ducts make their entry) (Figure 10-18A). The chronic obstruction of urinary outflow into the amniotic cavity grossly distends the urinary bladder and results in oligohydramnios. There may or may not be concomitant hydroureter or hydronephrosis. Megacystis may also be present.

Associated Abnormalities

The following abnormalities may be associated with prune belly syndrome:

- Pulmonary hypoplasia
- Trisomies 13 (Patau syndrome) and 18 (Edwards syndrome)
- Congenital cardiac anomalies
- Imperforate anus
- Polydactyly/syndactyly
- Talipes equinovarus (clubfoot)

Sonographic Signs

The following are the characteristic sonographic signs of prune belly syndrome:

- Hyperechoic renal parenchyma
- Clubbed, dilated calyces
- Dilated, tortuous ureters
- Large, megacystic bladder (Figure 10-19B)

GENITOURINARY NEOPLASMS

Several types of solid renal and adrenal masses may occur in utero, such as congenital adrenal neuroblastoma, Wilms tumor (nephroblastoma), and congenital mesoblastic nephroma (CMN). All are solid masses with robust hemodynamic characteristics that make them especially amenable to color Doppler evaluation. Because of their large size and the attendant distortion of adjacent anatomic architecture, differentiation of the pathologic type of a neoplasm is often not possible sonographically in these cases. While the high-volume hemodynamic shunting of blood via multiple small arteriovenous fistulae creates dramatic color Doppler images, it is also the major cause of morbidity and mortality during the prenatal period. Volume overload of the right heart ultimately leads to cardiac failure and the hydropic sequelae that can ensue from any type of fetal genitourinary neoplasm.

Congenital Adrenal Neuroblastoma

A *neuroblastoma* is a sarcoma consisting of malignant neuroblasts that arises from the adrenal medulla in more than 93% of cases.[13] Other sites of origin include the cervical and thoracic regions, and metastasis can occur locally or via the fetal circulation to the umbilical cord or placenta. Tumors can be so large that they

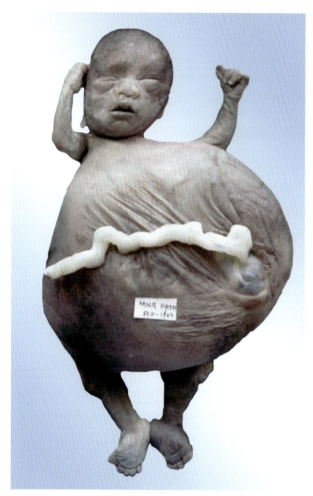

A

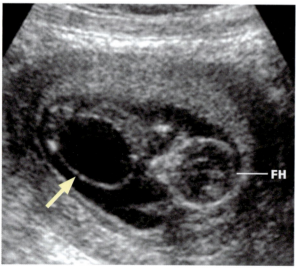

B

Figure 10-19. Prune belly syndrome. **A** Gross pathology of a fetus with prune belly syndrome demonstrating the classic appearance of the anterior abdominal wall. **B** Coronal section through a fetus at 15 weeks with a large, megacystic bladder (arrow). FH = fetal head.

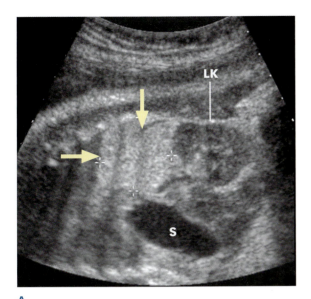

A

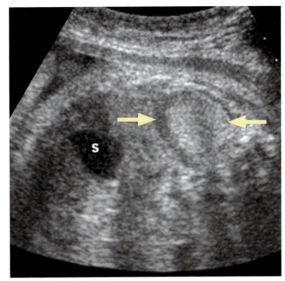

B

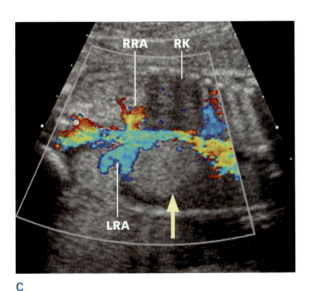

C

Figure 10-20. Neuroblastoma (arrows)—three sonographic images from the same fetus. **A** Left parasagittal section demonstrating an echogenic mass superior to the left kidney (LK) and posterior to the stomach (S). **B** Axial section through a mass in the left retroperitoneum. S = stomach. **C** Coronal color Doppler image showing flow through both right (RRA) and left (LRA) renal arteries, the right kidney (RK), and an echogenic mass (arrow) in the left renal fossa.

result in dystocia during delivery.[14] The sonographic demonstration of a solid mass sharing the same renal fossa with a normal-appearing kidney is strong evidence that the neoplasm is adrenal in origin; however, it is not pathognomonic—an exophytic renal tumor may create the same appearance (Figures 10-20A–C).

Wilms Tumor (Nephroblastoma)

Wilms tumor, also known as *nephroblastoma*, is a genitourinary malignancy that arises from the tissue of the primitive metanephros. It is the most common renal neoplasm found in neonates and children and accounts for more than 85% of all pediatric renal masses.[15] It occurs sporadically in about 1 in 10,000 live births, but it also has autosomal dominant familial tendencies. Tumors arising from a genetic source are more likely to be present bilaterally.

Congenital Mesoblastic Nephroma

Congenital mesoblastic nephroma (CMN), also called *fetal renal hamartoma*, is a usually benign tumor arising from within the kidney. It is not dissimilar to a uterine fibroid in its gross pathologic composition and sonographic characteristics. The solid, whorling bands of fibrous fascia attenuate the acoustic beam and create the appearance of an ill-defined, hypoechoic mass in the renal fossa.

Associated Abnormalities

The following abnormalities may be associated with all types of genitourinary neoplasm:

- Beckwith-Wiedemann syndrome
- Trisomy 18
- Turner syndrome
- External genital abnormalities

Sonographic Signs

Characteristic sonographic signs of all types of genitourinary neoplasm include the following:

- Solid mass in the renal fossa (Figure 10-21A)
- Complex mass; may contain cystic components
- Hemorrhage into the mass, with echogenicity varying over time
- Distortion of adjacent anatomic architecture (Figure 10-21B)
- Color Doppler may show:
  ‣ Central feeding vessel (Figure 10-21C)
  ‣ Diffuse vascularity throughout the mass
- Nonimmune hydrops fetalis (see Chapter 12, pages 302–304)

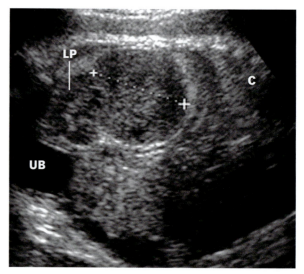

A

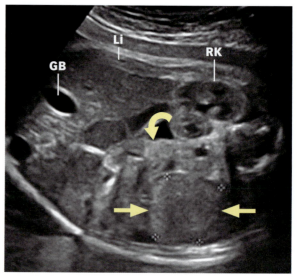

B

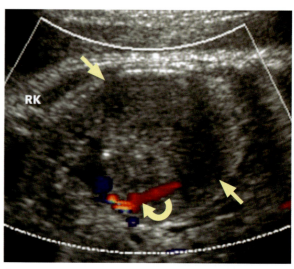

C

Figure 10-21. Genitourinary neoplasms. **A** Coronal section through the fetal retroperitoneum with cursors placed on the margins of a solid complex mass (arrow). LP = lower pole of kidney, UB = urinary bladder, C = chest. **B** Distortion of adjacent anatomic architecture in a fetus with genitourinary tumors. GB = gallbladder, Li = liver, RK = right kidney, straight arrows = solid mass, curved arrow = displaced retroperitoneal anatomy. **C** Color Doppler shows an artery (curved arrow) feeding a solid genitourinary tumor (straight arrows). RK = right kidney.

CHAPTER 10 REVIEW QUESTIONS

1. The fetal kidneys begin to develop at the:
   A. Beginning of the 5th menstrual week
   B. Beginning of the 6th menstrual week
   C. End of the 6th menstrual week
   D. Beginning of the 7th menstrual week

2. The first, nonfunctional buds of tissue that appear in the embryo as precursors to the kidneys are the:
   A. Pronephroi
   B. Metanephroi
   C. Mesonephroi
   D. Nephrons

3. The functioning, well-developed excretory organs that form immediately before the development of the permanent kidneys in the embryo are the:
   A. Pronephroi
   B. Metanephroi
   C. Mesonephroi
   D. Nephrons

4. Fetal kidneys can be identified as early as:
   A. 6–8 menstrual weeks
   B. 8–10 menstrual weeks
   C. 10–12 menstrual weeks
   D. 12–14 menstrual weeks

5. A rule of thumb for normal renal growth is approximately:
   A. 1 mm per week of gestation
   B. 2 mm per week of gestation
   C. 3 mm per week of gestation
   D. 4 mm per week of gestation

6. The fetal urinary bladder empties and fills in cycles of how many minutes?
   A. 10–25
   B. 20–35
   C. 30–45
   D. 45–60

7. Fetal external genitalia can be sonographically differentiated as early as:
   A. 8 menstrual weeks
   B. 10 menstrual weeks
   C. 12 menstrual weeks
   D. 14 menstrual weeks

8. The absence of one or both fetal kidneys is called:
   A. Renal agenesis
   B. Renal aplasia
   C. Renal dysplasia
   D. Renal ectopia

9. What is the term for the chronic absence of amniotic fluid in a severely oligohydramniotic sac that causes structural and developmental abnormalities with the fetus?
   A. Bilateral renal agenesis
   B. Potter sequence
   C. Beckwith-Wiedemann syndrome
   D. Zellweger syndrome

10. Potter sequence is characterized by all of the following EXCEPT:
    A. Pulmonary hypoplasia
    B. Hydrops fetalis
    C. Limb abnormalities
    D. Abnormal facies

11. Potter sequence results from:
    A. Severe oligohydramnios
    B. Severe polyhydramnios
    C. Placental insufficiency
    D. Nuchal cord

12. Unilateral renal agenesis is associated with all of the following EXCEPT:
    A. Trisomy 21
    B. Turner syndrome
    C. Müllerian duct anomalies
    D. Bladder exstrophy

13. Sonographic findings associated with unilateral renal agenesis include all of the following EXCEPT:
    A. Down syndrome
    B. Normal amount of amniotic fluid
    C. Potter sequence
    D. Obstructive uropathies

14. The presence of a kidney outside its expected position in the renal fossa is called:
    A. Ectopic ureterocele
    B. Renal agenesis
    C. Renal ectopia
    D. Renal dysplasia

15. Infantile polycystic renal disease (Potter type I) is characterized sonographically by all of the following EXCEPT:
    A. Multiple large cysts replacing renal parenchyma
    B. Large echogenic kidneys
    C. Nonfilling of the urinary bladder
    D. Loss of corticomedullary differentiation

16. Multicystic renal dysplasia (Potter type II) is characterized by all of the following EXCEPT:
    A. Multiple large cysts replacing renal parenchyma
    B. Large hyperechoic kidneys bilaterally
    C. Echogenic renal parenchyma
    D. Lobulated renal contour

17. Obstructive cystic renal dysplasia (Potter type IV) may be associated with all of the following EXCEPT:
    A. Posterior urethral valves
    B. Duplex collecting system
    C. Ureterovesicular obstruction
    D. Renal agenesis

18. Any congenital or acquired process that results in disruption of the normal outflow of the fetal urinary tract may result in:
    A. Renal agenesis
    B. Obstructive uropathy
    C. Renal ectopia
    D. Polycystic renal disease

19. The failure of complete canalization of the renal pelvis and proximal ureter in the embryo at about 10–12 weeks' gestation may result in:
    A. Renal agenesis
    B. Bladder exstrophy
    C. Ureteropelvic junction obstruction
    D. Multicystic dysplastic kidney

20. Chronic dilatation of a ureter related to abnormalities of the ureter per se, rather than distal obstructive pathology, is termed:
    A. Congenital primary megaureter
    B. Ectopic ureterocele
    C. Hydronephrosis
    D. Hydroureter

21. The sonographic findings seen in this image are most consistent with:

    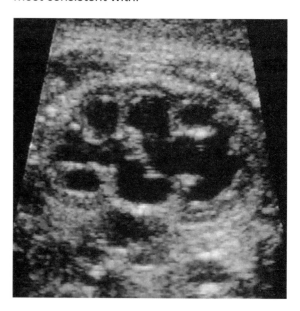

    A. Hydronephrosis
    B. Multicystic dysplastic kidney
    C. Polycystic kidney disease
    D. Intestinal atresia

22. The sonographic findings seen in this image are most consistent with:

    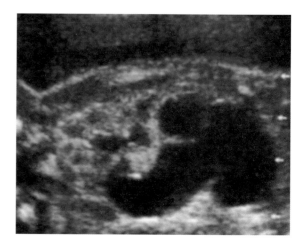

    A. Ectopic ureterocele
    B. Primary megaureter
    C. Ureteropelvic junction obstruction
    D. Posterior urethral valves

23. The sonographic findings seen in this image are most consistent with:

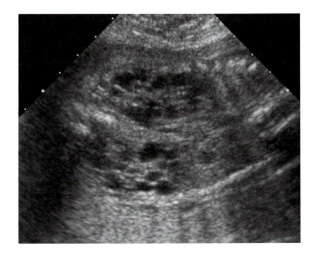

A. Polycystic kidney disease
B. Hydronephrosis
C. Multicystic dysplastic kidney disease
D. UPJ obstruction

24. The sonographic findings seen in this image are most consistent with:

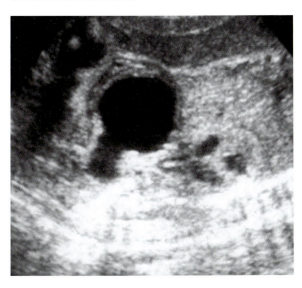

A. Prune belly syndrome
B. Ectopic ureterocele
C. Primary megacystis
D. Posterior urethral valves

ANSWERS

See Appendix A on page 481 for answers.

REFERENCES

1. Emanuel B, Nachman RP, Aronson N, et al: Congenital solitary kidney: a review of 74 cases. Am J Dis Child 127:17–19, 1974.

2. Cascio S, Paran S, Puri P: Associated urological anomalies in children with unilateral renal agenesis. J Urol 162:1081–1083, 1999.

3. Chang PL, Mrazek-Pugh B, Blumenfeld YJ: Prenatal diagnosis of cross-fused ectopia: does color Doppler and 3-dimensional sonography help? J Ultrasound Med 30:578–580, 2011.

4. Lonergan GJ, Rice RR, Suarez ES: Autosomal recessive polycystic kidney disease: radiologic-pathologic correlation. RadioGraphics 20:837–855, 2000.

5. Aslam M, Watson AR: Unilateral multicystic dysplastic kidney: long term outcomes. Arch Dis Child 91:820–823, 2006.

6. Nahm AM, Henriquez DE, Ritz E: Renal cystic disease (ADPKD and ARPKD). Nephrol Dial Transplant 17:311–314, 2002.

7. Blane CE, Barr M, DiPietro MA, et al: Renal obstructive dysplasia: ultrasound diagnosis and therapeutic implications. Pediatr Radiol 21:274–277, 1991.

8. Blachar A, Schachter M, Blachar Y, et al: Evaluation of prenatally diagnosed hydronephrosis by morphometric measurements of the kidney. Pediatr Radiol 24:131–134, 1994.

9. Blews DE: Sonography of the neonatal genitourinary tract. Radiol Clin North Am 37:1199–1208, 1999.

10. González R, De Filippo R, Jednak R, et al: Urethral atresia: long-term outcome in 6 children who survived the neonatal period. J Urol 165:2241–2244, 2001.

11. Blews DE: Sonography of the neonatal genitourinary tract. Radiol Clin North Am 37:1199–1208, 1999.

12. Routh JC, Huang L, Retik AB, et al: Contemporary epidemiology and characterization of newborn males with prune belly syndrome. Urology 76:44–48, 2010.

13. Acharya S, Jayabose S, Kogan S, et al: Prenatally diagnosed neuroblastoma. Cancer 80:304–310, 1997.

14. Jennings RW, LaQuaglia MP, Leong K, et al: Fetal neuroblastoma: prenatal diagnosis and natural history. J Pediatr Surg 28:1168–1174, 1993.

15. Lowe LH, Isuani BH, Heller RM, et al: Pediatric renal masses: Wilms tumor and beyond. RadioGraphics 20:1585–1603, 2000.

SUGGESTED READINGS

Avni FE, Maugey-Lalom B, Cassart M, et al: The fetal genitourinary tract. In Callen PW (ed): *Ultrasonography in Obstetrics and Gynecology*, 5th edition. Philadelphia, Saunders Elsevier, 2008, pp 640–675.

Fong KW, Robertson JE, Maxwell CV: The fetal urogenital tract. In Rumack CM, Wilson SR, Charboneau JW (eds): *Diagnostic Ultrasound*, 4th edition. Philadelphia, Elsevier Mosby, 2011, pp 1353–1388.

Roberts M: The fetal urogenital system. In Hagen-Ansert SL (ed): *Textbook of Diagnostic Ultrasonography*, 7th edition. St. Louis, Elsevier Mosby, 2012, pp 1350–1379.

CHAPTER 11
The Prenatal Genetic Workup

Indications for Prenatal Genetic Testing

Maternal Serum Testing

Invasive Procedures

Genetic Sonographic Fetal Anatomic Survey

Genetic Abnormalities

Nonaneuploidic Syndromes, Associations, and Sequences

A routine part of prenatal care for the past several decades has been the integration of genetic medicine into the comprehensive evaluation of a pregnancy. The advent of maternal serum markers used in conjunction with more invasively obtained biochemical assays and karyotype mapping (by means of amniocentesis and chorionic villus sampling) permits the early prenatal diagnosis of many significant congenital genetic abnormalities.

After amniocentesis and chorionic villus sampling, the third leg of the prenatal genetic diagnostic triad is high-resolution sonographic imaging of the fetus and of pertinent maternal gestational elements. The standard of practice in most locales in the United States is to perform, with the mother's assent, a routine but comprehensive sonogram at 18–20 weeks, which yields a great deal of useful information in the management of both normal and complicated pregnancies. This "screening" sonogram can:

- Establish fetal viability
- Establish baseline fetal biometric measurements
- Establish the number of fetuses present
- Provide a detailed anatomic survey of all fetal organ systems
- Assess the integrity of the placenta, cervix, and amount of amniotic fluid present

In the years when high-risk obstetric sonography and maternal-fetal medicine were evolving into their own subspecialties, there was a trend in some ob/gyn ultrasound centers to use a two-tiered approach with prenatal ultrasound. "Level II" became synonymous with a higher level of attention to more specific fetal anatomic details than in a "Level I" exam. This distinction has fallen into disuse as the ubiquitous availability of accurate, sophisticated, high-resolution ultrasound equipment in the hands of highly trained and experienced examiners has made a complete, detailed survey of fetal anatomic minutiae broadly available.

The community standard of care and recommendations from several national medical organizations mandate a complete and comprehensive assessment of the fetus during its first presentation after 14 weeks. Patients at risk for fetal abnormalities benefit from the enhanced examination provided by an obstetric *sonologist* (physician-sonographer). High-risk obstetric centers have sonologists on staff who, in addition to training in their primary specialty (obstetrics, maternal-fetal medicine, radiology), have completed a fellowship in directed obstetric sonographic examination.

INDICATIONS FOR PRENATAL GENETIC TESTING

A prenatal genetic workup is indicated in those pregnancies that carry an increased risk of a diagnosable fetal disorder. The most common indications include:

- Maternal age ≥ 35 at delivery
- Family history of congenital abnormalities
- Prior pregnancy with congenital abnormality
- Prenatal exposure to noxious substances (e.g., teratogens)
- Maternal diabetes

Patients identified as "at risk" are offered a genetic workup that typically includes referral to a specialized team of physicians, geneticists, and sonologists who provide a tiered battery of prenatal tests geared toward identifying prenatally diagnosable fetal anomalies. The goal of this methodology is to identify these abnormalities early enough in gestation to allow for a discussion and consideration of management options by the patient, her family, and her care providers. The major components of the *diagnostic triad* in a prenatal genetic testing program include:

- Maternal serum testing
- Invasive procedures
- Genetic sonographic fetal anatomic survey

MATERNAL SERUM TESTING

The goal of maternal serum testing is to identify variations in the levels of several pregnancy-produced substances circulating in the maternal blood that are statistically associated with the presence of concomitant congenital genetic abnormalities. A variety of substances can be tested for singly or in combination. In current practice, it is common to run a *triple* or *quad screen* on a single sample of maternal blood.

The *triple screen* consists of:

- Maternal serum alpha-fetoprotein (MSAFP)
- Human chorionic gonadotropin, beta subgroup (beta-hCG)
- Estriol (µE3)

A *quad screen* adds to this battery:

- The hormone inhibin A (inhA)

The most accurate maternal serum testing results are obtained when blood is drawn between 16 and 18 weeks' gestation.

As with all screening methods, there are advantages and pitfalls in looking for abnormalities in the absence of clinical findings or objective evidence:

- *False-positive results* are those that indicate the presence of an anomaly or pathologic condition when, in fact, it is not present. Several factors can skew maternal serum levels in a false-positive direction so that they suggest the presence of a congenital abnormality. These include maternal age, maternal weight, inaccurate gestational age, and the presence of diabetes.

- *False-negative results* are those that indicate normality when, in fact, abnormalities or pathologic conditions are present. Factors that may yield inaccurately normal (false-negative) maternal serum values are rare, the most common being inaccurate gestational age.

The data derived from the triple and quad screens can be interpreted in several ways. One is to extrapolate the risk of all chromosomal abnormalities that may affect the fetus as a function of serum level versus maternal age. Another is to identify patients who may benefit from further diagnostic testing, such as genetic amniocentesis, chorionic villus sampling, and/or sonographic fetal anatomic assessment. It is this second category that is most germane to sonography practitioners. The association of specific maternal serum markers with the most common prenatal conditions that they test for is presented in Table 11-1.

The results for both triple and quad screening programs are about the same in detecting trisomy conditions. In a large study (>550,000 patients) published by the California Prenatal Screening Program (PNS) of the California Department of Public Health in 2011, the detection rate for trisomy 21 (Down syndrome) was 77% with the triple screen and 76% with the quad screen. Both methods carried a 95% confidence interval.[1]

MATERNAL SERUM ALPHA-FETOPROTEIN

Alpha-fetoprotein (AFP) is a glycoprotein produced by the fetal liver, yolk sac, and developing fetal gastrointestinal tract. It crosses the fetal membranes and is normally found in maternal serum (MS) and amniotic fluid (AF). In a normally progressing gestation, MSAFP levels rise predictably with gestational age and peak at around 14 weeks. By 30 weeks, the fetal liver stops AFP production and both serum and amniotic fluid levels begin to decline. As both MSAFP and AFAFP levels are dependent on gestational age, it is critical that a pregnancy be properly and accurately dated before interpreting the results of maternal serum testing. In a patient with an unreliable menstrual history, sonographic biometry plays an important role in determining the correct gestational age.

Open fetal anatomic abnormalities—such as neural tube defects and gastroschisis—allow an increased volume of AFP to seep into the amniotic cavity. The excess glycoprotein crosses into maternal blood, elevating the bioassayed serum levels. Elevated MSAFP levels are typically reported as multiples of the median (MoM), a statistical methodology that measures how much a test result deviates from the average. While specific numeric test results vary from lab to lab, MSAFP levels of 2–2.5 MoM heighten concern about concomitant fetal genetic abnormalities and are an indication to refer the patient for additional prenatal diagnostic testing.

Table 11-1. Maternal serum markers.

Anomaly	MSAFP	beta-hCG	μE3	inhA
Trisomy 13 (Patau syndrome)	Low	—	Low	—
Trisomy 18 (Edwards syndrome)	Low	Low	Low	Low/normal
Trisomy 21 (Down syndrome)	Low	High	Low	High
Neural tube defects (open)	High	Normal	Low	Normal
Turner syndrome	Low	Low	Low	Low/normal
Cardiac defects	High	Low	Low	—
Abdominal wall defects	High	—	—	—

Elevation may result from:
- Incorrect gestational age
- Multiple gestations
- Open neural tube defects
- Open abdominal wall defects
- Esophageal and duodenal atresia
- Placental abruption
- Maternal comorbidity

Reduced levels may be associated with:
- Trisomy 21
- Trisomy 18

HUMAN CHORIONIC GONADOTROPIN

Human chorionic gonadotropin (beta-hCG) is another glycoprotein produced during pregnancy (see Chapter 1). Unlike AFP, which is produced by the conceptus, beta-hCG is produced by the syncytiotrophoblastic cells in developing placental tissue. As an isolated indicator of nonchromosomal congenital anomalies it is not very sensitive. However, in conjunction with the "soft" sonographic markers discussed later in this chapter, elevated serum levels of beta-hCG are associated with a high incidence of chromosomal anomalies, even in the presence of otherwise normal biochemical triple screen values.[2] The particular utility of beta-hCG levels in prenatal genetic testing is closely related to the sonographic component of the diagnostic triad.

ESTRIOL

Estriol (μE3) is one of the three primary types of estrogen produced by the human body. It occurs in significant amounts only during pregnancy, as it is produced by the placenta, fetal liver, and fetal adrenal cortex. As a prenatal maternal serum marker, unconjugated estriol levels can be used in conjunction with other biochemical markers to assess the risk of fetal anomalies, genetic abnormalities, or poor pregnancy outcomes.

In general, diminished levels of μE3 are associated with an increased frequency of adverse obstetric outcomes. Specifically, when serum μE3 levels are diminished by 25%–30% over normal values (<0.5 MoM) there is an increased risk for trisomies 18 and 21. As an individual predictor, reduced μE3 levels are the strongest indicator of trisomy 18.

INVASIVE PROCEDURES

When maternal serum testing is abnormal or when clinical indications warrant, invasive prenatal genetic testing may be employed. Chorionic villus sampling (CVS) and amniocentesis are two methods of obtaining additional biochemical data and fetal genetic material for standard and definitive karyotype mapping and analysis.

CHORIONIC VILLUS SAMPLING

Procedure

Chorionic villus sampling (CVS) is a method of prenatal assessment that permits the diagnosis of many genetic disorders in the first trimester. A needle or biopsy catheter is advanced into the chorion frondosum under ultrasound guidance. The introducer-needle approach can be either transabdominal or transcervical (Figure 11-1). The specific approach is determined by a pre-procedure ultrasound examination that identifies the location of villi in the uterus. The examiner takes a small sample of tissue that contains placental cells derived from the same fertilized egg as the fetus and submits the sample for karyotype mapping.

Risks and Complications

While chorionic villus sampling remains an available tool in the prenatal diagnostic armamentarium, its use has diminished under the shadow of the less risky but equally accurate second trimester amniocentesis. While morbidity and mortality statistics vary greatly

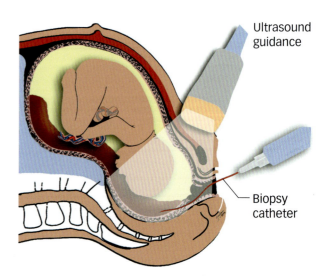

Figure 11-1. Chorionic villus sampling, transcervical approach: Under ultrasound guidance, a needle or biopsy catheter is advanced into the chorion frondosum and a small sample of tissue is retrieved for karyotype mapping.

from center to center, the risk of pregnancy loss from amniocentesis at 15–18 weeks' gestation is approximately 0.06%–0.5% (depending on the study)[3] whereas the overall risk of miscarriage from chorionic villus sampling is approximately 0.5%. It is slightly less using the transabdominal approach.[4] The sole advantage of chorionic villus sampling over amniocentesis is its earlier detection of the same genetic anomalies; chorionic villus sampling is performed between 10 and 14 weeks, whereas genetic amniocentesis is performed at 15–18 weeks.

Potential risks of the transcervical approach in chorionic villus sampling include:[5]

- Spontaneous abortion
- Maternal sepsis
- Perforation of the amniotic sac
- Unexplained mid-trimester oligohydramnios
- Limb reduction defects
- Rh sensitization

AMNIOCENTESIS

Procedure

Genetic *amniocentesis* is an invasive procedure in which a needle is advanced transabdominally into the amniotic cavity under ultrasound guidance and a small amount of amniotic fluid is withdrawn and sent to the lab for a variety of biochemical and genetic tests (Figure 11-2). Amniocentesis can also be performed later in gestation to test for fetal lung maturity; however, at 15–18 weeks its primary indication is the prenatal detection of fetal congenital abnormalities that may affect the subsequent management of the pregnancy.

Two categories of testing are performed on amniotic fluid during the second trimester: biochemical assays and chromosomal analysis.

Biochemical assays test for the presence and quantitated level of several substances that are elevated in the presence of certain congenital abnormalities. The substances most commonly tested for are:

- *Amniotic fluid alpha-fetoprotein* (AFAFP): elevated in the presence of open neural tube defects
- *Acetylcholinesterase*: elevated in the presence of open neural tube defects
- *Gamma-glutamyl transpeptidase* (GGTP): elevated in the presence of esophageal atresia or gastrointestinal abnormalities
- *Bilirubin*: elevated in the presence of Rh disease

Chromosomal analysis detects chromosomal abnormalities through the direct visualization and analysis of fetal DNA. Amniotic fluid contains cells that are sloughed off from fetal skin, bladder, gastrointestinal tract, and amnion. DNA present in these fetal cells can be mapped through a laboratory process called *karyotyping*; the normal human karyotype is seen in Figure 11-3. While advanced genetic analytic techniques are

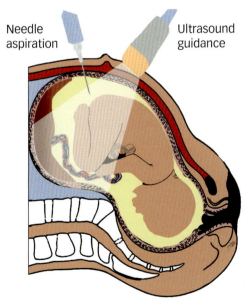

Figure 11-2. Amniocentesis: Under ultrasound guidance, a needle is advanced into the amniotic cavity and a small amount of amniotic fluid is withdrawn for biochemical and genetic tests.

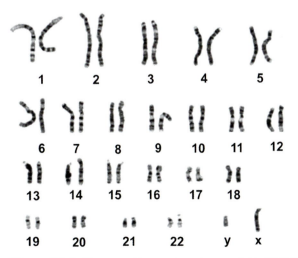

Figure 11-3. The normal human karyotype contains 23 pairs of chromosomes (46 individual ones), including the Y (male) and X (female) chromosomes.

useful in the prenatal detection of a wide range of congenital abnormalities, routine karyotyping performed on amniotic fluid obtained during the second trimester typically tests for aneuploidy conditions such as trisomies 13, 18, and 21.

Indications
Indications for amniocentesis in the early second trimester include:
- Advanced maternal age (≥35 years)
- Previous fetus with aneuploidy
- Parental balanced translocation
- X-linked recessive disorders
- Other genetic disorders
- Fetal anomaly
- Confirmation of lung maturity
- Evaluation for intrauterine infection
- Rh isoimmunization
- Polyhydramnios
- Fetal sex identification
- Paternity testing

Risks and Complications
The risks and complications from amniocentesis include:
- Miscarriage (0.06%–0.5%, depending on the study)[6]
- Cramping
- Bleeding
- Amniotic fluid leakage (1%–2%)
- Needle injuries (rare)
- Rh sensitization (rare)

GENETIC SONOGRAPHIC FETAL ANATOMIC SURVEY

In addition to the routine *screening sonogram* recommended at 16–20 weeks for all pregnancies, the *genetic sonogram* provides a useful adjunct in the earlier detection of some fetal conditions in patients at increased risk for congenital abnormalities. The identification of *soft sonographic markers*—minor ultrasound abnormalities, considered variants of normal, that do not constitute frank structural defects—can substantially increase detection rates for both chromosomal and nonchromosomal abnormalities, particularly Down syndrome.[7, 8]

Several methodologies for integrating the results of a genetic sonogram into overall risk assessment for aneuploidy and other congenital abnormalities have been proposed; however, the best estimate of risk seems to be achieved through the combined use of ultrasound, maternal serum screening, and maternal age. The genetic sonogram relies on the discovery of soft sonographic markers. Generally, the efficacy of soft sonographic markers applies only to a high-risk pregnancy, where the prevalence of congenital anomalies is increased. If the same information is applied to a low-risk pregnancy, especially as isolated findings encountered during a routine screening sonogram, the lower prevalence of aneuploidy makes the positive predictive value too low to be of any value in counseling patients.[9] Also, the absence of soft sonographic markers does not reduce the risk for the presence of aneuploidy. Like most screening tests, genetic sonograms occasionally miss the diagnosis, a potential shortcoming that should be made clear to participating patients.

A number of soft sonographic markers have been identified and reported in the medical literature since the early 1990s. The most widely studied and utilized include:
- Nuchal translucency
- Nuchal thickening
- Hyperechoic bowel
- Echogenic intracardiac focus
- Choroid plexus cysts
- Pyelectasis
- Nasal bone length

NUCHAL TRANSLUCENCY

The *nuchal translucency* is a hypoechoic area located in the interstitial space between the skin and the soft tissue overlying the posterior aspect of the fetal cervical spine. A small amount of fluid normally accumulates in this location until about 14 weeks, by which time the lymphatic system has developed enough to drain the area adequately. However, an increase in the amount of fluid in the nuchal region will elevate its anteroposterior (AP) diameter. In addition to serving as a soft marker for specific congenital anomalies, the nuchal translucency measurement, when significantly increased, is generally associated with an increase in perinatal morbidity and mortality.[10] Specifically, an increased nuchal translucency value, when used in conjunction with maternal serum screening and maternal age, is useful in predicting:

- Aneuploidy (trisomies)
- Turner syndrome
- Diaphragmatic hernia
- Congenital heart disease
- Omphalocele
- Skeletal dysplasias
- VACTERL association

Nuchal translucency is measured when crown-rump length (CRL) is 45–84 mm. The measurement is made in a sagittal plane of section, ideally with the fetal spine toward the bottom of the image. The head should not be hyperextended or hyperflexed and amniotic fluid should surround the fetal head and upper torso. The measurement is made of the translucent area only, placing the digital calipers on the inner-to-inner boundaries at the translucency's widest dimension; a normal measurement is less than 2.5 mm (Figure 11-4A). Soft tissue overlying the nuchal translucency should be excluded from the measurement.

Sonographic Signs

Sonographic signs and methods for demonstrating nuchal translucency include the following:

- Normal value is <2.5 mm (matched to maternal age and crown-rump length).
- There should be no septations within the translucent region.
- Abnormal values are ≥6 mm (Figure 11-4B)

The efficacy of nuchal translucency measurement in identifying fetuses at risk for congenital abnormalities is contingent upon its proper and accurate measurement. When correctly obtained and correlated with maternal age and crown-rump length, the detection rate for aneuploidic anomalies using nuchal translucency approaches 80%–90% with a false-positive rate of approximately 5%.[11] The incidence of abnormal measurements varies widely with the study population screened. The risk estimates for presence of Down syndrome calculated from a large group studied by Pandya et al. in 1995 are summarized in Table 11-2.[12] When correlated with maternal age, nuchal translucency measurements can be useful in predicting other trisomies as well.

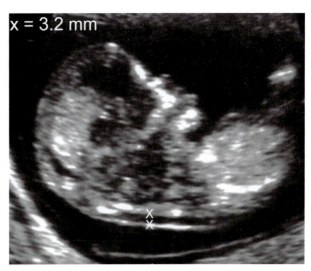

A

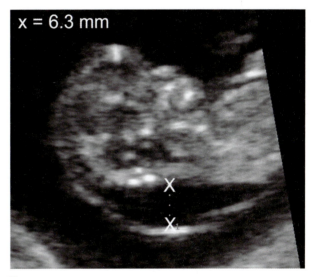

B

Figure 11-4. Nuchal translucency. **A** Sagittal image at 12 weeks showing a relatively lower-risk measurement of 3.2 mm. **B** Sagittal image at 10 weeks showing an abnormal measurement (≥6 mm). Note the cursor placement to exclude soft tissue overlying the translucency.

Table 11-2. Risk estimate for Down syndrome.

Nuchal Translucency Measurement	Risk Multiple
3 mm	3x
4 mm	18x
5 mm	28x
6 mm	36x

Source: Data from Pandya PP, Kondylios A, Hilbert L, et al: Chromosomal defects and outcome in 1015 fetuses with increased nuchal translucency. Ultrasound Obstet Gynecol 5:1, 15–19, 1995.

NUCHAL THICKENING

Nuchal thickness should not be confused with nuchal translucency. Nuchal thickness measurements are obtained in the second trimester and are not considered a part of a genetic sonogram. Nevertheless, there is good correlation between nuchal thickness measurements taken between 15 and 20 weeks, when adjusted for maternal age, and the risk of Down syndrome. In fact, an abnormally thickened nuchal fold is often considered the most sensitive and most specific second trimester marker for Down syndrome, with false-positive rates as low as 1%.[13] Other fetal anomalies associated with an increased nuchal thickness include Turner syndrome, cystic hygroma, other trisomies, congenital cardiovascular anomalies, skeletal dysplasia, and congenital infections.

Both normal (<6 mm) and increased (≥6 mm) values have useful predictive values; a normal measurement is associated with a reduced risk for Down syndrome and may obviate the need for follow-up amniocentesis, while an elevated value has a 95% sensitivity for detecting Down syndrome.[14] An increased nuchal fold thickness may also suggest fetal congenital cardiac heart disease and cystic hygroma.

Measurement of the nuchal fold is taken from an axial oblique section through the fetal head at the level of the posterior fossa. It is the same plane of section used when evaluating the cerebellum and cisterna magna. Other intracranial landmarks include the thalami and cavum septi pellucidi (Figure 11-5A). The measurement calipers should be placed on the outer edge of the occipital bone and the outer edge of the overlying soft tissue (Figure 11-5B).

Sonographic Signs and Diagnostic Criteria

It is important to note the following when demonstrating nuchal thickness:

- It is measured in an axial oblique plane of section.
- Normal value is <6 mm (although authors vary; some use 5 mm as the cutoff).

HYPERECHOGENIC BOWEL

The echogenicity of fetal bowel in the early second trimester is somewhat variable. It is typically more echogenic than adjacent solid visceral organs such as the liver and spleen and may consist of a single locus

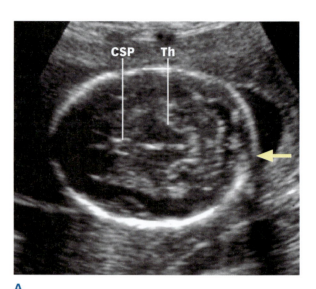

Figure 11-5. Nuchal thickening. **A** Axial oblique section showing a normal nuchal fold. Note the thalamus (Th) and cavum septi pellucidi (CSP). Arrow = nuchal soft tissue. **B** Abnormal nuchal thickening (≥6 mm) is demonstrated in this axial oblique section. Note proper placement of calipers: on the outer edge of the occipital bone and outer edge of the overlying soft tissue.

of bowel or may be multifocal in appearance. Several schemata have been suggested to grade fetal bowel echogenicity, with varying predictive results. A generally accepted rule of thumb is that normal bowel should not be as bright as or brighter than bone. However, technological advances that permit the use of higher frequencies and other imaging enhancements may be a potential source of false-positive interpretation of echogenic bowel.

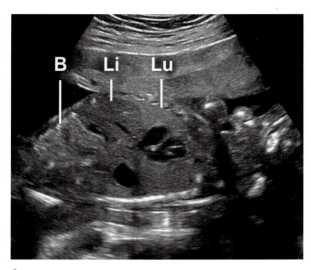
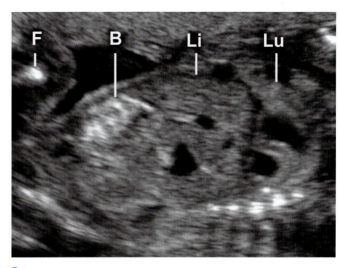

Figure 11-6. Echogenic fetal bowel. **A** Sagittal section through a fetus at 14 weeks demonstrating normal fetal bowel echogenicity; note that bowel (B) is slightly more echogenic than liver (Li) or lung (Lu). **B** Coronal section through a fetus at 14 weeks demonstrating abnormal fetal bowel (B) echogenicity, which is as bright as or brighter than bone. F = femur, Li = liver, Lu = lung.

Hyperechogenic bowel has been associated with an increased risk for:

- Aneuploidy: trisomies 13, 18, and 21
- Cystic fibrosis
- Congenital infections:
  - Cytomegalovirus
  - Herpes
  - Parvovirus
  - Rubella
  - Varicella
  - Toxoplasmosis
- Congenital malformations of the bowel
- Intra-amniotic hemorrhage
- Meconium ileus
- Perinatal complications, including intrauterine growth restriction

Sonographic Signs

Sonographic signs associated with fetal bowel include the following:

- *Normal bowel:* more echogenic than fetal liver, lung, and spleen but less echogenic than bone (Figure 11-6A)
- *Abnormal bowel:* echogenicity that is as bright as or brighter than bone (Figure 11-6B)

ECHOGENIC INTRACARDIAC FOCUS

An *echogenic intracardiac focus* (EIF) is a soft sonographic finding that can be seen in approximately 6% of all fetuses. Although more than 90% of the time there are no associated congenital or chromosomal abnormalities in these fetuses,[15] identification of a single echogenic focus in the fetal heart of a patient at risk for aneuploidy—which may represent mineralization within papillary muscle—is associated with a statistically significant probability of trisomy 13 or 21.[16] An echogenic intracardiac focus is most commonly seen as a bright, unilateral focus in the left ventricle of the heart; however, there may be foci in other chambers as well. There is some evidence that multiple echogenic intracardiac foci are associated with an increased risk of aneuploidy.[17] There is no association with structural cardiac abnormalities or cardiac function if the cardiac scan is otherwise normal in a low-risk fetus. In low-risk populations, most echogenic intracardiac foci disappear by term or a short time after delivery.

Sonographic Signs

An echogenic intracardiac focus is typically visualized as:

- A punctate, brightly echogenic focus in the heart (Figure 11-7)
- Located most commonly in the left ventricle

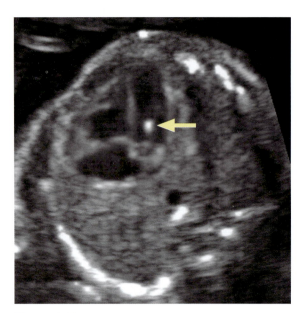

Figure 11-7. Echogenic intracardiac focus (arrow). Axial four-chamber view demonstrating a punctate, brightly echogenic focus within the left ventricle of this 20-week fetus.

CHOROID PLEXUS CYSTS

Choroid plexus cysts (CPCs) are discrete, well-circumscribed collections of fluid identified within the echogenic choroid plexus residing within the lateral cerebral ventricles. They generally measure less than 3 mm and are found in 1%–2% of all fetuses at 16 weeks, almost always regressing by 26 weeks.[18] The association with aneuploidy is small but statistically significant enough to warrant follow-up genetic testing in high-risk patients and in fetuses with other sonographically demonstrable anomalies. The presence of a choroid plexus cyst in association with other anatomic abnormalities is more suspicious of trisomy 18 than of other types of aneuploidy. There is a 1% risk for trisomy 18 if a choroid plexus cyst is the sole sonographic finding and a 4% risk if concomitant imaging findings are present.[19]

There is conflicting evidence on the significance of single versus multiple cysts in identifying fetal chromosomal abnormalities. Some studies demonstrate parity in risk between single and multiple cysts, while others suggest an increased risk when more than one cyst is present. However, in fetuses with trisomy 18, up to 50% present with a choroid plexus cyst.

Sonographic Signs

Sonographic signs associated with choroid plexus cysts include the following (Figures 11-8A and B):

- Single or multiple cysts
- Surrounded by an echogenic choroid plexus
- In a lateral cerebral ventricle

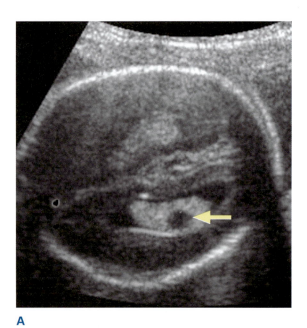
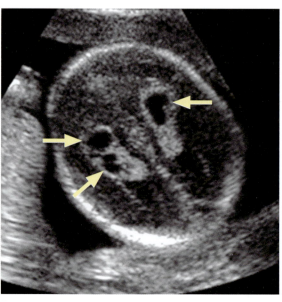

A B

Figure 11-8. Choroid plexus cysts (arrows). Axial sections through the lateral ventricles of two different fetuses demonstrating **A** a single choroid plexus cyst and **B** multiple choroid plexus cysts. Note the surrounding echogenic choroid plexus.

PYELECTASIS

Pyelectasis, generally, is the dilatation of the renal pelvis with urine. As a soft marker identified during prenatal sonographic screening during the second trimester, it is further quantified as dilatation of the renal pelvis measuring 5–10 mm without calyceal involvement. Pyelectasis can result from a number of factors. In the majority of cases identified in utero, it is physiologic and resolves spontaneously about 96% of the time.[20] Gross dilatation of the renal pelvis measuring more than 10 mm along with dilatation of the calyces and proximal ureter raises the diagnostic specter of obstructive uropathies and is not characteristic of the soft marker associated with aneuploidy risk. Sonographic identification of isolated, persistent pyelectasis in the third trimester is useful in predicting when a postnatal obstructive uropathy might require surgery, but it is not useful as an adjunctive sign in detecting aneuploidic fetuses.[21]

Mild pyelectasis is observed in the second trimester in 2% of normal fetuses. That incidence increases to 17%–25% in fetuses with trisomy 21. As an isolated finding, pyelectasis is associated with an incidence of 3.3% with Down syndrome.[22] In fetuses with pyelectasis, the presence of additional sonographic markers or an abnormal maternal serum screen significantly increases the risk of trisomies 13, 18, and 21.

Table 11-3. Renal pyelactasis values.

Menstrual Weeks	AP Renal Pelvis (mm)
18–20	>4.0–4.5
20–29	>5.0
30–32	>6.0
33–term	>7.0

Source: Data from Ahmad G, Green P: Outcome of fetal pyelectasis diagnosed antenatally. J Obstet Gynaecol 25:119–122, 2005.

Sonographic measurement of the renal pelvis is obtained from an axial plane through the kidneys at the level of the renal hilum. The cursors are placed at the inner surfaces of the anterior and posterior margins of the renal pelvis. The absolute anteroposterior (AP) measurement defining pyelectasis varies with gestational age and is presented in Table 11-3.

Sonographic Signs

Sonographic signs associated with pyelectasis include the following:

- Unilateral (Figure 11-9A) or bilateral (Figure 11-9B) renal pelvis dilatation
- Resolves spontaneously by 26 weeks
- No associated caliectasis or ureteral dilatation

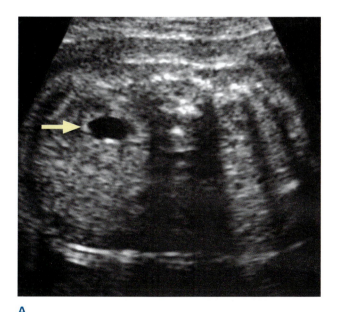
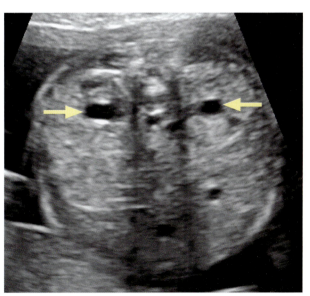

A   B

Figure 11-9. Renal pyelectasis (arrows = dilated renal pelvis). Axial sections through two different fetuses demonstrate **A** unilateral and **B** bilateral pyelectasis.

GENETIC ABNORMALITIES

DEFINITION OF TERMS

Several key genetic concepts are reviewed here before the discussion of genetic anomalies:

- *Karyotype:* A karyotype is the complete set of chromosomes that a species contains in its genetic makeup (genotype). The normal human karyotype contains 23 pairs of chromosomes (46 individual ones; see Figure 11-3, page 275). The first 22 pairs (autosomes) are numbered from 1 to 22 and are arranged from smallest to largest. The last (23rd) pair of chromosomes consists of the sex chromosomes and may be matched (in females) or mismatched (in males). Normal females have two X chromosomes; normal males, one X and one Y chromosome.

- *Single-gene disease:* Medical conditions arising from a single gene occur in about 1% of newborn infants. Approximately 10,000 single-gene diseases are known; about half are autosomal dominant, about a third are autosomal recessive, and the remainder are X-linked.

- *Aneuploidy:* A mismatch of any of the 22 autosomes creates *aneuploidy*, a condition characterized by an abnormal number of chromosomes, either excess or deficient. Aneuploidy originates during gamete cell division when, during meiosis, chromosomes are normally unzipped into two haploid halves. When this division proceeds abnormally, it can pull an extra half chromosome into the new gamete, creating a genetic excess, or leave behind a half chromosome, creating a genetic deficit.

- *Autosomal recessive disorder:* This is a condition in which a defective copy of the gene is contributed by each parent. If each parent carries one copy of the defective gene, the likelihood that the child will inherit two copies of the defective gene (one from each parent) and will contract the disease is 25%; the likelihood that the child will receive only one copy of the defective gene and become a carrier of the disorder is 50%. Every person in the population carries five or six recessive genes for significant diseases, and if the parents of the child are closely related, it is more likely that the child will contract a recessive disease. People who are carriers—who have one normal copy and one defective copy of a gene—will often have some decrease in enzymatic activity of the defective protein, but in recessive conditions that person is clinically normal.

- *Autosomal dominant disorder:* In autosomal dominant conditions, only one defective gene is required to cause the associated disease. A person who has an autosomal dominant disease usually possesses one copy of the defective gene and a normal copy of the gene. Assuming the other parent has normal copies of that particular gene, the risk of the child having the disease is 50%, for the child has a 50-50 chance of receiving either a defective copy or the normal copy of the gene from the affected parent. In many autosomal dominant diseases, the severity of the disease varies from individual to individual, and therefore it is difficult to predict the severity of the disease in a given case.

- *X-linked disease:* Most of these disorders are recessive. This means that a female who has one defective X chromosome and one normal X chromosome will be a carrier but will not manifest the disease. Because males possess only one copy of the X chromosome instead of two, a woman who has one normal and one abnormal copy of an X chromosome gene has a 50% chance of transmitting the abnormal gene to her offspring. If that offspring is male and inherits the abnormal X chromosome, he has a 100% chance of contracting the disease because the child will have only one abnormal X chromosome. In order to contract an X-linked disease from the father, the father must be affected by the disease (i.e., must carry an abnormal X chromosome), as he carries only one X chromosome.

ANEUPLOIDY

The following aneuploidies can occur:

- *Triploidy*, the presence of three chromosomes across the karyotype, for a total of 69 rather than the normal 46.

- *Trisomy*, the presence of three chromosomes instead of the normal two. The condition is further defined by identifying which numbered chromosome is aberrant; e.g., trisomy 21 is an extra chromosome in pair 21 on the karyotype.

- *Disomy*, the presence of two copies of a chromosome.

- *Monosomy*, the lack of one chromosome of the normal complement.

- *Tetrasomy* and *pentasomy*, the presence respectively of four and five copies of a chromosome.

Aneuploidic aberration in number of chromosomes may be present in all cells in an individual or in only a fraction of the cells. When only some cells are affected, the condition is called *mosaicism* and typically produces a less severe clinical manifestation of the syndrome. Most full aneuploidic conceptions spontaneously abort early in the first trimester. For many of the autosomal trisomies, only mosaic cases survive to term.

Triploidy

Triploidy (Figure 11-10) is a lethal genetic syndrome in which the conceptus receives an entire extra set of chromosomes. Rather than the normal two sets of 23 chromosomes (46 total), a triploidic conceptus has three sets (69 total). Similar to trisomies 13, 18, and 21, triploidy may be compatible with life; however, nearly 80% of these gestations end in early pregnancy failure and only anecdotal reports of live deliveries exist.[23] The anatomic abnormalities associated with triploidy span all organ systems, their breadth and severity responsible for the high mortality associated with this condition. Triploidy is also frequently associated with placental abnormalities, particularly partial hydatidiform mole, as both result from an extra set of, most commonly, paternal chromosomes.

Associated Abnormalities

Abnormalities characteristically associated with triploidy include the following:

- Central nervous system anomalies:
  - Spina bifida
  - Myelomeningocele
  - Holoprosencephaly
  - Agenesis of the corpus callosum
  - Hydrocephalus
- Cardiac anomalies:
  - Atrial septal defect
  - Ventricular septal defect
- Genitourinary anomalies:
  - Cystic renal dysplasia
  - Hydronephrosis
  - Hypospadias
  - Micropenis
  - Cryptorchidism

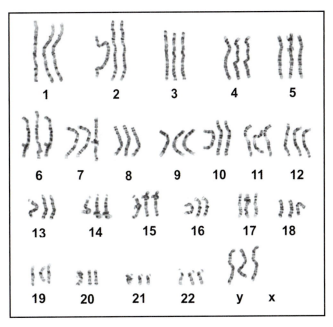

Figure 11-10. Triploidy karyotype: three (versus the normal two) sets of chromosomes, or 69 in all.

- Hand and foot anomalies:
  - Syndactyly
  - Talipes equinovarus
  - Splayed toes
- Craniofacial anomalies:
  - Hypertelorism
  - Microphthalmia
  - Micrognathia
  - Macroglossia
  - Low-set nasal bridge

Sonographic Markers

Sonographic markers associated with triploidy include the following:

- Molar placental changes
- Gross and extensive fetal anatomic abnormalities as listed above

Trisomy 21 (Down Syndrome)

Trisomy 21 (Figure 11-11), also known as *Down syndrome*, is the most common congenital syndrome observed in live births, with an overall incidence of approximately 1 in 600–800 newborns.[24] The incidence of Down syndrome increases with advancing maternal age. Among mothers 35 or older at term, the incidence of Down syndrome is approximately 1 in 275.[25] At a

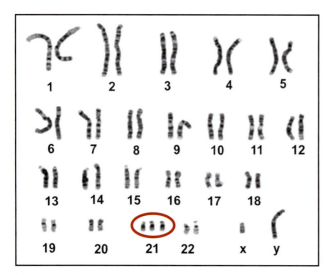

Figure 11-11. Karyotype for trisomy 21 (Down syndrome). Note the extra chromosome 21 (circled).

maternal age of 40, the incidence is approximately 1 in 75 pregnancies. Using sonography to diagnose Down syndrome is relatively difficult, as most of the findings observed in Down syndrome are subtle and nonspecific. However, the soft sonographic markers elucidated above do play a role in assessing the overall risk for Down syndrome when considered in association with maternal serum marker testing and maternal age.

Associated Abnormalities

Abnormalities that may be associated with trisomy 21 include the following:

- Cardiac anomalies:
  - Endocardial cushion defect
  - Ventricular septal defect
  - Patent ductus arteriosus
  - Atrial septal defect
- Gastrointestinal anomalies:
  - Tracheoesophageal fistula
  - Duodenal atresia
  - Omphalocele
  - Pyloric stenosis
  - Hirschsprung's disease
  - Imperforate anus
- Craniofacial anomalies:
  - Brachycephaly
  - Microcephaly
  - Absence or hypoplasia of the nasal bone
- Skeletal anomalies:
  - Short metacarpals and phalanges
  - Clinodactyly
  - Simian crease
  - Wide gap between first and second toes
  - Syndactyly of second and third toes
  - Plantar crease
  - Hip dysplasia

Sonographic Markers

Sonographic markers associated with trisomy 21 include the following:[26]

- Nuchal fold thickening
- Hyperechoic/echogenic bowel
- Mildly shortened femur and/or humerus
- Echogenic intracardiac foci (EIFs)
- Fetal pyelectasis
- Heart defects (including ventricular septal defects, atrial septal defects, and mild ventriculomegaly)
- Hypoplasia of the middle phalanx of the 5th digit
- Mild brachycephaly
- Underossification of the nasal bone
- Duodenal atresia
- Cystic hygroma
- Diaphragmatic hernia

Trisomy 18 (Edwards Syndrome)

Trisomy 18, or *Edwards syndrome* (Figure 11-12), is another of the three trisomy conditions that is compatible with live birth. After Down syndrome, it is the second most common autosomal trisomy condition, with an incidence estimated at 1 in 2500 pregnancies and about 1 in 6000 live births in the United States. The incidence of major structural anomalies is more common in trisomy 18 than in either trisomy 13 or trisomy 21, and multiple anomalies in multiple systems are not uncommon. More than 130 aberrant anatomic features have been reported in fetuses with trisomy 18; the most common ones, appearing in 90%–95% of cases, affect the heart. Choroid plexus cysts are present in a third of fetuses with trisomy 18, making them a soft sonographic marker that is statistically more likely to be predictive for this aneuploidy than others.

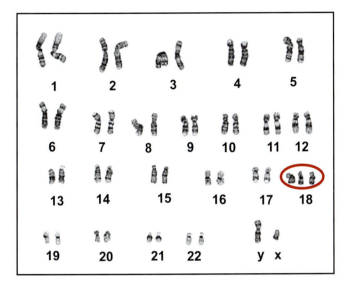

Figure 11-12. Karyotype for trisomy 18 (Edwards syndrome). Note the extra chromosome 18 (circled).

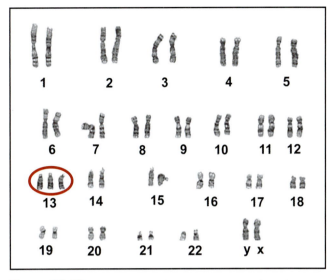

Figure 11-13. Karyotype for trisomy 13 (Patau syndrome). Note the extra chromosome 13 (circled).

Associated Abnormalities

Abnormalities characteristically associated with trisomy 18 include the following:

- Cardiac anomalies (90%–95%):
  - Atrial septal defects
  - Ventricular septal defects
  - Patent ductus arteriosus
  - Dextrocardia
- Central nervous system anomalies (70%):
  - Choroid plexus cysts
  - Agenesis of the corpus callosum
  - Dandy-Walker malformation
  - Neural tube defects
- Face and neck anomalies:
  - Micrognathia
  - Hypertelorism
  - Cleft lip/palate
  - Short neck
  - Prominent occiput
- Skeletal anomalies:
  - Arthrogryposis (clenched hand)
  - Radial ray anomalies
  - Absent thumb
  - Rocker bottom feet
  - Talipes equinovarus
- Gastrointestinal anomalies:
  - Omphalocele
  - Diaphragmatic hernia
- Genitourinary anomalies:
  - Hydronephrosis
  - Horseshoe kidney
- Other:
  - Intrauterine growth restriction (IUGR)
  - Single umbilical artery (80%)
  - Umbilical cord cysts
  - Cystic hygroma (20%)

Sonographic Markers

Sonographic markers associated with trisomy 18 include the following:[27]

- Choroid plexus cysts
- Brachycephaly
- Single umbilical artery

Trisomy 13 (Patau Syndrome)

The third most common congenital autosomal chromosomal abnormality is *trisomy 13*, or *Patau syndrome* (Figure 11-13). While this condition is technically compatible with life, only 13% of these infants are born live and only a few live more than several postnatal days.[28] There are extensive structural abnormalities associated with trisomy 13, the most common being congenital cardiac and central nervous system abnormalities.

Associated Abnormalities

Abnormalities characteristically associated with trisomy 13 include the following:

- Cardiac anomalies (50%–80%):
  - Hypoplastic left heart syndrome
  - Ventricular septal defect
- Central nervous system anomalies (70%):
  - Holoprosencephaly (40%–50%)
  - Agenesis of the corpus callosum
  - Hydrocephalus
  - Microcephaly
  - Spina bifida
  - Agenesis of the corpus callosum
  - Persistent stapedial artery
  - Retinal dysplasia
- Face and neck anomalies:
  - Cleft lip/palate
  - Micrognathia
  - Hypo-/hypertelorism
  - Cyclopia/proboscis
  - Increased nuchal thickness
- Skeletal anomalies:
  - Polydactyly
  - Rocker bottom feet
  - Arthrogryposis
- Gastrointestinal/genitourinary anomalies:
  - Omphalocele
  - Bladder exstrophy
  - Cystic renal dysplasia
  - Cryptorchidism
- Other:
  - Intrauterine growth restriction (IUGR)
  - Polyhydramnios or oligohydramnios

Sonographic Markers

Sonographic markers associated with trisomy 13 include the following:[29]

- Echogenic intracardiac foci (EIFs)
- Pyelectasis
- Echogenic bowel
- Mild ventriculomegaly
- Increased nuchal thickness
- Hydrops fetalis

Turner Syndrome

Turner syndrome (otherwise known as *XO syndrome*) is a form of monosomy, a congenital genetic condition in which one of the sex chromosomes is absent while the other is an X chromosome. Turner syndrome is not associated with advanced maternal age, and the missing sex chromosome is usually contributed by the father. Most fetuses with Turner syndrome are spontaneously aborted before 16 weeks' gestation, the incidence of Turner syndrome in newborns being 1 in 2500.[30] In Turner syndrome, the fetuses are phenotypically female. After delivery, the ovaries degenerate and at adolescence there is little functioning ovarian tissue, which precludes normal reproductive development. There is also a risk of mental retardation with Turner syndrome.

A nonaneuploidic condition that appears phenotypically similar to Turner but demonstrates a normal karyotype is called *Noonan syndrome*.

Associated Abnormalities

Abnormalities characteristically associated with Turner syndrome include the following:

- Cardiac anomalies:
  - Coarctation of aorta
  - Bicuspid aortic valve
- Genitourinary anomalies:
  - Horseshoe kidney
  - Unilateral renal agenesis
- Intrauterine growth restriction (IUGR)
- Shortened limbs

Sonographic Markers

Sonographic markers associated with Turner syndrome include the following:

- Cystic hygroma
- Increased nuchal translucency in the first trimester
- Increased nuchal thickness (14–21 weeks)

Disomy

Uniparental disomy (UPD) occurs when a person receives two copies of a chromosome, or of part of a chromosome, from one parent and no copies of that same chromosome from the other parent. This usually occurs when an embryo trisomic for a certain chromosome "self-corrects" by eliminating one of the extra chromosomes. There are no hallmark abnormalities, constellations of abnormalities, or specific sonographic markers associated with disomy. When uniparental disomy leads to duplication of lethal parental genes, UPD is incompatible with life.

Tetrasomy and Pentasomy

Tetrasomy is a condition characterized by the presence of four, while *pentasomy* is the presence of five, chromosomes of any one type in an otherwise diploid cell. Clinical manifestations of either type of aneuploidy are exceedingly rare. There are no characteristic sonographic signs of either condition and, depending on the severity of clinical manifestations, outcomes will vary.

NONANEUPLOIDIC SYNDROMES, ASSOCIATIONS, AND SEQUENCES

DEFINITION OF TERMS

A *syndrome* is the recognizable appearance of several clinical features, often occurring together, that serve as harbingers of the presence of other, less apparent anomalies. A syndrome consists of two or more embryologically unrelated anomalies occurring together with relatively high frequency and having the same etiology. The so-called syndromes related to aneuploidy—including Down, Edwards, Patau, Turner, and Noonan syndromes—are not, by strict definition, true syndromes because the hallmark congenital anomalies arise from a single abnormal chromosomal etiology. Hundreds of congenital syndromes have been identified; however, only a few are reliably diagnosed prenatally with sonography. Those for which sonography plays a diagnostic role are discussed in this chapter.

An *association* is the occurrence of two or more congenital traits, where at least one is known to be of genetic origin, observed in the same individual more often than can be readily explained by chance. Examples included in this chapter are VACTERL and CHARGE associations.

A *sequence* is a series of ordered consequences due to a single cause. It differs from a syndrome in that the physical traits occur sequentially—i.e., a primary defect cascades into secondary structural changes. For example, Potter sequence (the implications of which are described in Chapter 10) is a constellation of abnormal facies, intrauterine growth restriction, and limb anomalies resulting from chronic mechanical compression of the fetus in a severely oligohydramniotic sac. In this example, the single primary defect is bilateral renal agenesis, which is responsible for the secondary structural changes.

COMMON CONGENITAL SYNDROMES

Amniotic Band Syndrome

Amniotic band syndrome is the collection of multiple, bizarre anomalies—including in utero amputation of limbs, facial dysmorphia, abdominal wall defects, and other structural abnormalities—caused by constricting bands of amniotic tissue. Early rupture of the amniotic membrane can cause entanglement of fetal parts with the relatively inelastic sheets floating freely in the amniotic cavity. As the affected fetal part grows, the constricting band mechanically disrupts normal architectural development and strangulates its perfusion, creating the dramatic sonographic findings typically associated with amniotic band syndrome. Risk factors for amniotic band syndrome include genetic predisposition, maternal use of drugs or tobacco, maternal diabetes, and (some have suggested) iatrogenically induced amniotic tearing during invasive needle procedures such as amniocentesis or amnioreduction.[31] Minor strangulation amputations of fetal digits or distal extremities are certainly compatible with life; more severe disruptions of the fetal head, chest, and abdomen are not.

Syndromal Findings

Syndromal findings characteristically associated with amniotic band syndrome include the following:
- Limb defects:
  - Amputations (Figure 11-14)
  - Clubfeet
  - Constriction rings
  - Pseudosyndactyly
- Craniofacial defects:
  - Anencephaly
  - Encephalocele
  - Facial clefting
  - Severe facial dysmorphia
- Visceral defects:
  - Gastroschisis
  - Omphalocele

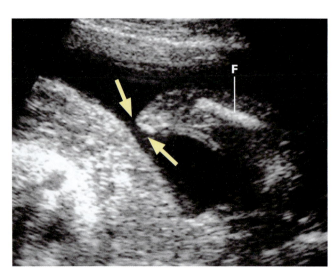

Figure 11-14. Amniotic band syndrome. Longitudinal scan through the fetal arm at 24 weeks, demonstrating a normal-appearing forearm (F) with hand amputation (arrows).

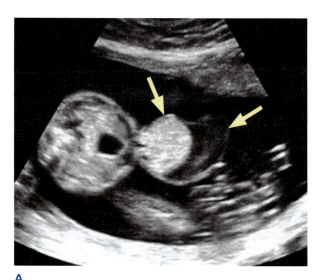

A

Figure 11-15. Beckwith-Wiedemann syndrome. **A** Axial section through the fetal lower abdomen at 14 weeks demonstrating a liver containing omphalocele. Left arrow = liver, right arrow = membranous sac. (Figure continues . . .)

Sonographic Signs

Sonographic signs associated with amniotic band syndrome include the following:

- Presence of two or more of the defects listed above
- Identification of an echogenic linear structure attached to fetal parts
- Fetal postural deformities

Beckwith-Wiedemann Syndrome

Beckwith-Wiedemann syndrome (BWS) is a congenital overgrowth syndrome that results in macroglossia, enlarged internal organs, and omphalocele. Defective genetic signals stimulate excessive production of growth hormone and insulin-like growth factor, which gives rise to overgrowth of individual organs and to the generally large size of both neonates and children afflicted with this syndrome. BWS is estimated to occur in 1 in 13,700 births. While some affected fetuses exhibit an increased prenatal growth rate in the latter half of pregnancy, clinical manifestations often do not appear until childhood or early adolescence.[32]

While the classic triad associated with Beckwith-Wiedemann syndrome consists of omphalocele, macroglossia, and visceromegaly, many other anatomic and developmental abnormalities may also be present. The diagnosis of Beckwith-Wiedemann syndrome may be suspected prenatally on the basis of omphalocele and large fetal size, but it is typically not confirmed until after birth with laboratory analysis and genetic testing.

Syndromal Findings

Syndromal findings characteristically associated with Beckwith-Wiedemann syndrome include the following:

- Omphalocele
- Macroglossia
- Visceromegaly, including the liver and kidneys

Associated Abnormalities

Abnormalities characteristically associated with Beckwith-Wiedemann syndrome include the following:

- Genitourinary neoplasia: Wilms tumor, neuroblastoma, adrenocortical carcinoma
- Gastrointestinal neoplasia: rhabdomyosarcoma, hepatoblastoma, pancreatoblastoma
- Cardiac anomalies
- Genital anomalies: cryptorchidism, hypospadias

Sonographic Signs

Sonographic signs associated with Beckwith-Wiedemann syndrome include the following:

- Omphalocele (Figure 11-15A)
- Macroglossia (Figure 11-15B)
- Hepatomegaly
- Nephromegaly
- Polyhydramnios
- Placentomegaly (Figure 11-15C)

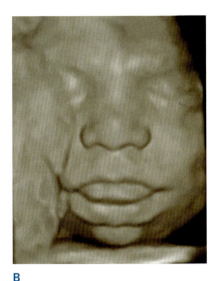
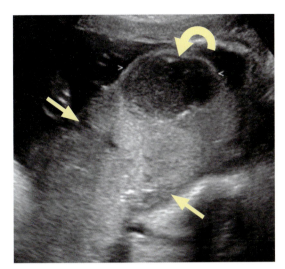

Figure 11-15, continued.
B 3D surface rendering showing a protruding tongue (macroglossia). **C** An enlarged, thickened placenta (straight arrows) with a concomitant chorioangioma (curved arrow).

B

C

Caudal Regression Syndrome

Caudal regression syndrome (CRS), also called *caudal dysplasia sequence*, is a varying constellation of anatomic abnormalities originating from a developmental disruption in the caudal region of the embryo. Early in gestation, a toxic, infectious, or ischemic insult stunts the primary neurulation process, resulting in dysplasia and underdevelopment of the lumbosacral vertebrae, posterior gluteal fascia, and distal portion of the spinal cord. Severity of the syndrome ranges from mild müllerian duct anomalies that remain undetected until adulthood to complete agenesis of the sacrum with sensorimotor paresis and lower limb abnormalities. Caudal regression syndrome occurs in approximately 1 per 25,000 live births. There is a strong antenatal association between caudal regression syndrome and maternal diabetes mellitus; both types I and II diabetes are present in up to 22% of cases.[33]

Associated Abnormalities

Abnormalities characteristically associated with caudal regression syndrome include the following:

- Genitourinary abnormalities:
  - Renal agenesis
  - Renal duplication
  - Hydronephrosis
  - Anorectal atresia
- Spinal anomalies:
  - Myelomeningocele
  - Anterior sacral meningocele
  - Diastematomyelia (split spinal cord)
  - Tethered cord
- Cardiac anomalies
- Pulmonary hypoplasia

Sonographic Signs

Sonographic signs associated with caudal regression syndrome include the following:

- Conus ending above expected level (Figure 11-16A)
- Blunted distal spinal cord
- Absent or hypoplastic sacrum
- Lower extremities hyperextended (Figure 11-16B) or in a "cross-legged" position

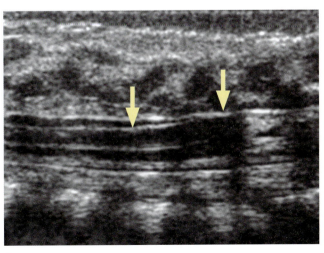

A

Figure 11-16. Caudal regression syndrome. **A** Sagittal scan through the lumbar spine demonstrating the conus medularis (arrows) terminating above the expected level. (Figure continues . . .)

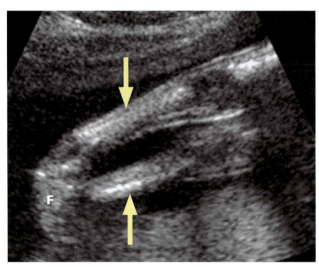

B

Figure 11-16, continued. B Lower extremities hyperextended (arrows) in a 13-week fetus. F = foot.

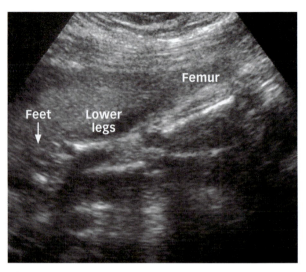

Figure 11-17. Sirenomelia (mermaid syndrome). Coronal section through the lower extremities demonstrating a single fused soft-tissue mass encompassing fused femurs, lower legs, and feet.

Sirenomelia

A congenital anomaly similar in gross pathologic and sonographic appearance to caudal regression syndrome is a rare malformation known as *sirenomelia*, more commonly known as *mermaid syndrome*. In this condition, concomitant with the caudal embryonic anomalies seen in caudal regression syndrome is the presence of a single, fused lower extremity. The degree of skeletal fusion is variable, but both hypoplastic and anomalously developed limbs are encased in a single mass of soft tissue and muscle, creating the hallmark "mermaid" appearance. It is the presence of the fused lower limbs that distinguishes sirenomelia from caudal regression syndrome.[34] Sirenomelia is also associated with aberrant abdominal vasculature, including a hypoplastic aorta, hypoplastic or single iliac artery, absent renal arteries, and almost always a single umbilical artery.[35] Isolated sirenomelia is rare, with a prevalence of less than 1 (0.98) case per 100,000 births, with fewer than 50% of fetuses being born alive.[36] There is some evidence, although controversial, that isolated sirenomelia may be associated with gestational diabetes.[37]

Associated Abnormalities

Abnormalities characteristically associated with sirenomelia include the following:

- Renal agenesis
- Single umbilical artery
- Imperforate anus
- Cardiac anomalies
- Abdominal wall defects

Sonographic Signs

Sonographic signs associated with sirenomelia include the following:

- Appearance of a single lower limb (Figure 11-17)
- Absent or fused feet
- Single umbilical artery
- Oligohydramnios

Ellis–van Creveld Syndrome

Ellis–van Creveld syndrome, also called *chondroectodermal dysplasia*, is a rare type of congenital skeletal dysplasia with only about 150 cases reported worldwide between 1940 and 2008. In addition to the more readily identifiable major syndromal abnormalities, there are changes in the hair, teeth, and nails, which are not usually seen sonographically. Postnatally, affected infants are managed symptomatically, particularly for complications associated with respiratory distress related to a narrow thoracic cavity and heart failure.[38]

Syndromal Findings

Syndromal findings characteristically associated with Ellis–van Creveld syndrome include the following:

- Rhizomelic shortening of the limbs
- Polydactyly (always present)
- Cleft lip/palate
- Cryptorchidism

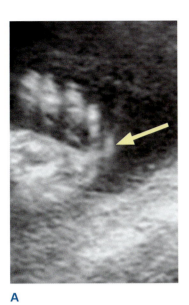
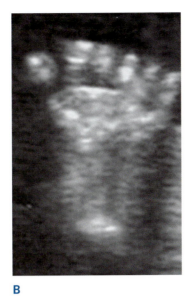
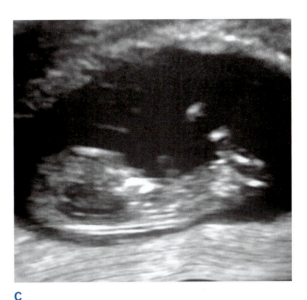

A　　　　　　　　　　B　　　　　　　　　　　　　C

Figure 11-18. Ellis–van Creveld syndrome. Demonstration of the hallmark sonographic signs of **A** polydactyly (arrow) in the hand, **B** polydactyly in the foot, and **C** a shortened forearm.

Associated Abnormalities

Abnormalities characteristically associated with Ellis–van Creveld syndrome include the following:

- Pulmonary hypoplasia
- Cardiac anomalies (present in up to 50% of cases)

Sonographic Signs

Sonographic signs associated with Ellis–van Creveld syndrome include the following:

- Polydactyly (Figures 11-18A and B)
- Limb shortening (Figure 11-18C)
- Cardiac anomalies (not always present)

Meckel-Gruber Syndrome

Meckel-Gruber syndrome is a lethal autosomal recessive disorder characterized by renal cystic dysplasia, central nervous system anomalies, developmental defects of the liver, and pulmonary hypoplasia secondary to chronic oligohydramnios. The incidence of this syndrome is 1 per 13,250–140,000 live births, with a higher incidence in some demographic groups, such as individuals of Finnish descent, Belgians, Bedouins in Kuwait, and some Western Indian populations.[39]

Sonographically, the appearance of the kidneys is similar to that in polycystic renal disease, although the causative pathology is more akin to that found in multicystic Potter type II disease. The renal parenchyma is replaced by cysts of varying size, eventually eliminating normal renal function. Lacking amniotic fluid, the fetal lungs fail to mature, leading to the pulmonary hypoplasia that is responsible for the assured mortality associated with this syndrome. As the sonographic findings resemble those for polycystic kidney disease (a reasonable differential diagnosis), the presence of concomitant central nervous system anomalies and postaxial polydactyly helps correctly identify fetuses with Meckel-Gruber syndrome.

Syndromal Findings

Syndromal findings characteristically associated with Meckel-Gruber syndrome include the following:

- Cystic dysplastic kidneys
- Holoprosencephaly/encephalocele
- Polydactyly

Associated Abnormalities

Abnormalities characteristically associated with Meckel-Gruber syndrome include the following:

- Central nervous system abnormalities:
  - Agenesis of the corpus callosum
  - Dandy-Walker malformation
  - Microcephaly
  - Ventriculomegaly
- Craniofacial dysmorphia:
  - Cleft lip/palate

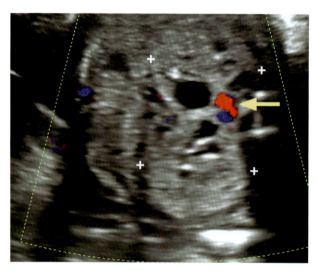

Figure 11-19. Meckel-Gruber syndrome. Axial section through the fetal abdomen at 20 weeks demonstrating grossly enlarged cystic dysplastic kidneys (cursors) that fill the retroperitoneum and encompass the abdominal aorta (arrow).

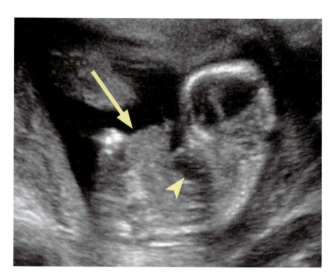

Figure 11-20. Pentalogy of Cantrell. Midline sagittal section through an embryo at 9 weeks demonstrating the hallmark sonographic signs of omphalocele (arrow) and ectopia cordis (arrowhead). Note the presence of a concomitant intracranial cystic abnormality.

- Cardiovascular abnormalities:
  - Ventricular septal defects
  - Aortic coarctation/hypoplasia
- Musculoskeletal abnormalities:
  - Talipes equinovarus (clubfoot)
  - Syndactyly
  - Clinodactyly

Sonographic Signs

Sonographic signs associated with Meckel-Gruber syndrome include the following:

- Enlarged, cystic, dysplastic, echogenic kidneys—bilateral (Figure 11-19)
- Central nervous system anomalies (e.g., holoprosencephaly, encephalocele)
- Oligohydramnios

Pentalogy of Cantrell

Pentalogy of Cantrell, also called *thoracoabdominal syndrome*, is a rare congenital syndrome characterized by a combination of five anatomic defects. It is caused by abnormal folding of the lateral mesoderm at the end of the 6th menstrual week and early in the 7th menstrual week. The lateral mesoderm gives rise to the anterior abdominal wall, the sternum, and portions of the diaphragm. If all five anomalies are present, the condition is referred to as a *complete* pentalogy of Cantrell. However, more commonly, only two or three defects are present in an *incomplete* type. It is extremely rare, with an incidence of approximately 6 per million live births, and carries a very poor prognosis for affected neonates.[40]

Syndromal Findings

The five main features of pentalogy of Cantrell include the following syndromal findings:

- Omphalocele (less commonly, gastroschisis) (Figure 11-20)
- Ectopia cordis (Figure 11-20)
- Diaphragmatic defect
- Pericardial defect or cleft sternum
- Cardiovascular abnormalities
  - Ventricular septal defects
  - Atrial septal defects
  - Tetralogy of Fallot

Associated Abnormalities

Abnormalities characteristically associated with complete pentalogy of Cantrell include the following:

- Cystic hygroma
- Cleft lip/palate
- Encephalocele
- Hydrocephalus
- Trisomies 13 and 18
- Vertebral anomalies
- Limb abnormalities

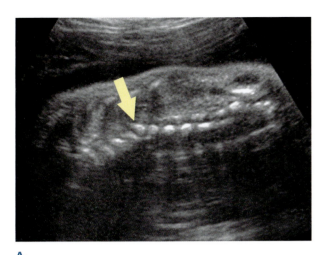 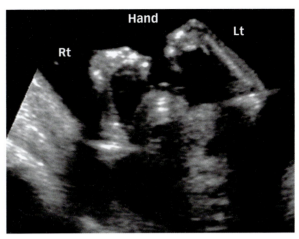

A **B**

Figure 11-21. VACTERL association. **A** Sagittal oblique section through the lower back with hemivertebrae (arrow). **B** Bilateral radial ray anomaly.

Sonographic Signs

Sonographic signs associated with complete pentalogy of Cantrell include the following:

- Omphalocele
- Ectopia cordis
- Cleft sternum
- Diaphragmatic hernia
- Cardiac abnormalities

COMMON ASSOCIATIONS

VACTERL Association

VACTERL association is a constellation of nonrandom congenital anomalies arising from the embryonic mesoderm that occur simultaneously in a fetus. The cause is unknown; however, the abnormalities all arise from the embryonic mesoderm.

The term *VACTERL* is an acronym for the six associated types of abnormalities:

- **V**—vertebral anomalies:
  - Hemivertebrae
  - Caudal regression
  - Spina bifida
- **A**—anorectal anomalies:
  - Anal atresia
- **C**—cardiac anomalies/cleft lip
- **TE**—tracheoesophageal fistula
- **R**—radial ray anomalies/renal anomalies
- **L**—limb anomalies (polydactyly)

Sonographic Signs

Sonographic signs characteristic of VACTERL association include the following:

- Polyhydramnios
- Lumbosacral hemivertebrae (Figure 11-21A)
- Radial ray anomaly (Figure 11-21B)
- Identification of other anomalies listed above

CHARGE Association

Sometimes classified as a syndrome, CHARGE is an acronym for its constituent features:

- **C**—coloboma (focal discontinuity in the structure of eye)
- **H**—heart defects
- **A**—atresia (choanal)
- **R**—retardation (mental)
- **G**—genital hypoplasia
- **E**—ear abnormalities/deafness

Associated Abnormalities

Abnormalities that characterize CHARGE association include the following:

- Microphthalmia/anophthalmia
- Facial clefts
- Intrauterine growth restriction (IUGR)
- Congenital renal anomalies
- Esophageal/tracheoesophageal fistula

Sonographic Signs

Sonographic signs characteristic of CHARGE association include the following:

- Microphthalmia (Figure 11-22A)
- Facial cleft (Figure 11-22B)
- Renal anomalies

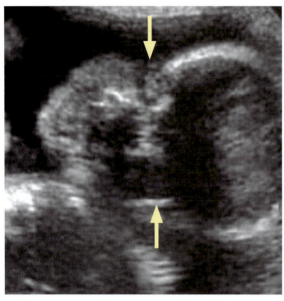

A

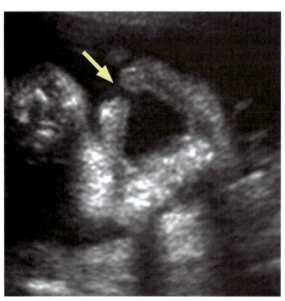

B

Figure 11-22. CHARGE association. **A** Coronal section through the fetal face at 14 weeks demonstrating small, close-set orbits (arrows). **B** Axial oblique upshot through the cleft upper lip (arrow) in a 16-week fetus.

CHAPTER 11 REVIEW QUESTIONS

1. All of the following are indications for prenatal genetic testing EXCEPT:
   A. Maternal age > 30 years
   B. Family history of congenital anomalies
   C. Prenatal exposure to noxious substances
   D. Maternal diabetes

2. The major components of the diagnostic triad in a prenatal genetic testing program include all of the following EXCEPT:
   A. Maternal serum testing
   B. Amniocentesis
   C. Sonographic fetal anatomic survey
   D. Serial serum beta-hCG titers

3. All of the following are components in a maternal serum triple test EXCEPT:
   A. Maternal serum AFP
   B. Serum beta-hCG
   C. Estriol
   D. Luteinizing hormone

4. All of the following may cause elevation of maternal serum beta-hCG EXCEPT:
   A. Esophageal atresia
   B. Multicystic dysplastic renal disease
   C. Open abdominal wall defects
   D. Spina bifida

5. Maternal serum AFP levels typically peak at around:
   A. 8 weeks' gestation
   B. 10 weeks' gestation
   C. 12 weeks' gestation
   D. 14 weeks' gestation

6. An abnormal decrease in MSAFP may be found in cases of:
   A. Trisomy 21
   B. Spina bifida
   C. Omphalocele
   D. Multiple gestations

7. All of the following biochemical assays are assessed on amniotic fluid EXCEPT:
   A. Alpha-fetoprotein
   B. Human chorionic gonadotropin
   C. Acetylcholinesterase
   D. Bilirubin

8. All of the following are "soft" sonographic markers that may be useful when performing a screening genetic sonogram EXCEPT:
   A. Nuchal thickening
   B. Choroid plexus cyst
   C. Echogenic bowel
   D. Hypotelorism

9. An increase in nuchal translucency measurement has been associated with all of the following EXCEPT:
   A. Diaphragmatic hernia
   B. Talipes equinovarus
   C. Omphalocele
   D. Congenital heart disease

10. Nuchal translucency should be obtained when the crown-rump length most closely measures:
    A. 20–40 mm
    B. 40–50 mm
    C. 40–80 mm
    D. 80–120 mm

11. A normal value for nuchal translucency measurement most closely approximates:
    A. <2.5 mm
    B. >2.5 mm
    C. <5.0 mm
    D. >5.0 mm

12. An abnormal nuchal translucency measurement is:
    A. ≥1 mm
    B. ≥2 mm
    C. ≥4 mm
    D. ≥6 mm

13. Nuchal thickness measurements should be obtained between:
    A. 6 and 8 weeks
    B. 8 and 10 weeks
    C. 12 and 16 weeks
    D. 15 and 20 weeks

14. A normal nuchal thickness measurement is:
    A. <2 mm
    B. <4 mm
    C. <6 mm
    D. <8 mm

15. All of the following conditions have been associated with echogenic fetal bowel EXCEPT:
    A. Spina bifida
    B. Cystic fibrosis
    C. CMV infection
    D. Trisomy 21

16. A congenital condition created when each parent contributes a defective copy of a gene is called:
    A. Aneuploidy
    B. Trisomy
    C. Autosomal dominant
    D. Autosomal recessive

17. The normal human karyotype contains:
    A. 23 pairs of chromosomes
    B. 46 pairs of chromosomes
    C. 23 pairs of genes
    D. 46 pairs of genes

18. A congenital condition characterized by the presence of three chromosomes instead of the normal two is called:
    A. Trisomy
    B. Disomy
    C. Monosomy
    D. Tetrasomy

19. All of the following soft sonographic markers may be associated with trisomy 21 EXCEPT:
    A. Nuchal thickening
    B. Echogenic bowel
    C. Pyelectasis
    D. Demineralized bone

20. Trisomy 18 is also called:
    A. Down syndrome
    B. Patau syndrome

C. Edwards syndrome
D. Meckel-Gruber syndrome

21. All of the following soft sonographic markers may be associated with trisomy 18 EXCEPT:
    A. Choroid plexus cysts
    B. Single umbilical artery
    C. Brachycephaly
    D. Echogenic bowel

22. A congenital genetic condition in which one of the sex chromosomes is absent while the other is an X chromosome, otherwise known as XO syndrome, is also called:
    A. Turner syndrome
    B. Down syndrome
    C. Edwards syndrome
    D. Meckel-Gruber syndrome

23. The recognizable appearance of several clinical features, often occurring together, that serve as harbingers for the presence of other, less apparent structural abnormalities is called a(n):
    A. Association
    B. Syndrome
    C. Anomaly
    D. Condition

24. All of the following anomalies are associated with Beckwith-Wiedemann syndrome EXCEPT:
    A. Omphalocele
    B. Hydrocephalus
    C. Macroglossia
    D. Hepatosplenomegaly

25. Caudal regression syndrome may be associated with all of the following fetal anomalies EXCEPT:
    A. Anencephaly
    B. Hydronephrosis
    C. Pulmonary hypoplasia
    D. Myelomeningocele

26. Sonographic findings in a fetus with sirenomelia may include all of the following EXCEPT:
    A. Absent feet
    B. Oligohydramnios
    C. Single umbilical artery
    D. Macroglossia

27. All of the following congenital anomalies may be associated with VACTERL EXCEPT:
    A. Holoprosencephaly
    B. Spina bifida
    C. Cleft lip
    D. Polydactyly

28. The sonographic findings demonstrated in this image are most consistent with:

    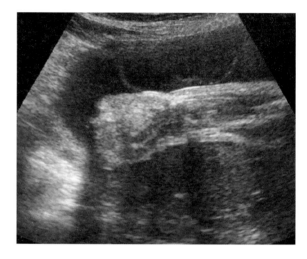

    A. Severe micromelia
    B. Homozygous achondroplasia
    C. Radial ray anomaly
    D. Amniotic band syndrome

29. The sonographic abnormality demonstrated in this image is more commonly associated with an increased risk for which of the following conditions:

    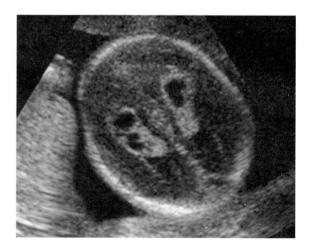

    A. Trisomy 18
    B. Trisomy 21
    C. Turner syndrome
    D. Sirenomelia

30. The sonographic abnormality demonstrated in this image is more commonly associated with which of the following syndromes:

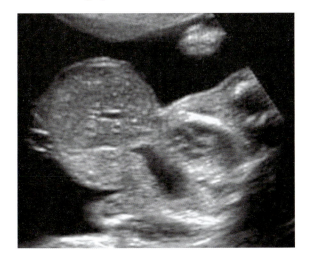

A. Caudal regression
B. Ellis–van Creveld
C. Meckel-Gruber
D. Beckwith-Wiedemann

31. The sonographic abnormality demonstrated in this image is more commonly associated with which of the following syndromes:

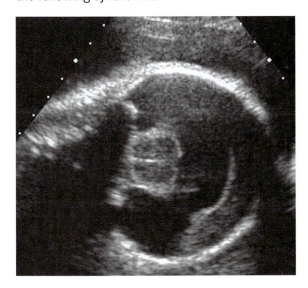

A. Caudal regression
B. Ellis–van Creveld
C. Meckel-Gruber
D. Beckwith-Wiedemann

32. The sonographic abnormality demonstrated in this image is more commonly associated with which of the following syndromes:

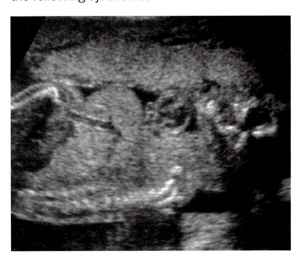

A. Tetralogy of Fallot
B. Pentalogy of Cantrell
C. VACTERL association
D. CHARGE association

33. The sonographic abnormality demonstrated in this image is more commonly associated with which of the following fetal conditions:

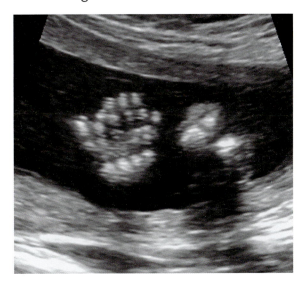

A. Amniotic band syndrome
B. VACTERL association
C. Caudal regression syndrome
D. CHARGE association

ANSWERS

See Appendix A on page 481 for answers.

REFERENCES

1. Kazerouni NN, Currier RJ, Flessel M, et al: Detection rate of quadruple-marker screening determined by clinical follow-up and registry data in the statewide California program, July 2007 to February 2009. Prenat Diagn 31:901–906, 2011.

2. Celentano C, Guanciali-Franchi PE, Liberati M, et al: Lack of correlation between elevated maternal serum hCG during second-trimester biochemical screening and fetal congenital anomaly. Prenat Diagn 25:220–224, 2005.

3. Ishiro BT, Gill KA: Invasive procedures. In Gill KA: *Ultrasound in Obstetrics and Gynecology: A Practitioner's Guide*. Pasadena, Davies Publishing, 2014, pp 444–445.

4. Verp MS: Prenatal diagnosis of genetic disorders. In Gleicher N (ed): *Principles and Practice of Medical Therapy in Pregnancy*, 2nd edition. Norwalk, Appleton and Lange, 1992, pp 159–170.

5. Olney RS, Moore CA, Khoury MJ, et al: Chorionic villus sampling and amniocentesis: recommendations for prenatal counseling. MMWR 44:1–12, 1995.

6. Ishiro BT, Gill KA: Invasive procedures. In Gill KA: *Ultrasound in Obstetrics and Gynecology: A Practitioner's Guide*. Pasadena, Davies Publishing, 2014, pp 444–445.

7. Aagaard-Tillery KM, Malone FD, Nyberg DA, et al: Role of second-trimester genetic sonography after Down syndrome screening. Obstet Gynecol 114:1189–1196, 2009.

8. Nyberg DA, Souter VL, El-Bastawissi A, et al: Isolated sonographic markers for detection of fetal Down syndrome in the second trimester of pregnancy. J Ultrasound Med 20:1053–1063, 2001.

9. Stewart TL: Screening for aneuploidy: the genetic sonogram. Obstet Gynecol Clin North Am 31:21–33, 2004.

10. Sonek J: First trimester ultrasonography in screening and detection of fetal anomalies. Am J Med Genet C Semin Med Genet 145C:45–61, 2007.

11. van Vugt JM, van Zalen–Sprock RM, Kostense PJ: First-trimester nuchal translucency: a risk analysis on fetal chromosome abnormality. Radiology 200:537–540, 1996.

12. Pandya PP, Kondylios A, Hilbert L, et al: Chromosomal defects and outcome in 1015 fetuses with increased nuchal translucency. Ultrasound Obstet Gynecol 5:15–19, 1995.

13. Locatelli A, Piccoli MG, Vergani P, et al: Critical appraisal of the use of nuchal fold thickness measurements for the prediction of Down syndrome. Am J Obstet Gynecol 182:192–197, 2000.

14. Bahado-Singh RO, Goldstein I, Uerpairojkit B, et al: Normal nuchal thickness in the midtrimester indicates reduced risk of Down syndrome in pregnancies with abnormal triple-screen results. Am J Obstet Gynecol 173:1106–1110, 1995.

15. Cho RC, Chu P, Smith-Bindman R: Second trimester prenatal ultrasound for the detection of pregnancies at increased risk of trisomy 18 based on serum screening. Prenat Diagn 29:129–139, 2009.

16. Manning JE, Ragavendra N, Sayre J, et al: Significance of fetal intracardiac echogenic foci in relation to trisomy 21: a prospective sonographic study of high-risk pregnant women. Am J Roentgenol 170:1083–1084, 1998.

17. Carriço A, Matias A, Areias JC: How important is a cardiac echogenic focus in a routine fetal examination? Rev Port Cardiol 23:459–461, 2004.

18. Nyberg DA, McGahan JP, Pretorius DH: *Diagnostic Imaging of Fetal Anomalies*. Philadelphia, Lippincott Williams & Wilkins, 2003.

19. Peleg D, Yankowitz J: Choroid plexus cysts and aneuploidy. J Med Genet 35:554–557, 1998.

20. Yamamura Y, Swartout JP, Anderson EA, et al: Management of mild fetal pyelectasis: a comparative analysis. J Ultrasound Med 26:1539–1543, 2007.

21. Thornburg LL, Pressman EK, Chelamkuri S, et al: Third trimester ultrasound of fetal pyelectasis: predictor for postnatal surgery. J Pediatr Urol 4:51–54, 2008.

22. Benacerraf BR, Mandell J, Estroff JA, et al: Fetal pyelectasis: a possible association with Down syndrome. Obstet Gynecol 76:58–60, 1990.

23. Lakovschek IC, Streubel B, Ulm B: Natural outcome of trisomy 13, trisomy 18, and triploidy after prenatal diagnosis. Am J Med Genet A 155A:2626–2633, 2011.

24. Adams M, Erikson J, Layde P, et al: Down's syndrome: recent trends in the United States. JAMA 246:758–760, 1981.

25. Benacerraf BR: Ultrasound evaluation of chromosomal abnormalities. In Callen PW (ed): *Ultrasonography in Obstetrics and Gynecology*, 4th edition. Philadelphia, Saunders Elsevier, 2000, p 52.

26. Nyberg DA, Souter VL: Sonographic markers of fetal trisomies: second semester. J Ultrasound Med 20:655–674, 2001.

27. Nyberg DA, Souter VL: Sonographic markers of fetal trisomies: second semester. J Ultrasound Med 20:655–674, 2001.

28. Lakovschek IC, Streubel B, Ulm B: Natural outcome of trisomy 13, trisomy 18, and triploidy after prenatal diagnosis. Am J Med Genet A 155A:2626–2633, 2011.

29. Nyberg DA, Souter VL: Sonographic markers of fetal trisomies: second semester. J Ultrasound Med 20:655–674, 2001.

30. Davee MA, Weaver DD: Turner syndrome. In Buyse ML (ed): *Birth Defects Encyclopedia*. Cambridge, Blackwell Scientific Publications, 1990, pp 1717–1719.

31. Cignini P, Giorlandino C, Padula F, et al: Epidemiology and risk factors of amniotic band syndrome, or ADAM sequence. J Prenatal Med 6:59–63, 2012.

32. Weksberg R, Shuman C, Beckwith JB: Beckwith-Wiedemann syndrome. Eur J Hum Genet 18:8–14, 2010.

33. Stroustrup Smith A, Grable I, Levine D: Case 66: caudal regression syndrome in the fetus of a diabetic mother. Radiology 230:229–233, 2004.

34. Thottungal AD, Charles AK, Dickinson JE, et al: Caudal dysgenesis and sirenomelia—single centre experience suggests common pathogenic basis. Am J Med Genet A 152A:2578–2587, 2010.

35. Stevenson RE, Jones KL, Phelan MC, et al: Vascular steal: the pathogenetic mechanism producing sirenomelia and associated defects of the viscera and soft tissues. Pediatrics 78:451–457, 1986.

36. Orioli IM, Amar E, Arteaga-Vazquez J, et al: Sirenomelia: an epidemiologic study in a large dataset from the International Clearinghouse of Birth Defects Surveillance and Research, and literature review. Am J Med Genet C Semin Med Genet 157C:358–373, 2011.

37. Al-Haggar M, Yahia S, Abdel-Hadi D, et al: Sirenomelia (symelia apus) with Potter's syndrome in connection with gestational diabetes mellitus: a case report and literature review. Afr Health Sci 10:395–399, 2010.

38. Baujat G, Le Merrer M: Ellis–van Creveld syndrome. Orphanet J Rare Dis 2:27, 2007.

39. Parelkar SV, Kapadnis SP, Sanghvi BV, et al: Meckel-Gruber syndrome: a rare and lethal anomaly with review of literature. J Pediatr Neurosci 8:154–157, 2013.

40. van Hoorn JH, Moonen RM, Huysentruyt CJ, et al: Pentalogy of Cantrell: two patients and a review to determine prognostic factors for optimal approach. Eur J Pediatr 167:29–35, 2007.

SUGGESTED READINGS

Benacerraf BR: *Ultrasound of Fetal Syndromes*, 2nd edition. Philadelphia, Churchill Livingstone, 2008.

Malone FD: First trimester screening for aneuploidy. In Callen PW (ed): *Ultrasonography in Obstetrics and Gynecology*, 5th edition. Philadelphia, Saunders Elsevier, 2008, pp 60–69.

Milunsky A, Milunsky J: *Genetic Disorders of the Fetus: Diagnosis, Prevention and Treatment*, 6th edition. Oxford, Wiley-Blackwell, 2010.

Norton ME: Genetics and prenatal diagnosis. In Callen PW (ed): *Ultrasonography in Obstetrics and Gynecology*, 5th edition. Philadelphia, Saunders Elsevier, 2008, pp 26–59.

Paladini D, Volpe P: *Ultrasound of Congenital Fetal Anomalies: Differential Diagnosis and Prognostic Indicators*, 2nd edition. Boca Raton, Taylor and Francis, 2014.

Simpson JL, Holzgreve W, Driscoll DA: Genetic counseling and genetic screening. In Gabbe SG, Niebyl JR, Simpson JL, et al (eds): *Obstetrics: Normal and Problem Pregnancies*, 6th edition. Philadelphia, Elsevier Saunders, 2012, pp 210–236.

Simpson JL, Richards DS, Otaño L, et al: Prenatal genetic diagnosis. In Gabbe SG, Niebyl JR, Simpson JL, et al (eds): *Obstetrics: Normal and Problem Pregnancies*, 6th edition. Philadelphia, Elsevier Saunders, 2012, pp 210–236.

Yeo L, Vintzileos AM: The second trimester genetic sonogram. In Callen PW (ed): *Ultrasonography in Obstetrics and Gynecology*, 5th edition. Philadelphia, Saunders Elsevier, 2008, pp 70–111.

CHAPTER 12

At-Risk and Multiple-Gestation Pregnancies

Fetal Complications

Multiple Gestations

Maternal Complications

Antepartum/Postpartum Risks

Fetal Therapy

Pregnancy outcomes can be adversely affected by a variety of both fetal and maternal factors. When one or more of these conditions are present, the pregnancy is considered to be at-risk (or high-risk). While only about 6%–8% of pregnancies are complicated by such concomitant maternal and/or fetal conditions, these pregnancies require special care to ensure the best possible outcomes. The major classifications of maternal and fetal complicating conditions are listed in Table 12-1.

FETAL COMPLICATIONS

HYDROPS FETALIS

Hydrops fetalis is the excessive accumulation of fluid in at least two locations within the fetus. It is characterized by diffuse interstitial edema (*anasarca*), pleural and/or pericardial effusions, and ascites resulting from prenatal cardiac failure. The pathophysiologic problem is an imbalance in fluid homeostasis whereby more fluid is produced than is resorbed by normal physiologic processes. There are two categories of hydrops fetalis, immune and nonimmune.

Immune Hydrops Fetalis

Immune hydrops fetalis (IHF) results from an immune response to foreign antigens (*alloantigens*) encountered by the fetal circulatory system. Alloimmune hemolytic disease and Rh isoimmunization are the predominant causes of immune hydrops.

Hemolytic disease in the fetus (a condition characterized by the destruction of fetal red blood cells) is caused by maternal immunoglobulin (IgG) antibodies acting on paternally inherited antigens present on fetal red cells but absent on the maternal red cells. The maternal immunoglobulin antibodies are transmitted across the placenta and bind to fetal red blood cells, causing their destruction (*erythroblastosis fetalis*) and the subsequent severe fetal anemia that creates the cardiac failure responsible for systemic fluid overload—*hydrops fetalis*.

In *Rh isoimmunization*, an Rh-negative mother, who has been sensitized by exposure to a prior fetus's Rh-positive blood, develops Rh antibodies. During a subsequent pregnancy in which the fetus carries Rh antigens, maternal antibodies perceive those antigens as invaders and attack and destroy them. Large numbers of fetal red blood cells are destroyed in the process, resulting in severe anemia and its hydropic sequelae.

Nonimmune Hydrops Fetalis

Nonimmune hydrops fetalis (NIHF) is the result of a pathologic condition that disrupts the normal homeostatic mechanisms that control the fetal body's ability to manage fluid. Fetal cardiac anomalies are the most common cause of nonimmune hydrops, chromosomal anomalies the second.

Risk Factors/Etiologies

The wide range of fetal and maternal conditions that can induce hydropic changes in the fetus include:

- Chromosomal anomalies:
  - Turner syndrome
  - Trisomies 13, 18, 21
- Fetal cardiothoracic abnormalities:
  - Cardiac anatomic abnormalities
  - Cardiac arrhythmias
  - Cardiac tumors
  - Cystic adenomatoid malformations of the lung
  - Diaphragmatic hernias
- Maternal disease:
  - TORCH infections (toxoplasmosis, "other" infections, rubella, cytomegalovirus, herpes)
  - Parvovirus

Table 12-1. Major classifications of maternal and fetal complicating conditions.

Classification	Condition
Fetal conditions	Hydrops fetalis
	Intrauterine growth restriction
	Fetal anemia
	Intracranial calcifications
	Fetal demise
Multiple gestations	Various maternal and fetal
Maternal conditions	Incompetent cervix
	Maternal diabetes
	Hypertensive disorders of pregnancy
	TORCH infections
	Uterine rupture
	Coexisting masses
Antepartum/postpartum risks	Fetal malposition
	Preterm labor
	Premature rupture of membranes
	Postpartum bleeding
	Puerperal infection
	Abscesses
	Cesarean section
	Hematomas
	Venous thrombosis

- Maternal diabetes
- Pre-eclampsia
• Fetal malformations:
  - Obstructive vascular problems
  - Neoplasms, e.g., teratomas
  - Genitourinary abnormalities and disease
  - Skeletal abnormalities
  - Cord/placental abnormalities

Sonographic Signs

The following sonographic signs are associated with both immune and nonimmune hydrops fetalis:

- Polyhydramnios
- Pericardial effusion (Figure 12-1A)
- Ascites, hepatomegaly (Figure 12-1B)
- Pleural effusions (Figure 12-1C)
- Subcutaneous edema (anasarca > 5 mm) (Figure 12-1D)

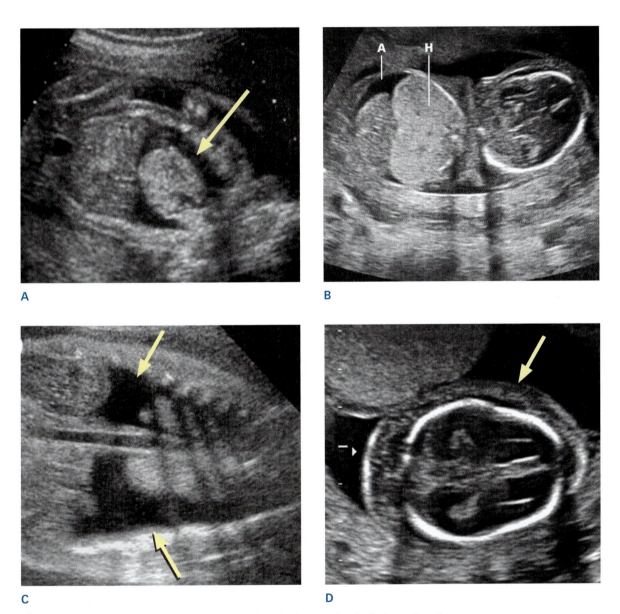

Figure 12-1. The constellation of sonographic signs for hydrops fetalis. **A** Coronal section through the chest and abdomen demonstrating pericaridal effusion (arrow). **B** Axial oblique section through the upper abdomen showing ascites (A) and hepatomegaly (H). **C** Coronal section through a chest with bilateral pleural effusions (arrows). **D** Anasarca (arrow) with gross scalp edema. (Figure continues . . .)

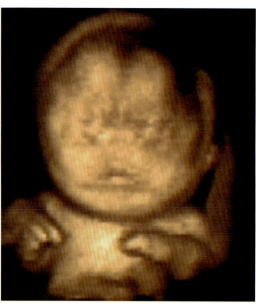
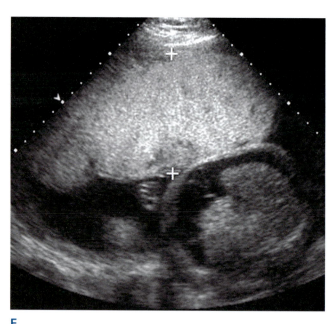

Figure 12-1, continued. E 3D surface rendering demonstrates hydropic facies in a 10-week embryo. **F** Calipers measuring an abnormally thickened and echogenic placenta (>4 cm).

- Hydropic facies (Figure 12-1E)
- Cardiomegaly
- Dilated umbilical vein
- Abnormally thickened placenta >4 cm (Figure 12-1F)

INTRAUTERINE GROWTH RESTRICTION

Intrauterine growth restriction (IUGR) is a general term that applies to a wide spectrum of fetal physiologic conditions that result in a neonate weighing below the 10th percentile. Some fetuses are constitutionally but not pathologically small for gestational age (SGA, which is <10th percentile). In IUGR, pathologic condition(s) prevent the fetus from achieving its genetically determined growth potential. A fetus may be SGA because of IUGR; most are not.

The causes are many and varied, but most are related to the conditions of the uterus and placenta, amniotic fluid volume, and placental transfer rate. Decrease in uterine plasma volume is thought to be a major physiologic factor in IUGR. When the developing fetus does not receive enough nutrition to provide for normal metabolic needs, growth slows. Growth-restricted infants are born with diminished stores of fat and glycogen and are likely to be hypoglycemic. Nutritional support is needed until the infant increases glycogen and fat deposits.

There are several approaches to clinically defining IUGR, but all rely on sonographic estimations of fetal weight. The most common reason for intrauterine growth restriction is a uteroplacental abnormality or anomaly of placental perfusion. Subtle changes in the umbilical arterial Doppler waveforms are often the first recognizable physiologic indicator of fetal compromise. This change is followed by decreased resistance in middle cerebral arterial Doppler as a manifestation of *brain sparing* (the process whereby the fetal circulatory system increases delivery of oxygenated blood to the brain at the expense of other organs). As compromise worsens, resistance in the umbilical artery increases. In the end stage of fetal compromise, the middle cerebral arterial Doppler waveforms will be noted to return to an apparently normal pattern. This is accompanied by profoundly abnormal umbilical waveforms and overtly identifiable venous changes.

Etiologic Spectrum and Risk Factors

Causative mechanisms for intrauterine growth restriction are vast and varied but can be grouped into three major categories: maternal conditions, placental insufficiency, and fetal contributing factors:

- Maternal conditions:
  - Poor nutritional status
  - Smoking

- Multiple gestation
- TORCH infections
- Alcohol/substance abuse
- Severe anemia
- Diabetes
- Chronic renal disease
- Rh sensitization
- Severe chronic asthma
- Age ≤ 17 or ≥ 35 years
- Heart disease
- Residing at high altitude
- Placental insufficiency:
  - Placental infarcts and hemangiomas
  - Small placenta
  - Single umbilical artery
  - Abruptio placentae (placental abruption)
- Fetal contributing factors:
  - Multifetal pregnancy
  - Intrauterine infections
  - Chromosomal defects
  - Trisomy conditions
  - Syndromic anomalies

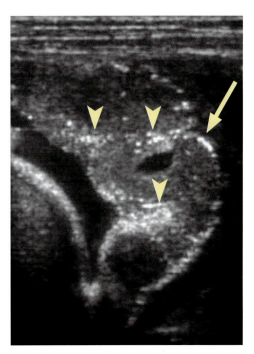

Figure 12-2. Symmetric intrauterine growth restriction, with mature grade III placenta earlier than expected at 32 weeks. Note calcifications along the basal plate (arrow) and interspersed between the cotyledons (arrowheads).

Symmetric Intrauterine Growth Restriction

The etiology of *symmetric intrauterine growth restriction* is usually genetic. Since the condition begins earlier in gestation, fetal growth is universally stunted. Symmetric intrauterine growth restriction is characterized by all fetal biometric parameters measuring less than expected (below the 10th percentile) for the given gestational age. It accounts for about 10% of all cases of IUGR.

Associated Abnormalities

- Trisomy 18 (Edwards syndrome)
- Trisomy 21 (Down syndrome)
- Neural tube defects
- Potter sequence

Sonographic Signs

The following sonographic signs are associated with symmetric intrauterine growth restriction:

- All measurements > 2 weeks below expected gestational age
- Transcerebellar diameter consistent with dates when other parameters are less than expected
- Mature placenta earlier than expected (Figure 12-2)
- Oligohydramnios
- Low biophysical profile

Asymmetric Intrauterine Growth Restriction

Asymmetric intrauterine growth restriction is characterized by the disproportionate reduction in some biometric growth parameters while others remain normal for gestational age. Typically, the abdominal circumference measures below the 10th percentile while the biparietal diameter (BPD), head circumference (HC), and femur length (FL) remain appropriate for dates. Asymmetric intrauterine growth restriction occurs in the last 8–10 weeks of pregnancy and accounts for approximately 90% of cases. The most common etiologic factors are those listed on pages 304–305 that are external to the fetus, i.e., maternal and placental factors. Hemodynamic patterns in the fetus assure that the brain receives the most nutrient-rich blood first and provide for brain sparing in cases of intrauterine growth restriction. As a result, there is an asymmetry between the head size and the abdominal size.

Sonographic Signs

The following sonographic signs are associated with asymmetric intrauterine growth restriction:

- Head circumference to abdominal circumference (HC/AC) ratio > 2 standard deviations
- Abdominal circumference (AC) > 2 weeks behind head circumference (HC)
- Oligohydramnios
- Advanced maturity of the placenta

Doppler Evaluation of IUGR

A great deal of information on the use of Doppler ultrasound in obstetrics has been published since the 1990s. Unfortunately, no single technique has proven to be diagnostic of intrauterine growth restriction, and all have a very low predictive value (20%–40%).[1] When Doppler findings suggest an abnormality, additional prenatal monitoring, such as biophysical profile and/or a nonstress test, should be performed. While many protocols interrogating a wide variety of fetal arteries have been studied, measurements of the umbilical artery and the middle cerebral artery are most widely used and accepted.

Umbilical Artery Doppler

Umbilical artery (UA) Doppler provides an indirect measure of the resistance of blood flow into the placenta. The normal, uncompromised placenta is a low-resistance vascular bed that permits large volumes of blood to flow across both its maternal and its fetal sides. When structural anomalies or pathologic conditions increase the resistance to flow of fetal blood into the placenta, the altered hemodynamic state is reflected in changes in the Doppler spectral waveform. In a normal gestation, the umbilical artery will yield a low-resistance spectral waveform (Figure 12-3A) that becomes marginally less resistant as a result of the progressive maturation of the placenta and the increase in the number of tertiary stem villi.

As Doppler diagnostic criteria are measures of placental resistance, nomograms for standard measures of distal vascular bed resistance—i.e., for systolic/diastolic (S/D) ratios, resistivity indices (RI), and pulsatility indices (PI)—have been established (some simplified examples are presented in Figures 12-3B–D). When identified, abnormal Doppler diagnostic criteria provide a useful indicator of fetal compromise. When used in correlation with a third trimester biophysical profile

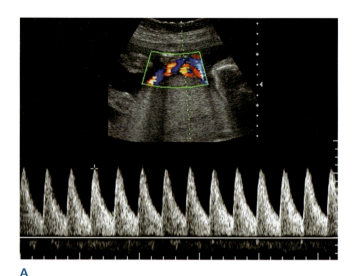

A

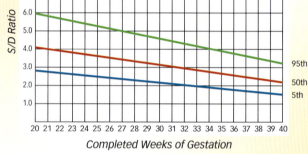

B

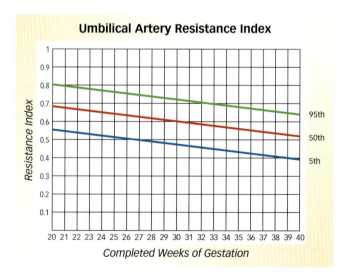

C

Figure 12-3. **A** Triplex (color flow) ultrasound imaging demonstrates a normal low-resistance spectral waveform. **B** Example of an umbilical atery (UA) standard deviation (S/D) ratio nomogram. **C** Example of a UA resistivity index nomogram. (Figure continues . . .)

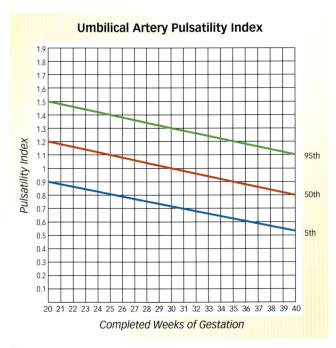

D

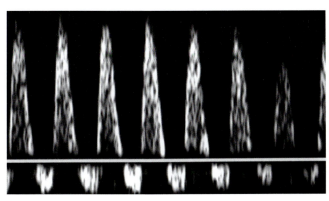

E

Figure 12-3, continued. D Example of a UA pulsatility index nomogram. **E** Highly resistive waveform obtained from the umbilical artery demonstrating flow reversal during diastole, a finding associated with perinatal mortality in more than a quarter of cases.

score (BPS) they provide tools to prepare for a potentially complicated remaining course of the pregnancy. Unfortunately, abnormal umbilical artery Doppler findings are present in only about 30% of compromised or growth-restricted fetuses.[2] While correlating specific Doppler diagnostic criteria with severity of clinical outcomes has not held up to statistical scrutiny, the presence of highly resistive flow in the umbilical artery, particularly when presenting a flash of reverse flow during fetal diastole, is a uniformly pessimistic finding (Figure 12-3E). This particular finding is associated with significant perinatal mortality (27%–64%)[3] and with overall mortality (>50%).[4]

Doppler evaluation of umbilical vein hemodynamics provides insight on the flow through the right of the fetal circulation via the ductus venosus. A normal pregnancy yields a monophasic, nonpulsatile flow pattern with a mean velocity of 10–15 cm/sec. In early pregnancy up to 13 weeks, there is the appearance of normal fetal movements such as breathing and hiccups.

> *Note:* Fetal Doppler interrogation should not be used as a screening tool in healthy pregnancies. It has not been shown to be of value in this group, and the unnecessary acoustic exposure is inconsistent with the ALARA standard (i.e., to keep exposure to ultrasound waves "as low as reasonably achievable").

Middle Cerebral Artery (MCA) Doppler

Doppler interrogation of the middle cerebral arteries (MCAs) is an indirect method of assessing brain sparing, the hemodynamic phenomenon whereby compromised and growth-restricted fetuses preferentially shunt blood to the brain, heart, and adrenal glands at the expense of the visceral and peripheral circulation. Blood flow in the middle cerebral arteries of a normally progressing fetus demonstrates a relatively high resistance with little antegrade flow during diastole (Figure 12-4A). With brain sparing, vasodilatation of the intracranial vasculature reduces flow resistance and is reflected on the spectral waveform as increased diastolic flow (Figure 12-4B). In cases of severe cerebral edema, blood flow can paradoxically revert to a high-resistance pattern. Doppler of the middle cerebral arteries is also useful as a noninvasive method for detecting fetal anemia, obviating the need for invasive cordocentesis to make the same diagnosis.[5]

Like Doppler studies of the umbilical artery, MCA Doppler has limited value as a sole indicator of fetal compromise or as a predictor of gestational complications or poor pregnancy outcomes. Studies correlating MCA spectral measurement criteria with birth weight outcomes show that Doppler interrogation can provide useful information in the clinical management of a fetus with suspected intrauterine growth restriction. However, Doppler criteria are not independent predictors of outcomes and are frequently (49% of the time, according to one study) normal in fetuses with postnatally confirmed intrauterine growth restriction.[6]

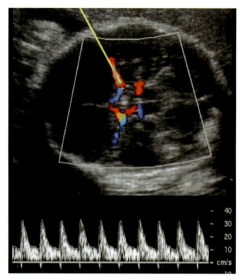

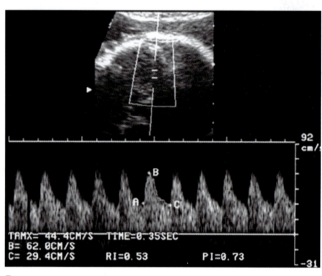

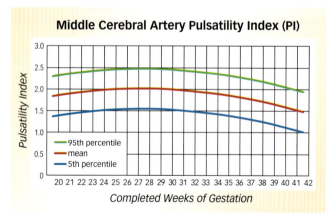

Figure 12-4. A MCA Doppler demonstrates a relatively high-resistance flow pattern with diminished antegrade flow during diastole in a normal fetus. **B** By comparison, abnormal MCA Doppler shows increased diastolic flow, suggestive of brain sparing. **C** Example of a pulsatility index for the middle cerebral artery.

Percentile charts correlating pulsatility index (PI) with gestational age have been published (Figure 12-4C). As PI values fall further below the 50th percentile, the probability of adverse outcomes increases. Another useful ratio is the ratio of MCA-RI to UA-RI (UA is the umbilical artery here), which normally measures ≥1. A value of <1 is suggestive of intrauterine growth restriction.

Fetal Weight Estimation

Estimation of fetal weight is a useful biometric method for helping to predict fetal, maternal, and neonatal complications. While the absolute value obtained by applying any of a number of estimation algorithms rarely coincides with the actual birth weight of the neonate, comparison with standard fetal-growth curves provides valuable information about potential complications (Figure 12-5).[7] There are several limitations to the use of these curves:

- They apply only to "typical" fetuses of normal size for gestational age.
- Gestational age must be accurately known.
- Curves are highly population- and author-dependent.
- The standard deviation is broad, typically exceeding 450–500 grams.[8]
- The 95% confidence intervals (CI) for fetal-weight estimates are > 1600 grams at term (i.e., ±800 grams or ±23%).[9]
- Several different curves exist in the literature, with concomitant variations in what is considered "normal" and "abnormal."

Weight changes in growth-restricted fetuses are less than expected for gestational age; in macrosomic fetuses, weight estimations are greater than expected. Both are associated with increased perinatal morbidity and mortality. For low-birth-weight infants—currently defined as weighing less than 5 pounds, 8 ounces—increased morbidity and mortality are usually associated with preterm delivery. The vast majority of low-birth-weight children have normal outcomes; however, as a group they generally have higher rates of subnormal growth, illnesses, and neurodevelopmental problems.

For macrosomic fetuses, potential postpartum complications include shoulder dystocia, brachial plexus injuries, bony injuries, intrapartum fetal asphyxia, and maternal risks that include birth canal injuries,

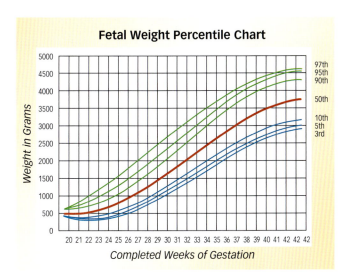

Figure 12-5. Example of a fetal weight percentile chart.

pelvic floor trauma, and postpartum hemorrhage. (See "Maternal Diabetes" on pages 322–324.)

A variety of weight-estimation algorithms have been developed and validated over decades of clinical research. The simplest relies solely on the abdominal circumference (AC) measurement plotted against gestational age; the most complex incorporates all standard biometric measurements (BPD, HC, AC, and FL) and maternal weight, each modified by trigonometric delimiters. As a rule, however, all currently utilized algorithms are generally comparable in their predictive value for fetal birth weight.[10]

Two generally accepted quantitative criteria for defining intrauterine growth restriction are:

- An estimated fetal weight, at any one point in the pregnancy, that falls at or below the 10th percentile for gestational age[11]
- Fetal biometric parameters that fall at or below the 5th percentile or below 2 standard deviations for gestational age[12]

Sonographic Signs

The following sonographic signs are associated with abnormal fetal weight:

- Estimated fetal weight at or below the 10th percentile
- HC/AC ratio above the normal range
- Oligohydramnios
- Umbilical artery Doppler abnormalities (see Chapter 3)
- Middle cerebral artery pulsatility index > 2 standard deviations below mean for gestational age[13]

FETAL ANEMIA

Fetal anemia is a reduction in the number of red blood cells (RBCs) being carried through the fetal circulatory system. Red blood cells transport oxygen to the cells and organs in the body; an inadequate quantity or reduced functionality of these cells results in hypoxia, a reduction of oxygen supply to a tissue below physiologically necessary levels. In response to diminished oxygen levels, physiologic regulatory mechanisms increase cardiac output; if persistent, this increased cardiac output can cause in utero cardiac failure and the hallmark hydrops fetalis associated with it (see pages 302–304).

Risk Factors

Causes of and risk factors for fetal anemia include:

- Hemolytic disease:
  ▸ ABO incompatibility
  ▸ Rh incompatibility
- Fetal infections (e.g., parvovirus B19)
- Rare hematologic syndromes (Aase syndrome, Fanconi anemia)
- Tumors:
  ▸ Placental chorioangioma
  ▸ Sacrococcygeal teratoma

Sonographic Signs

The following sonographic signs are associated with fetal anemia:

▸ Hydrops fetalis (see "Hydrops Fetalis" on pages 302–304)
▸ Hepatosplenomegaly
▸ Doppler findings of elevated MCA velocity as measured by peak systolic velocity (PSV) and time-averaged mean velocity (TAMV)[14]

INTRACRANIAL CALCIFICATIONS

Focal intracranial calcifications detected in the fetus can arise from a number of pathologic conditions in the mother, including in utero infections (toxoplasmosis, rubella, and cytomegalovirus), intracranial tumors (particularly teratomas), and neurocutaneous disorders called *phakomatoses* (neurofibromatosis, tuberous sclerosis, and other rare diseases). They may also be associated with in utero intracranial hemorrhage.

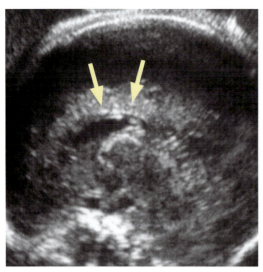 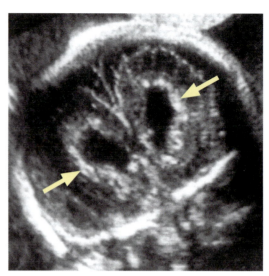

Figure 12-6. Intracranial calcifications. **A** Sagittal section through the lateral ventricle with periventricular intracranial calcifications (arrows) visualized as punctate echogenic foci without acoustic shadowing. **B** Coronal section through a different fetus with bilateral periventricular hyperechogenic calcifications (arrows) associated with cytomegalovirus infection.

Sonographic Signs

Intracranial calcifications are visualized as follows:

- They are punctate echogenic foci found either in groups or in isolation.
- Because of their small size, they frequently do not exhibit posterior acoustic shadowing, otherwise the sonographic hallmark of calcific structures (Figure 12-6A).
- Periventricular hyperechogenic foci are most often associated with cytomegalovirus infection[15] (Figure 12-6B).

FETAL DEMISE

The in utero death of a fetus, at any stage of gestation, is called *fetal demise*. A death that occurs prior to 20 weeks is usually classified as a *spontaneous abortion*. Fetal demise can be caused by maternal, fetal, or placental factors. In many instances, however, the cause cannot be identified.

Risk Factors

Risk factors for fetal demise include:

- Maternal factors:
  - Diabetes (poorly controlled)
  - Systemic lupus erythematosus
  - Infection
  - Hypertension (poorly controlled)
  - Pre-eclampsia
  - Eclampsia
  - Hemoglobinopathy
  - Advanced maternal age
  - Rh isoimmunization
  - Uterine rupture
  - Maternal trauma
- Fetal factors:
  - Multiple gestations
  - Intrauterine growth restriction
  - Congenital abnormalities
  - Infection
  - Hydrops fetalis
- Placental factors:
  - Cord accident
  - Abruption
  - Premature rupture of membranes (PROM)
  - Vasa previa
  - Fetomaternal hemorrhage
  - Placental insufficiency

Sonographic Signs

Diagnosis of fetal demise is usually straightforward: the absence of fetal cardiac activity on real-time ultrasound examination. In later gestation, the mother will

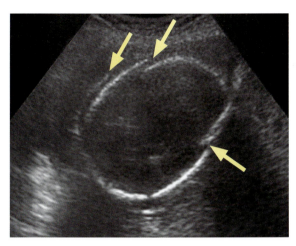

Figure 12-7. Spalding's sign—overriding skull bones (arrows)—indicating fetal demise.

frequently report the sudden absence of previously experienced fetal movements. Other ultrasound findings, particularly in late detection of fetal demise, include:

- Overriding skull bones (Spalding's sign) (Figure 12-7)
- Abnormal angulation of the spine
- Oligohydramnios
- Air in pulmonary and/or biliary vasculature

MULTIPLE GESTATIONS

Multiple gestations are covered in this chapter with at-risk pregnancies because multiple pregnancies are always at higher risk than singleton pregnancies. Twin and other multiple gestations have become increasingly common in the past several decades. As more women are delaying pregnancy until midlife, the use of assisted reproductive technologies (ART) has become widespread, carrying with it the increased probability of multiple dizygotic gestations.

The incidence of naturally occurring twin pregnancy varies by race (10–40 per 1000 live births in black women, 7–10 per 1000 live births in whites, and approximately 3 per 1000 live births in Asians); by maternal age (more common in women over 40 years old); and by some genetic factors. In the general, non-ART population, twinning occurs in approximately 1 in 30 pregnancies. Births of naturally occurring triplets take place in approximately 1 in 7000–10,000 births, and naturally occurring quadruplet births take place in approximately 1 in 600,000 births. With increased prevalence and use of ART, the incidence of twinning or higher-order multiple gestations can be as great as 60%.[16]

COMPLICATIONS

Increased perinatal morbidity and mortality are associated with multifetal gestations for both mothers and fetuses. Twin births account for almost 10% of all perinatal morbidity and mortality. The perinatal mortality rate for twins is approximately 4–6 times as high as it is for singletons, and the morbidity rate is twice as high.[17] The perinatal death rate for twins is 5–10 times greater than for singletons.[18]

Maternal Complications

The maternal complications associated with multiple gestations include the following:

- Hypertensive diseases
- Anemia
- Preterm labor
- Premature rupture of membranes
- Hyperemesis gravidarum
- Polyhydramnios
- Delivery complications:
  - Cesarean delivery
  - Placental abruption
  - Postpartum endometriosis

Fetal Complications

The fetal complications associated with multiple gestations include the following:

- Premature delivery
- Malpresentation
- Cord accidents (prolapse, entanglement)
- Hypoxia of the second twin or another multiple due to premature separation of the placenta
- Intrauterine growth restriction
- Fetal death
- Developmental anomalies
- Polyhydramnios

CLINICAL FINDINGS IN TWIN PREGNANCY

In addition to the typical signs of pregnancy, signs of twin and other multiple pregnancies include these:

- Earlier and more severe pressure problems in the maternal pelvis such as hemorrhoids, constipation, or backaches
- Increased fetal activity

- Increased uterine size; uterus larger than expected (>4 cm) for dates
- Maternal shortness of breath and/or difficulty breathing
- Excessive maternal weight gain not explained by edema or obesity

PLACENTATION/MEMBRANES

The placentation type of a multiple pregnancy refers to its chorionicity (number of placentas) and its amnionicity (number of amniotic sacs). A variety of placental and membrane combinations can occur in monozygotic twinning. The specific configuration is determined by the timing of the division of the embryonic disk; a variable number of chorionic and amniotic membranes may result. There may be two placentas implanted discretely and separately from each other or there may be a single mass of placental tissue. Dizygotic twins, on the other hand, will always have two amnions, two chorions, and two placentas.

MONOZYGOTIC TWINS

Monozygotic twins, also known as identical twins, result from the fertilization of a single ovum by a single sperm. The co-twins are always of the same gender; however, they develop differently depending on the time of preimplantation division. Normally, monozygotic twins have the same physical characteristics (skin/hair/eye color and body build) and genetic features (gender, blood characteristics such as ABO and serum group, histocompatible genes), and they are often mirror images of each other (one left-handed, the other right-handed, etc.). Monozygotic twin births occur world over at a constant rate of 3.5 in 1000 live births.

There are three types of monozygotic twinning: monochorionic/monoamniotic (MM), which are single-placenta, single-sac gestations; monochorionic/diamniotic (MD), which are single-placenta, two-sac gestations; and dichorionic/diamniotic (DD), which are double-placenta, two-sac gestations.

Monochorionic/Monoamniotic Gestations

Monochorionic/monoamniotic (MM, or "mono, mono") single-placenta, single-sac gestations result when division of the conceptus occurs after differentiation of the syncytiotrophoblast (conceptual days 7–8). Two embryos sharing a single amnion and a single chorion result (Figure 12-8).

MM gestation is the least common type of monozygotic twinning, accounting for just 1%–2% of monozygotic twins. Whenever multiple fetuses share a single placenta (i.e., when a multiple pregnancy is monochorionic), anomalous arteriovenous vascular communications in the placental mass may cause hemodynamic complications such as twin-to-twin transfusion syndrome, twin embolization syndrome, twin anemia polycythemia sequence, twin reversed arterial perfusion sequence, and acardiac twins. Sharing the same sac also increases the risk of umbilical cord entanglement and its usually lethal sequela, umbilical vein thrombosis. Conjoined twinning, although rare, is also a complication of MM pregnancies. The mortality rate in MM pregnancies has improved over the past few decades but still approximates 20%, particularly in gestations with concomitant complications.[19]

Monochorionic/Diamniotic Gestations

Monochorionic/diamniotic (MD) twin gestations are the most common type of monozygotic twinning, accounting for approximately 70%–75% of live births. An MD gestation results when the division of the conceptus occurs following differentiation of the amnion (conceptual days 5–10) after the cells destined to become the chorion have already differentiated. Consequently, two embryos, two amnions, and two yolk sacs will be formed within a single chorion (Figure 12-9). MD twins share a single placenta.

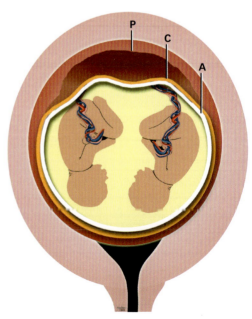

Figure 12-8. Schematic of monozygotic, monochorionic/monoamniotic twins. P = placenta, A = amnion, C = chorion.

Dichorionic/Diamniotic Gestations

Dichorionic/diamniotic (DD) monozygotic twin gestations result when division of the conceptus occurs before implantation. Each conceptus has its own implantation site and therefore its own placenta; two embryos form, each with its own amnion and chorion. Like dizygotic twins (which are all DD), monozygotic DD twins have two fused or partially fused placentas (Figure 12-10). They constitute about 20%–25% of monozygotic twins and on sonographic interrogation appear morphologically identical to twins in dizygotic pregnancies, with the same risk factors.

DIZYGOTIC TWINS

Dizygotic (fraternal) twins arise from two separately fertilized ova (zygotes). The two zygotes develop into blastocysts that implant independently, each forming an embryo with its own amnion, chorion, and yolk sac, resulting in a dichorionic/diamniotic pregnancy. Dizygotic dichorionic/diamniotic twins have two visibly separate placentas, unless implantation of the two blastocysts is close enough to result in the fusing of the two placentas, which on sonography can appear as one placental mass. As they arise from two separately fertilized ova, dizygotic twins may be the same or different in gender. Factors associated with an increased incidence of dizygotic twinning include recent cessation of long-term oral contraceptives, maternal family history of twinning, and maternal age of 35–40 years.

HIGHER-ORDER MULTIPLE GESTATIONS

Higher-order multiple gestations, defined as three or more fetuses associated with a single pregnancy, have also become more prevalent with the increased use of ART. The zygosity of so-called supertwins can range from identical monozygotic triplets arising from the repeated division of a single conceptus to trizygotic triplets arising from three separate fertilizations (Figure 12-11A). Similarly, quadruplets may be monozygotic, paired dizygotic, or quadrizygotic; i.e., they may arise

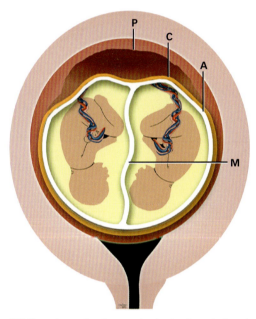

Figure 12-9. Schematic of monochorionic/diamniotic twins. P = placenta, A = amnion, C = chorion, M = separating amniotic membranes.

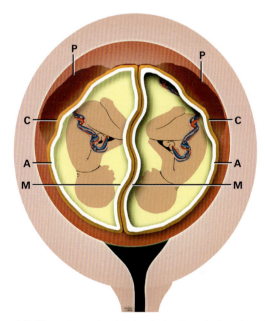

Figure 12-10. Schematic of dichorionic/diamniotic twins with two fused (or partially fused) placentas. P = placenta, A = amnion, C = chorion, M = separating chorionic and amniotic membranes.

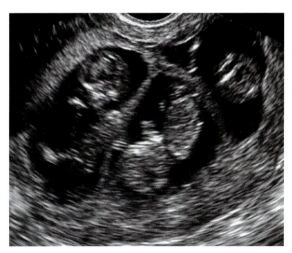

A

Figure 12-11. A Multiple gestation: triplets. (Figure continues . . .)

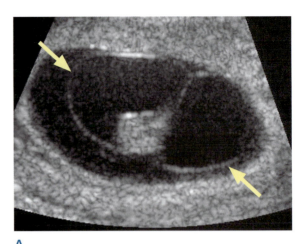

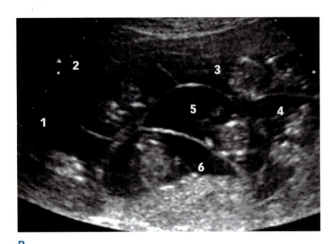

B

Figure 12-11, continued. B Sextuplets (numbers 1–6) identified in a patient undergoing ART treatment with multiple individual fertilizations.

from one to four fertilized ova. Any combination of monozygotic and dizygotic implantations can occur in higher-order multiple gestations. In most cases, particularly when ART methods such as in vitro fertilization are employed, supertwins are the result of multiple individual fertilizations (Figure 12-11B).

SONOGRAPHIC EVALUATION

Sonographic evaluation of the membranes and placenta provides valuable information in planning for and managing the potential perinatal morbidity and mortality associated with a multiple gestation.

First Trimester

The first trimester is the ideal time to count the number of gestational sacs and to assess the chorionicity and amnionicity of a multiple gestation. If a single gestational sac is identified but two amniotic sacs and two embryos are present, the pregnancy is monochorionic/diamniotic (Figure 12-12A). If two embryos are identified lying within a single amniotic cavity, the pregnancy is monochorionic/monoamniotic (Figure 12-12B).

If two separate sacs are identified sonographically, each with its own primitive placenta (chorion frondosum) and separated by a relatively thick echogenic wall, the pregnancy is either dichorionic/diamniotic monozygotic or DD dizygotic (Figure 12-12C).

Second and Third Trimesters

After the first trimester, accurate determination of chorionicity and amionicity becomes more challenging. However, the single most important sonographic

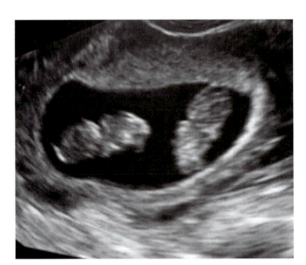

Figure 12-12. A A single gestational sac with two amniotic sacs (arrows) indicates a monochorionic/diamniotic pregnancy. **B** First trimester axial image of two embryos lying in a single amniotic cavity, absent a separating membrane; the pregnancy is monochorionic/monoamniotic. **C** Two separate sacs are identified, each with its own primitive placenta (chorion frondosum), separated by a relatively thick echogenic wall representing the fused chorion and amnion (arrow); this pregnancy is dichorionic/diamniotic and, most likely, dizygotic.

finding during the mid and late trimesters is simply the identification of a membrane separating the gestations. Absence is strong evidence of a monochorionic/monoamniotic pregnancy and raises the specter of the complications and attendant morbidity and mortality associated with this type of multiple gestation.

Sonographic Tips and Signs

The following sonographic guidelines and signs are associated with evaluation of membranes in multiple gestations:

- Identify the presence of a membrane (Figure 12-13A). The presence of a membrane indicates a diamniotic pregnancy (two separate amniotic cavities).
- An interfetal membrane measuring > 2 mm is suggestive of dichorionicity (Figure 12-13B).
- Determine fetal sex. If the examination indicates clearly that one fetus is male and the other female, it can be deduced that the pregnancy is dizygotic and therefore dichorionic/diamniotic. If the fetuses are the same sex, then zygosity cannot be inferred.
- The projection of chorionic tissue whose appearance and echogenicity are similar to those of the placenta, extending into the intertwin membrane and tapering to a point within this membrane, is called the *twin peak* or *lambda* sign (Figure 12-13C). The presence of a chorionic peak is diagnostic of a dichorionic/diamniotic twin pregnancy.[20] However, nonvisualization of a chorionic peak cannot be used as a predictor of chorionicity.

ABNORMALITIES OF MULTIPLE GESTATIONS

Complications specific to multiple gestation depend primarily on placentation type. Monochorionic twins may develop complications resulting from vascular anastomoses through the common placenta. Monoamniotic twins are also at high risk for umbilical cord entanglement and cord accidents within their common amniotic cavity.

Vanishing Twin

The term *vanishing twin* refers to the disappearance of a nonviable gestation initially demonstrated on routine first trimester endovaginal sonography. Follow-up sonographic examination reveals the presence of a singleton gestation, strongly suggesting the demise of the co-twin and its complete or partial resorption. If the resorption is complete, the subsequent sonographic

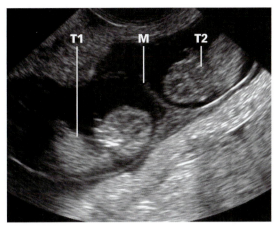

A

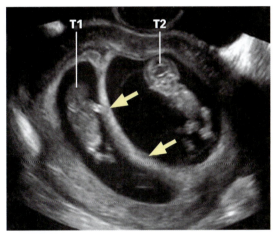

B

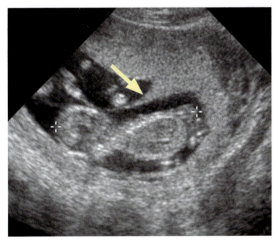

C

Figure 12-13. **A** A membrane (M) separates twin 1 (T1) from twin 2 (T2) in this pregnancy, indicating that the pregnancy is not monochorionic/monoamniotic. **B** Interfetal membrane (arrows) measuring > 2 mm, suggesting dichorionicity. T1 = twin 1, T2 = twin 2. **C** The projection of chorionic tissue of appearance and echogenicity similar to those of the placenta, extending into the intertwin membrane and tapering to a point within this membrane, is called the twin peak or lambda sign (arrow).

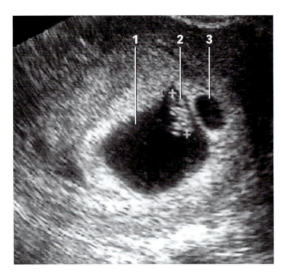

Figure 12-14. Vanishing twin. Endovaginal sagittal section through the uterus at 6 weeks demonstrating (1) a normal gestational sac containing (2) a living embryo (calipers) and (3) a small adjacent, nonviable gestational sac.

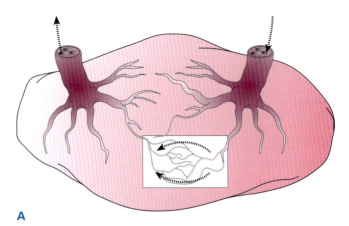

A

Figure 12-15. A In twin-twin transfusion syndrome, excess blood volume is directed toward the recipient (larger) twin through anomalous vascular anastomoses in the placenta seen in the schematic; this excess blood volume overloads the recipient's circulatory system, resulting in hypervolemia, hypertension, ascites, organomegaly, and polyhydramnios. (Figure continues . . .)

appearance will be that of a normal singleton pregnancy; if the resorption is partial, the demised embryo may be seen as a flattened echogenic structure compressed against the inner uterine wall, a state known as *fetus papyraceus*.

Sonographic Signs

The following sonographic signs are associated with vanishing twin (Figure 12-14):

- Sonographic identification of twin gestation in the early first trimester
- Failure to demonstrate multiple gestations on subsequent sonograms
- Failure of sac growth in a twin
- Irregularly marginated sac

Twin-Twin Transfusion Syndrome

Twin-twin transfusion syndrome (TTTS)—also referred to as *twin-to-twin transfusion syndrome, cross-transfusion,* or *twin oligohydramnios-polyhydramnios sequence* (TOPS)—is a complication of monochorionic twinning in which an unbalanced volume of blood is exchanged between co-twins via aberrant anastomotic vascular channels in a shared placenta. Significant artery-to-vein anastomoses shunt blood away from the *donor twin*, diminishing perfusional volume, which stunts fetal growth and creates myriad physiologic complications, including intrauterine growth restriction, severe anemia, hypovolemia, hydrops fetalis, oligohydramnios, and fetal heart failure. The excess blood volume directed toward the *recipient twin*, on the other hand, overloads its circulatory system and results in hypervolemia, hypertension, ascites, organomegaly (enlargement of the liver, kidneys, and spleen), and polyhydramnios (Figure 12-15A).

Twin-twin transfusion syndrome in the United States occurs in approximately 15%–20% cases of monochorionic/diamniotic twinning. If it is left untreated, the outcome is grim, with a 60%–100% mortality rate, particularly for the donor twin.

Sonographic Signs

The sonographic features of twin-twin transfusion syndrome include a dramatic discrepancy in the amniotic fluid volumes and discordant fetal sizes. Increased pressure from the polyhydramniotic sac of the recipient twin may compress the donor twin in the oligohydramniotic sac against the uterine wall, creating a phenomenon called *stuck twin* (page 318). If such twins are able to arrive at the neonatal intensive care unit, the recipient twin (not the donor) is often first at risk for demise due to the stress and overload on the heart. The recipient twin can go into heart failure, the stress on its system causing demise prior to any demise happening with the donor twin. Quantification of amniotic fluid may be performed using the amniotic fluid index (AFI), although the preferred method for multiples is to use the maximum vertical pocket (MVP) measurement in each sac.

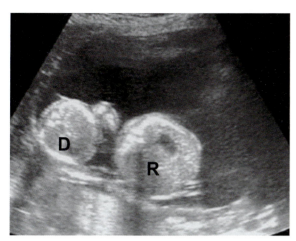

B

Figure 12-15, continued. B Axial section through the abdomens of both twins demonstrating a significant discrepancy in girth between the growth-retarded donor twin (D) in an oligohydramniotic sac and the recipient twin (R) in a polyhydramniotic sac.

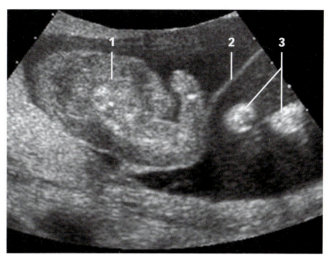

Figure 12-16. Twin reversed arterial perfusion (TRAP) sequence. A grossly malformed acardiac twin (1) separated by a membrane (2) from the pump twin. 3 = pump twin's extremities.

The following sonographic signs are associated with twin-twin transfusion syndrome:

General sonographic criteria:[21]

- Gender concordance
- Monochorionic placentation
- AFI discrepancy:
  - Donor twin MVP < 2 cm
  - Recipient twin MVP > 8 cm
- Significant growth discordance (>20%)

Twin-specific criteria (Figure 12-15B):

- Donor twin:
  - Small for dates
  - Oligohydramnios
  - "Stuck twin" with empty bladder and restricted movement
- Recipient twin:
  - Hydropic changes
  - Ascites
  - Enlarged liver, heart, and kidneys
  - Polyhydramnios

Twin Reversed Arterial Perfusion Sequence

Twin reversed arterial perfusion (TRAP) *sequence* is an unusual variant of twin-twin transfusion syndrome in which a severely malformed twin (more specifically, a hydropic mass) is maintained by a normal co-twin. Perfusion is accomplished through two anastomoses, one vein-to-vein and one artery-to-artery, causing a flow reversal in which blood flows to one twin via the umbilical arteries. The arterial perfusion pressure in the *pump twin* exceeds that in the *recipient twin*, which results in perfusion of the recipient with only deoxygenated blood. Chronic oxygen deficiency in the developing fetus results in varying degrees of upper-body reduction abnormalities, including the most dramatic anomaly associated with TRAP sequence, the absence of a heart, or acardia.

Other anatomic abnormalities commonly present in the recipient twin include anencephaly, holoprosencephaly, other intracranial anomalies when a head is present, absent or hypoplastic upper torso and limbs, multiloculated dorsal cystic hygroma, and a two-vessel umbilical cord. The increased cardiac burden on the pump twin leaves it at risk for high-output congestive heart failure. Left untreated in utero, the donor twin is at risk for demise.

Sonographic Signs

The following sonographic signs are associated with TRAP sequence:

Grossly malformed recipient twin:

- Acardia (Figure 12-16)
- Absent upper body
- Absent head or intracranial malformations when head is present
- Cystic hygroma

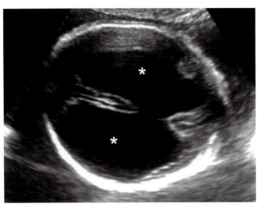 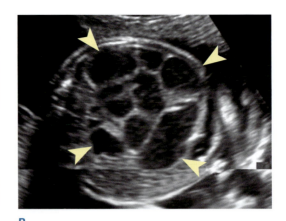

Figure 12-17. **A** Hydranencephaly (asterisks) in twin embolization syndrome. **B** Gastrointestinal atresia in twin embolization syndrome. Note multiple, fluid-filled bowel loops filling the fetal abdominal cavity (arrowheads).

Pump twin:
- Frequently normal-appearing
- Signs of heart failure (e.g., hydrops fetalis)
- Polyhydramnios
- Umbilical artery flow reversal demonstrated with Doppler ultrasound

Twin Embolization Syndrome

Twin embolization syndrome (TES) is a rare complication of monozygotic twinning in which a living twin incurs serious, life-threatening sequelae secondary to sharing the uterus with a demised co-twin. Traditionally, the etiology of twin embolization syndrome was explained as the transfusion of thromboplastin-rich blood or the embolization of clot and necrotic debris across placental vascular anastomoses into the surviving twin. More recent thinking points to an acute hemodynamic shift of blood away from the living fetus to the now parasitic dead fetus, resulting in severe hypoperfusion that creates widespread, systemic ischemia in the living twin. A broad spectrum of central nervous system and somatic abnormalities in the surviving twin can result from this rapid onset of hemodynamic deficiency.

Associated Abnormalities

The following abnormalities are associated with twin embolization syndrome in the living twin:
- Central nervous system:
  - Ventriculomegaly
  - Porencephalic cysts
  - Diffuse cerebral atrophy
  - Hydranencephaly (Figure 12-17A)
  - Microcephaly
  - Cystic encephalomalacia
- Somatic:
  - Hepatic and splenic infarcts
  - Gastrointestinal atresia (Figure 12-17B)
  - Gastroschisis
  - Fetal hydrothorax
  - Enlarged, echogenic kidneys
  - Terminal limb defects

Sonographic Signs

The following sonographic signs are associated with twin embolization syndrome:
- Intrauterine death of co-twin
- Surviving twin:
  - Central nervous system abnormalities listed above
  - Somatic abnormalities listed above
  - Hydrops
  - Polyhydramnios

Stuck Twin (Fetus Papyraceus)

In scenarios characterized by significant growth restriction or death of a co-twin, the affected fetus may be compressed, or "stuck," against the uterine wall by the volume of the surviving twin's amniotic sac (Figure 12-18A). If the stuck twin remains viable, the sonographic appearance is that of a small fetus in an oligohydramniotic sac sharing the uterine cavity with a fetus in a normal or polyhydramniotic sac. If there is

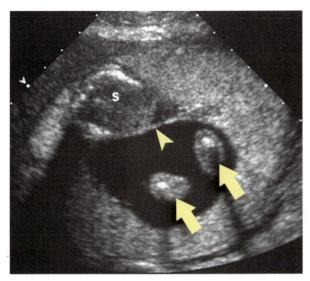

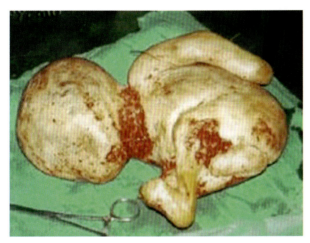

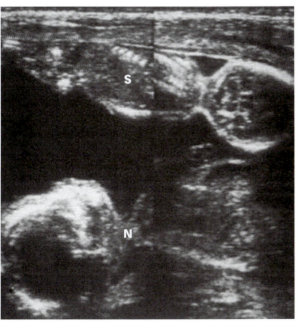

demise of the affected twin, it may retract and desiccate, remaining adherent to the uterine wall until it is delivered as a small, blighted, mummified fetus. The gross pathologic appearance resembles a small doll made of papyrus—thus the moniker *fetus papyraceus* (Figure 12-18B).

Sonographic Signs

The following sonographic signs are associated with stuck twin syndrome:

- Twin pregnancy
- One twin in sac with normal fluid
- One twin in sac with oligohydramnios
- Smaller twin compressed against uterine wall (Figure 12-18C)
- Restricted movement of stuck twin

Cord Entanglement

Monoamniotic twins and their umbilical cords reside in a common amniotic sac, potentially leading to intertwining of the two cords that may create kinks and knots cutting off blood flow to one or both fetuses (Figure 12-19A). This complication is a substantial contributor to the high mortality rate in monoamniotic twinning. While there is some cord entanglement present in virtually all monoamniotic twin pregnancies, perinatal outcomes worsen only when there is compression of the umbilical blood vessels to a hemodynamically significant level. Mortality rates from cord entanglement are higher in pregnancies complicated by TRAP sequence, conjunction, and other discordant anomalies.[22]

Color Doppler imaging is the modality of choice for investigating umbilical cord entanglement. It provides an immediate and global display of all the blood flow patterns present in the large, complicated vascular mass that typically occupies a prominent portion of the amniotic cavity. Observation of two arterial segments pulsating out of sync is evidence of the two separate heartbeats powering flow through the intertwined cords. In the event of a single fetal demise,

Figure 12-18. A Stuck twin (S) in a 16-week gestation with the severely growth-restricted co-twin confined against the uterine wall in a grossly oligohydramniotic sac. A membrane (arrowhead) separates it from the pump twin; arrows = pump twin extremities. **B** Gross pathologic specimen of a stuck twin (fetus papyraceus). Note the papyrus-like skin. **C** Restricted mobility of the stuck donor twin (S) is evident in this image. N = normal twin.

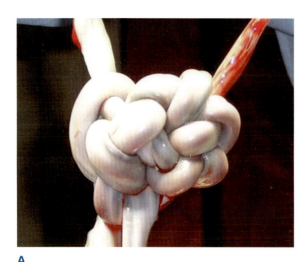 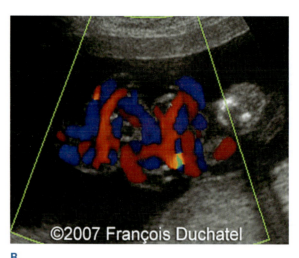

Figure 12-19. Cord entanglement. **A** Gross pathologic specimen. **B** Color Doppler image demonstrating continued blood flow through a mat of knotted and kinked umbilical vessels. © 2007 François Duchatel; reprinted with permission from TheFetus.net.

color Doppler imaging demonstrates quickly and accurately the absence of blood flow in a portion of the blood vessels (Figure 12-19B).

Spectral Doppler findings may also assist in detecting impaired or deteriorating umbilical artery flow reflecting increasing cord compression prior to the onset of adverse and potentially irreversible effects upon the fetus. Extremely elevated peak systolic velocities in a cord segment and the presence of a notch in the spectral Doppler waveform are both associated with an increased risk of perinatal sequelae.[23, 24]

Sonographic Signs

The following sonographic signs are associated with cord entanglement:

- B-mode demonstration of a convoluted, intertwined mass of cord
- Color Doppler demonstration of arterial and venous blood flow within the mass
- Notch in the umbilical artery velocity waveform with spectral Doppler
- Evidence of two different heart rates in the two segments of the vascular mass

Conjoined Twins

Conjoined twins are rare, occurring in approximately 1 in 50,000 live births. They arise only when the twinning event occurs at about the primitive streak stage of development (about 13–14 days following conception) and are exclusively associated with the monoamniotic/monochorionic type of placentation. Conjoined twinning is caused by the incomplete splitting of the embryonic axis; the inner cell mass of the blastocyst fails to separate, establishing a point of conjunction between the two emerging embryos. With the exception of parasitic conjoined twins, all are symmetric and the anatomic part(s) of one twin are always united to the same anatomic part(s) of the other.

The nomenclature for conjoined twinning is based on the location of the conjunction.

- Thoracopagus: conjoined at the thorax (~40%)
- Omphalopagus: conjoined at the abdominal wall (~33%)
- Craniopagus (cehalopagus): conjoined at the head (~2%)
- Pygopagus: conjoined at the sacrum (<1.0%)
- Ischiopagus: conjoined at the pelvis (<1.0%)
- Other types (~25%)

Sonographic Signs

The following sonographic signs are associated with conjoined twinning:

- Dramatically abnormal fetal appearance
- Movement in unison; no independent major movements
- Single thorax: thoracopagus (Figure 12-20A) and thoraco-omphalopagus
- Fused abdomen: omphalopagus (Figure 12-20B) and thoraco-omphalopagus

- Fused head: craniopagus (Figure 12-20C)
- Fused sacrum: pygopagus
- Fused pelvis: ischiopagus

MATERNAL COMPLICATIONS

Many maternal diseases may adversely affect a pregnancy. Outcomes of these maternal complications include early pregnancy loss, late fetal demise, and major congenital fetal malformations and syndromes. There are two broad categories of maternal complications: those resulting from *structural pathology* (such as an incompetent cervix and extrinsic masses) and those induced by *pathologic physiology* (such as diabetes, hypertension, maternal infections, and pharmaceutical insult). Such conditions can take their toll on the healthy progression of a pregnancy.

INCOMPETENT CERVIX

An *incompetent cervix* is one that cannot support an intrauterine gestation to term. Clinically, it is the painless spontaneous dilatation of the cervix that ultimately leads to preterm delivery of the uterine contents. Typically manifesting in the second trimester, cervical incompetence is more commonly seen in patients with certain risk factors, which include:

- Uterine anatomic anomalies
- Exposure to diethylstilbestrol (DES)
- Prior cervical trauma or surgery
- Recurrent spontaneous or elective abortions
- Previous preterm deliveries
- Multifetal pregnancy

Sonographic evaluation of the cervix can be performed using endovaginal, translabial, and transperineal methods. Endovaginal ultrasound examination should be avoided in patients who have experienced premature rupture of the membranes (PROM) or who are actively bleeding vaginally.

Sonographic Signs

Diagnosis of incompetent cervix is based on a combination of patient history and the following sonographic signs:

- Cervical length < 2.5 cm before 34 weeks (compare Figures 12-21A and B)
- Cervical width > 2 cm in the second trimester (Figure 12-21C)

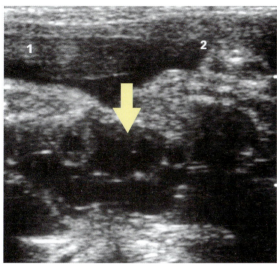

A

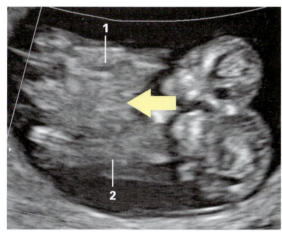

B

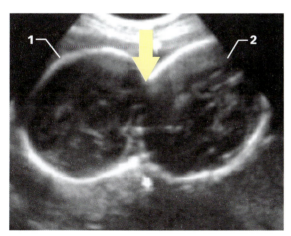

C

Figure 12-20. A Thoracopagus conjoined twins—twins conjoined at the thorax. 1 = thorax of twin 1; 2 = thorax of twin 2; arrow = conjoined heart. **B** Omphalopagus conjoined twins—twins conjoined at the abdomen. 1 = abdomen of twin 1; 2 = abdomen of twin 2; arrow = site of conjunction. **C** Craniopagus conjoined twins—twins conjoined at the head. 1 = cranium of twin 1; 2 = cranium of twin 2; arrow = site of conjunction.

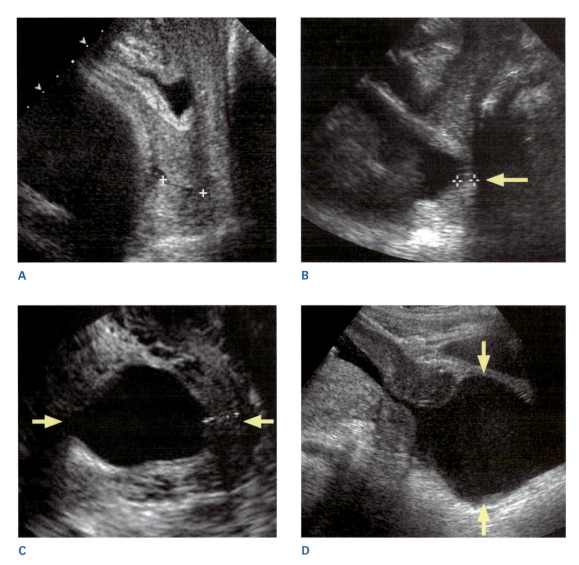

Figure 12-21. Incompetent cervix. **A** Calipers measure normal cervical length of >3 cm before 34 weeks, suggesting absence of incompetence. **B** Translabial sagittal scan demonstrating a diminished cervical length (arrow/calipers) in a 32-week pregnancy, suggesting cervical incompetence. **C** Axial section through a cervix measuring > 2 cm (arrows) maximum lateral dimension in the second trimester, suggesting cervical incompetence. **D** Sagittal scan through the cervix and vagina demonstrating membranes bulging (arrows) into the vaginal vault. (Figure continues . . .)

- Bulging cervical membranes (Figure 12-21D)
- Bladder distention that may cause false-negative findings

Cervical Cerclage

Cervical cerclage is the method of treating cervical incompetence. The cervix is sutured (sometimes using a cervical ring pessary) to mechanically cinch the cervix shut, usually early in the second trimester (12–14 weeks). The sutures are removed toward the end of pregnancy when the risk of miscarriage has passed. Alternatively, the cervix can be cinched shut using a transabdominal approach when other methods of treating cervical incompetence have failed. The disadvantages of this approach include the necessity for two laparotomies during pregnancy—one to place the cerclage and the other to remove it. A cerclage can be identified sonographically as interrupted, curvilinear, brightly echogenic foci emanating from the cervix (Figure 12-21E).

MATERNAL DIABETES

Diabetes during pregnancy, whether a preexisting medical condition (*diabetes mellitus*) or a complication that arises from the pregnancy itself (*gestational*

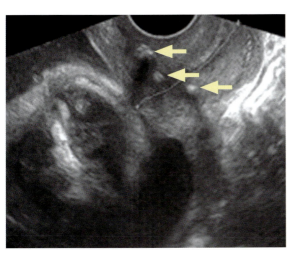

E

Figure 12-21, continued. E Cervical cerclage; sutures (arrows) are identifiable as interrupted, curvilinear, brightly echogenic foci emanating from the cervix.

diabetes), poses a significant risk of complications to both fetus and mother. Episodic surges of maternal serum glucose levels induce episodic fetal hyperinsulinemia, which generates a cascade of physiologic aberrations potentially resulting in myriad structural, medical, and growth-related fetal abnormalities. Maternal complications typically result from excess fetal growth and the increased hemodynamic and metabolic burden associated with it.

Diabetes Mellitus

Diabetes mellitus (DM) is a spectrum of disorders involving compromised carbohydrate, lipid, and protein metabolism due to an absolute or relative paucity of insulin. Diabetes mellitus may occur spontaneously (90%) or may be secondary to pancreatic disease, hormonal imbalances, or drug reactions. Poorly managed, preexisting diabetes mellitus is the type most frequently associated with many of the fetal anatomic abnormalities known to occur in babies born to diabetic mothers. In fact, a fetus gestating in a diabetic mother has a three- to eightfold increased risk of congenital anatomic abnormalities.[25]

The two general classifications of spontaneous, preexisting diabetes can be summarized as follows:

Type I:
- Results from insufficient insulin production by the pancreas
- Insulin-dependent (IDDM)
- Juvenile onset

Type II:
- Metabolic disorder characterized by elevated blood glucose resulting from insulin resistance and relative insulin insufficiency
- Non–insulin-dependent (NIDDM), although poor response to treatment with diet, exercise, and oral medication may necessitate insulin administration
- Adult onset

Gestational Diabetes

Hormonal and metabolic changes associated with pregnancy can result in a condition characterized by elevated maternal glucose levels, referred to as *glucose intolerance of pregnancy* (GIP) or, more commonly, *gestational diabetes*. While it usually resolves after pregnancy, during gestation this form of diabetes can induce fetal growth–related deviations (intrauterine growth restriction and macrosomia) that increase the risk of complications in both mother and neonate.

Fetal Effects

As a rule of thumb, preexisting diabetes mellitus is the type responsible for anatomic abnormalities; gestational diabetes is responsible for macrosomia and intrauterine growth restriction. However, there may be significant crossover in individual cases. Certainly fetuses with serious structural defects can also exhibit growth-related aberrations, and fetuses with significant growth restriction or excessive somatic growth may present with structural abnormalities, particularly of the cardiovascular and central nervous systems.

Specific fetal *anatomic abnormalities* associated with maternal diabetes include:
- Caudal regression
- Inguinal hernias
- Neural tube defects
- Clubfoot (talipes equinovarus)
- Cardiac anomalies
- Single umbilical artery
- Renal anomalies
- Polydactyly
- Gastrointestinal anomalies
- Skeletal anomalies

Fetal *metabolic abnormalities* associated with maternal diabetes include:
- Intrauterine growth restriction
- Macrosomia

- Hypoglycemia
- Hypocalcemia

Macrosomia is usually defined as fetal weight greater than 4500 grams or a birth weight above the 90th percentile for gestational age. It typically presents in the third trimester and is commonly referred to as *large for gestational age* (LGA). While its most common association is with gestational diabetes, macrosomia may also appear in pregnancies complicated by maternal obesity, advanced maternal age (≥35 years), and a variety of fetal congenital syndromes.

Maternal Effects

Gestational diabetes, as it is usually responsible for significant growth aberrations, can cause complications at delivery. Because of the disproportionately large size and weight of the fetus, birth trauma to mother and neonate (see above) are the morbidities of primary concern. In addition to macrosomia, an enlarged placenta, polyhydramnios, excessive anasarca, and organomegaly may be observed in a diabetic pregnancy.

In a well-managed pregnancy that is complicated by diabetes, maternal morbidities such as perineal tears and hemorrhage are uncommon. However, there is an increased probability that the pregnancy will be delivered via cesarean section.[26] The detection of macrosomia in the third trimester is helpful for clinical management and for planning the delivery. Gestational diabetes also predisposes the mother to a gamut of metabolic complications, which include:

- Pre-eclampsia
- HELLP syndrome (hemolysis, elevated liver enzymes, low platelets)
- Renal dysfunction (diabetic nephropathy)
- Diabetic retinopathy
- Hypoglycemia
- Peripheral vascular disease

Sonography in the Management of Diabetic Complications

Sonography plays an important role in the management of a pregnant patient with diabetes. Three categories of sonographic findings provide useful information to the managing clinician: fetal anatomic abnormalities, placental changes, and growth-related changes.

- Fetal anatomic abnormalities:
    - Identification of specific anatomic abnormalities
    - Single umbilical artery
    - Oligo- or polyhydramnios
- Placental changes:
    - Thickened placenta
    - Premature aging
    - Doppler ultrasound evidence of placental insufficiency
- Growth-related changes:
    - Macrosomia
    - Intrauterine growth restriction

HYPERTENSIVE DISORDERS OF PREGNANCY

Hypertension is the most common medical problem encountered during pregnancy, complicating 2%–3% of all gestations.[27] Various schemata have been used over the years to categorize pregnancy-related hypertensive disorders; the one currently in widespread use employs three categories: *preexisting hypertension, gestational hypertension,* and *pre-eclampsia* (preferred over the older term *pregnancy-induced hypertensive disorder* [PIHD]). Hypertensive disorders of pregnancy increase the risk of maternal and fetal morbidity.

The definitions for chronic hypertension are the same across all classifications:

- Systolic pressure > 140 mmHg
- Increase in systolic pressure > 30 mmHg (over the pre-pregnant state)
- Diastolic pressure > 90 mmHg
- Diastolic pressure increase > 15 mmHg (over the pre-pregnant state)

Preexisting and Gestational Hypertension

Preexisting hypertension, as its name suggests, is the chronic elevation of blood pressure before the onset of pregnancy; *gestational hypertension* refers to persistent elevation of blood pressure that begins after 20 weeks' gestation and resolves postpartum. Preexisting and gestational hypertension, if controlled well, are generally associated with good outcomes.

Pre-eclampsia

Pre-eclampsia is hypertension complicated by proteinuria and, in some cases, generalized edema. Unlike preexisting or gestational hypertension, it is the result of structural, functional, and hemodynamic alterations of the placenta and is associated with placental insufficiency, diffuse placental thrombosis, decidual vasculopathy, and/or abnormal trophoblastic invasion of the endometrium. These underlying organic causes make control of maternal blood pressure difficult, if not impossible, and are responsible for the increased morbidity partnered with pre-eclampsia. When uncontrolled, pre-eclampsia (formerly *toxemia of pregnancy*) can evolve into *eclampsia* (*eclamptic toxemia*), an acute, life-threatening complication whose clinical hallmarks, in addition to hypertension, proteinuria, and edema, are tonic-clonic seizures, coma, and ultimately death.

Risk factors associated with the onset of pre-eclampsia include:

- Maternal age ≤18 years and ≥35 years
- History of pre-eclampsia
- Obesity
- Preexisting diabetes
- Renal disease
- Multiple gestations
- Gestational trophoblastic disease
- Hydrops fetalis
- Triploidy

Sonography in the Management of Hypertensive Disorders

Sonography plays a role in monitoring pregnancies complicated by hypertensive disorders, primarily by monitoring the pregnancy and tracking fetal growth. Serial surveillance with spectral Doppler is the method of choice for monitoring placental vascular resistance, a key predictor of poor outcomes. A variety of sonographic findings may be observed in pregnancies complicated by hypertensive disorders:

- Intrauterine growth restriction
- Oligohydramnios
- Decreased placental volume
- Accelerated placental aging
- Fetal demise
- Increased placental resistance

MATERNAL TORCH INFECTIONS

Any severe, systemic maternal infection may result in untoward outcomes, including spontaneous abortion, premature labor and delivery, and fetal death. A group of specific viral, bacterial, and protozoan infections that gain access to the fetal bloodstream via chorionic villi in the placenta and are associated with predictable complications are known as *TORCH infections*. Hematogenous transmission of these infectious agents may occur at any time during gestation or, in some cases, at the time of delivery via maternal-to-fetal transfusion.

TORCH is an acronym for the following:

- **T**—toxoplasmosis
- **O**—other
- **R**—rubella
- **C**—cytomegalovirus
- **H**—herpes infections

Sonographic fetal abnormalities may be indicative of fetal infections, but these signs are generally neither sensitive nor specific. Prenatal detection of infection is based less on fetal sonographic findings than on polymerase chain reaction studies, which can identify the specific agent. In fact, most affected fetuses exposed to infection in utero appear sonographically normal; serial scanning may, however, reveal evolving findings.

Toxoplasmosis

Congenital *toxoplasmosis* results from the transplacental transmission of the protozoan *Toxoplasma gondii* following maternal infection acquired during pregnancy. One of the major consequences of pregnant women becoming infected by *T. gondii* is vertical transmission to the fetus. Although rare, congenital toxoplasmosis can cause severe neurologic or ocular disease (leading to blindness) as well as cardiac and cerebral anomalies. *T. gondii*, which is commonly found in cat feces and uncooked meat, is transmitted to the mother by oral ingestion of microscopic *T. gondii* oocytes after handling infected substances.[28] It is for this reason that pregnant women are advised not to clean cat litter or otherwise expose themselves to feline fecal matter.

Sonographic Signs

The following sonographic signs are associated with toxoplasmosis:[29]

- Ventriculomegaly/hydrocephalus (Figure 12-22)
- Microcephaly
- Focal intracranial calcifications
- Increased periventricular echogenicity

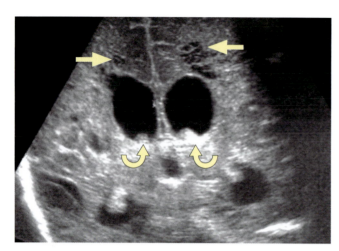

Figure 12-22. Coronal section demonstrating periventricular cysts (straight arrows) and ventriculomegaly (curved arrows) associated with toxoplasmosis in a term fetus.

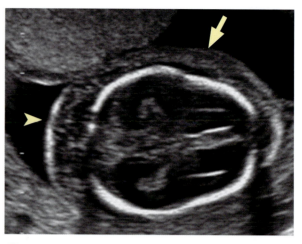

Figure 12-23. Axial section through the fetal skull showing hydropic gross scalp edema (arrow) associated with parvovirus. Note the concomitant presence of ventriculomegaly in this fetus (arrowhead).

- Periventricular cysts (Figure 12-22)
- Ascites
- Hepatosplenomegaly
- Severe intrauterine growth restriction

"Other" Infections in TORCH

"Other" (and less common) maternal TORCH infections that can complicate a pregnancy include coxsackievirus, syphilis, varicella-zoster virus, human immunodeficiency virus, and parvovirus B19. Of these, only parvovirus has characteristic sonographic findings reported in the medical literature.

Parvovirus

Parvovirus B19 infection is a common and highly contagious childhood ailment, sometimes called *slapped-cheek disease* because of the distinctive face rash that it induces. Primary maternal infection has been associated with nonimmune fetal hydrops and intrauterine fetal demise. The pathogenic sequence begins with the transplacental transfer of the B19 virus with infection of fetal red blood cell (RBC) precursors. As a result, there is arrested production of red blood cells and subsequent severe anemia, which cascades into congestive heart failure and fetal hydrops.

Fetal complications include:

- Anemia
- Hydrops fetalis
- Cardiomyopathy
- Spontaneous abortion
- Fetal demise

Sonographic Signs

The following sonographic signs are associated with parvovirus:

- Signs of fetal hydrops
- Soft tissue/scalp edema (Figure 12-23)
- Pleural effusion
- Ascites
- Hepatosplenomegaly
- Cardiomyopathy

Rubella

Also known as *German measles*, in utero *rubella* infection is extremely teratogenic to the fetus, especially when exposure occurs during the first 16 weeks of pregnancy. Many women who contract this viral disease will spontaneously miscarry; those who carry the gestation to viability may deliver a neonate with *congenital rubella syndrome* (CRS)—a constellation of cardiac, cerebral, ophthalmic, and auditory defects. The classic triad and most common manifestations of congenital rubella syndrome include:

- Cataracts, retinopathy, microphthalmia
- Congenital heart disease, particularly patent ductus arteriosus
- Deafness

Sonographic Signs

The following sonographic signs are associated with rubella:

- Microcephaly (Figure 12-24)
- Intrauterine growth restriction

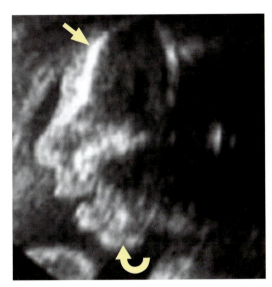

Figure 12-24. Sagittal profile view showing the microcephaly (straight arrow) and micrognathia (curved arrow) associated with rubella.

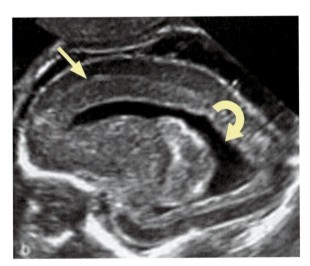

Figure 12-25. Sagittal section through the lateral ventricle demonstrating the increased periventricular echogenicity (straight arrow) and ventriculomegaly (curved arrow) associated with cytomegalovirus in a 34-week fetus.

- Hepatomegaly
- Micrognathia (Figure 12-24)

Cytomegalovirus

Cytomegalovirus (CMV) is a ubiquitous herpes-family virus that, in healthy immunocompetent individuals, produces few if any symptoms or sequelae following infection. However, the virus remains dormant in the exposed individual and may be transmitted to a fetus if a recurrent maternal cytomegalovirus infection occurs during pregnancy. The vertical transmission rate to the fetus is around 30%–50%; about 10% of infected fetuses will present with associated abnormalities, which include the following:[30, 31]

- Spontaneous abortion
- Intrauterine growth restriction
- Abdominal abnormalities:
  - Ascites
  - Hepatomegaly
  - Splenomegaly
  - Jaundice
- Central nervous system abnormalities:
  - Microcephaly
  - Chorioretinitis
  - Intracranial calcifications
  - Hearing loss

Sonographic Signs

The following sonographic signs are associated with cytomegalovirus:[32]

- Increased periventricular echogenicity (Figure 12-25)
- Ventriculomegaly (Figure 12-25)
- Intraventricular adhesions
- Increased thalamic echogenicity
- Enlarged cisterna magna
- Lissencephaly
- Cerebellar cysts

Herpes

The *herpes simplex virus* (HSV) *type 2* is a common sexually transmitted infectious agent found in approximately 16% of all Americans aged 16–49.[33] Antibodies to herpes simplex virus have been detected in approximately 20% of pregnant women.[34] This infectious agent is rarely transmitted transplacentally to a fetus in utero. When it is, fetal sepsis may result in multiorgan failure including fetal brain death and ultimate demise. Infection is more commonly transmitted during vaginal delivery, when the neonate is exposed to secretions from maternal herpetic genital lesions. If active herpes simplex virus infection is present at time of delivery, cesarean section is recommended.

Neonatal herpes manifests in three ways: as skin, eyes, and mouth (SEM) herpes; as disseminated (DIS) herpes; and as central nervous system (CNS) herpes. Specific complications include:[35]

- Neonatal encephalitis
- Seizures

- Psychomotor retardation
- Spasticity
- Blindness
- Learning disabilities
- Death

Sonographic Signs

The following sonographic signs are associated with herpes:[36]

- Asymmetric ventriculomegaly
- Increased cerebral parenchymal echogenicity

UTERINE RUPTURE

Uterine rupture is a rare but potentially catastrophic obstetric emergency. In most cases, increased intrauterine pressure associated with pregnancy forces dehiscence of the endpoints of a prior cesarean scar. Uterine rupture associated with pregnancy is more likely to occur with the lower-uterine-segment scars from "bikini cut" cesarean sections. The rupture may remain limited to the endpoints with an intact overlying serosal layer, or it may extend to the full thickness of the uterus. In the latter case, direct communication between the uterine and peritoneal cavities can result in a massive hemoperitoneum with the attendant high risk of fetal and maternal morbidity and mortality. Clinically, patients present with acute uterine pain and hemodynamic instability.

Maternal complications include:

- Hemorrhage
- Shock
- Postoperative infection
- Ureteral damage
- Amniotic fluid embolism
- Disseminated intravascular coagulopathy
- Death of mother and/or child

Sonographic Signs

The following sonographic signs are associated with uterine rupture (Figure 12-26):

- Oligohydramnios
- Large amount of peritoneal fluid (hemoperitoneum)
- Extrauterine hematoma
- Identification of a protruding portion of the amniotic sac

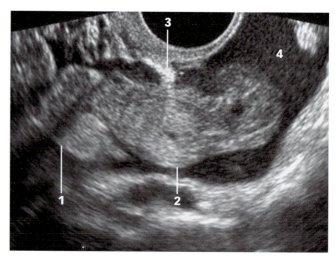

Figure 12-26. Dramatic appearance of uterine rupture complicating an anomalous twin pregnancy. 1 = twin A, 2 = twin B with omphalocele, 3 = rupture site, 4 = hemoperitoneum.

COEXISTING MASSES

The presence of a mass sharing the pelvic cavity with an intrauterine pregnancy presents several management concerns, depending on the size, location, and histopathologic nature of the mass:

- There may be hemodynamic shunting of blood away from the gravid uterus with subsequent fetal growth restriction.
- The mass may interfere with a normal vaginal delivery (dystocia).
- Malignant masses present other clinical concerns such as timing of oncologic treatment and/or termination of the pregnancy.

Most persistent adnexal masses move well out of the pelvis or resolve spontaneously as pregnancy progresses. However, if the mass persists in its location, if the mass continues to grow during gestation, or if the mass is malignant, prepartum intervention may be necessary. Obviously, the patient and her physician must weigh the benefit of prompt surgical intervention against the risk to the pregnancy. The most common types of coexisting masses are summarized below.

Fibroids

Fibroids, or *uterine leiomyomas*, are common, benign uterine muscular tumors. Their position relative to the cervix should be ascertained. They may increase in size during the second and third trimesters under the influence of altered hormone levels or because of degenerative changes and hemorrhage into the

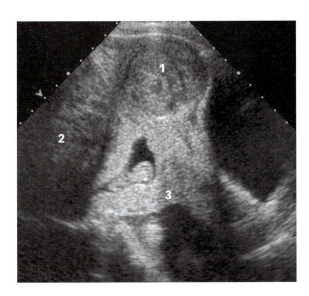

Figure 12-27. Fibroids as coexisting masses during pregnancy. Sagittal section through a first trimester gestation demonstrating (1) an anterior lower uterine segment fibroid and (2) a large fundal fibroid. 3 = gravid uterus.

mass. During delivery, fibroids may be responsible for decreased intensity of uterine contractions; they may also cause fetal malpresentation and/or obstruct delivery. In some cases, cesarean section is indicated.

Sonographic Signs

The following sonographic signs are associated with fibroids (Figure 12-27):

- Hypoechoic mass distorting normal uterine contours
- Sonolucent center associated with degeneration
- May be confused with myometrial contraction

Ovarian Cysts

Ovarian cystic masses are frequently found in pregnancy. Two types of cysts are associated with pregnancy itself: progesterone-producing *corpus luteum cysts*, which usually regress by 16–18 weeks but may persist; and *theca-lutein cysts*, the large, bilateral, multiseptated cysts seen in association with ovarian hyperstimulation syndrome and gestational trophoblastic disease (Figures 12-28A and B). Regardless of the type of cyst, its location and size should be documented; if it persists and is large enough it may cause dystocia. Other cystic lesions that may coexist with a pregnancy include benign cystadenomas (Figure 12-28C) and benign cystic teratomas.

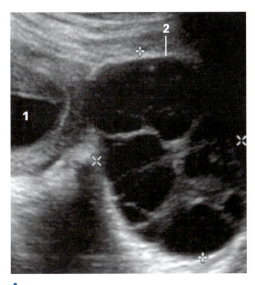

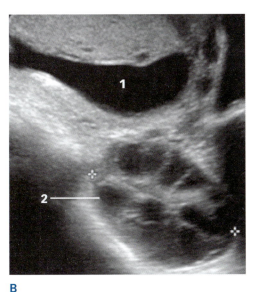

Figure 12-28. A A transverse section during pregnancy showing a large, space-occupying theca-lutein ovarian cyst and a large, multiseptated cystic structure lying lateral to the gravid uterine cornu. 1 = gravid uterus, 2 = theca-lutein cyst. **B** Longitudinal section through the lateral aspect of (1) the gravid uterus showing (2) a theca-lutein cyst lying posteriorly. **C** A large coexisting cystadenoma lying posterior to the maternal urinary bladder and filling the pelvic outlet is demonstrated in this sagittal section. 1 = gravid uterus, 2 = maternal urinary bladder, 3 = multiloculated cyst.

Sonographic Signs

The following sonographic signs are associated with ovarian cysts:

- Presence of a cystic mass in the adnexa
- May be simple, septated, or complex
- Possible distortion of uterine and cervical contour

Malignancies

The occurrence of cancer in pregnant women is uncommon, with the incidence ranging from 0.07% to 0.1%. The most common malignancies associated with pregnancy include cervical cancer, breast cancer, melanoma, lymphomas, and leukemia.[37]

Sonographic Signs

As most concomitant malignancies are not in the pelvis, there are no diagnostic sonographic signs associated with malignancies during pregnancy.

Solid Masses

Other solid masses found in the pelvis during pregnancy may also cause dystocia and clinical symptoms. Common pathologic types of solid masses are usually related to the ovary and include benign *teratomas* (dermoids) and *endometriomas*. Anatomic variations and abnormalities can also present as coexisting pelvic masses. These include:

- Pelvic kidney
- Wandering (ectopic) spleen
- Nongravid horn of a bicornuate uterus (Figure 12-29)

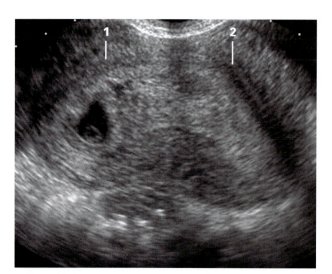

Figure 12-29. Coronal endovaginal section demonstrating a nongravid horn of a bicornuate uterus acting as a coexisting mass during pregnancy. 1 = gravid horn, 2 = nongravid horn.

- Feces-filled colon
- Dilated ureter

Sonographic Signs

The following sonographic signs are associated with solid masses:

- Presence of a solid mass in the adnexa
- Presence of a kidney in the adnexa
- Possible distortion of uterine and cervical contour

ANTEPARTUM/POSTPARTUM RISKS

FETAL POSITION

Fetal position refers to the position of the fetus relative to the maternal pelvis. Correct sonographic determination of fetal position requires knowledge of the relational anatomy between the long axis of the fetus and the long axis of the mother.

Fetal position is determined by two factors: fetal lie and fetal presentation. Fetal *lie* describes the relationship of the longitudinal axis of the fetus to the longitudinal axis of the mother and can be any one of the following:

- Transverse lie (Figure 12-30A): The long axis of the fetus is positioned horizontal to the long axis of the mother.
- Longitudinal lie: The long axis of the fetus is positioned parallel to the long axis of the mother.
- Oblique lie: The long axis of the fetus is positioned at an angle to the pelvic inlet.

Fetal *presentation* describes the part of the fetus that is expected to be delivered first. There are many variations, only the more common of which are listed here:

- Cephalic presentation (Figure 12-30B): The fetus is in a longitudinal lie with the head in the maternal pelvis:
  - Vertex presentation: parietal bones presenting
  - Face presentation: chin and nose presenting
  - Brow presentation: forehead presenting
- Shoulder presenting: There are four types based on the location of the fetal scapula.
- Breech (Figures 12-30C–E): The fetal head is located in fundus of the uterus:
  - Footling: hips extended, foot or feet presenting
  - Frank: thighs flexed, lower legs extended
  - Complete: thighs flexed, lower extremities flexed

Determination of fetal position is generally reported as a part of a complete obstetric ultrasound examination throughout the second and third trimesters. While it may be of marginal interest in the second trimester, it attains clinical significance as the pregnancy approaches term. Abnormal position—i.e., any position other than fetal head within the pelvic inlet—increases the risk of a complicated delivery and may necessitate a cesarean delivery. As noted above (page 311), malpresentation is a particular risk in multiple pregnancies.

PRETERM DELIVERY

Preterm delivery is defined as spontaneous delivery regardless of birth weight that occurs before 37 weeks' gestation. This diagnosis is made when the mother enters *labor* (regular uterine contractions accompanied by changes in the cervix or rupture of the amniotic membranes) at this early stage.

Clinical factors associated with preterm delivery include:
- Previous uterine surgery
- Uterine anomalies
- Maternal stress
- Heavy cigarette smoking
- Multiple gestations
- Polyhydramnios
- Antepartum bleeding (from previa, abruption)
- Systemic infections (e.g., appendicitis with sepsis)
- Idiopathic factors

Methods used to assess those at risk for preterm delivery include:
- Visual/digital cervical examination
- Monitoring uterine activity measured by tocodynamometer
- Evaluating levels of salivary estriols
- Sonographic evaluation of cervical length, with a cervical length of <2.5 cm in the latter part of pregnancy suggesting risk for preterm delivery

PREMATURE RUPTURE OF MEMBRANES

Premature rupture of membranes (PROM) is the spontaneous rupture of membranes prior to the onset of labor. PROM that occurs prior to 37 weeks' gestation is called *preterm premature rupture of membranes* (or PPROM). If rupture occurs prior to 26 weeks, there is an increased risk of fetal demise.

PROM is the cause of approximately one-third of preterm deliveries, and it can lead to significant perinatal morbidity, including respiratory distress syndrome, neonatal sepsis, umbilical cord prolapse, placental abruption, and fetal death. Generally, the treatment of pregnancies complicated by PROM is directed toward conserving the pregnancy and reducing perinatal morbidity due to prematurity while monitoring closely for evidence of infection, placental abruption, labor, or fetal compromise due to umbilical cord compression.

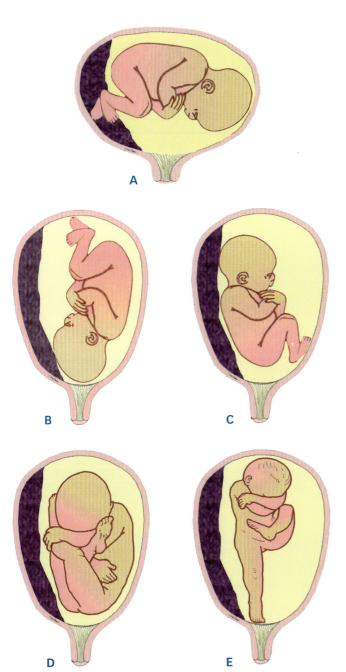

Figure 12-30. **A** Transverse fetal lie. **B** Cephalic fetal presentation. **C** Complete breech presentation. **D** Frank breech presentation. **E** Footling breech presentation.

THE PUERPERIUM

The *puerperium* is the period after delivery that begins with the expulsion of the placenta and ends when maternal anatomy and physiology return to a normal "nonpregnant" state. Indications for sonographic examination during this period include attempts to identify:

- Retained products of conception
- Postpartum hemorrhage
- Postsurgical hematomas
- Abscesses
- Ovarian vein thrombosis

Normal Anatomy

The uterus may assume a variety of positions following either vaginal or cesarean delivery. Typically it remains large and boggy for the first week, after which it quickly reduces in size. It should return to normal size within 6 weeks after delivery. *Uterine involution* is the process by which the uterus returns to its normal size.

Sonographic Signs

The following sonographic signs are associated with normal postpartum uterine anatomy:

- Large, hypoechoic uterus with irregular contours (Figure 12-31A)
- Fluid identified within the endometrial cavity representing residual blood (Figure 12-31B)
- Varying shape and position
- Possibly open internal os

Postpartum Bleeding

Postpartum hemorrhage (PPH) is one of the most significant causes of maternal morbidity after childbirth. It can be classified according to the timing of the hemorrhage as primary or secondary.

Primary Postpartum Hemorrhage

Primary postpartum hemorrhage is bleeding that occurs during the first 24 hours after delivery as a result of acute clinical problems, such as:

- Coagulopathies
- Chorioamnionitis
- Abnormal placental implantation such as previa or accreta
- Bilobed placenta
- Uterine relaxation due to such agents as halothane or magnesium sulfate
- Retained placenta

Secondary Postpartum Hemorrhage

Secondary postpartum hemorrhage is bleeding that occurs more than 24 hours after delivery. The cause is usually retained placental tissue. Sonographically it is difficult to differentiate hemorrhage from retained products of conception (RPOCs). Doppler assessment has not proven to be successful.

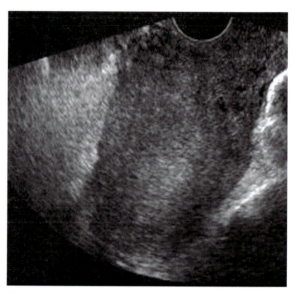

A

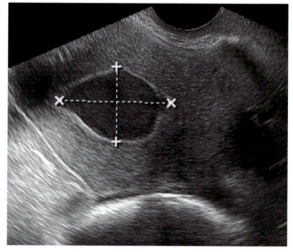

B

Figure 12-31. A Sagittal section demonstrating an irregularly contoured, hypoechoic uterus. **B** Sagittal section demonstrating residual blood in the endometrial cavity (cursors).

Sonographic Signs

The following sonographic signs are associated with postpartum hemorrhage:

- Fluid-filled uterine cavity (in patients with active bleeding) (Figure 12-32A)
- Echogenic masses in the endometrial cavity with an anteroposterior (AP) diameter > 1.5 cm, which is consistent with retained products of conception (Figure 12-32B)
- Doppler evidence of retained placental tissue (Figure 12-32C)

Puerperal Infection

Puerperal infection is suspected when the postpartum patient experiences elevated body temperatures (>100.4° Fahrenheit or 38° Celsius) on any two of the first ten postpartum days. It is a clinical diagnosis characterized by fever, elevated white cell count, tachycardia, and uterine tenderness; sonography plays little role in the diagnosis of puerperal infection. The vagina is the most common route of infection into the uterine cavity.

Risk of postpartum infections is increased with:

- Poor nutrition and hygiene
- Anemia
- Vaginitis or cervicitis
- Delayed rupture of membranes
- Use of invasive fetal and maternal monitoring devices
- Cesarean section
- Prolonged labor

Abscesses

Puerperal infections that persist or that do not respond to antimicrobial therapy may produce an *abscess*, a localized collection of pus and fluid. Abscesses may be located anywhere in the abdominal or pelvic cavity and are more common in patients who have had a cesarean section.

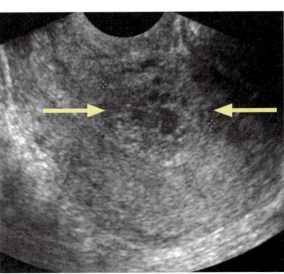

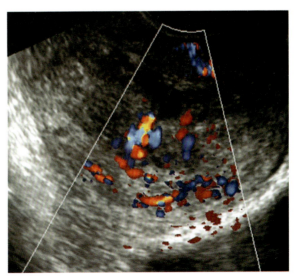

Figure 12-32. A Postpartum hemorrhage. Sagittal section through a postpartum uterus in a patient with active bleeding demonstrates a blood-filled uterine cavity (arrows). **B** Coronal endovaginal B-mode section of retained products of conception (arrows) shows the uterine cavity filled with echogenic material. **C** Doppler color flow shows hyperemic flow in retained placental tissue.

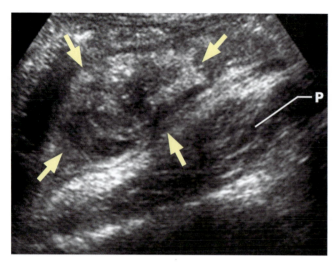

Figure 12-33. Sagittal section through the right lower quadrant demonstrating a complex echogenic postpartum abscess (arrows) anterior to the psoas muscle (P).

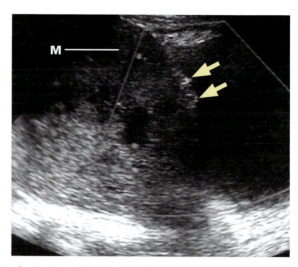

Figure 12-34. Sagittal section through the lower uterine segment following cesarean section showing sutures as highly reflective focal echoes (arrows). M = hypoechoic myometrium.

Sonographic Signs

The following sonographic signs are associated with abscesses (Figure 12-33):

- Complex or anechoic fluid collections anywhere in pelvis
- Presence of internal debris
- Acoustic shadowing when gas bubbles are present

Cesarean Section

A *cesarean section* (*c-section*) is the delivery of the fetus, placenta, and membranes through an incision in the abdominal wall. Cesarean section is indicated when vaginal delivery is not feasible or would pose undue risk to mother and/or infant. A transverse incision through the lower uterine segment (commonly known as a "bikini cut") is the most common type, although an incision through the body of the uterus (*classic cesarean section*) can also be utilized.

Common indications for cesarean section include:

- Central placenta previa
- Cephalopelvic disproportion
- Uterine inertia
- Premature separation of the placenta
- Malpresentation
- Pre-eclampsia/eclampsia
- Fetal distress
- Cord prolapse
- Maternal genital infection

Sonographic Signs

The following sonographic signs are associated with cesarean section during the puerperium (Figure 12-34):

- Presence of highly reflective focal echoes representing sutures
- Decreased echogenicity in the myometrium surrounding the sutures
- Anechoic area anterior to the uterine incision and the posterior bladder wall

Hematomas

A postpartum *hematoma* is most commonly related to cesarean section and is located anterior to the uterine incision and posterior to the bladder wall (*bladder flap*). Hematomas are the result of failure to stop bleeding after the uterine incision has been closed.

Sonographic Signs

The following sonographic signs are associated with hematomas:

- Presence of a complex mass between the anterior lower uterine segment and the posterior bladder wall (bladder flap) (Figure 12-35)
- Poorly defined borders
- Possible presence of internal septations

Venous Thrombosis

Vascular changes associated with pregnancy, labor, and delivery increase the risk of blood clotting during the postpartum state. During the first 6 weeks postpartum,

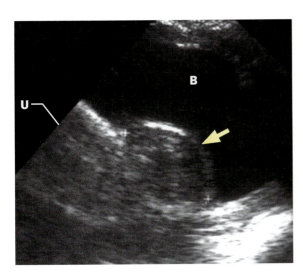

Figure 12-35. Sagittal section through the full urinary bladder demonstrating a complex mass between the anterior lower uterine segment and the posterior bladder wall (bladder flap). U = uterus, B = bladder, arrow = hematoma.

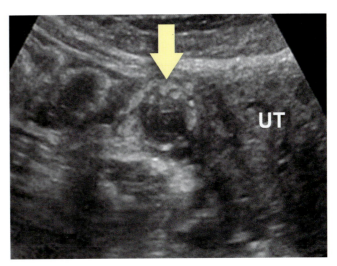

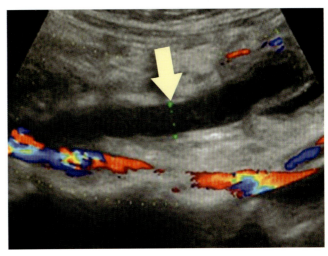

Figure 12-36. A Transverse section through the right adnexa showing a dilated thrombosed ovarian vein (arrow) adjacent to the uterus (UT). **B** Color Doppler imaging demonstrates absent flow in a thrombosed iliac vein (arrow). Flow is identified in the iliac artery. Courtesy of Ultrasoundcases.info.

a woman's risk of venous thromboembolism increases substantially (84-fold) compared to that of nonpregnant, nonpostpartum women, although the incidence of venous thromboembolism declines quickly after delivery.[38]

The three physiologic factors that contribute to this increased risk are called *Virchow's triad* and consist of:

- Hypercoagulability of blood
- Venous stasis
- Alterations of the venous endothelium (endothelial damage)

Predisposing factors for venous thrombosis include:

- Endometritis
- Increased age or parity
- Obesity
- Administration of high-dose estrogens
- Heart disease
- Anemia

The most common locations of postpartum venous thrombosis are in the lower extremity, manifesting as deep venous thrombosis (DVT), and in the ovarian veins. DVT poses the additional risk of pulmonary embolism, venous insufficiency, postphlebitic syndrome, and other chronic lower extremity venous disorders. Ovarian venous thrombosis is rare but is associated with serious sequelae, including septic pelvic thrombophlebitis. It occurs on the right side in 80%–90% of cases; patients present with clinical signs including pelvic pain, fever, and a right-sided pelvic mass.[39]

Sonographic Signs

The following sonographic signs are associated with venous thrombosis:

- Anechoic or hypoechoic oval mass extending superiorly from the adnexa (Figure 12-36A)
- Contiguous with ovarian vessel
- Doppler evaluation that reveals limited or absent blood flow[40] (Figure 12-36B)

FETAL THERAPY

Although intrauterine fetal diagnosis and therapy constitute an emerging field, several forms of therapy have been developed for various fetal conditions.

CORDOCENTESIS

Cordocentesis—also known as *fetal blood sampling* or *percutaneous umbilical blood sampling* (PUBS)—is an invasive method of obtaining a fetal blood sample using ultrasound guidance.

Procedure

A fine-gauge (typically 20-gauge) spinal needle is inserted transabdominally under direct sonographic guidance and is directed toward the umbilical vein (Figures 12-37A and B). With an anterior placenta, the needle is advanced through the anterior uterine wall, through the placenta, and toward the umbilical vein at its insertion site on the placental surface. Puncturing the cord at the placental insertion stabilizes the vein, preventing it from moving or rolling significantly during the puncture. After puncture of the vein is achieved, blood is aspirated from the umbilical cord and sent for appropriate laboratory testing. If the placenta is located posteriorly, cordocentesis is more difficult, as the fetus may lie between the anterior abdominal wall and the cord insertion point or move into the path of the advancing needle. An initial sonogram will establish the accessibility of the cord insertion on the placenta from an anterior approach.

Before cordocentesis can be performed, the fetus must be immobilized to minimize the risk of traumatic needle injury. Usually a muscle relaxant is injected into the fetal buttock or thigh. After observing the effects of the medication on the fetus for a few minutes, the physician may administer additional injections if the desired effect has not been achieved. If the placenta is located posteriorly and the cord insertion is not accessible, puncturing a loose loop of umbilical cord may be attempted. This can be rather difficult, as the cord tends to move away from the needle during the puncture. Another possible cordocentesis site is the fetal cord insertion. If either a loose loop of cord or a fetal cord insertion puncture is attempted, it is advisable to paralyze the fetus before the procedure.

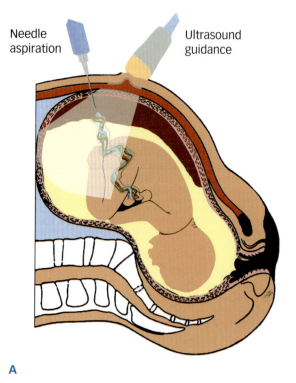

A

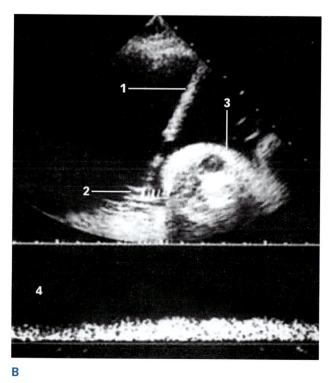

B

Figure 12-37. **A** Schematic of cordocentesis. **B** Ultrasound needle guidance image demonstrating the cordocentesis needle (1) present in the amniotic cavity cannulating the umbilical vein (2). A spectral Doppler venous waveform (4) confirms presence in the correct vessel. 3 = fetal abdomen.

Indications

Indications for cordocentesis include:

- Assessment of the degree of fetal anemia
- Further investigation of genetic disease or chromosomal anomalies
- Diagnosis of congenital infection
- Determination of fetal blood type in anticipation of neonatal transplantation
- Rapid karyotyping
- Red blood cell alloimmunization
- Neonatal alloimmune thrombocytopenia
- Rh disease
- Other blood problems
- Administration of medications

Risks and Complications

Risks and complications for cordocentesis include:

- Bleeding
- Fetal bradycardia
- Cord hematoma
- Infection
- Preterm labor
- Rupture of membranes
- Fetal demise

INTRAVASCULAR FETAL TRANSFUSION

Procedure

Intravascular fetal transfusion (also known as *intrauterine transfusion*) is the treatment of choice in fetuses with severe hemolytic anemia due to maternal red-blood-cell isoimmunization. It is performed by using the same technique described above in the section on cordocentesis. Once the needle is inserted into the umbilical cord, a sample of blood is aspirated. Usually some clinical estimate of the degree of fetal anemia, based on middle cerebral artery velocity or amniotic bilirubin levels, is available, and the fetal transfusion is begun while the fetal blood sample is being evaluated. It is important to proceed promptly with the transfusion, for the transfusion needle may be dislodged at any time and would require a lengthy repositioning.

Typically, a 20-gauge needle is used for fetal transfusion. Packed red blood cells travel slowly through the needle; therefore, 15–25 minutes of transfusion time may be required. During the transfusion, the positions of the needle tip and the umbilical vein and adjacent umbilical cord are observed sonographically. In most cases, bright speckles can be observed within the umbilical vein during the transfusion. These speckles are observed during injection but not between injections. Once the fetal blood sample has been analyzed for hematocrit, a calculation is made to determine how much additional blood should be transfused into the fetus, and the transfusion is completed. If the transfusing needle has not been dislodged, a post-transfusion blood sample may be taken to establish post-transfusion hematocrit.

After withdrawing the needle, the physician should observe the puncture site on the umbilical vein for several minutes to establish whether blood is leaking into the amniotic fluid from the site. If so, it usually will cease within 1–2 minutes. A few investigators have reported using direct intracardiac transfusion with the needle in rare instances when severe hemorrhage after transfusion or cordocentesis has occurred.

Indications

Indications for intravascular fetal transfusion include fetal anemia/hemolytic disease due to:

- Red blood cell alloimmunization
- Parvovirus infection
- Other causes

Risks and Complications

Risks and complications for intravascular fetal transfusion include:

- Bleeding
- Fetal bradycardia
- Hemorrhage
- Post-procedure fetal demise

INTRAPERITONEAL FETAL TRANSFUSION

Before intravascular fetal transfusion techniques were perfected, another procedure, *intraperitoneal fetal transfusion*, was used. The physician advanced a needle directly into the fetal peritoneal cavity, taking care to avoid major organs in the abdomen such as the liver, spleen, and kidneys, and blood was transfused directly into the peritoneal cavity of the fetus. Intraperitoneal fetal transfusion usually was not successful if the fetus had ascites or subcutaneous edema, and for this reason as well as its risks the technique is rarely used today.

CHAPTER 12 REVIEW QUESTIONS

1. The excessive accumulation of fluid in at least two anatomic locations within a fetus is called:
   A. Anasarca
   B. Ascites
   C. Hydrops fetalis
   D. Hydrocephalus

2. All of the following fetal conditions may result in immune hydrops fetalis EXCEPT:
   A. Fetal anemia
   B. Hemolytic diseases
   C. Rh isoimmunization
   D. Turner syndrome

3. Pathologic conditions that disrupt the normal homeostatic mechanisms that control the body's ability to manage fluid may result in:
   A. Immune hydrops
   B. Nonimmune hydrops
   C. Erythroblastosis fetalis
   D. Fetal anemia

4. All of the following are sonographic findings in a fetus with hydrops fetalis EXCEPT:
   A. Pericardial effusion
   B. Ascites
   C. Subcutaneous edema
   D. Abnormally small and mature placenta

5. A spectrum of fetal physiologic conditions that result in an infant weighing below the 10th percentile is referred to as:
   A. Intrauterine growth restriction
   B. Hydrops fetalis
   C. Erythroblastosis fetalis
   D. Fetal anasarca

6. What is the term for a fetal condition characterized by all biometric parameters measuring less than expected for a given gestational age?
   A. Asymmetric intrauterine growth restriction
   B. Symmetric intrauterine growth restriction
   C. Beckwith-Wiedemann syndrome
   D. Trisomy 21

7. All of the following sonographic findings are consistent with asymmetric intrauterine growth restriction EXCEPT:
   A. AC measuring > 2 weeks behind HC
   B. HC measuring > 2 weeks behind AC
   C. Normal femur length measurement
   D. Early grade III placenta

8. All of the following conditions may cause fetal anemia EXCEPT:
   A. Rh incompatibility
   B. Hemolytic disease
   C. Fetal parvovirus infection
   D. Intrauterine growth restriction (IUGR)

9. A monochorionic/monoamniotic twin pregnancy will have:
   A. A single amnion and a single chorion
   B. Two amnions and a single chorion
   C. A single amnion and two chorions
   D. Two amnions and two chorions

10. A twin gestation arising from two separately fertilized ova is called:
    A. Monoamniotic/dizygotic
    B. Diamniotic/monozygotic
    C. Dizygotic
    D. Monozygotic

11. A complication of monochorionic twinning in which an unbalanced volume of blood is exchanged between co-twins via aberrant anastomotic vascular channels in a shared placenta is called:
    A. Stuck twin
    B. Twin embolization syndrome
    C. Twin-twin transfusion syndrome
    D. Fetus papyraceus

12. All of the following sonographic findings are consistent with twin-twin transfusion syndrome EXCEPT:
    A. Significant growth discordance
    B. AFI discrepancy between two sacs
    C. Double placentation
    D. Gender concordance

13. The recipient fetus in a twin-twin transfusion syndrome gestation may demonstrate all of the following sonographic findings EXCEPT:
    A. Oligohydramnios
    B. Hydropic changes
    C. Hepatosplenomegaly
    D. Ascites

14. The recipient fetus in twin reversed arterial perfusion (TRAP) sequence may demonstrate all of the following sonographic findings EXCEPT:
    A. Acardiacus
    B. Cystic hygroma
    C. Hydrops fetalis
    D. Absent upper body

15. Conjoined twins attached at the head are called:
    A. Omphalopagus
    B. Craniopagus
    C. Pygopagus
    D. Ischiopagus

16. Twins conjoined at the anterior abdominal wall are referred to as:
    A. Omphalopagus
    B. Craniopagus
    C. Pygopagus
    D. Ischiopagus

17. Conjoined twins occur only in:
    A. Dizygotic twinning
    B. Dichorionic/diamniotic twinning
    C. Monochorionic/diamniotic twinning
    D. Monochorionic/monoamniotic twinning

18. The findings demonstrated in this image of the fetal chest are consistent with:

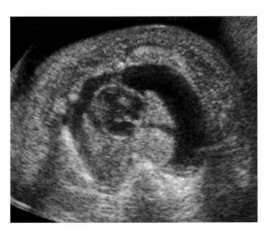

    A. Intrauterine growth restriction
    B. Rh isoimmunization
    C. Maternal hypertension
    D. Stuck twin syndrome

19. This image is of Twin A. Twin B appeared small and growth restricted. These findings are consistent with:

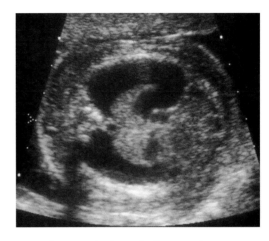

    A. Twin-to-twin transfusion syndrome
    B. Conjoined twins
    C. Vanishing twin
    D. Twin demise

20. This image demonstrates:

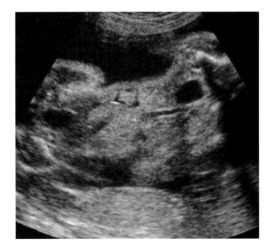

    A. Stuck twin
    B. Omphalocele
    C. Conjoined twins
    D. Acardiacus

21. This image demonstrates which type of twinning?

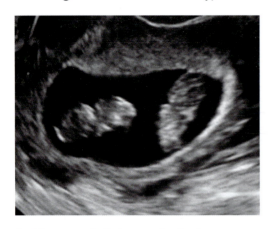

A. Monoamniotic/monochorionic
B. Monoamniotic/dichorionic
C. Diamniotic/monochorionic
D. Diamniotic/dichorionic

ANSWERS

See Appendix A on page 482 for answers.

REFERENCES

1. Baschat AA, Gembruch U, Reiss I, et al: Relationship between arterial and venous Doppler and perinatal outcome in fetal growth restriction. Ultrasound Obstet Gynecol 16:407–413, 2000.

2. Baschat AA, Galan HL, Bhide A, et al: Doppler and biophysical assessment in growth restricted fetuses: distribution of test results. Ultrasound Obstet Gynecol 27:41–47, 2006.

3. Mandruzzato GP, Bogatti P, Fischer L, et al: The clinical significance of absent or reverse end-diastolic flow in the fetal aorta and umbilical artery. Ultrasound Obstet Gynecol 1:192–196, 1991.

4. Brar HS, Platt LD: Reverse end-diastolic flow velocity on umbilical artery velocimetry in high-risk pregnancies: an ominous finding with adverse pregnancy outcome. Am J Obstet Gynecol 159:559–561, 1988.

5. Gagnon R, Van den Hof M: The use of fetal Doppler in obstetrics. J Obstet Gynaecol Can 25:601–614, 2003.

6. Nehal S, Nandita M, Ragini V, et al: Umbilical and cerebral arterial flow velocity waveforms and neonatal outcome in high risk pregnancy. J Obstet Gynecol India 57:216–220, 2007.

7. Kierans J, Kendall P, Foster LT, et al: New birth weight and gestational age charts for the British Columbia population. BC Med J 48:28–32, 2006.

8. Amini SB, Catalano PM, Hirsch V, et al: An analysis of birth weight by gestational age using a computerized perinatal data base, 1975–1992. Obstet Gynecol 83:342–352, 1994.

9. Gruenwald P: Growth of the human fetus: I. normal growth and its variation. Am J Obstet Gynecol 94:1112–1119, 1966.

10. Nahum GG, Pham KQ, McHugh JP: Ultrasonic prediction of term birth weight in Hispanic women: accuracy in an outpatient clinic. J Reprod Med 48:13–22, 2003.

11. Smith-Bindman R, Chu PW, Ecker JL, et al: US evaluation of fetal growth: prediction of neonatal outcomes. Radiology 223:153–161, 2002.

12. Merz E, Bahlmann F: *Ultrasound in Obstetrics and Gynecology*. New York, Thieme, 2005.

13. Baschatt AA, Galan HL, Bhide A, et al: Doppler and biophysical assessment in growth restricted fetuses: distribution of test results. Ultrasound Obstet Gynecol 27:41–47, 2006.

14. Mari G, Adrignolo A, Abuhamad AZ, et al: Diagnosis of fetal anemia with Doppler ultrasound in the pregnancy complicated by maternal blood group immunization. Ultrasound Obstet Gynecol 5:400–405, 1995.

15. Malinger G, Lev D, Zahalka N, et al: Fetal cytomegalovirus infection of the brain: the spectrum of sonographic findings. Am J Neuroradiol 24:28–32, 2003.

16. Sunderam S, Kissin DM, Flowers L, et al: Assisted reproductive technology surveillance—United States, 2009. MMWR Surveill Summ 61:1–23, 2012.

17. Crane JP: Sonographic evaluation of multiple pregnancy. Semin Ultrasound CT MR 5:144–156, 1984.

18. Naeye RL: Causes of fetal and neonatal mortality by race in a selected U.S. population. Am J Public Health 69:857–861, 1979.

19. Hack KE, Derks JB, Schaap AH, et al: Perinatal outcome of monoamniotic twin pregnancies. Obstet Gynecol 113(2 Pt 1):353–360, 2009.

20. Sepulveda W, Sebire NJ, Hughes K, et al: Evolution of the lambda or twin-chorionic peak sign in dichorionic twin pregnancies. Obstet Gynecol 89:439–441, 1997.

21. Quintero RA, Morales WJ, Allen MH, et al: Staging of twin-twin transfusion syndrome. J Perinatol 19(8 Pt 1):550–555, 1999.

22. Dias T, Mahsud-Dornan S, Bhide A, et al: Cord entanglement and perinatal outcome in monoamniotic twin pregnancies. Ultrasound Obstet Gynecol 35:201–204, 2010.

23. Abuhamad AZ, Mari G, Copel JA, et al: Umbilical artery flow velocity waveforms in monoamniotic twins with cord entanglement. Obstet Gynecol 86(4 Pt 2):674–677, 1995.

24. Nehal S, Nandita M, Ragini V, et al: Umbilical and cerebral arterial flow velocity waveforms and neonatal outcome in high risk pregnancy. J Obstet Gynecol India 57:216–220, 2007.

25. Sheffield JS, Butler-Koster EL, Casey BM, et al: Maternal diabetes mellitus and infant malformations. Obstet Gynecol 100(5 Pt 1):925–930, 2002.

26. Weissmann-Brenner A, Simchen MJ, Zilberberg E, et al: Maternal and neonatal outcomes of macrosomic pregnancies. Med Sci Monit 18:PH77–PH81, 2012.

27. Report of the National High Blood Pressure Education Program Working Group on High Blood Pressure in Pregnancy. Am J Obstet Gynecol 183:S1–S22, 2000.

28. Paquet C, Yudin MH: Toxoplasmosis in pregnancy: prevention, screening, and treatment. J Obstet Gynaecol Can 35:78–81, 2013.

29. Malinger G, Werner H, Rodriguez-Leonel JC, et al: Prenatal brain imaging in congenital toxoplasmosis. Prenat Diagn 31:881–886, 2011.

30. Benoist G, Leruez-Ville M, Magny JF, et al: Management of pregnancies with confirmed cytomegalovirus fetal infection. Fetal Diagn Ther 33:203–214, 2013.

31. Munro SC, Trincado D, Hall B, et al: Symptomatic infant characteristics of congenital cytomegalovirus disease in Australia. J Paediatr Child Health 41:449–452, 2005.

32. Dogan Y, Yuksel A, Kalelioglu IH, et al: Intracranial ultrasound abnormalities and fetal cytomegalovirus infection: report of 8 cases and review of the literature. Fetal Diagn Ther 30:141–149, 2011.

33. National Center for HIV/AIDS, Viral Hepatitis, STD, and TB Prevention, Centers for Disease Control and Prevention: CDC study finds U.S. herpes rates remain high. March 9, 2010.

34. Fleming DT, McQuillan GM, Johnson RE, et al: Herpes simplex virus type 2 in the United States, 1976 to 1994. N Engl J Med 337:1105–1111, 1997.

35. Rudnick CM, Hoekzema GS: Neonatal herpes simplex virus infections. Am Fam Physician 65:1138–1142, 2002.

36. O'Reilly MA, O'Reilly PM, de Bruyn R: Neonatal herpes simplex type 2 encephalitis: its appearances on ultrasound and CT. Pediatr Radiol 25:68–69, 1995.

37. Pavlidis NA: Coexistence of pregnancy and malignancy. Oncologist 7:279–287, 2002.

38. Jackson E, Curtis KM, Gaffield ME: Risk of venous thromboembolism during the postpartum period: a systematic review. Obstet Gynecol 117:691–703, 2011.

39. Salomon O, Apter S, Shaham D, et al: Risk factors associated with postpartum ovarian vein thrombosis. Thromb Haemost 82:1015–1019, 1999.

40. Giraud JR, Poulain P, Renaud-Giono A, et al: Diagnosis of post-partum ovarian vein thrombophlebitis by color Doppler ultrasonography: about 10 cases. Acta Obstet Gynecol Scand 76:773–778, 1997.

SUGGESTED READINGS

Ball RH, Deprest J: The prenatal management of the fetus with a correctable defect. In Callen PW (ed): *Ultrasonography in Obstetrics and Gynecology*, 5th edition. Philadelphia, Saunders Elsevier, 2008, pp 867–886.

Egan JFX, Borgida AF: Ultrasound evaluation of the multiple pregnancies. In Callen PW (ed): *Ultrasonography in Obstetrics and Gynecology*, 5th edition. Philadelphia, Saunders Elsevier, 2008, pp 266–296.

Fleischer AC, Toy E, Lee W, et al (eds): *Sonography in Obstetrics and Gynecology: Principles and Practice*, 7th edition. New York, McGraw-Hill, 2011, ch 13.

Foy PM: Ultrasound of the cervix during pregnancy. In Gill KA: *Ultrasound in Obstetrics and Gynecology: A Practitioner's Guide*. Pasadena, Davies Publishing, 2014, pp 215–228.

Gill KA: Maternal disorders and pregnancy. In Gill KA: *Ultrasound in Obstetrics and Gynecology: A Practitioner's Guide*. Pasadena, Davies Publishing, 2014, pp 313–334.

Gill KA: Multiple gestations and their complications. In Gill KA: *Ultrasound in Obstetrics and Gynecology: A Practitioner's Guide*. Pasadena, Davies Publishing, 2014, pp 291–312.

Levine D: Fetal hydrops. In Rumack CM, Wilson SR, Charboneau JW, et al (eds): *Diagnostic Ultrasound*, 4th edition. Philadelphia, Elsevier Mosby, 2011, pp 1424–1454.

Mehta TS: Multifetal pregnancy. In Rumack CM, Wilson SR, Charboneau JW, et al (eds): *Diagnostic Ultrasound*, 4th edition. Philadelphia, Elsevier Mosby, 2011, pp 1145–1165.

Mitchell C, Trampe B: Sonography and high-risk pregnancy. In Hagen-Ansert SL (ed): *Textbook of Diagnostic Ultrasonography*, 7th edition. St. Louis, Elsevier Mosby, 2012, pp 1170–1189.

PART II

Gynecology

Chapter 13 | Pelvic Anatomy and Physiology

Chapter 14 | Pelvic Pathology

Chapter 15 | Infertility

Chapter 16 | Pediatric and Postmenopausal Gynecologic Sonography

CHAPTER 13

Pelvic Anatomy and Physiology

Pediatric Development and Sonographic Appearance

Adult Anatomy and Sonographic Appearance

Physiology

The pelvic anatomic structures include skeletal, muscular, ligamentous, and vascular components as well as the urinary tract and the internal organs of reproduction. These can be visualized at various stages of postnatal development. A mastery of this pelvic anatomy and physiology is essential for anyone performing gynecologic ultrasound. It is the underpinning of the successful utilization of this widely used diagnostic imaging modality. Without a command of normal anatomic and hemodynamic sonographic appearances, it is impossible to recognize abnormalities and, more specifically, how they deviate from normal—the essence of the diagnostic process.

PEDIATRIC DEVELOPMENT AND SONOGRAPHIC APPEARANCE

UTERUS

The fetal uterus responds to maternal hormones; it assumes a more cylindrical or hourglass configuration than its adult counterpart and may measure up to 4 cm in length. At birth, because of this in utero hormonal stimulation, the typical neonatal uterus is quite prominent, measuring approximately 3.5 cm

Table 13-1. Mean uterine size across the life span.

Age Group	Diameter in cm (L × W × AP)
Neonatal	3.5 × 1.0 × 1.4
Prepubertal	4.0 × 1.0 × 1.1
Parity = 0	7.3 × 4.0 × 3.2
Parity = 1	8.3 × 4.6 × 3.9
Parity ≥ 2	9.2 × 5.1 × 3.9
Postmenopausal	5.6 × 3.1 × 2.5

Table 13-2. Ovarian volume across the life span.

Age Group	Mean Volume (cc)
Neonatal*	1.06 (±0.96)
4–12 months	1.05 (±0.67)
13–24 months	0.67 (±0.35)
3–4 years	0.7–0.8 (±0.4)
5 years	0.9 (±0.02)
6–8 years	1.2 (±0.4)
9–10 years	2.1 (±0.7)
11 years	2.5 (±1.3)
12 years	3.8 (±1.4)
13 years	4.2 (±2.3)
Menstrual	9.8 (±5.8)
Postmenopausal	1.2–5.8**

*1 day to 3 months.
**A volume of ≥8 cc is considered abnormal.

Table 13-3. Average ovarian dimensions across the life span.

Age Group	Dimensions in cm (L × W × AP)
Pediatric	2.5 × 1.5 × 0.5
Menstrual	3.0 × 2.0 × 1.0
Postmenopausal	2.0 × 1.0 × 0.5

in length. As the effects of the hormones of pregnancy subside, the neonatal uterus regresses in size and by age 2 measures about 3.2 cm long on average. In the pediatric patient, the uterine corpus is usually smaller in anteroposterior (AP) dimension and shorter in cephalocaudal length than the cervix. At about 9–10 years of age, the uterus enlarges to approximately 4 cm in length, and by age 13 it measures approximately 5.4 cm in maximum length. During menarche, the uterus also begins to assume the adult configuration in terms of the relation between the uterine corpus and the cervix. (See Table 13-1.[1,2])

OVARIES AND ADNEXA

Like the fetal uterus, fetal ovaries respond to maternal hormonal stimulation in utero. In fact, ovarian cysts are not an uncommon finding during routine sonographic examination of the fetal pelvis and may persist after birth. (See Chapter 9, page 240.) In the neonate, the mean ovarian volume of 1.06 cc is considerably larger than in the pediatric patient, reflecting the prevalence of residual in utero hormonal stimulation and persistent ovarian cysts.[3] As with the fetal uterus, when the effects of maternal hormones subside pediatric ovarian volume regresses to the typical early childhood size of approximately 0.7–0.8 cc. By age 6 the ovarian volume has increased to 1.0–1.2 cc, and by 8–11 years the ovarian volume has increased to 2.0–2.5 cc. At age 13 the ovarian volume is approximately 4 cc (Table 13-2).[4,5] Benchmark values for ovarian dimensions throughout the life span based on the author's professional experience are summarized in Table 13-3.

ADULT ANATOMY AND SONOGRAPHIC APPEARANCE

PELVIC FRAMEWORK

The structural framework of pelvic anatomy is provided by the bony skeleton, supporting musculature, and ligaments.

Skeletal Structures

The maternal bony pelvis serves several structural functions: It provides a weight-bearing bridge between the spinal column and the lower extremities; it directs the pathway of the fetal head during birth; and it protects the internal organs of reproduction. The paired bones of the pelvis are the *ischia*, which form the inferior and posterior part of the hip bones, and the

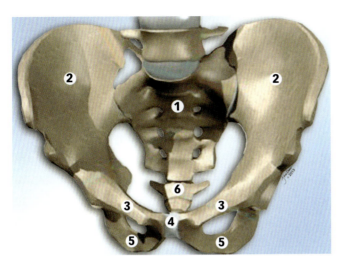

Figure 13-1. Pelvic skeletal structures. 1 = sacrum, 2 = ilium, 3 = pubic ramus, 4 = pubic symphysis, 5 = ischium, 6 = coccyx.

large *ilia* (iliac bones), which form the posterolateral boundary of the pelvis. The posteriorly located *sacrum* connects the pelvis to the lumbar spine and ends in the tail-like *coccyx*. The *pubic bones* form the anteroinferior border of the bony pelvis, with the lateral portions fusing into the acetabulum and the medial portions. The *pubic rami* (medial aspects of the pubic bones) articulate in the midline to form the *symphysis pubis*. (See Figure 13-1.)

Pelvic Musculature

The musculature both protects and supports the internal visceral organs of the pelvis. The paired muscles consist of the following (see Figure 13-2 for visualization of the posterior musculature):

- *Rectus abdominis*: Forms the anterior margin of the abdominal and pelvic spaces. It extends from the costal margin to the symphysis pubis.
- *Psoas major*: Originates at the lower thoracic vertebrae and extends anteriorly and laterally as it courses through the retroperitoneal space. It separates from the vertebral column at the level of the fifth lumbar vertebra (L5) and continues through the pelvis to insert on the lesser trochanter on each side. Just below the iliac crest it merges with the *iliacus* muscle, creating the *iliopsoas* muscle. It forms part of the lateral margins of the pelvic basin.
- *Iliacus*: Arises at the iliac crest and extends inferiorly until it merges with the psoas major.
- *Levator ani*: Formed by the *coccygeus, iliococcygeus,* and *pubococcygeus* muscles. (Some anatomists

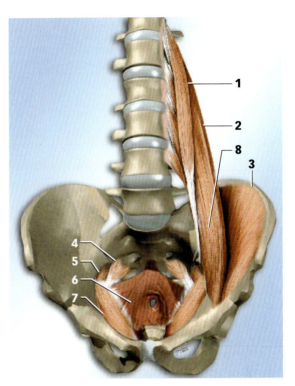

Figure 13-2. Schematic illustration of pelvic musculature. 1 = psoas minor, 2 = psoas major, 3 = iliacus, 4 = coccygeus, 5 = piriformis, 6 = levator ani group (iliococcygeus and pubpococcygeus internus not distinguishable here), 7 = obturator internus, 8 = iliopsoas.

consider the puborectalis part of this group, although it is not typically included in sonographic images.) On each side, this muscle group attaches to the side of the true pelvis and extends medially, where it fuses with its lateral counterpart to form the floor of the pelvic cavity.

- *Obturator internus*: A triangular muscle located along the pelvic sidewall. It extends from the brim of the true pelvis inferior to the levator ani muscles and exits the pelvis through the lesser sciatic foramen.
- *Piriformis*: A triangular muscle located along the lateral wall of the pelvis. It extends from the brim of the true pelvis inferior to the levator ani muscles, exits the pelvis through the greater sciatic foramen, and inserts on the greater trochanter of the femur.

Pelvic Cavities

The pelvis can be divided into two spaces (Figure 13-3) defined in relation to the *linea terminalis*—an imaginary line drawn from the superior aspect of the sacral promontory to the superior aspect of the symphysis pubis. The space superior to this line is called the

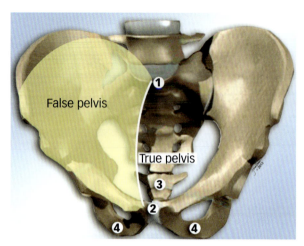

Figure 13-3. The pelvic cavities: The false pelvis sits superior to the *linea terminalis*—an imaginary line drawn from the superior aspect of the sacral promontory to the superior aspect of the symphysis pubis (white line). The true pelvis sits inferior to the linea terminalis. 1 = sacral promontory, 2 = superior aspect of the symphysis pubis, 3 = coccyx, 4 = ischial tuberosities.

false pelvis and houses mostly small bowel; the space inferior to this line is called the *true pelvis*, where the urinary bladder and the internal organs of reproduction reside. The true pelvis is further classified into the horizontally oriented *pelvic inlet*, bounded by the pubic rami anteriorly and the sacral promontory posteriorly,

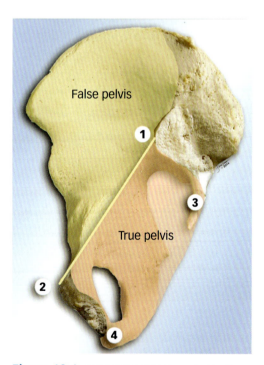

Figure 13-4. The pelvic inlet is bounded by the sacral promontory posteriorly (1) and the pubic bones anteriorly (2), while the pelvic outlet sits below this and is bounded by the coccyx (3) and the ischial tuberosities (4).

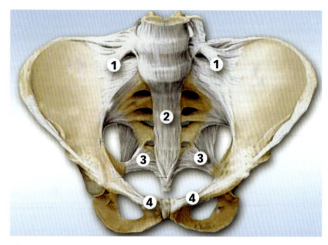

Figure 13-5. Osseous pelvic ligaments. 1 = sacroiliac, 2 = sacrococcygeal, 3 = sacrosciatic, 4 = pubic.

and the vertically oriented *pelvic outlet*, bounded by the ischial tuberosities ("sitting bones") laterally and by the coccyx (tailbone) posteriorly (Figure 13-4).

Osseous Ligaments

The osseous ligaments serve to bind the pelvic bones together. They consist of the following (Figure 13-5):

- *Sacroiliac ligaments*: Bind the sacrum and iliac bones.
- *Sacrococcygeal ligaments*: Bind the sacrum and coccyx.
- *Sacrosciatic* (also called the *sacrospinous*) *ligaments*: Bind the sacrum, iliac bones, and coccyx.
- *Pubic ligament*: Binds the paired pubic rami.

Ovarian Suspensory Ligaments

Several ligaments support and stabilize the position of the ovaries and fallopian tubes. They include the following (Figure 13-6):

- *Mesovarium ligament*: Attaches the ovary posteriorly to the broad ligament. It consists of a short, double layer of peritoneum and supports the primary route of access for blood vessels traveling into and out of the ovarian hilum.
- *Ovarian* (also called the *utero-ovarian*) *ligament*: A flattened, fibromuscular band that connects the inferior pole of the ovary with the uterine cornu.
- *Suspensory* (also called the *infundibulopelvic*) *ligament*: A fold of peritoneum that suspends the superior pole of the ovary from the posterolateral pelvic wall at the brim of the true pelvic space.

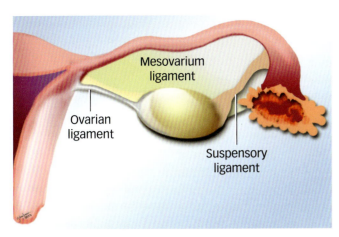

Figure 13-6. Ovarian suspensory ligaments: ovarian, mesovarium, and suspensory.

Uterine Ligaments

The uterus is suspended and anchored in the pelvic cavity by several peritoneal ligaments. They include the following (Figure 13-7):

- *Uterosacral* (also called the *rectouterine*) *ligament*: The posterior edge of the cardinal ligament that extends from the cervix to the sacrum. It anchors the cervix and orients its axis parallel to the central axis of the uterine corpus.
- *Cardinal* (also called the *lateral cervical*) *ligament*: The primary supporting ligament of the uterus. It arises from the lateral aspect of the cervix and uterus and inserts along the lateral pelvic wall.
- *Round ligaments*: The fibromuscular bands arising from the uterine cornua and anchoring the uterine fundus to the anterior pelvic wall. They normally tilt the uterus forward (anteflexion).
- *Pubovesicular ligament*: Extends from the neck of the bladder to the inferior aspect of the pubic bones, anchoring the lower portion of the bladder to the bony pelvis.
- *Broad ligament*: A double fold of peritoneum that arises from the lateral aspect of the uterus on each side. It contains fat, vessels, and nerves between layers of peritoneum and divides the true pelvis into anterior and posterior compartments. The ovaries are attached to the posterior surface of the broad ligament.

URINARY BLADDER

The *urinary bladder* is a musculomembranous, highly distensible sac located between the symphysis pubis and the vagina. It serves as the reservoir for urine prior to *micturition* (urination). The *ureters*, which propel urine into the bladder by peristaltic action, insert along the inferior third of the posterior wall on either side. The superior concavity above the insertion of the ureters is called the *dome*—the most distensible region of the bladder. The *trigone* is the triangular area residing along the posterior wall of the bladder and is defined by the orifices of both ureters and the urethra. The *urethra*, which allows for the excretion of urine, arises along the inferior middle portion of the urinary bladder. At its point of exit it is surrounded by a thickened region of bladder wall referred to as the *internal urethral sphincter*.

The walls of the bladder are composed of three layers of tissue: the outer *epithelial*, the middle *muscularis*, and the inner *mucosal* layers (Figure 13-8). When the bladder is empty, the mucosal layer is quite thick and can be demonstrated sonographically. When the urinary bladder is distended, the mucosa is stretched and can no longer be recognized as a distinct layer. The urinary bladder provides the transabdominal acoustic window through which pelvic anatomy can be visualized sonographically.

UTERUS

Gross Uterine Anatomy

The *uterus* is a hollow, pear-shaped, muscular organ located deep in the pelvic cavity posterior to the urinary bladder and anterior to the rectum (Figure 13-9).

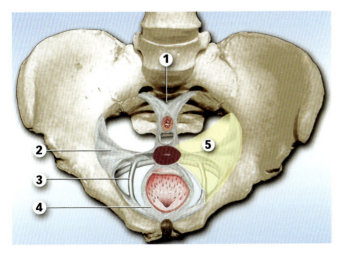

Figure 13-7. Uterine ligaments. 1 = uterosacral, 2 = cardinal, 3 = round, 4 = pubovesicular, 5 = broad.

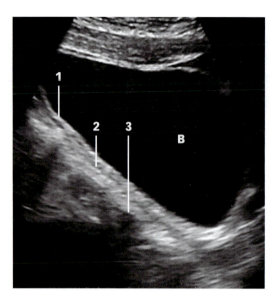

Figure 13-8. Sagittal section through the full urinary bladder (B) with demonstration of the thinned echogenic inner mucosal layer (1), the middle hypoechoic muscularis layer (2), and the outer echogenic epithelial layer (3).

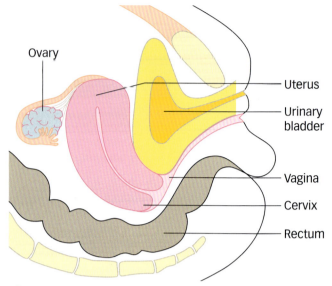

Figure 13-9. Sagittal schematic representation of uterine relational anatomy.

It is suspended and anchored in place by several ligaments and normally flexes anteriorly along the midline. Uterine size varies markedly with age and parity (see Table 13-1).[2,3]

The uterus is divided into the following anatomic regions (Figure 13-10):

- *Fundus*: The uterine *fundus* (Latin for "bottom" or "base") is the rounded, superior aspect located superior to the insertion of the fallopian tubes and opposite the opening of the uterus (the cervix). The narrowed lateral portions of the fundus form the *cornua*, or *horns*, of the uterus.
- *Corpus*: The largest portion of the uterus, the *corpus* (Latin for "body"), contains the uterine cavity.
- *Isthmus*: The *isthmus* (Latin for "neck") is the transitional portion between the corpus above and the cervix below; in the gravid uterus it is called the *lower uterine segment* (LUS) and is the point at which the uterus is most flexible.
- *Cervix*: The cylindrical neck of the uterus located posterior to the urinary bladder. It is more fibrous and less muscular than the uterine body. It measures 2–3 cm in length in the normal nulliparous patient. The mucosa-lined *endocervical canal* is contiguous with the uterine cavity at the *internal cervical os* and opens into the upper vagina at the *external cervical os*.

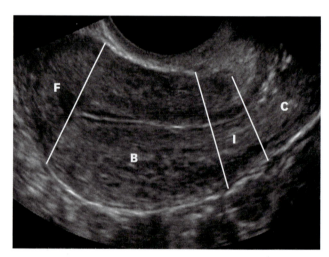

Figure 13-10. Sagittal endovaginal view of the major segments of the uterine anatomy. F = fundus, B = body (corpus), I = isthmus, C = cervix.

The uterus comprises the following fascial layers:

- *Serosa*: Also called the *perimetrium*, the thin outer layer of the uterus. The serosal layer is continuous with the visceral peritoneum and covers the fundus and posterior corpus.
- *Myometrium*: The middle fascial layer, composed of smooth muscle cells interspersed with connective tissue fibers.
- *Endometrium*: The specialized, inner mucosal layer, which varies in thickness and appearance based on the influence of the hormones estrogen and progesterone.

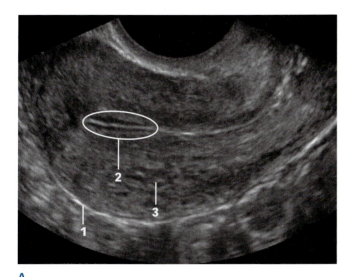 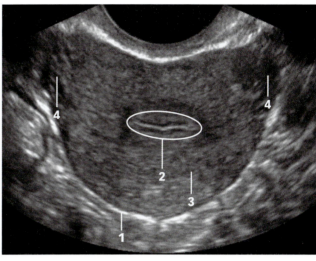

Figure 13-11. Normal uterine sonographic anatomy in **A** sagittal and **B** axial sections demonstrating the outer echogenic serosal layer (1), the multilayered endometrium (2), the solid vascularized myometrium (3), and both cornua (4).

Sonographic Appearance of Uterine Anatomy

The normal uterus in a postmenarcheal, premenopausal patient has a smooth contour and on sonography (Figures 13-11A and B) is surrounded by a thin, echogenic line representing the serosal layer. The normal myometrium is homogeneously echogenic, although varying degrees of homogeneity and echogenicity may be present based on many anatomic and physiologic factors. However, the myometrium is hypoechoic relative to the brighter endometrial layer. The normal endometrium varies significantly in size and appearance based on hormonal status. Sonographic measurements of the uterus are obtained in orthogonal planes, measuring in longitudinal section from the uterine fundus to the external cervical os and transversely from the lateral borders at the level of the broad ligament.

Endometrium

The *endometrium* lines the uterine cavity, a triangular space defined by the openings of the fallopian tubes superiorly and the internal cervical os inferiorly. In premenopausal women, the sonographic appearance of the endometrium varies with the menstrual cycle; in postmenopausal women, the appearance varies with hormonal status related to clinical management. Clinicians rely on a detailed sonographic examination of the endometrium to manage a variety of gynecologic scenarios, from the prediction of ovulation to patient response to therapeutic hormone regimens.

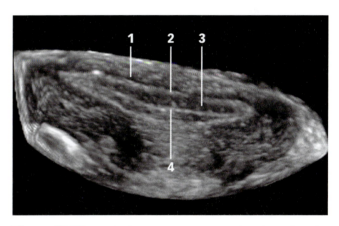

Figure 13-12. Axial volumetric scan through the mid portion of the uterine body demonstrates (1) the outer basalis layer in apposition to the myometrium; (2) the inner, thicker echogenic functionalis layer; (3) the hypoechoic "inner ring"; and (4) the apposition of the endometrial surfaces.

Endovaginal sonography is the modality of choice in evaluating the endometrium. The normal endometrium demonstrates several distinct sonographic layers (Figure 13-12):

- the innermost echogenic line (apposition of anterior and posterior endometrial surfaces)
- the hypoechoic layers just below the surface ("inner ring"), whose presence may confirm that ovulation has occurred
- the middle, echogenic *functionalis layer*
- the outer, hypoechoic *basalis layer*

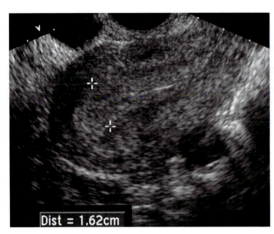

Figure 13-13. Proper cursor placement for measuring the endometrium in this sagittal midline image. The patient is in her menstrual years, at the beginning of the secretory phase.

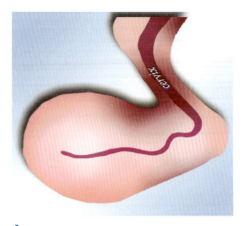

A

Figure 13-14. Normal uterine position. **A** Anteverted/anteflexed uterus: both the uterine corpus and the cervix are tilted anteriorly. (Figure continues . . .)

Normal endometrial sonographic texture should be diffusely homogeneous with smooth margins.[6]

Sonographic measurements correlate well with actual endometrial thickness, and overall thickness varies with the menstrual cycle. These measurements properly include both anterior and posterior surfaces of the endometrium, which are measured from echogenic border to echogenic border across the endometrial cavity on a sagittal midline image (Figure 13-13). The outermost (deepest), hypoechoic rim (*basalis layer*) around the endometrium should *not* be measured, as it represents myometrium. Thickness and texture are influenced by the amount of estrogen and progesterone present. Normal endometrial measurements are summarized in Table 13-4.[7]

Uterine Positional Variants

The typical uterus lies along the pelvic midline with the body (uterine corpus) tilted anteriorly at the cervix. In this normal orientation, called *anteflexion*, the angle between the uterine corpus and the cervix is acute (i.e., anteverted); ordinarily, it is no greater than 90° (Figure 13-14A).

Malposition occurs when this angular configuration is altered by laxity of the cervical and round ligaments that allows a backward tilting of the uterus, cervix, or both. In a *retroverted* uterus (Figure 13-14B), the axis of the cervix is directed toward the hollow of the sacrum without a marked bend in the endometrial stripe. In a *retroflexed* uterus (Figure 13-14C), the uterine corpus tilts backward while the cervix maintains normal anterior flexion. A *retroverted/retroflexed* uterus (Figure 13-14D) is characterized by extreme backward tilting of both uterine corpus and cervix. Differentiation between retroversion and retroflexion is based on the angular relationship between the long axis of the cervix and that of the uterine corpus (Figures 13-15A–D).

On transabdominal imaging, uterine retroflexion creates imaging challenges because beam axis is not perpendicular to the long axis of the uterus, which diminishes axial resolution. This oblique beam path through the muscular myometrium also results in increased acoustic attenuation and subsequent drop-off of echoes within the uterine parenchyma.

CERVIX

The *cervix* is the cylindrical neck of the uterus. Located posterior to the urinary bladder, it is more fibrous, less muscular, and narrower than the uterine body. The normal cervix measures 2–3 cm in length in the

Table 13-4. Endometrial thickness across the life span.

Age Group	Range (mm)
Menstrual: proliferative phase	3–6
Menstrual: secretory phase	6–10
Postmenopausal: no HRT	<5
Postmenopausal: with HRT	<8

HRT = hormone replacement therapy.

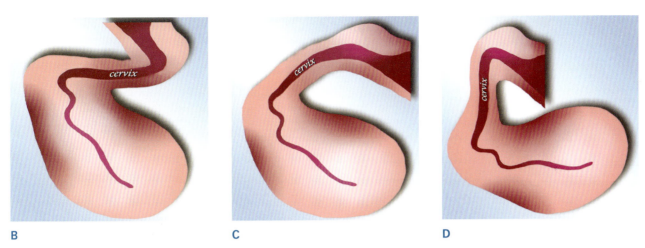

Figure 13-14, continued. B Retroverted uterus: backward-tilted cervix with uterine corpus in normal position. **C** Retroflexed uterus: backward-tilted uterine corpus with cervix in normal position. **D** Retroverted/retroflexed uterus: both uterus and cervix are tilted backward.

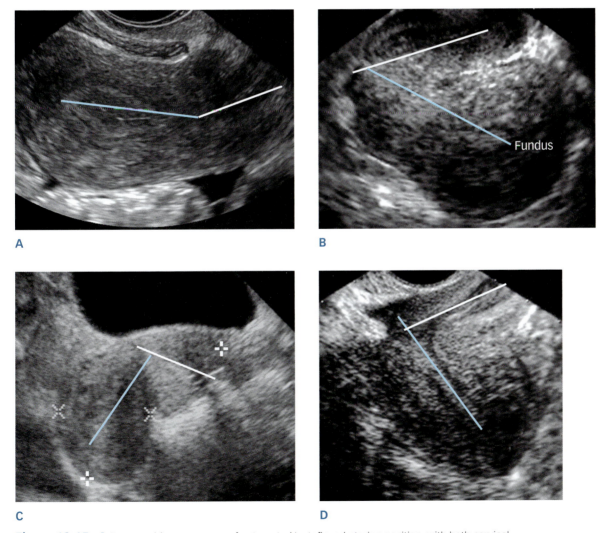

Figure 13-15. A Sonographic appearance of anteverted/anteflexed uterine position, with both cervical and uterine axes in normal orientation. **B** Retroverted uterus, with posterior angulation of the cervical axis and an anterior angulation of the uterine corpus. **C** Retroflexed uterus, with normal anterior cervical angulation and a posteriorly directed uterine axis. **D** Retroverted/retroflexed uterus, with posterior angulation of both the cervix and uterine corpus. White lines = long axis of the cervix, blue lines = long axis of the uterus.

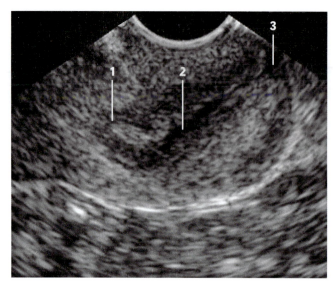

Figure 13-16. Sagittal endovaginal sonographic appearance of cervical anatomy demonstrating (1) the internal cervical os, (2) the endocervical canal, and (3) the external cervical os.

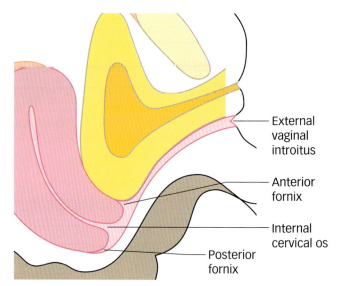

Figure 13-17. Schematic representation of vaginal relational anatomy.

nulliparous female. The mucosa-lined *endocervical canal* is contiguous with the uterine cavity at the *internal cervical os* and opens into the upper vagina at the *external cervical os* (Figure 13-16).

Sonographic Appearance of the Cervix

The cervix may be examined sonographically using a transabdominal, endovaginal, or translabial approach. In longitudinal section both the internal and external cervical ora (plural of *os*) can be identified. The sonographic texture of the cervix is similar to that of the myometrium superior to it. Surrounding the exterior aspect of the cervix is a thin, echogenic line that represents the serosal layer. Coursing through the central portion is the cervical canal, which assumes a variable sonographic appearance—from a smooth, thin, brightly echogenic line in a closed cervix to a multilayered appearance in a cervix containing fluid and/or mucous secretions. Adjacent to both sides of the cervix, the large terminal branches of the uterine artery can be seen as they insert distally and course cephalad along its lateral aspect. Sonographic measurements of the cervix are obtained in orthogonal sections longitudinally from the internal to the external os and transversely at its widest portion.

VAGINA

The *vagina* (Figure 13-17) is a fibromuscular tube extending from the external cervical os to the *external vaginal introitus* (the entrance into the vaginal canal).

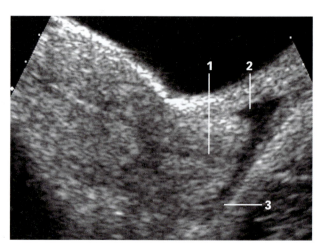

Figure 13-18. Sagittal transabdominal image showing normal sonographic appearance of the vagina with fluid present in the anterior and posterior fornices. 1 = cervix, 2 = anterior fornix, 3 = posterior fornix.

It has two primary functions: to accommodate sexual intercourse and to serve as the birth canal. Its circumferential attachment to the cervix creates angular spaces called the *vaginal fornices*: anterior, posterior, and two lateral (Figure 13-18). The posterior fornix is a frequent site of fluid accumulation.

Sonographic Appearance of the Vagina

The vagina is best examined sonographically using a transabdominal or transperineal approach. Proximally the vaginal fornices can be visualized as triangular sonolucent zones anteriorly and posteriorly just above the external cervical os. The vaginal vault itself is a

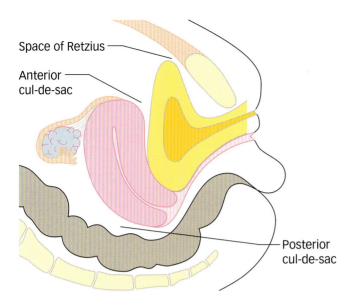

Figure 13-19. Schematic representation of the pelvic recesses. The space of Retzius lies between the anterior abdominal wall and the anterior bladder surface. The anterior cul-de-sac lies between the posterior bladder wall and the anterior uterine surface. The posterior cul-de-sac lies between the posterior uterine surface and the anterior surface of the rectum.

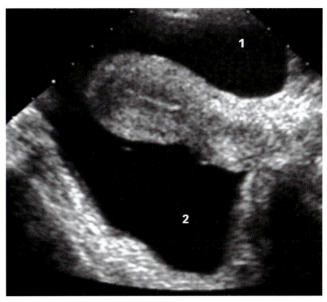

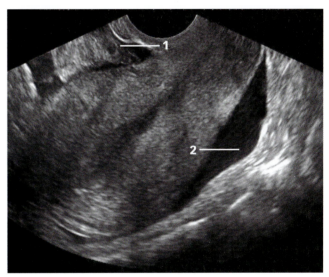

Figure 13-20. Sonographic demonstration of the pelvic recesses. **A** Sagittal transabdominal section through the pelvis in a patient with gross ascites. The (1) anterior and (2) posterior cul-de-sacs are filled with anechoic fluid. **B** Sagittal endovaginal section demonstrating smaller amounts of free fluid in the (1) anterior and (2) posterior cul-de-sacs.

potential space that, in the absence of an intraluminal fluid collection, appears as a thin hypoechoic structure with an echogenic central stripe.

PELVIC RECESSES

Several *potential spaces*, called pelvic recesses, are formed by the draping of the peritoneum over the uterus (Figure 13-19). They include the following:

- *Space of Retzius*: Between the anterior abdominal wall and the anterior bladder surface.
- *Anterior cul-de-sac* (*uterovesical space*): Between the posterior bladder wall and the anterior uterine surface.
- *Posterior cul-de-sac* (*pouch of Douglas*): Between the posterior uterine surface and the anterior surface of the rectum.

Sonographic Appearance of the Pelvic Recesses

In the absence of free fluid in the pelvic cavity, the pelvic recesses are potential spaces that do not appear as discrete structures sonographically. However, when blood, pus, or serous fluid accumulates in the pelvis, these potential spaces expand and can be easily identified (Figures 13-20A and B).

Because gravity pulls free fluid to the dependent portion of the pelvis, the posterior cul-de-sac is the most frequently identified site of fluid accumulation. However, this finding is not always pathologic in origin. A small amount of fluid is normally visualized during the menstrual cycle, the greatest amount of free fluid being observed at mid cycle after ovulation. Fluid associated with normal ovulation should be anechoic. Debris or septations in the fluid are abnormal, suggesting hemorrhage, infection, or neoplasm.

FALLOPIAN TUBES

The *fallopian tubes*, also called *oviducts* or *salpinges*, are musculomembranous tubes extending laterally from each uterine cornu to the corresponding ovary. They lie within the broad ligament and serve to transport ova from the *paraovarian space* to the uterine cavity. When fertilization occurs, which normally takes place within the ampullary portion of the fallopian tube, the conceptus is conveyed from there into the endometrial cavity by means of ciliated epithelium lining the inner surface of the tube.

Gross Fallopian Anatomy

Fallopian tubes consist of three tissue layers: the outer *serosal layer*, which is continuous with the peritoneum; the *muscular* middle layer; and the inner *mucosal* layer. The anatomic regions of the tube are the following (Figure 13-21):

- *Intramural (interstitial) portion*: The narrowest portion of the tube, which traverses the cornu of the uterus.
- *Isthmic portion*: The longest portion of the tube, connecting the intramural and ampullary portions.
- *Ampullary portion*: The trumpet-shaped, open portion of the tube adjacent to the ovary. Here, small finger-like projections called *fimbria* surround the ovary and capture the released ovum following ovulation.
- *Infundibulum*: The inner, funnel-shaped cavity of the ampullary portion.

Sonographic Appearance of the Fallopian Tubes

The normal fallopian tube is not typically demonstrable sonographically as a discrete adnexal structure. Rather, it appears as part of the adnexal hypoechoic triangle that is contiguous with the uterine horn medially and the ovary laterally (Figure 13-22). When the fallopian tube is visible, it is usually because a pathology fills the tube with serous exudate or pus.

OVARIES

The *ovaries* are the female pelvic reproductive organs (gonads) that house and release *ova* (eggs). They are also responsible for the production of the two main sex hormones, estrogen and progesterone, and to a lesser extent relaxin, inhibin A, and a small amount of testosterone.

Gross Ovarian Anatomy

The paired ovaries lie posterior to the broad ligament on each side of the uterus, tucked into the *ovarian*

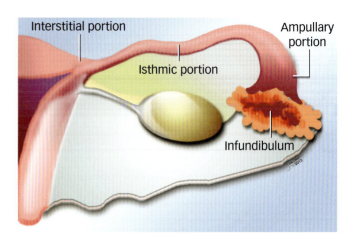

Figure 13-21. Schematic representation of the anatomy of the fallopian tube.

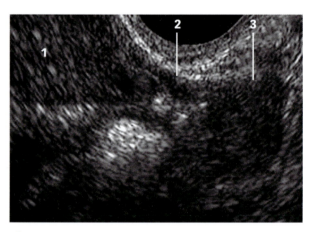

Figure 13-22. The normal fallopian tube appears as part of the adnexal hypoechoic triangle, formed by (1) the uterine fundus and (2) the broad ligament. The ovary (3) is seen laterally.

fossa—a space bounded by the external iliac vessels and the ureters (Figures 13-23A and 13-26 on pages 357 and 358). Architecturally, the ovary is divided into an outer *cortex*, which contains a large number of primordial follicles—the source of ova at ovulation—and an inner *medulla*, which consists primarily of blood vessels and connective tissue (Figure 13-23B). The histologic layers of the ovary are the following:

- *Germinal epithelium*: The outer layer of epithelial cells covering the ovary.
- *Tunica albuginea (ovarian capsule)*: A layer of fibrous connective tissue between the germinal epithelium and the ovarian parenchyma.
- *Ovarian cortex*: The external layer that comprises the bulk of the ovarian substance. It is composed of connective tissues within which are scattered primary and secondary follicles.

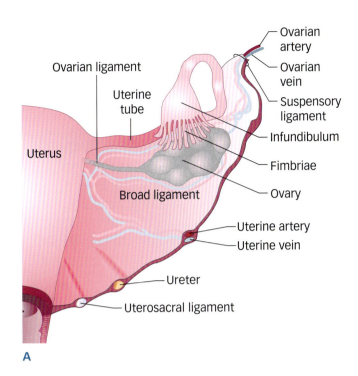

A

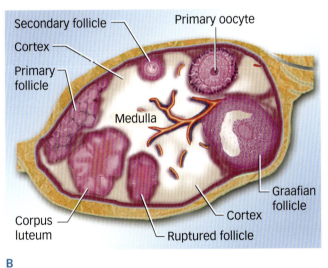

B

Figure 13-23. A Ovarian relational anatomy. **B** Schematic representation of the outer, follicle-containing ovarian cortex encompassing the inner vascular supply in the medulla.

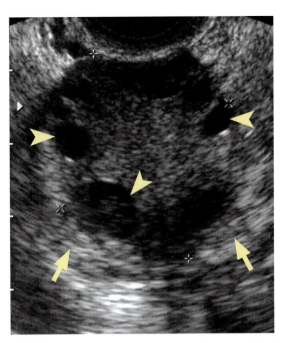

Figure 13-24. Sonographic anatomy of a normal (right) ovary demonstrating solid echogenic parenchyma (arrows) surrounding well-circumscribed fluid-containing follicles (arrowheads).

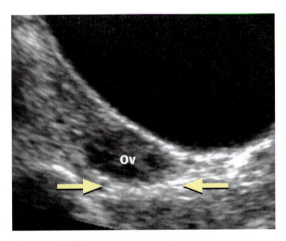

Figure 13-25. Posterior acoustic enhancement (arrows) helps differentiate the ovary (Ov) from adjacent pelvic structures in this view.

- *Medulla*: The central portion of the ovary, which contains blood vessels, lymphatic vessels, and nerves entering through the *ovarian hilum* (the point where vessels and nerves enter the ovary).

Sonographic Appearance of the Ovaries

During the reproductive years, ovaries contain multiple follicles of varying degrees of development and maturity. Solid parenchyma can be visualized as a moderate to highly echogenic stroma surrounding well-circumscribed, fluid-filled foci with varying degrees of echogenicity (Figure 13-24). The fluid content of these structures, in conjunction with the highly vascularized nature of the ovarian cortex, creates an organ that, while considered solid by anatomists, possesses a sonographic appearance more consistent with a cystic structure. One of the clinical pearls in differentiating the sonographic appearance of the ovary from that of adjacent pelvic anatomic structures is the identification of the posterior acoustic enhancement (Figure 13-25) commonly seen behind the ovary.

Ovaries vary significantly in size, shape, and configuration based on age and hormonal status. Ovarian volume measurement is the preferred method of assessing normality of size. It is calculated using the formula for the volume of a prolate ellipsoid: length × width × anteroposterior height × 0.52. (Size by age group is summarized in Tables 13-2 and 13-3.)

PELVIC VASCULAR ANATOMY

Gross Arterial Anatomy

Blood supply to the pelvic organs (Figure 13-26) is provided by major branches of the distal abdominal aorta, which bifurcates at the level of the third lumbar vertebra (L3) into the right and left *common iliac arteries* (CIAs). The *internal iliac (hypogastric) artery* gives rise to most of the branches that supply the reproductive tract. These arteries and the vascular beds that they supply are the:

- *Obturator artery*: Supplies the pelvic bone and muscles, bladder, and external genital organs.
- *Vesicular arteries*: Supply the urinary bladder.
- *Vaginal artery*: Supplies the vagina, bladder neck, and part of the rectum.
- *Uterine artery*: Courses medially from the pelvic sidewall and attaches to the uterus at about the level of the cervix. Ascends along the lateral uterine wall between layers of the broad ligament, with branches that perforate the uterine substance. Supplies the uterus, cervix, round ligament, part of the fallopian tube, and vagina.
- *Ovarian artery*: Arises directly from the abdominal aorta or, less commonly, from the main renal artery. Courses into the pelvis and passes between two layers of the broad ligament. Courses along the superior aspect of the ovary; some of its branches supply the fallopian tube. Near the cornu of the uterus, it anastomoses with the ascending uterine artery. It is the main source of blood supply to the ovary.

The anastomoses of uterine and ovarian arterial branches near the uterine cornu provide for collateral flow to both organs in the event the primary perfusional source is obliterated by disease and anatomic variation.

Sonographic Appearance of Pelvic Arterial Anatomy

As it is with all vascular structures, color Doppler imaging is a useful adjunct in identifying and assessing patency and normality of the pelvic vessels, particularly of small parenchymal arteries and their branches. The use of endovaginal transducers allows high-resolution imaging and enhanced sensitivity to even low-flow states and is the method of choice for sonographic assessment of pelvic visceral vasculature.

The *uterine artery* can best be appreciated sonographically as it inserts on the lateral aspect of the uterus just above the cervix (Figure 13-27).

The impedance to blood flow into the uterine parenchyma varies across the menstrual cycle, but to a much lesser degree than found in the ovary. In a normal menstrual cycle that does not result in pregnancy, the pulsatility and resistivity in the uterine artery demonstrate only mild to moderate changes. Normal values for uterine artery Doppler resistivity (RI) and pulsatility (PI) indices vary widely based on hormonal status. Uterine RI values are summarized in Table 13-5. Uterine artery Doppler studies have little clinical utility outside research protocols and evaluation of early pregnancy.

The *ovarian artery* can be identified coursing along the margin of each ovary, giving rise to small penetrating

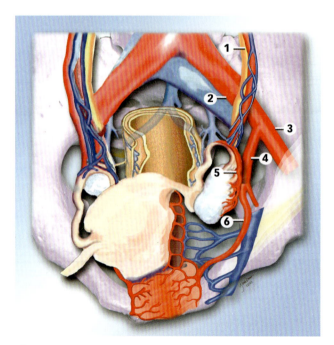

Figure 13-26. Schematic illustration of pelvic vascular anatomy. 1 = gonadal artery, 2 = common iliac artery, 3 = external iliac artery, 4 = internal iliac (hypogastric) artery, 5 = ovarian artery, 6 = uterine artery.

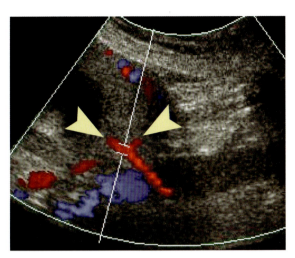

Figure 13-27. Color Doppler imaging demonstrates the uterine artery giving rise to smaller parenchymal branches (arrowheads) as it inserts on the lateral aspect of the cervix.

Table 13-5. Uterine artery resistivity indices.

Patient Status	Resistivity Index
On HRT	0.82
Normal cycles	0.88
Postmenopausal	0.92

parenchymal branches (Figure 13-28A). Resistance of arterial flow through an ovarian artery, as demonstrated with spectral Doppler, varies with the metabolic status of the ovary being examined. As a rule of thumb, the ovary containing the dominant follicle requires more blood flow to accommodate the increase in metabolic activity present; therefore the Doppler signal will be low-resistance. The nondominant ovary typically requires less perfusion and the Doppler signal appears more resistive (Figures 13-28B–D). Typical ovarian resistivity values are presented in Table 13-6.

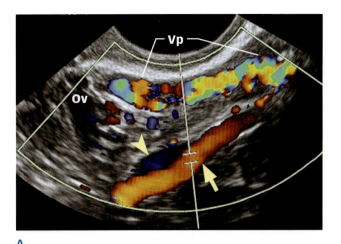

A

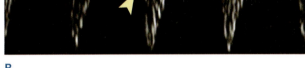

B

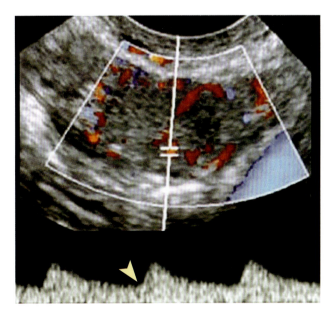

C

Figure 13-28. **A** Color Doppler image demonstrating the anatomy of the ovarian vasculature. Ov = ovary, Vp = uterine venous plexus, arrowhead = ovarian vein, arrow = ovarian artery. Note smaller penetrating intraparenchymal branches in the ovary. **B** Doppler demonstration of highly resistive hemodynamic pattern seen in the nondominant ovary with flow almost returning to baseline during diastole (arrowhead). **C** Increased diastolic flow (arrowhead) during the early follicular phase with maintenance of spectral contour. (Figure continues . . .)

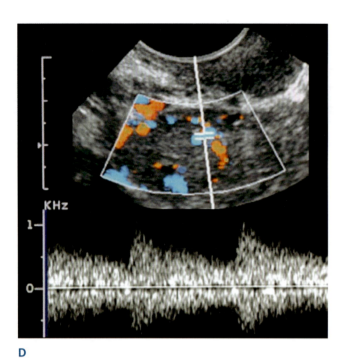

Figure 13-28, continued. D Very low-resistance hyperemic flow with loss of spectral contour during the ovulatory phase.

Table 13-6. Ovarian artery resistivity indices.

Distal Vascular Bed—Ovary	Resistivity Index
Nondominant ovary	0.96
Dominant ovary during follicular phase	0.86
Dominant ovary during luteal phase	0.83

Gross Venous Anatomy

The anatomy of the pelvic veins (Figure 13-29) parallels that of its arterial counterparts. Venous outflow from the uterus begins in the mat of veins coursing laterally along its margins, the *uterine venous plexus*. These small veins empty into the larger *uterine vein*, which drains sequentially into the *internal iliac vein*, the *common iliac vein*, and finally the *inferior vena cava*. Venous outflow from the ovary originates in the *ovarian venous plexus* (Figures 13-30A and B), situated in the broad ligament near the ovary and fallopian tube. From here blood empties into the *ovarian vein*, which drains either into the internal iliac vein and inferior vena cava or into a variant *gonadal vein*, which courses upward through the retroperitoneum and drains directly into the *renal vein*.

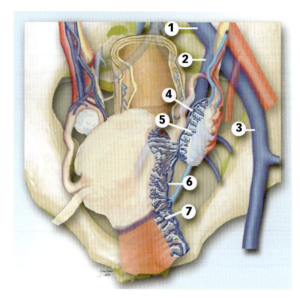

Figure 13-29. Schematic illustration of the pelvic venous anatomy. 1 = common iliac vein, 2 = internal iliac vein, 3 = external iliac vein, 4 = ovarian vein, 5 = ovarian venous plexus, 6 = uterine vein, 7 = uterine venous plexus.

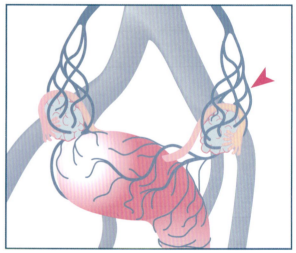

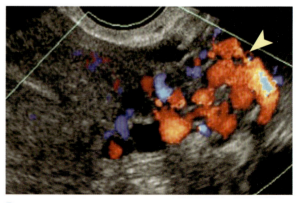

Figure 13-30. A Schematic of the ovarian venous plexus (arrowhead). **B** Doppler imaging of the ovarian venous plexus (arrowhead).

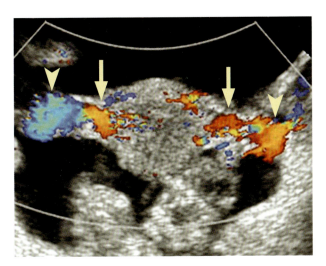

Figure 13-31. Color Doppler demonstration of both uterine venous plexuses (arrows) emptying into the uterine vein (arrowheads).

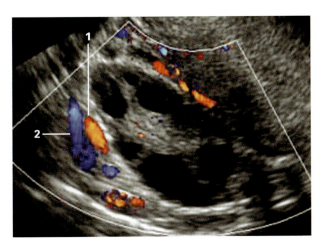

Figure 13-32. The ovarian vein (2) is seen running parallel to the ovarian artery (1).

Sonographic Appearance of Pelvic Venous Anatomy

Uterine and ovarian veins may be difficult to visualize sonographically, as normally they are small, may collapse with respiratory phasicity, and channel low-velocity, low-amplitude blood flow. However, in the presence of increased venous pressure—as occurs with conditions causing pelvic venous congestion—they are more readily seen.

The *uterine venous plexus* (Figure 13-31) may be seen originating in the uterine parenchyma, pooling on the area of the broad ligament and emptying into the *uterine vein*. The normal ovarian vein can usually be identified running parallel to the artery coursing around the periphery of the ovary (Figure 13-32).

PHYSIOLOGY

THE MENSTRUAL CYCLE

Menstruation is bleeding and physiologic shedding of the uterine endometrium that occurs at approximately monthly intervals from menarche to menopause. It is a catabolic process under control of the anterior pituitary gland and ovarian hormones. The onset of the years during which a woman experiences menstrual cycles, *menarche*, usually occurs between 11 and 14 years of age; its termination, *menopause*, normally occurs between 45 and 55 years of age. Surgery, irradiation, chemotherapy and other medications, various diseases, and abnormalities of the X chromosome can induce premature menopause (before age 40).

The monthly *menstrual cycle* begins as the pituitary gland responds to low levels of *estradiol* by secreting *follicle-stimulating hormone* (FSH). This initial increase in follicle-stimulating hormone is essential for follicular growth and the production of *estrogens* (in a process known as *steroidogenesis*). As the follicles continue to grow, estradiol production within the follicles enhances their sensitivity to *luteinizing hormone* (LH) and FSH by activating FSH receptors. The combined action of LH/FSH and estradiol increases the number of LH receptors, allowing *luteinization* and *ovulation* to occur. Ovulation is triggered by the surge in luteinizing hormone, which is a response to the rising levels of estradiol. A rise in *progesterone* follows ovulation, along with a second rise in estradiol, inducing the 14-day luteal phase characterized by low FSH and LH levels. The demise of the *corpus luteum*, with a fall in hormone levels, allows the gonadotropins to increase again, initiating a new cycle. The changes in hormone levels that take place during a normal menstrual cycle are shown in Figures 13-33A and B.

UTERINE RESPONSE

There are three phases in the uterine response of the menstrual cycle: the menstrual phase, the proliferative phase, and the secretory phase. The endometrium responds directly to stimulation or withdrawal of estrogen and progesterone. As serum estradiol level begins to rise at the beginning of the proliferative phase, endometrial thickness and echogenicity begin to increase until the thickness of the endometrium reaches its maximum dimension just before ovulation, followed by sloughing of myometrium after ovulation. Histologic and sonographic correlates are shown in Figure 13-34.

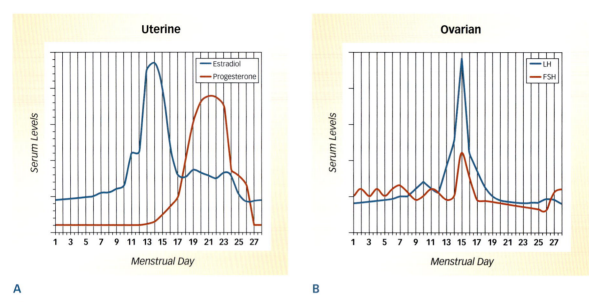

Figure 13-33. Changes in hormone levels during a normal menstrual cycle. **A** Hormones affecting a uterine response include estradiol and progesterone. **B** Hormones that target the ovary are luteinizing hormone (LH) and follicle-stimulating hormone (FSH).

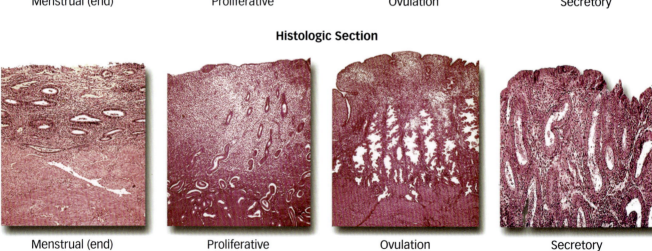

Figure 13-34. Uterine response to the menstrual cycle, including the three uterine phases—menstrual, proliferative, and secretory—along with changes seen at ovulation. Sonographic images through the endometrium (above) are paired with corresponding histologic sections (below). Endometrial changes observed at ovulation are demonstrated in transverse section; the other images are in sagittal section.

Menstrual Phase (Days 1–5)

The endometrium becomes ischemic, degenerates, sloughs off the myometrium, and is expelled as menses. The pattern of menstrual bleeding is varied but typically begins with 12–24 hours of heavy flow followed by scanty flow for another 4–7 days.

Summary of Sonographic Signs

The following sonographic signs are associated with the menstrual phase:

- Thickened, echogenic endometrium prior to start of menses
- Complex appearance at the beginning of menses
- Thin, slightly irregular endometrium after shedding from the myometrium (Figure 13-35)
- Maximum anteroposterior diameter (post menses) of 2 mm

Proliferative Phase (Days 6–14)

The regrowth of the endometrium in response to estrogen released by ovarian follicles begins on the fourth or fifth day after the beginning of a period and typically lasts about 10 days, ending at ovulation. Under the influence of estrogen, the endometrium becomes increasingly thicker and more echogenic in anticipation of the implantation of a conceptus. As the proliferative phase progresses, the endometrium metamorphoses sonographically from a homogeneously echogenic central uterine collection to a multilayered stack representing the distinct histologic layers of the uterine lining.

Summary of Sonographic Signs

The following sonographic signs are associated with the proliferative phase:[7]

- *Early proliferative phase*: hyperechoic endometrium with a faint central echo (5–7 mm) (Figure 13-36)
- *Late proliferative (periovulatory) phase*: thickened (up to 11 mm), isoechoic endometrium with a multilayered pattern[8] (Figure 13-37)

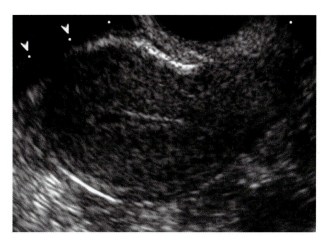

Figure 13-36. Early proliferative phase: Sagittal endovaginal section on day 7 of a normal menstrual cycle demonstrates a faint linear central endometrial echo, commonly called the *endometrial stripe*.

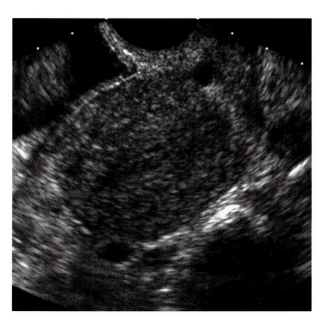

Figure 13-35. Sagittal endovaginal section immediately following menstruation shows a thin, slightly irregular endometrial appearance.

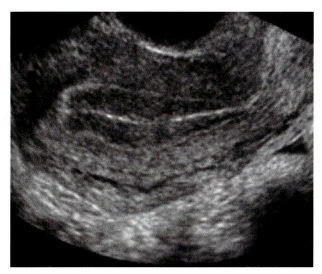

Figure 13-37. Late proliferative (periovulatory) phase: Sagittal endovaginal section on day 13 of a normal menstrual cycle demonstrates a thickened, isoechoic endometrium with a multilayered pattern.

Secretory Phase (Days 15–28)

The *secretory phase*, also called the *luteal phase*, begins at ovulation and ends about 14 days later. It coincides with the formation of the *corpus luteum*, which secretes the progesterone responsible for final endometrial thickening and maturation in preparation for implantation. In the absence of fertilization and implantation, the corpus luteum begins to regress, estrogen and progesterone secretion declines, and the uterine lining begins to slough off.

Summary of Sonographic Signs

Sonographically, the secretory phase is characterized by increased and more homogeneous echogenicity of the endometrium (7–16 mm) (Figure 13-38).[9]

OVARIAN RESPONSE

The ovarian response during the menstrual cycle results from physiologic processes that stimulate an immature *primary follicle* to grow and develop into a mature *Graafian follicle* that will become the dominant follicle and ultimately extrude an ovum ready for fertilization (see Figure 13-23). When fertilization occurs, the feedback mechanism continues with the development of the *corpus luteum*, the transient ovarian hormone-producing structure that is responsible for retention of the uterine lining. A conceptus implanted in the secretory endometrium produces the *human chorionic gonadotropin, subunit beta* (beta-hCG), which signals the corpus luteum to continue the progesterone production that induces decidualization of the endometrium (the response to progesterone that prepares the endometrium for pregnancy).

When fertilization does not occur, the corpus luteum stops secreting progesterone and decays after approximately 14 days. It subsequently degenerates into the *corpus albicans*, a small, whitish, fibrous scar that can be visually identified near the surface of an ovary. The three ovarian phases of the menstrual cycle are the *follicular*, *ovulatory*, and *luteal* phases.

Follicular Phase (Days 1–14)

The *follicular phase* of the menstrual cycle begins on the first day of menstruation and continues until ovulation. It is characterized primarily by the development of multiple follicles within both ovaries. Under the influence of follicle-stimulating hormone (FSH), primary follicles begin the process of maturation that typically

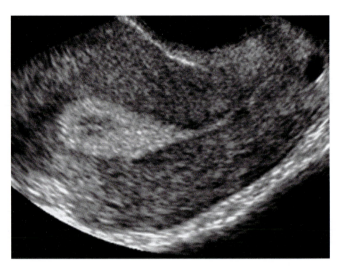

Figure 13-38. Secretory endometrium: Sagittal endovaginal section on day 18 of a normal menstrual cycle shows an increased and more homogeneous echogenic appearance of the endometrium.

results in the development of a single mature Graafian follicle—the *dominant follicle*. The laterality of the Graafian follicle typically rotates between the two ovaries from month to month, but individual variations are common. Between 3 and 30 follicles may respond to FSH during each cycle. Ovarian follicles are best demonstrated sonographically with endovaginal imaging. They appear as smoothly marginated, anechoic, cystic foci of varying sizes (1–9 mm in diameter) arrayed around the periphery of the ovary (Figure 13-39). The dominant follicle is characterized by its greater size (>10 mm in diameter) early in the cycle and by its continued growth to approximately 25 mm in diameter at ovulation (Figure 13-40).

Summary of Sonographic Signs

Other sonographic characteristics of a dominant follicle include the following:

- Any follicle measuring >11 mm in diameter will most likely ovulate.
- It grows linearly (approximately 2–3 mm/day).
- Its maximum diameter ranges between 15 and 30 mm.
- A line of decreased reflectivity around the follicle suggests that ovulation will occur within 24 hours.
- The presence of a *cumulus oophorus* (a mass of follicular cells surrounding the ovum) suggests that ovulation will occur within 36 hours (Figures 13-41A and B).

Pelvic Anatomy and Physiology CHAPTER 13

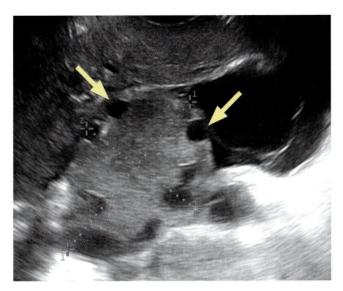

Figure 13-39. Follicular phase: Sagittal endovaginal section through the ovary shows the normal sonographic appearance of multiple small, smoothly marginated, anechoic primary ovarian follicles (arrows) arrayed around the periphery of the ovary.

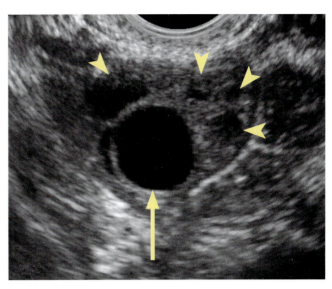

Figure 13-40. Early in the follicular phase the dominant follicle (arrow) is characterized by its size, greater than that of the surrounding nondominant follicles (arrowheads).

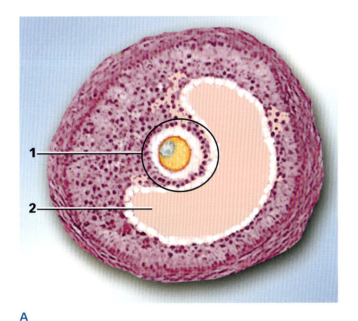

A

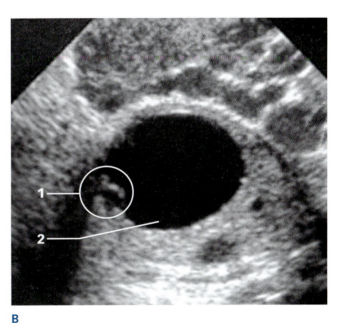

B

Figure 13-41. A Schematic representation of the cumulus oophorus with B correlative sonographic image. 1 = cumulus oophorus, 2 = antrum with follicular fluid.

Ovulation (Day 14)

Ovulation is the extrusion of an ovum from the dominant follicle in anticipation of fertilization. It occurs approximately 10–12 hours after the *LH peak* (highest concentration of luteinizing hormone). At ovulation, the wall of the mature follicle ruptures, releasing the oocyte and a small amount of follicular fluid into the peritoneal cavity.

Summary of Sonographic Signs

There are several sonographic signs that suggest that ovulation has occurred:

- Sudden decrease in follicular size
- Fluid in the posterior cul-de-sac (Figure 13-42A)
- Hemorrhage into the dominant follicle (Figure 13-42B)

Luteal Phase (Days 15–28)

The *luteal phase* is the process during which a ruptured dominant follicle involutes into a *corpus luteum* (Latin for "yellow body"). The corpus luteum produces progesterone, which maintains the secretory endometrium should implantation occur. In the absence of the beta-hCG produced by the trophoblastic tissue of a conceptus, the corpus luteum begins to atrophy and by the end of the luteal phase is completely regressed.

Summary of Sonographic Signs

The following sonographic signs are associated with the luteal phase:

- Replacement of dominant, cystic follicle with an echogenic structure (2–5 cm in diameter) (Figure 13-43A)
- Thrombus present within the antral lumen
- Thick-walled cyst with characteristic "ring of fire" peripheral vascularity (Figure 13-43B)

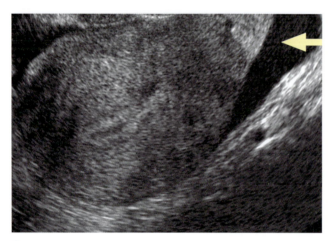

A

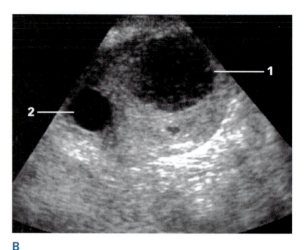

B

Figure 13-42. A Sonographic appearance of ovulation: a normal amount of free fluid in the posterior cul-de-sac (arrow). **B** Sonographic appearance of ovulation: low-level internal echoes representing hemorrhage into the dominant follicle (1) compared with a simple anechoic non-dominant Graafian follicle (2).

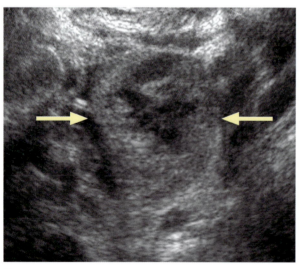

A

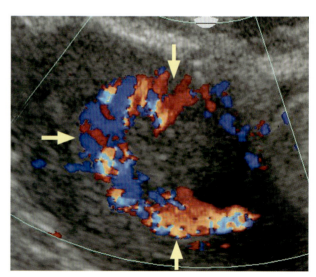

B

Figure 13-43. A Sonographic appearance of the corpus luteum (arrows), showing replacement of a dominant cystic follicle with a complex echogenic structure. **B** Color Doppler imaging demonstrating a thick-walled corpus luteum cyst with characteristic "ring of fire" peripheral vascularity.

CHAPTER 13 REVIEW QUESTIONS

1. The anterior margin of the abdominal and pelvic spaces is formed by the:
   A. Psoas major
   B. Rectus abdominis
   C. Obturator internus
   D. Piriformis

2. The false pelvis is that portion of the pelvic cavity located superior to the:
   A. Rectus abdominis
   B. Umbilicus
   C. Linea terminalis
   D. Linea alba

3. The suspensory ligament that attaches the ovary to the broad ligament is the:
   A. Mesovarium ligament
   B. Ovarian ligament
   C. Infundibulopelvic ligament
   D. Pubic ligament

4. The fibromuscular bands arising from the uterine cornua and extending into the inguinal canal are called the:
   A. Round ligament
   B. Broad ligament
   C. Uterosacral ligament
   D. Cardinal ligament

5. The primary supporting ligament of the uterus that arises from the lateral aspect of the cervix and uterus and inserts along the lateral pelvic wall is the:
   A. Round ligament
   B. Broad ligament
   C. Uterosacral ligament
   D. Cardinal ligament

6. The double fold of peritoneum that arises from the lateral aspect of the uterus and divides the true pelvis into anterior and posterior compartments is called the:
   A. Round ligament
   B. Broad ligament
   C. Uterosacral ligament
   D. Cardinal ligament

7. The rounded, superior aspect of the uterus located above the insertion of the fallopian tubes is called the:
   A. Corpus
   B. Body
   C. Fundus
   D. Cornu

8. The largest portion of the uterus, which contains the uterine cavity, is called the:
   A. Isthmus
   B. Fundus
   C. Corpus
   D. Cornu

9. A normal cervical length in a nulliparous woman measures:
   A. 1–2 cm
   B. 2–3 cm
   C. 1–2 mm
   D. 2–3 mm

10. The thin outer layer of the uterus is the:
    A. Serosa
    B. Myometrium
    C. Endometrium
    D. Exometrium

11. The outermost (deepest) tissue layer of the normal endometrium is called the:
    A. Functionalis layer
    B. Basalis layer
    C. Decidual layer
    D. Intimal layer

12. A uterus whose body is directed toward the hollow of the sacrum without a marked bend in the endometrial stripe is called:
    A. Anteverted
    B. Retroverted
    C. Retroflexed
    D. Involuted

13. A uterus in which the uterine corpus tilts backward while the cervix maintains normal anterior flexion is called:
    A. Anteverted
    B. Retroverted

C. Retroflexed
D. Involuted

14. The potential space created by the circumferential attachment of the vagina around the cervix is called the:
    A. Fornix
    B. Space of Retzius
    C. Pouch of Douglas
    D. Cul-de-sac

15. The potential space between the anterior abdominal wall and anterior bladder surface is called the:
    A. Fornix
    B. Space of Retzius
    C. Pouch of Douglas
    D. Cul-de-sac

16. The potential space between the posterior uterine surface and the anterior surface of the rectum is called the:
    A. Fornix
    B. Space of Retzius
    C. Pouch of Douglas
    D. Cul-de-sac

17. The narrowest portion of the fallopian tube that traverses the uterine cornu is called the:
    A. Isthmic portion
    B. Ampullary portion
    C. Infundibulum
    D. Interstitial portion

18. The longest portion of the fallopian tube, connecting the intramural and ampullary portions, is called the:
    A. Isthmic portion
    B. Ampullary portion
    C. Infundibulum
    D. Fimbrial portion

19. The outer portion of the ovary, which contains the primordial follicles, is called the:
    A. Medulla
    B. Cortex
    C. Germinal epithelium
    D. Tunica albuginea

20. The layer of fibrous connective tissue between the germinal epithelium and the ovarian parenchyma is called the:
    A. Medulla
    B. Cortex
    C. Germinal epithelium
    D. Tunica albuginea

21. The ovarian artery arises from the:
    A. Internal iliac artery
    B. External iliac artery
    C. Abdominal aorta
    D. Vesicular artery

22. The uterine artery arises from the:
    A. Internal iliac artery
    B. External iliac artery
    C. Abdominal aorta
    D. Vesicular artery

23. The uterine artery inserts on the uterus:
    A. Laterally, superior to the cervix
    B. Laterally, inferior to the cervix
    C. Medially, at the cornu
    D. Anteriorly, at the fundus

24. As a rule, Doppler findings in the ovarian artery supplying the dominant ovary will demonstrate:
    A. High resistance
    B. Low resistance
    C. High pulsatility
    D. A dicrotic notch

25. The onset of menstruation, usually occurring between 11 and 14 years of age, is called:
    A. Menopause
    B. Menarche
    C. Thelarche
    D. Pubarche

26. A transient ovarian hormone-producing structure that is responsible for retention of the uterine lining is the:
    A. Primordial follicle
    B. Graafian follicle
    C. Theca-lutein cyst
    D. Corpus luteum

27. The phase of the menstrual cycle that begins on the first day of menstruation and continues to ovulation is called the:
    A. Follicular phase
    B. Ovulatory phase
    C. Luteal phase
    D. Secretory phase

28. A dominant ovarian follicle typically will grow at the rate of:
    A. 1–2 mm/day
    B. 2–3 mm/day
    C. 3–4 mm/day
    D. 4–5 mm/day

29. All of the following sonographic signs are evidence that ovulation has occurred EXCEPT:
    A. Sudden decrease in follicular size
    B. Presence of a cumulus oophorus
    C. Fluid in the posterior cul-de-sac
    D. Hemorrhage into the dominant follicle

30. Regression of the corpus luteum in a nonpregnant patient should be complete by:
    A. 24 hours
    B. 7 days
    C. 14 days
    D. 28 days

31. The arrows in this image point to:

    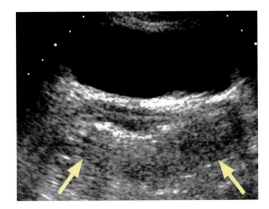

    A. Psoas muscle
    B. Levator ani muscle group
    C. Piriformis muscle
    D. Obturator internus muscle

32. This image was obtained in patient undergoing infertility treatment. The salient finding here is evidence that:

    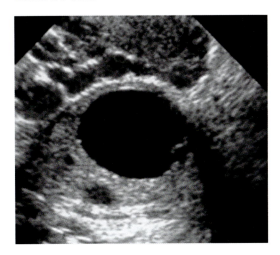

    A. Ovulation will occur within 36 hours
    B. Ovulation has already occurred
    C. Hormonal therapy has failed
    D. An ectopic pregnancy has implanted on the ovary

ANSWERS

See Appendix A on page 482 for answers.

REFERENCES

1. Merz E, Miric-Tesanic F, Bahlmann G, et al: Sonographic size of uterus and ovaries in pre- and postmenopausal women. Ultrasound Obstet Gynecol 7:38–42, 1996.

2. Garel L, Dubois J, Grignon A, et al: US of the pediatric female pelvis: a clinical perspective. RadioGraphics 21:1393–1407, 2001.

3. Cohen HL, Shapiro MA, Mandel FS, et al: Normal ovaries in neonates and infants: a sonographic study of 77 patients 1 day to 24 months old. Am J Roentgenol 160:583–586, 1993.

4. Rosenberg HK, Chaudhry H: Pediatric pelvic sonography. In Rumack CM, Wilson SR, Charboneau JW, et al (eds): *Diagnostic Ultrasound*, 4th edition. Philadelphia, Elsevier Mosby, 2011, pp 1928–1929.

5. Salem S: Gynecology. In Rumack CM, Wilson SR, Charboneau JW, et al (eds): *Diagnostic Ultrasound*, 4th edition. Philadelphia, Elsevier Mosby, 2011, pp 574–575.

6. Dubinsky TJ, Stroehlein K, Abu-Ghazzeh Y, et al: Prediction of benign and malignant endometrial disease: hysterosonographic-pathologic correlation. Radiology 210:393–397, 1999.

7. Nalaboff KM, Pellerito JS, Ben-Levi E: Imaging the endometrium: disease and normal variants. RadioGraphics 21:1409–1424, 2001.

8. Cohen BM, Berry L, Roethemeyer V, et al: Sonographic assessment of late proliferative phase endometrium during ovulation induction. J Reprod Med 37:685–690, 1992.

9. Grunfeld L, Walker B, Bergh PA, et al: High-resolution endovaginal ultrasonography of the endometrium: a noninvasive test for endometrial adequacy. Obstet Gynecol 78:200–204, 1991.

SUGGESTED READINGS

Gill KA: Gynecology. In Gill KA: *Ultrasound in Obstetrics and Gynecology: A Practitioner's Guide*. Pasadena, Davies Publishing, 2014, pp 25–88.

Goldstein C, Hagen-Ansert SL: Normal anatomy and physiology of the female pelvis. In Hagen-Ansert SL (ed): *Textbook of Diagnostic Ultrasonography*, 7th edition. St. Louis, Elsevier Mosby, 2012, pp 938–954.

Levi CS, Lyons EA, Holt SC, et al: Normal anatomy of the female pelvis and transvaginal sonography. In Callen PW (ed): *Ultrasonography in Obstetrics and Gynecology*, 5th edition. Philadelphia, Saunders Elsevier, 2008, pp 887–918.

Rosenberg HK, Chaudhry H: Pediatric pelvic sonography. In Rumack CM, Wilson SR, Charboneau JW, et al (eds): *Diagnostic Ultrasound*, 4th edition. Philadelphia, Elsevier Mosby, 2011, pp 1925–1981.

Salem S: Gynecology. In Rumack CM, Wilson SR, Charboneau JW, et al (eds): *Diagnostic Ultrasound*, 4th edition. Philadelphia, Elsevier Mosby, 2011, pp 613–638.

CHAPTER 14
Pelvic Pathology

Vaginal Pathology

Uterine Pathology

Endometrial Pathology

Ovarian Pathology

Adnexal Pathology

Gynecologic pelvic pathologies can be broadly categorized according to the anatomic structures from which they arise: the vagina, uterus, endometrium, ovary, or adnexa. These sites can develop their own sonographically unique and specific types of pathology as well as other categories of human pathology that are characterized by the sonographic hallmarks that generally accompany congenital or acquired anatomic and physiologic abnormalities, neoplastic lesions, and inflammatory processes. This chapter presents an overview of the types of pathology that are most commonly encountered by sonographers in a gynecologic sonography practice.

VAGINAL PATHOLOGY

Most congenital vaginal anomalies are first detected by physical examination and, secondarily, by pelvic sectional imaging modalities such as computed tomography (CT) and magnetic resonance imaging (MRI). Sonography is not useful in evaluating patients with known or suspected vaginal anatomic abnormalities.

Commonly encountered anomalies of the vagina include:

- *Agenesis*: Congenital absence of the vagina due to incomplete or failed development.
- *Atresia*: A spectrum of congenital anomalies characterized by imperforation, occlusion, or a failed formation of part or all of the vagina. Isolated vaginal atresia is an extremely rare finding. Most cases occur as müllerian agenesis or are associated with the more common Mayer-Rokitansky-Küster-Hauser (MRKH) syndrome.
- *Imperforate hymen*: A completely closed hymen, which may be the result of congenital maldevelopment or the result of inflammatory occlusion after perforation.
- *Persistent uterovaginal septum*: The presence of a complete or partial septum within the vaginal cavity resulting from incomplete resorption of the embryonic uterovaginal septum.
- *Gartner's duct cyst*: A mesonephric duct remnant that forms a cyst along the lateral or anterolateral wall of the vagina (Figure 14-1). Gartner's duct cysts may be associated with other congenital genitourinary anomalies, such as renal agenesis, renal dysplasia, and cross-fused renal ectopia.[1]
- *Hydrometrocolpos*: An expanded, fluid-filled vaginal cavity with associated distention of the uterine cavity. It may present in infancy with a lower abdominal mass or may not appear until menarche. Most commonly caused by imperforate hymen, it also can be caused by vaginal stenosis/transverse vaginal septum, lower vaginal atresia, and cervical stenosis.

UTERINE PATHOLOGY

CONGENITAL ANOMALIES

Cervical Anomalies

Anomalies of the cervix can be congenital or acquired. Congenital anomalies include:

- *Atresia (stenosis)*: An uncommon finding occasionally encountered in an infertile couple. The diagnosis is made clinically by attempting and failing to pass a small catheter or probe into the cervical canal.
- *Nabothian cysts*: Inclusion cysts caused by the obstruction of an endocervical gland (Figure 14-2).
- *DES-related anomalies*: Diethylstilbestrol (DES) was used from the 1940s to the 1970s as treatment for threatened abortion. The most common anomalies associated with exposure to DES in utero include:[2]
  - T-shaped uterus
  - Constricting bands within the uterine cavity
  - Hypoplastic uterus

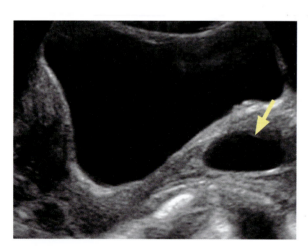

Figure 14-1. Sagittal transabdominal section through the cervix and vagina demonstrating a smoothly marginated, anechoic Gartner's duct cyst (arrow).

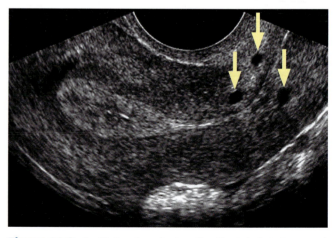

Figure 14-2. Sagittal endovaginal section through the uterus and cervix demonstrating three nabothian cysts (arrows).

- Intrauterine polyps
- Synechiae (adhesions found within the uterine cavity)

Sonographic Signs

The following are the characteristic sonographic signs of cervical anomalies:

- Reduced uterine volume
- Increased uterine artery pulsatility index
- T-shaped uterus

Müllerian Duct Anomalies

Müllerian duct anomalies (Figure 14-3) comprise a spectrum of congenital anatomic abnormalities resulting from the failed fusion of the paired embryonic paramesonephric (müllerian) ducts. While these anomalies are relatively common, patients are usually asymptomatic. There is, however, an association with an increased risk of pregnancy failure with most types of müllerian duct anomalies and other congenital genitourinary abnormalities. The most common subtypes include:

- *Uterine agenesis*: Congenital absence of the uterus, cervix, and vagina.
- *Arcuate uterus* (Figure 14-3B): Mild (<1 mm) indentation of the endometrium into the uterine fundus. This may be considered a normal variant and is usually not associated with pregnancy failure.
- *Unicornuate uterus* (*uterus unicornis*) (Figure 14-3C): The presence of a single uterine horn that may or may not communicate with the cervix. Unicornuate uterus has been implicated as a cause of infertility in 5%–20% of cases.[3]
- *Bicornuate uterus* (*uterus bicornis*) (Figure 14-3D): The presence of two uterine horns contained within a single uterine body communicating with a single cervix and vagina.
- *Didelphic uterus* (*uterus didelphys*) (Figure 14-3E): The presence of two separate uterine bodies and two separate cervices, usually with the presence of a vaginal septum. Didelphic uterus is associated with concomitant renal agenesis.
- *Septate uterus* (*uterus subseptus*) (Figure 14-3F): The presence of two distinct intrauterine cavities separated by a septum. This is the most common uterine anomaly, associated with pregnancy failure in 67% of patients.[4]

Sonographic Signs

Subtle müllerian duct anomalies, such as arcuate uterus and unicornuate uterus, may not be demonstrable during routine sonographic examination. However,

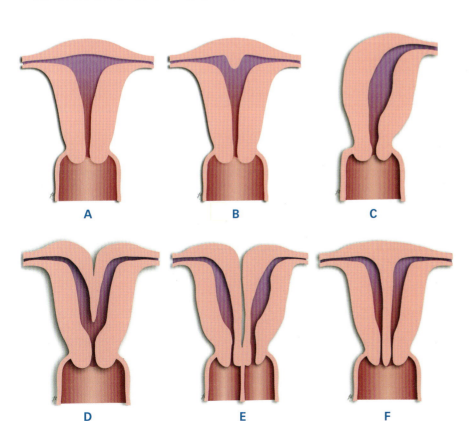

Figure 14-3. Müllerian duct anomalies. **A** Schematic of a normal uterus. **B** Arcuate uterus. **C** Unicornuate uterus. **D** Bicornuate uterus. **E** Didelphic uterus. **F** Septate uterus.

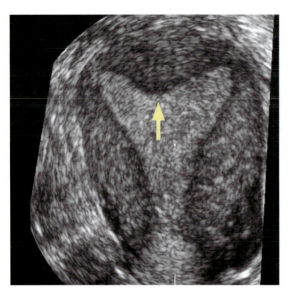

Figure 14-4. Coronal volumetric section demonstrating an arcuate uterus. Note the indentation (arrow) of the uterine fundus.

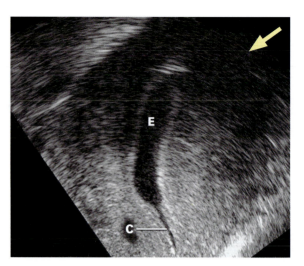

Figure 14-5. Unicornuate uterus: endovaginal coronal section demonstrating lateral deviation of the uterine fundus (arrow) relative to the midline of the pelvis. E = fluid in endometrial cavity, C = cervix.

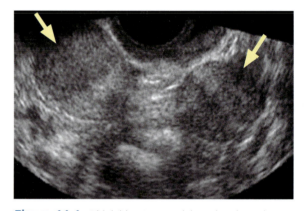

Figure 14-6. Didelphic uterus: axial section through two separated uterine horns (arrows).

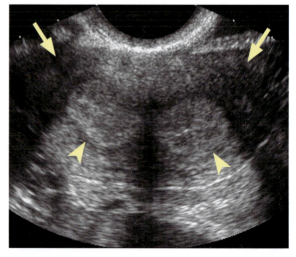

Figure 14-7. Bicornuate uterus: axial section demonstrating widely divergent uterine horns (arrows) and two separate endometrial cavities (arrowheads).

the more apparent anomalies demonstrate the following characteristics:

- Arcuate uterus:
  - Normal uterine contour
  - Indentation of the fundal endometrium into the uterine cavity (Figure 14-4)
  - No division of uterine horns
  - Increased transverse diameter of the uterine fundus
- Unicornuate uterus:[5]
  - Lateral displacement of the uterine fundus (Figure 14-5)
  - Asymmetric appearance
  - Loss of pear shape
- Didelphic uterus:
  - Separate divergent uterine horns identified with a large fundal cleft (Figure 14-6)
  - Separate endometrial cavities with no evidence of communication
  - Two separate cervices
- Bicornuate uterus:
  - Widely divergent uterine horns with a fundal cleft >1 cm deep (Figure 14-7)
  - Single, heart-shaped external uterine contour
  - Caudally fused symmetric uterine cavities with some degree of communication between them (usually at the uterine isthmus)

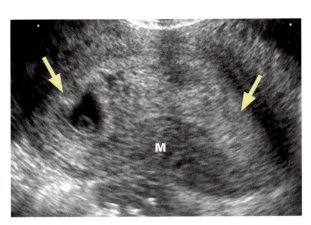

Figure 14-8. Septate uterus: axial section demonstrating discrete endometrial cavities (arrows) separated at the fundus by myometrium (M).

- Septate uterus:
  - Endometrial cavities separated at the fundus by myometrium (Figure 14-8)
  - Widened fundus
  - Convex, flat, or mildly concave external uterine contour
  - Color Doppler imaging showing vascularity in the septum in 70% of cases

ACQUIRED ANOMALIES

Acquired uterine anomalies are those that arise after prenatal life as the result of pathologic processes or toxic or mechanical insult to the uterus. Acquired anomalies include endometrial polyps, uterine fibroids, and a host of other pathologic conditions that are considered separately in this chapter.

Asherman Syndrome

Asherman syndrome (also known as *intrauterine adhesions* or *uterine synechiae*) is the obliteration of the endometrial cavity as a result of excessive or traumatic uterine instrumentation. Endometrial tissue is replaced with fibromuscular connective tissue, resulting in the development of uterine adhesions, or synechiae, that can significantly interfere with pregnancy. The reproductive outcomes of women with Asherman syndrome are generally poor. In the absence of treatment, approximately 40% of pregnancies in these women appear to end in spontaneous abortion, and another 23% result in preterm deliveries.[6] While endovaginal sonographic examination may yield suspicious findings for Asherman syndrome, more direct endometrial imaging methods—such as hysteroscopy (with or without biopsy), hysterosalpingography, and hysterosonography—are required for a confirmatory diagnosis.

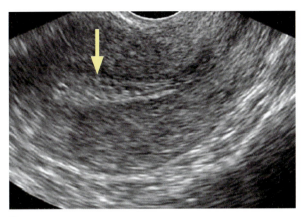

A

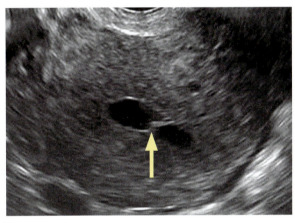

B

Figure 14-9. A Sagittal endovaginal section demonstrating a thickened, heterogeneous endometrium (arrow) in a patient with Asherman syndrome. **B** Hysterosonogram demonstrating an intrauterine synechia (arrow) in Asherman syndrome.

Clinical Signs and Symptoms

Presenting signs and symptoms associated with Asherman syndrome include the following:

- Amenorrhea or hypomenorrhea
- Pelvic pain
- Infertility
- Recurrent spontaneous abortions

Sonographic Signs

The following are the characteristic sonographic signs of Asherman syndrome:

- Thickened endometrium apparent on routine B-mode sonography (Figure 14-9A)
- Intrauterine synechiae on hysterosonography (Figure 14-9B)

Uterine Masses

While myometrial malignancies are extremely rare, benign neoplasms are fairly common.

Fibroids (Leiomyomas, Myomas)

By far the most common type of uterine mass is the *fibroid*, also called a *leiomyoma* or *myoma*. Benign uterine tumors arising from muscular tissue in the myometrium, discrete myomas, or diffuse myomatous changes have been found to some degree in approximately 60% of women.[7] Only 20%–30%, however, have clinical signs and symptoms; most are asymptomatic.

The prevalence of fibroids is increased in:

- Black women (incidence is three times higher than in Caucasians)[8]
- Older women (incidence increases as a woman moves through her reproductive years)
- Perimenopausal women
- Obese women
- Diabetic women

While the exact etiology for fibroids is not understood, it is postulated that genetic predisposition, prenatal hormone exposure, and the effects of growth factors and estrogen-mimicking hormones induce myomatous changes in uterine muscular tissue. Under the continued influence of cyclical estrogen and progesterone, these diffusely affected areas grow into focal masses.

The gross pathologic appearance of a uterine fibroid is that of a well-circumscribed, round or irregularly lobulated, nonencapsulated mass. Although myomas have only a false capsular covering, they are clearly demarcated from the surrounding myometrium and can be easily and cleanly enucleated from the surrounding tissue. On gross cross-sectional examination, they are buff-colored, rounded, smooth, and characterized by a whorling tissue pattern (Figure 14-10A).

Fibroids can occur anywhere in the uterus, cervix, or broad ligament but are most commonly found in the uterine corpus (Figure 14-10B). Description of the location of a fibroid is based on its relationship to uterine layer and anatomic part:

- *Pedunculated*: arising from a stalk
- *Intramural*: having an interstitial location within the myometrium
- *Submucosal*: lying directly beneath the endometrium and frequently projecting into the uterine cavity, most commonly producing vaginal bleeding

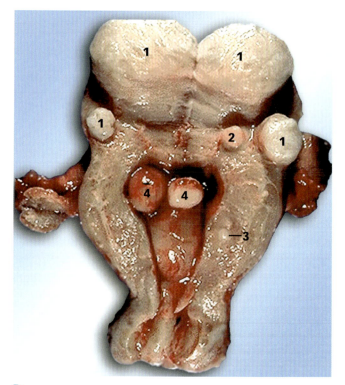

Figure 14-10. A Cross-sectional gross pathology of uterine fibroids (3x magnification); note the whorling pattern of tissue planes within the masses. **B** Fibroids can be located anywhere in the uterus, cervix, or broad ligament. They are most commonly located in the uterine corpus as (1) exophytic (also seen in the broad ligament), (2) subserosal, (3) intramural, and (4) submucosal solid masses.

- *Subserosal*: lying beneath the outer peritoneal surface of the uterus
- *Interligamentous*: occurring within the broad ligament
- *Cervical*: occurring within the cervix
- *Exophytic*: growing out of and away from the uterus

Clinical Signs and Symptoms

Four categories of presenting symptoms are associated with fibroids:

- Abnormal uterine bleeding:
  - Heavy periods
  - Alteration in normal menstrual flow
  - Intermenstrual flow
- Pelvic mass palpable on pelvic exam
- Sensations of pressure in the pelvis
- Frequent urination
- Pain:
  - Chronic pelvic pain
  - Mid-cycle pelvic pain
  - Dyspareunia (painful intercourse)
  - Pain associated with torsion or degeneration of a fibroid

Clinical complications of fibroids may include:

- *Torsion*: The twisting of a pedunculated myoma on its pedicle. Torsion results in interruption of blood flow to the mass and typically causes sudden-onset, acute pelvic pain with tenderness localized to the myoma. If the torsion is not reduced, ischemia of the myoma results.
- *Prolapse*: Extrusion of a submucosal myoma through the vagina.
- *Degeneration*: Inadequate perfusion of a fibroid can cause chronic ischemic changes that result in breakdown of the tissue (necrosis). This degeneration of the mass typically results in liquefaction of the central portion of the fibroid. Calcific changes can also occur as calcium salts precipitate within the tumor. Changes in sonographic appearance on serial examinations may reflect these alterations in gross appearance of the fibroid.
- *Pregnancy-related complications*: During pregnancy, myomas can change due to the altered hormonal status. About 20% increase in size, 20% decrease in size, and 60% remain unchanged.
- *Dystocia*: Difficult vaginal delivery. Malpresentation of the fetus may occur if the fibroid lies in the lower uterine segment. Fibroids of the lower uterine segment and/or cervix may prevent normal cervical dilatation.
- *Placental abruption*: If a portion of the placenta is implanted over a submucosal fibroid, there may be defective implantation, resulting in an increased risk of premature separation of the placenta from the uterine wall (placental abruption).

Sonographic Signs

The specific sonographic appearance of fibroids depends on the size and number of the masses present and the type and extent of degeneration present. The most common sonographic findings of an individual fibroid include:

- A well-circumscribed, hyperattenuating mass in or arising from the uterus (Figure 14-11A)
- Calcification within or on the periphery of the mass (Figure 14-11B)
- Distortion of the normal uterine contour and echo texture (Figure 14-11C)

Uterine Leiomyosarcoma

A *leiomyosarcoma* is the rare and malignant relative of the benign fibroid. Leiomyosarcomas arise from smooth muscle cells and can occur anywhere in the

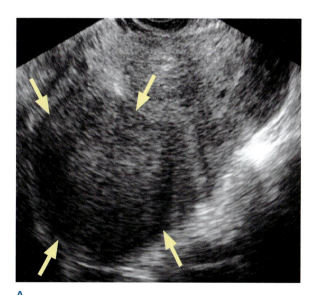

A

Figure 14-11. A Sagittal endovaginal section demonstrating the typical sonographic findings of a fibroid—a well-circumscribed, hyperattenuating mass (arrows), in this case occupying the fundus of the uterus. (Figure continues . . .)

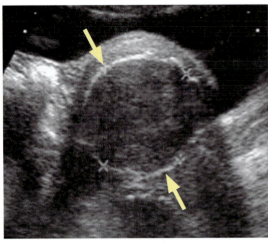
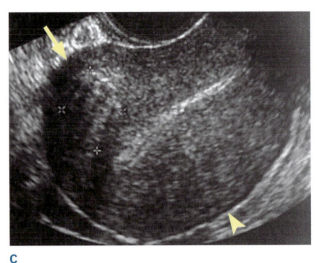

Figure 14-11, continued. B Calcific degeneration of a fibroid with a thin, echogenic rim of calcium (arrows) around the periphery of the mass. **C** Sagittal endovaginal section demonstrating alterations of the uterine contour created by fibroids in the anterior fundal region (arrow) and along the posterior corpus (arrowhead).

body where smooth muscle tissue resides. The uterus is the most common site for leiomyosarcomas, and they can spread from the myometrium to pelvic blood vessels, lymphatics, adjacent pelvic structures, and then distantly, most often to the lungs.

Clinical Signs and Symptoms

Clinical signs and symptoms associated with uterine leiomyosarcoma are nonspecific and usually do not present until the disease has progressed to an advanced stage.

- Postmenopausal vaginal bleeding
- Irregular intermenstrual bleeding in premenopausal patients
- Pelvic discomfort or pain
- Palpable uterine mass on pelvic exam

Sonographic Signs

The following are the characteristic sonographic signs of leiomyosarcoma:[9]

- Large, heterogeneous, hypoechoic uterine mass (Figures 14-12A and B)
- Indistinguishable from benign fibroid with sonography alone
- Rapid growth on serial examinations
- High-velocity, low-resistance Doppler waveforms in feeding vessels

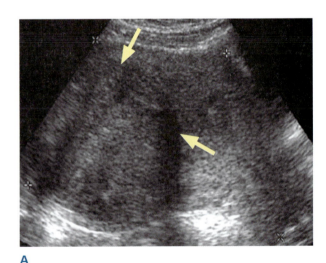
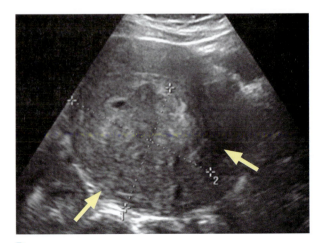

Figure 14-12. Leiomyosarcoma: sagittal endovaginal sections showing **A** a large, hypoechoic fundal mass (arrows) and **B** a large, heterogeneous mass (arrows), both in the body of the uterus.

Adenomyosis

Adenomyosis is the benign overgrowth of endometrial tissue into the myometrium. It is relatively common in women of reproductive age, reportedly occurring in approximately 36% of women undergoing hysterectomy for any clinical indication.[10]

Risk factors that significantly increase the incidence of adenomyosis include age, gravidity, pelvic endometriosis, and presence of uterine fibroids.[11] While the exact etiology is unknown, the most commonly accepted theory posits that a compromise of the natural barrier between the endometrial and myometrial layers occurs, allowing the growth of ectopic endometrial glands and stromata into the myometrium. Excessive growth of the endometrium with progressive penetration of the myometrium results in uterine enlargement. Pathologically, adenomyosis may present with either diffuse or focal involvement of the myometrium. Most commonly, the uterus is grossly enlarged and somewhat globular, with involvement of both anterior and posterior uterine walls. There is usually greater involvement of the posterior wall.

Clinical Signs and Symptoms

Adenomyosis is a frequent cause of dysmenorrhea and menorrhagia in about 60% of women. While typically vague and nonspecific, clinical symptoms include:

- Secondary dysmenorrhea (15%–30% of cases)
- Menorrhagia (40%–50%)
- Midline dyspareunia (in advanced cases)

Sonographic Signs

While not all cases of adenomyosis are demonstrable sonographically, frequently reported ultrasound findings include:[12, 13]

- Symmetrically enlarged uterus with normal contours
- Focal or diffuse bulkiness, particularly of the posterior wall (Figures 14-13A and B)
- Heterogeneous uterine myometrial texture (Figure 14-13C)
- Focal cystic areas within the myometrium (Figure 14-13C)
- Indistinct endometrial/myometrial interface

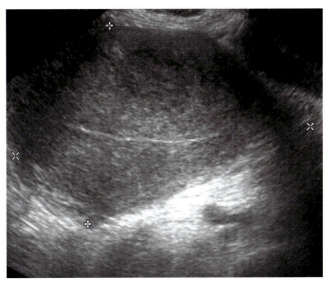

A

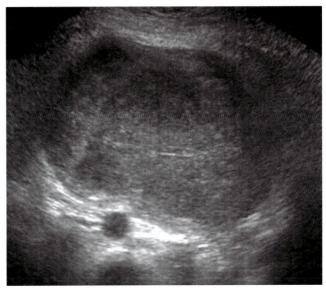

B

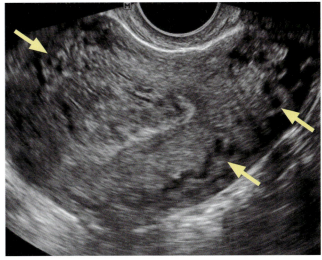

C

Figure 14-13. Adenomyosis. Diffuse bulkiness of the uterus demonstrated in **A** sagittal and **B** axial sonographic sections. **C** Heterogeneous uterine myometrial texture; note the cystic areas (arrows) within the myometrium.

ENDOMETRIAL PATHOLOGY

ENDOMETRIAL HYPERPLASIA

Endometrial hyperplasia is the excessive proliferation of endometrial glandular tissue. There are several histologic types, including adenomatous and atypical forms, but the most common and most benign type is *cystic endometrial hyperplasia*, in which small cystic changes produce a classic "Swiss-cheese" appearance of the endometrium.

Some types of endometrial hyperplasia are considered "premalignant." Endometrial hyperplasia is associated with hyperestrogenic states such as tamoxifen and unopposed estrogen administration (e.g., with hormone replacement therapy), estrogen-producing tumors, persistent anovulatory cycles, and polycystic ovary syndrome (PCOS).

Clinical Signs and Symptoms

Presenting signs and symptoms associated with endometrial hyperplasia include the following:

- Vaginal bleeding: intermenstrual, hypermenorrheal, or postmenopausal
- Hyperestrogenism—conditions with possible alterations in estrogen metabolism, such as:
  - Ovarian granulosa cell tumor
  - Polycystic ovary syndrome
  - Obesity
  - Late menopause

Sonographic Signs

The sonographic appearance of endometrial hyperplasia is nonspecific; the differentiation between it and malignant *endometrial carcinoma* can be made only with biopsy. Nonspecific signs include:

- Increased thickness of the endometrial stripe (>6 mm) in postmenopausal patients[14] (Figure 14-14A)
- Endometrial circumference (EC) > 14 mm in premenopausal women
- Smooth, well-defined borders
- Homogeneous appearance of the endometrium, including possible cystic changes (Figure 14-14B)

DYSFUNCTIONAL UTERINE BLEEDING

Dysfunctional uterine bleeding (DUB) is abnormal vaginal bleeding present without demonstrable structural abnormalities or pathologic causes. It usually results from hormonal imbalances, either deficient progesterone or excess estrogen. Sonographic evidence of increased endometrial thickness may be grounds for initiating treatment. As a rule of thumb, a thick, secretory-looking endometrium may be associated with inadequate progesterone levels, while a thin endometrium may indicate a need for combined estrogen and progesterone therapy. Diagnostic tools—such as ultrasound, endometrial sampling, sonohysterography, and diagnostic hysteroscopy—are useful in the prompt

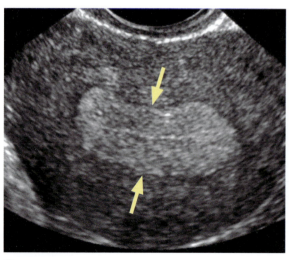

A

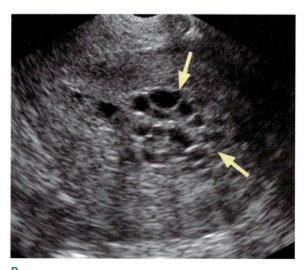

B

Figure 14-14. Endometrial hyperplasia. **A** Increased homogeneous thickening of the endometrial stripe (arrows) in a postmenopausal patient. **B** Cystic appearance (arrows) of the endometrium in a patient with endometrial hyperplasia.

diagnosis and treatment of an increasing number of menstrual disorders. There are, however, no specific sonographic findings solely associated with or pathognomonic for dysfunctional uterine bleeding.

Clinical Signs and Symptoms

The only clinical sign of dysfunctional uterine bleeding is bleeding *per vaginam* unexplained by structural abnormalities or other pathologic causes.

Sonographic Signs

There are no specific sonographic correlates for dysfunctional uterine bleeding.

ENDOMETRITIS

Endometritis is any acute or chronic inflammatory reaction of the uterine lining (endometrium). It may spread to the myometrium and, on occasion, the parametrium.

The etiologies for endometritis can be categorized as pregnancy-related or non–pregnancy-related. When the condition is not related to pregnancy or a gestational event, it is typically referred to as pelvic inflammatory disease (PID; see page 398) and is frequently associated with concomitant inflammation of the fallopian tubes and pelvic peritonitis. Pregnancy-related endometritis can result from prolonged labor, premature rupture of membranes, and retained intrauterine clots or products of conception. The diagnosis is usually made based on history and clinical findings.

Clinical Signs and Symptoms

Presenting signs and symptoms associated with endometritis include the following:

- Fever
- Uterine tenderness
- Leukocytosis

Sonographic Signs

Characteristic sonographic signs of endometritis are the following:[15]

- May be normal in early stages
- Thickened, heterogeneous endometrium (Figure 14-15A)
- Fluid in the endometrial cavity
- Air bubbles in the endometrial cavity (Figure 14-15B)

ENDOMETRIAL CARCINOMA

Endometrial carcinoma, also referred to as *uterine cancer*, is the most common type of gynecologic malignancy. It usually occurs in women 60–70 years of age, although about 12% of cases occur in premenopausal women.[16] The most common histologic type is adenocarcinoma of the endometrium, which accounts for approximately 90% of cases, while papillary serous carcinoma, clear cell carcinoma, and adenosquamous carcinoma constitute most of the remaining 10% of cases. The malignancy arises from the endometrium, and initially the tumor mass grows into the uterine cavity. Myometrial invasion is the first indication of continued spread

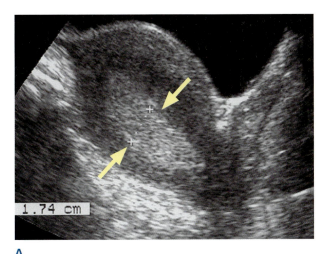

A

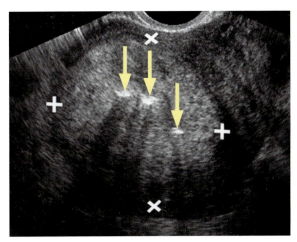

B

Figure 14-15. Endometritis. **A** Sagittal transabdominal scan demonstrating a thickened, heterogeneous endometrium (arrows). **B** Sagittal endovaginal section demonstrating punctate echogenic foci (arrows) within the endometrial cavity consistent with air bubbles. Calipers are placed at the periphery of the echogenic endometrium.

of the disease. Without treatment, the malignancy may spread to the cervix, uterus, and adnexa (including the fallopian tubes and ovaries). Distant metastases may occur if the pelvic lymphatic system is infiltrated. Risk factors for endometrial carcinoma include:

- Hormone replacement therapy (HRT)
- Obesity
- Early menarche
- Late menopause
- Diabetes mellitus
- Strong familial history of uterine cancer
- Tamoxifen therapy

Tamoxifen is an antiestrogen agent used in the treatment of early and late breast cancer. It has proestrogenic effects on the endometrium and induces histologic effects that are demonstrable sonographically. Its use is also associated with an increased risk of endometrial hyperplasia, polyps, and adenocarcinoma.[17] (See Chapter 16, page 430.)

Clinical Signs and Symptoms

Presenting signs and symptoms associated with endometrial carcinoma include:

- Postmenopausal vaginal bleeding
- Hypermenorrhea and intermenstrual flow in patients still having periods
- Pain as the result of uterine distention

Sonographic Signs

Endovaginal ultrasound imaging plays a critical role in the early diagnosis of endometrial carcinoma. While first presentation in advanced cases is often associated with dramatic sonographic appearances, early detection is based on the relationship between endometrial thickness, hormone status of the patient, and clinical presentation.

- Early detection:
  ▸ Thickening of endometrial echoes (>5 mm) in any postmenopausal patient
  ▸ Poorly defined endometrium with irregular contours (Figure 14-16A)
- Late detection:
  ▸ Alteration in size, shape, and sonographic texture of the myometrium
  ▸ Polypoid mass extending into the uterine cavity (Figure 14-16B)

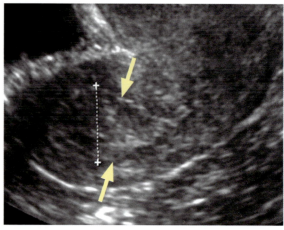

A

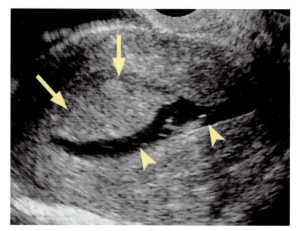

B

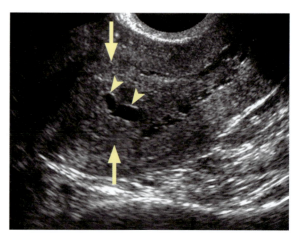

C

Figure 14-16. **A** Early sonographic appearance of endometrial carcinoma: Sagittal endovaginal section demonstrates a poorly defined, thickened, heterogeneous endometrium with irregular borders (arrows). **B** Later-stage endometrial carcinoma: Sagittal endovaginal section demonstrates a solid polypoid mass (arrows) growing into the endometrial cavity, which contains fluid and debris (arrowheads). **C** Sagittal endovaginal section demonstrates a thickened, irregular endometrium (arrows) with cystic changes (arrowheads) consistent with malignant transformation in a patient on tamoxifen.

- Increased uterine size
- Fluid in the endometrial cavity (Figure 14-16B)
• Effects of tamoxifen (Figure 14-16C):
  - Thickened endometrium
  - Irregular, cystic appearance

ENDOMETRIAL POLYPS

Endometrial polyps are benign masses of endometrial tissue projecting out from the surface of the endometrium into the endometrial cavity (Figures 14-17A and B). Sessile polyps grow exophytically from a wide base while pedunculated polyps arise from a stalk-like pedicle. They may be single or multiple and range in size from small, 1 mm excrescences to masses that fill or distend the entire uterine cavity. Endometrial polyps most commonly arise in the fundal region and may undergo malignant transformation. They are common in the endometrial cavity, particularly in women between the ages of 29 and 59, with the greatest incidence occurring in women after age 50 and in women on tamoxifen. Endocervical polyps can originate from the surface of the endocervical canal or can prolapse through the cervical os.

Clinical Signs and Symptoms

Presenting signs and symptoms associated with endometrial polyps include the following:

- Often asymptomatic
- Vaginal bleeding, either intermenstrual flow or heavy periods (menorrhagia)
- Infertility
- Occasionally postmenopausal bleeding
- Usually discovered incidentally during dilatation and curettage (D&C)

Sonographic Signs

The following are the characteristic sonographic signs of endometrial polyps:

- Nonspecific endometrial thickening that may be indistinguishable from endometrial hyperplasia
- Discrete mass in the endometrium (Figure 14-18A)
- Smooth, intracavitary masses, outlined by fluid, that are isoechoic, with myometrium demonstrated on hysterosonography (Figure 14-18B)
- Vascular pedicle demonstrated with color Doppler (pedunculated polyps) (Figure 14-18C)

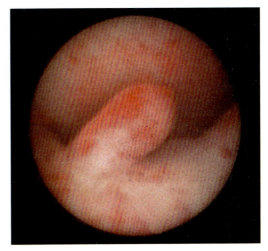

A

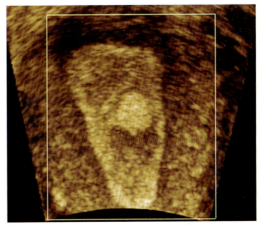

B

Figure 14-17. A Endometrial polyps: Hysteroscopy demonstrates the gross pathologic appearance of a sessile endometrial polyp. **B** B-mode volumetric reconstruction of the image in Figure 14-17A.

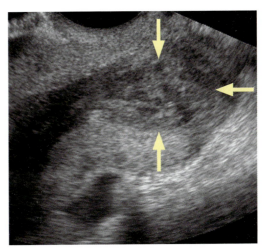

A

Figure 14-18. A A large, discrete heterogeneous mass (arrows) filling the endometrial cavity. (Figure continues . . .)

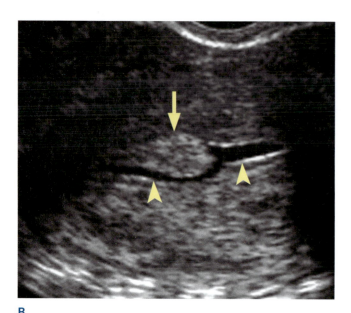
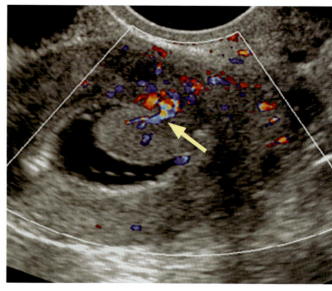

Figure 14-18, continued. B On hysterosonography, this endometrial polyp (arrow) appears as a smooth, intracavitary mass outlined by instilled fluid (arrowheads). **C** The vascular pedicle (arrow) of an endometrial polyp is demonstrated with color Doppler imaging.

OVARIAN PATHOLOGY

NON-NEOPLASTIC LESIONS—FUNCTIONAL CYSTS

Functional (*physiologic*) *cysts* are generic types of hormonally active cysts that result from the stimulation of the ovary by hormones. They present as the most common type of ovarian enlargement in young women. The general appearance of a functional cyst may change over the course of the menstrual cycle. Several clinical pearls can serve in the quick bedside assessment of cystic structures identified in an ovary:

- Most cysts are small and clinically unimportant; however, each cyst potentially represents an early manifestation of a benign or malignant neoplasm.
- Simple cysts in the premenopausal woman are common; however, clinical follow-up is necessary to rule out malignant changes.
- Simple functional cysts measuring less than 3 cm are considered normal and usually spontaneously resolve over the course of one or two menstrual cycles. Persistence of a cyst for more than 60 days in a patient with normal menstrual cycles probably indicates that the cyst is *not* functional and must be considered neoplastic.
- Any ovarian cystic mass measuring more than 3 cm should be reevaluated sonographically 6–8 weeks later. Persistence, enlargement, or change in appearance of the lesion is usually an indication for further workup and treatment, such as laparoscopy or surgical excision.

Clinical Signs and Symptoms

Presenting signs and symptoms associated with functional cysts include the following:

- Frequently asymptomatic
- Presence of a palpable adnexal mass
- Usually unilateral
- Acute pelvic pain (produced by bleeding into the cyst)

Sonographic Signs

The following are the characteristic sonographic signs of functional cysts:

- Smoothly marginated mass in the ovarian fossa
- Unilocular
- Absent internal echoes (anechoic)
- Absent nodules or solid components
- Posterior acoustic enhancement

Follicular Cysts

Follicular cysts arise when the dominant follicle fails to rupture or when the fluid in an incompletely developed follicle fails to be resorbed. They are typically larger

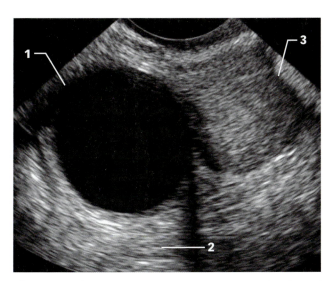

Figure 14-19. Endovaginal axial section demonstrating the typical sonographic findings associated with a simple follicular cyst: (1) a smooth-walled, anechoic mass with (2) posterior acoustic enhancement. 3 = uterus.

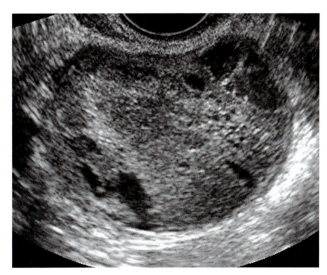

Figure 14-20. A large, hemorrhagic corpus luteum cyst. The lumen is filled with complex, heterogeneous thrombotic material that complicates sonographic evaluation.

than normal follicles and measure between 3 and 8 cm. Simple cystic structures in the ovary measuring less than 3 cm are consistent with normal follicles.

Clinical Signs and Symptoms

Presenting signs and symptoms associated with follicular cysts include the following:

- Typically asymptomatic
- Pelvic pain, dyspareunia, and occasionally vaginal bleeding (may be caused by large cysts)
- Differential diagnoses include salpingitis and endometriosis

Sonographic Signs

The following are the characteristic sonographic signs of a follicular cyst (Figure 14-19):

- Smoothly marginated mass in the ovarian fossa
- Unilocular
- Absent internal echoes (anechoic)
- Absent nodules or solid components
- Posterior acoustic enhancement
- Measures > 3 cm

Corpus Luteum Cyst

A *corpus luteum cyst* is the functional, non-neoplastic enlargement of an ovary caused by failure of the dominant follicle to regress after ovulation. (It should not be confused with the normal corpus luteum cyst that forms during the secretory phase of the menstrual cycle or during pregnancy, the latter regressing after 16–18 menstrual weeks.) If there is hemorrhage into the central lumen of a ruptured follicle, it expands into a fluid-filled mass on the ovary. The blood components are resorbed first, leaving residual serous fluid to fill the cystic cavity. Corpus luteum cysts are unilateral and frequently asymptomatic; however, when they do cause symptoms, diagnostic studies are indicated to rule out ectopic pregnancy. Corpora lutea are not considered to be corpus luteum cysts until they reach at least 3 cm in diameter.

Clinical Signs and Symptoms

Presenting signs of persistent corpus luteum cysts may include the following:

- Frequently asymptomatic
- Local pain and tenderness
- Amenorrhea
- Delayed menstruation

Sonographic Signs

The following are the characteristic sonographic signs of a corpus luteum cyst:

- Cystic mass in ovarian fossa
- Either simple or complex cystic appearance
- Hemorrhage into a corpus luteum cyst (common, complicating the sonographic evaluation) (Figure 14-20)
- Measures > 3 cm

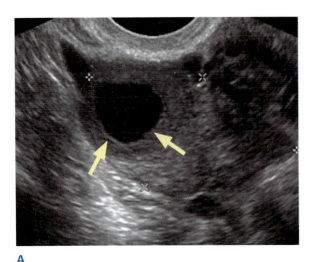 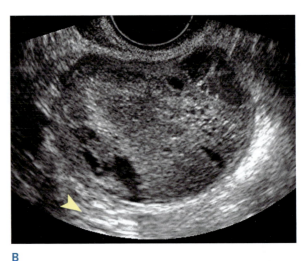

Figure 14-21. A A corpus luteum cyst of pregnancy appears as a well-circumscribed, anechoic ovarian mass (arrows). **B** Pathologic corpus luteum cyst demonstrated as a large, hemorrhagic adnexal mass exhibiting posterior acoustic enhancement (arrowhead).

Corpus Luteum Cyst of Pregnancy

A *corpus luteum cyst of pregnancy* is the normal cystic enlargement of the ruptured follicle in the presence of beta-hCG secreted by a conceptus. The corpus luteum is necessary for the production of progesterone and maintenance of the endometrium in normal early pregnancy. It typically regresses by week 18; however, cystic dilatation may persist well into the second trimester (Figure 14-21A). Failure of the corpus luteum to regress may encourage torsion of the ovary, causing severe pain, or the cyst may rupture, requiring laparoscopic or open surgical intervention. Hemorrhage into the cyst is also common and dramatically complicates the sonographic picture.

Clinical Signs and Symptoms
- Amenorrhea or delayed menses
- Localized pain and tenderness in the ovary

Sonographic Signs
The following are the characteristic sonographic signs of a persistent corpus luteum cyst:
- Hemorrhagic, large adnexal mass exhibiting posterior acoustic enhancement (Figure 14-21B)
- Complex internal architecture
- Thickened, irregular borders

Theca-Lutein Cysts

Theca-lutein cysts arise in response to excessive levels of circulating gonadotropins, particularly beta-hCG. The high level of hormones reactivates atretic follicles, which become cystically enlarged. They are typically found in association with medical conditions that hyperstimulate ovarian follicles, such as choriocarcinoma, polycystic ovary syndrome (PCOS), gestational trophoblastic disease, multifetal pregnancy, and hyperstimulated ovaries in patients on infertility drugs.

Clinical Signs and Symptoms
Clinical signs and symptoms that may be associated with the presence of theca-lutein cysts include:
- Pelvic fullness
- Dull aching
- Elevated serum beta-hCG
- Hyperemesis gravidarum
- Breast paresthesias

Sonographic Signs
The following are the characteristic sonographic signs of theca-lutein cysts:
- Multiple large cysts (2–3 cm) (Figure 14-22A)
- Multilocular, septated internal architecture
- Typical "spoke-wheel" distribution (Figure 14-22A)
- Generous vascular stromata (Figure 14-22B)
- Bilateral (if both ovaries are present)

Hemorrhagic Cysts

Bleeding into the lumen of an ovarian cyst, known as a *hemorrhagic cyst*, may occur spontaneously or may be the result of torsion that causes disruption of normal hemodynamic patterns. Blood flows into the cystic lumen and begins the sonographic metamorphosis from diffuse, low-level echoes swirling within the cavity to complex, solid architectural thrombus adherent to the walls. Hemorrhage can occur into any type of ovarian functional cyst, thus confusing the sonographic appearance. Clinical correlation provides diagnostic direction.

Clinical Signs and Symptoms

Presenting signs and symptoms associated with a hemorrhagic cyst include the following:

- Sudden onset of pelvic pain
- Palpable adnexal mass

Sonographic Signs

Characteristic sonographic signs of a hemorrhagic cyst include the following:

- Acute hemorrhagic cysts (Figure 14-23A):
  - Typical characteristics of a cystic mass: thin-walled, smoothly marginated, posterior acoustic enhancement
  - Diffuse low-level echoes within the lumen that may swirl
- Chronic hemorrhagic cysts (Figure 14-23B):
  - Complex, predominantly cystic mass with thick walls
  - Solid internal architecture representing organized thrombus
  - Absent blood flow within the internal solid components

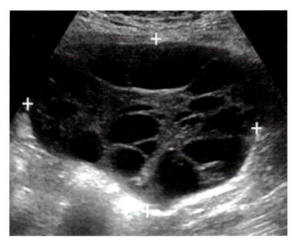

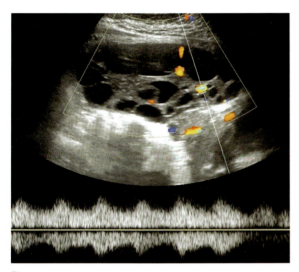

Figure 14-22. A Theca-lutein cysts appear as large, multiple cystic areas in a "spoke-wheel" distribution. **B** Color Doppler demonstrates robust low-resistance flow in the generous vascular stromata associated with theca-lutein cysts.

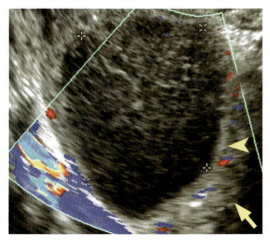

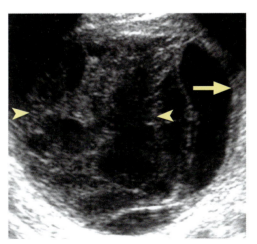

Figure 14-23. A Acute hemorrhagic ovarian cyst demonstrating a thin-walled (arrowhead) mass filled with diffuse low-level echoes and posterior acoustic enhancement (arrow). **B** Chronic hemorrhagic ovarian cyst: a complex, predominantly cystic mass with thickened walls (arrow) and organized thrombus (arrowheads).

Paraovarian Cysts

Paraovarian cysts occur in the broad ligament, not in the ovary. They account for 10%–20% of all adnexal masses and are most common in the third and fourth decades of life.[18] Sonographically they have an appearance typical of cysts but do not lie within the ovary. They frequently are located superior to the uterine fundus. Like functional cysts, paraovarian cysts may hemorrhage, complicating the sonographic picture.

Clinical Signs and Symptoms

Presenting signs and symptoms associated with paraovarian cysts include the following:

- Generally asymptomatic
- Pelvic pain if cyst is large

Sonographic Signs

The following are the characteristic sonographic signs of paraovarian cysts (Figure 14-24):

- Single, unilocular cystic mass
- Papillary projections present in 30% of lesions
- Located outside the ovarian fossa—superior and lateral to uterine fundus

Polycystic Ovaries

Polycystic ovary is a term used to describe the imaging appearance of an ovary. Some women who have polycystic ovaries may have bona fide polycystic ovary syndrome (PCOS), but diagnosis of PCOS requires additional clinical and laboratory correlates. Hormonal imbalances and unknown causes induce follicular growth that results in multiple cysts developing within both ovaries. Polycystic ovaries may be seen in approximately 20% of women of reproductive age.[19] Regardless of etiology, the sonographic appearance of polycystic ovaries is similar.

Polycystic Ovary Syndrome

Polycystic ovary syndrome (PCOS) is an endocrine disease characterized by chronic anovulation. While sonographic evidence of polycystic ovaries is one of three criteria for diagnosis, it alone is not specific. The other two criteria are oligo-ovulation or anovulation and laboratory-demonstrated hyperandrogenism. *Stein-Leventhal syndrome* consists of polycystic ovaries concomitant with the classic clinical triad of oligomenorrhea, hirsutism, and obesity. (See Chapter 15, page 411.)

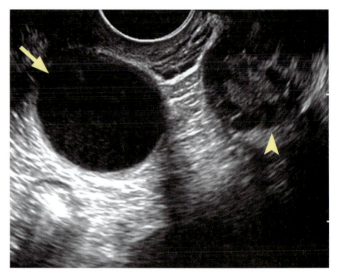

Figure 14-24. Paraovarian cyst: axial endovaginal section through the adnexa demonstrating a simple cystic mass (arrow) located adjacent to the ovary (arrowhead). There are no papillary projections demonstrated in this case.

Clinical Signs and Symptoms

Presenting signs and symptoms associated with polycystic ovary syndrome include the following:

- Amenorrhea or oligomenorrhea
- Infertility
- Hirsutism
- Obesity

Sonographic Signs

The following are the characteristic sonographic signs of both polycystic ovary syndrome and polycystic ovaries (Figure 14-25):

- Enlarged multicystic ovaries
- Presence of more than 10 follicles
- Ovarian enlargement (volume > 10 cc)[20]
- May be bilateral or unilateral

NEOPLASTIC OVARIAN MASSES

Neoplasia of the ovary can be categorized histologically or by sonographic appearance. While some masses demonstrate certain typical sonographic findings, the overall specificity of ultrasound in identifying particular histologic types is quite low. Any non-simple cystic mass of the ovary is usually an indication for surgical or laparoscopic intervention, as its malignant or benign nature can be determined only in the pathology

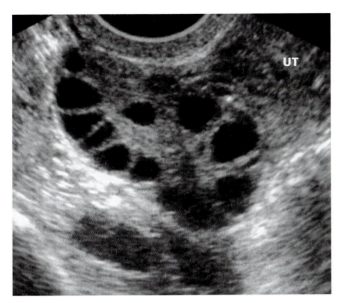

Figure 14-25. Axial endovaginal section through the adnexa demonstrating an enlarged polycystic ovary containing multiple dilated follicles. UT = uterus.

laboratory. Many of the malignant neoplastic masses can be scored using criteria in Table 14-1.

Sonographically, ovarian neoplastic masses can be categorized as cystic, solid, or complex—a mixture of both types of tissue. Similarly, the specific imaging characteristics of a mass, even in conjunction with clinical and laboratory findings, are rarely pathognomonic.

Clinical Signs and Symptoms

Clinical signs and symptoms for most types of ovarian tumors, whether benign or malignant, are nonspecific and frequently do not manifest themselves in a sufficiently robust manner to concern the patient until the disease has achieved an advanced stage.

Clinical signs and symptoms common to most histologic types of ovarian neoplasia include:

- Bloating, abdominal distention, discomfort
- Malaise
- Pressure effects on bladder and rectum
- Constipation
- Digestive disorders
- Weight changes
- Increased girth
- Infertility

Table 14-1. Ovarian mass scoring system.

Feature	Finding	Points
Inner wall structure	Smooth	1
	Irregularities ≥3 mm	2
	Papillarities ≥3 mm	3
Wall thickness	Thin (≤3 mm)	1
	Thick (>3 mm)	2
Echogenicity	Sonolucent	1
	Low echogenicity	2
	Low echogenicity with echogenic core	3
	Mixed echogenicity	4
	High echogenicity	5

Interpretation:

- Minimum ultrasound score = 4.
- Maximum ultrasound score = 15.
- A score < 9 indicated a low risk of malignancy.
- A score ≥ 9 was associated with an increased risk of malignancy.
- Mature teratomas (dermoid cysts) and other benign cysts may have a score ≥ 9.

Source: Data from Sassone AM, Timor-Tritsch IE, Artner A, et al: Transvaginal sonographic characterization of ovarian disease: evaluation of a new scoring system to predict ovarian malignancy. Obstet Gynecol 78:70–76, 1991.

Scoring Chart

In 1991, a method of determining the malignancy or benignity of an ovarian mass based on select sonographic criteria was developed by Drs. Sassone and Timor-Tritsch (Table 14-1).[21] This method is applicable to all ovarian masses detected sonographically, not just epithelial tumors. Endovaginal ultrasound, of course, is the examination method of choice because of the enhanced resolving capabilities inherent in intracavitary imaging probes. The performance of this scoring system, while not perfect, is impressive, with a sensitivity of 100%, a specificity of 83%, a positive predictive value of 37%, and a negative predictive value of 100%. Its primary strength lies in its ability to virtually exclude malignancy should the mass rate a score less than 9. Masses with a score of 9 or more carry an increased risk of malignancy and can be used

Table 14-2.	Common malignant ovarian neoplasms.
Type	Frequency
Epithelial neoplasms	65%–75%
Germ cell neoplasms	15%–20%
Metastases to the ovary	5%–10%
Sex cord stromal tumors	5%–10%

Source: Data from Bolger DM: Malignant diseases of the ovary. In Raatz Stephenson S (ed): *Diagnostic Medical Sonography: Obstetrics and Gynecology*, 3rd edition. Philadelphia, Lippincott Williams & Wilkins, 2012, table 10-2, pp 240–241.

as a foundation for gynecologic intervention. Common malignant ovarian neoplasms are listed in order of frequency in Table 14-2.

Epithelial Tumors

Epithelial ovarian tumors arise in the tissue covering the ovary. They are the most prevalent type of ovarian tumor, accounting for nearly 90% of cases. Both malignant types of epithelial tumors (*cystadenocarcinomas*) and those with low malignant potential (*cystadenomas*) exist. There are several histologic malignant types, listed here from most to least common: serous cystadenocarcinoma, mucinous cystadenocarcinoma, undifferentiated adenocarcinoma, endometrioid carcinoma, clear cell carcinoma, and Brenner's tumor. Tumors can grow quite large if not detected early and when mature demonstrate a gross pathologic appearance of a partially cystic mass with solid internal components and papillary projections. The sonographic appearances of different types of ovarian tumors are similar and therefore are not specific in rendering a final diagnosis.

Clinical Signs and Symptoms

In addition to the general signs and symptoms listed above, presenting signs and symptoms associated more specifically with epithelial tumors include the following:
- Vaginal bleeding
- Elevated serum CA-125 levels in > 90% of cases
- Symptoms of abnormal endocrine activity, such as:
  - Cushing's syndrome
  - Hypoglycemia
  - Hypercalcemia
  - Hyperthyroidism

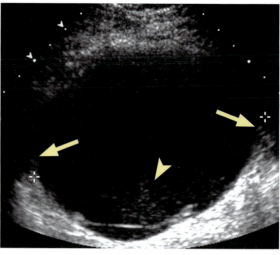

A

Figure 14-26. **A** A benign serous cystadenoma demonstrating typical sonographic characteristics of a unilocular mass with smooth borders (arrows) and some low-level echoes within (arrowhead). (Figure continues . . .)

Sonographic Signs

The sonographic characteristics of epithelial ovarian tumors cover a broad spectrum of appearances and are rarely pathognomonic. The mass may be predominantly cystic, hyperechoic, hypoechoic, and/or heterogeneous. The internal architecture may show central anechoic necrosis, hemorrhage, homogeneous and nonhomogeneous solid components, papillary excrescences, and mural irregularities.

The following criteria provide a generalized approach to differentiating a benign from a malignant ovarian mass—but again, sonography alone is not pathognomonic of either state:

- Benign criteria (Figure 14-26A):
  - Smooth borders
  - Unilocular or multilocular cysts
  - Anechoic with low-level echoes within
  - Internal calcifications
  - Absent internal Doppler evidence of blood flow
- Malignant criteria:
  - Irregular borders (Figure 14-26B)
  - Solid components (Figure 14-26B)
  - Mixed solid/cystic
  - Doppler evidence of blood flow to internal components (Figure 14-26C)
  - Ascites

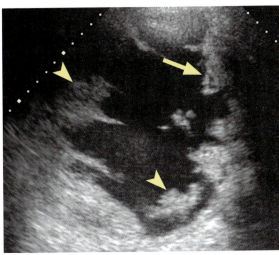
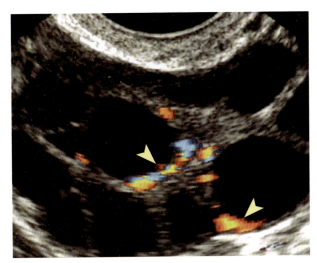

B
C

Figure 14-26, continued. B A cystadenocarcinoma demonstrating the more complex sonographic appearance associated with malignant ovarian tumors: irregular walls (arrow) with several solid internal components (arrowheads). **C** Doppler color imaging demonstrates blood flow (arrowheads) through the internal components of a complex malignant ovarian mass.

Pseudomyxoma Peritonei

A characteristic of epithelial ovarian tumors is their propensity to form large, multiseptated cystic masses filled with serous or mucinous fluid. When a mucin-filled cyst ruptures or leaks, the peritoneal cavity fills with sticky, gelatinous fluid and copious amounts of ascites, a condition called *pseudomyxoma peritonei*. Rupture of a mucinous neoplasm of the appendix is another common cause. Dissemination of bits of neoplastic tissue into the peritoneal cavity can seed tumorous growth on the surface of bowel, liver, spleen, omentum, and peritoneal walls.

Sonographic Signs

The following are the characteristic sonographic signs of pseudomyxoma peritonei (Figure 14-27):

- Echogenic peritoneal masses
- Ascites with echogenic particulate matter
- Displaced small bowel loops

Transitional Cell (Brenner) Tumor

A *transitional cell* or *Brenner tumor* is an uncommon, usually benign, solid ovarian tumor of epithelial origin. It is typically found in women between 50 and 60 years old and is most frequently found incidentally during pelvic examination or at operative laparotomy. These tumors are frequently bilateral and may be associated with another epithelial tumor on either the ipsi- or contralateral ovary in about 30% of cases. As is true

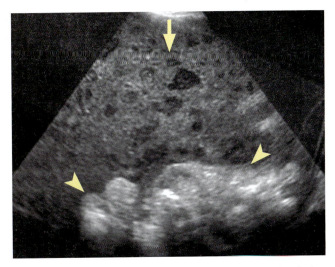

Figure 14-27. Pseudomyxoma peritonei: axial transabdominal section through the lower abdomen demonstrating ascites with echogenic particulate matter (arrow) and displaced small bowel loops (arrowheads).

with all ovarian tumors, sonographic findings are not specific for Brenner tumor; likely differential diagnoses include ovarian fibroma and thecoma.

Sonographic Signs

The following are the characteristic sonographic signs of Brenner tumor (Figure 14-28):

- Solid, hypoechoic ovarian mass
- May cast an acoustic shadow
- Calcifications present in 50% of cases

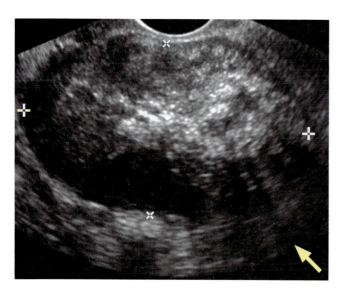

Figure 14-28. Endovaginal image of a Brenner tumor (cursors) presenting as a delineated solid hypoechoic mass with posterior acoustic shadowing (arrow).

Germ Cell Tumors

Germ cell tumors of the ovary account for approximately 15%–20% of all ovarian tumors.

They are believed to arise from ectopic embryonic cells that migrate from the yolk sac and attach to the ovary. Because they originate as pluripotent stem cells, they have the potential to grow and differentiate into masses carrying a broad spectrum of neoplastic potential and gross pathologic appearance.

Histologic types of germ cell tumors include the *teratoma, dysgerminoma, yolk sac tumor, ovarian choriocarcinoma,* and *malignant mixed germ cell tumor.* Although most germ cell tumors are benign, they do carry a malignant potential. As a rule of thumb, cystic germ cell tumors tend to be benign; solid ones tend to be malignant. However, the ultimate determination must be made histologically. Germ cell tumors are not confined to the ovary but can be found widely throughout the body.

Teratomas

The most common type of ovarian germ cell tumor is the *mature cystic teratoma,* a typically benign, complex tumor comprising tissue components from all three germ cell layers—ectoderm, mesoderm, and endoderm. The name derives from the Greek combining form *terato*, meaning "monster"—which attests to the typical dramatic and bizarre gross pathologic appearance of these ovarian masses. Teratomas have a wide and varied sonographic appearance based on the gross pathologic composition of the mass. It is not possible to differentiate a benign mature teratoma from its malignant counterpart, the immature variety.

Teratomas can be divided into three major subtypes:

- Mature (cystic) teratoma (generally benign)
- Immature teratoma (generally malignant)
- Struma ovarii (a rare tumor in which thyroid tissue comprises more than 50% of the mass)

Mature (Cystic) Teratomas

Mature teratomas are the most common benign tumor of the ovary and usually occur in women aged 20–30.[22] These masses are also frequently referred to as *dermoids*, but there is a fundamental histologic distinction between the two: Dermoids that contain dermal and epidermal tissue types are always benign, whereas *teratomas*, which contain mesodermal and ectodermal tissue components as well, maintain a malignant potential.

As these tumors arise from all three germ cell layers, they grow into encapsulated, complex cystic masses that may contain developmentally mature bits of skin, cartilage, bone, teeth, eyes, and fingernails. Free-floating fat, which has a lower specific gravity than the sebaceous fluid filling the locules of the mass, may rise to the top, creating a sonographic "tip of the iceberg" sign. Mature cystic teratomas are bilateral in 10%–15% of cases.[23] A variety of sonographic appearances are associated with these pathologically variable and complex masses.

Sonographic Signs

The following are the characteristic sonographic signs of cystic teratomas:

- Cystic mass with dense, echogenic tubercle (Rokitansky nodule) projecting into lumen (Figure 14-29A)
- Diffuse or partially echogenic mass with posterior acoustic or refractory shadowing (Figure 14-29B)
- Cystic mass with complex internal architecture that may include:
  - Calcifications (teeth, bone)
  - Thin echogenic bands (hair)
  - "Tip of the iceberg" sign created by fat/fluid level (Figure 14-29C)

Immature Teratomas

Immature ovarian teratomas differ from the mature variety by the presence of immature tissue contained within the mass and their higher malignant potential. They are also typically larger, measuring up to 25 cm in diameter. Immature teratomas are relatively uncommon and generally affect a younger population, occurring most often in the first two decades of life. The gross pathologic appearance is that of a large, encapsulated mass with a prominent solid component. There may be internal components similar to those found in the mature teratoma, such as hair, cartilage, bone, and calcifications. Immature teratomas are associated with concomitant mature cystic teratomas on the ipsilateral ovary in 26% of cases and an immature teratoma on the contralateral ovary in 10% of cases.[24]

Sonographic Signs

As with all complex ovarian masses, sonography provides a sensitive method of detecting the pathology but a very limited specificity in calling the tumor by name. The following are the characteristic sonographic signs of immature ovarian teratomas:

- Solid or mixed heterogeneous adnexal mass (Figure 14-30A)
- Possible presence of calcifications (Figure 14-30B)
- Hemorrhage into cystic component (Figure 14-30C)
- Contralateral ovarian mass (10% of cases)

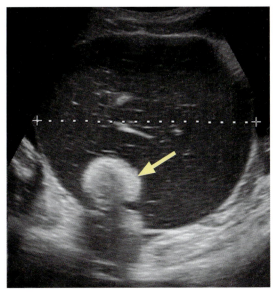

A

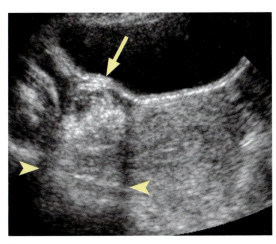

B

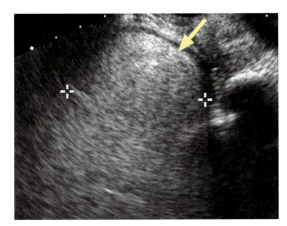

C

Figure 14-29. Mature (cystic) teratomas. **A** A predominantly cystic mass with a dense, echogenic tubercle, or Rokitansky nodule (arrow), projecting into the lumen. **B** A partially echogenic mass (arrow) with posterior acoustic or refractory shadowing (arrowheads). **C** The "tip of the iceberg" sign (arrow).

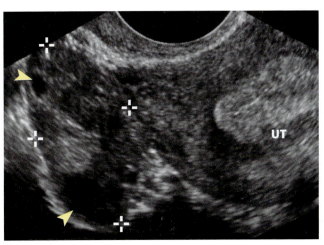

A

Figure 14-30. A Immature (cystic) teratoma: a predominantly solid adnexal mass (cursors) with small cystic components (arrowheads). UT = uterus. (Figure continues . . .)

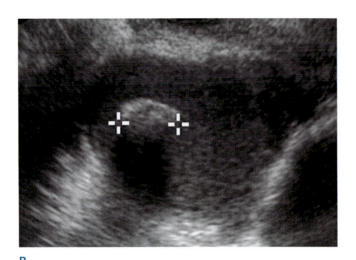

B

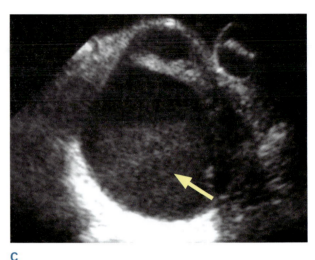

C

Figure 14-30, continued. B Immature (cystic) teratoma: focal calcification (cursors). **C** Immature (cystic) teratoma: internal hemorrhage (arrow).

Struma Ovarii

Struma ovarii is a mature cystic teratoma that is composed entirely or predominantly (at least 50%) of thyroid tissue. Although the tumor is composed mainly of thyroid tissue, thyrotoxicosis is seen in only 5% of all cases. Pathologically, these tumors present as large, multiloculated cystic masses with areas of solid thyroid tissue, hemorrhage, and necrotic debris.

Sonographic Signs

The following are the characteristic sonographic signs of struma ovarii:[25]

- Smoothly marginated, multiloculated cystic and solid mass (Figure 14-31)
- Complex internal architecture (hemorrhage, necrosis)
- Well-vascularized solid component in the central portion of the mass
- Ascites in 30% of cases

Dysgerminoma

A *dysgerminoma* is a rare type of ovarian germ cell tumor comprising about 1% of ovarian cancers.[24] As dysgerminomas arise from primordial germ cells, they are considered the ovarian counterparts to testicular seminomas in men. Dysgerminomas occur primarily in young women under 30 years old and are bilateral in approximately 15% of cases. All dysgerminomas are considered malignant; however, only one-third behave aggressively. The gross pathologic appearance is typically that of a large, solid, encapsulated mass with central hemorrhage and necrosis.

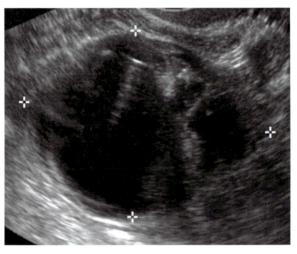

Figure 14-31. Struma ovarii appearing as a complex, multiloculated mass (cursors).

Sonographic Signs

The following are the characteristic sonographic signs of dysgerminoma:

- Solid ovarian mass that may have focal cystic areas within
- Varying internal echotexture
- Color Doppler demonstration of vascular flow within solid components (Figure 14-32)

Yolk Sac Tumor

An ovarian *yolk sac tumor* is a rare type of germ cell tumor that typically appears in the second decade of life. These tumors may arise from a preexisting dermoid cyst and are most often unilateral. Grossly, the

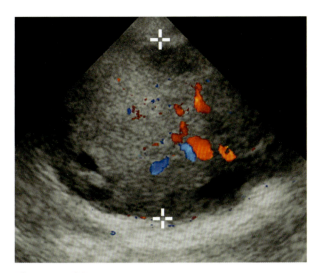

Figure 14-32. Doppler color flow imaging demonstrates vascularization of a solid dysgerminoma (cursors).

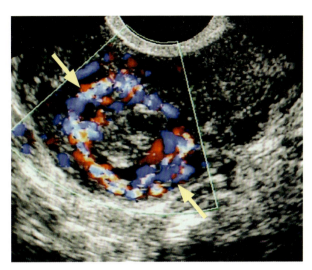

Figure 14-33. Ovarian choriocarcinoma: endovaginal image of a well-defined mixed solid and cystic ovarian mass (arrows) with robust vascularization, as demonstrated with color Doppler imaging.

mass is well encapsulated and complex, consisting of both cystic and solid components. These tumors have a tendency to become quite large and can extend into the abdominal cavity.

Sonographic Signs

There are no specific or characteristic sonographic findings that allow differentiation of this type of lesion from other ovarian tumors.

Ovarian Choriocarcinoma

An *ovarian choriocarcinoma* may be primary, arising from germ cells, or metastatic, arising from a uterine choriocarcinoma. In either case, this tumor type is rare, accounting for less than 1% of all ovarian cancers.[26] As these tumors have trophoblastic tissue components, an elevated serum beta-hCG often accompanies ovarian choriocarcinoma. They are typically solid, vascularized masses.

Sonographic Signs

The following are the characteristic sonographic signs of ovarian choriocarcinoma (Figure 14-33):

- Well-defined, solid adnexal mass
- Highly vascularized on color Doppler imaging
- Cystic, hemorrhagic, and necrotic areas present

Malignant Mixed Germ Cell Tumor

Another rare subtype of ovarian germ cell tumor is the *malignant mixed* variety. These are composed of a combination of tissue types found in other germ cell tumors, such as yolk sac tumors, dysgerminomas, immature teratomas, and ovarian choriocarcinomas. Gross pathology demonstrates a typically solid vascularized tumor that may contain cystic, hemorrhagic, and/or necrotic elements.

Sonographic Signs

Sonographic findings for malignant mixed germ cell tumors vary with the gross pathology present.

Sex Cord Stromal Tumors

Sex cord stromal tumors account for approximately 8% of all ovarian tumors. The plethora of subtypes can generally be categorized based on the cell type from which they originate. These include *granulosa cells*, *theca cells*, *Sertoli* and *Leydig cells*, and *fibroblasts* of stromal origin.

Granulosa Cell Tumors

Granulosa cell tumors vary in size from tiny lesions to large masses that fill the entire abdominal cavity. They are rarely (in only 2% of cases) bilateral.[27] They may be entirely solid, mixed cystic and solid, or predominantly cystic with internal hemorrhage and necrosis present. Cystic tumors may be uni- or multiloculated and filled with moderately echogenic proteinaceous material and lysed blood.

Sonographic Signs

There are no specific or characteristic sonographic findings that allow differentiation of granulosa cell tumors from other ovarian tumors.

Fibromas and Thecomas

Fibromas are the most common subtype of sex cord stromal tumors and account for almost 70% of this pathologic category of neoplasms. They typically occur in older women, with a mean age at detection of 48 years. Ascites is present in approximately 10% of all patients with ovarian fibromas and up to 50% of patients when the mass measures more than 5 cm. Abdominal distention from the ascitic fluid is a common initial clinical presentation. A fibroma is usually a hard, solid mass with a smooth surface. Like its relative, the thecoma, the fibroma may cast a posterior acoustic shadow on ultrasound examination.

A *thecoma* is a solid, benign, estrogen-producing tumor of the ovary. Thecomas account for 1% of all ovarian tumors and can occur at any age; they are most common, however, in women over 40 years of age. Estrogenic manifestations are the typical clinical presentation, which usually takes the form of menstrual irregularities or postmenopausal bleeding. The tumors range in size from small nodules to large, solid, firm tumors measuring several centimeters in diameter and are usually unilateral.

Sonographic Signs

The following are the characteristic sonographic signs of fibromas and thecomas (Figure 14-34):

- Hypoechoic adnexal mass
- Enhanced acoustic attenuation resulting in an acoustic shadow

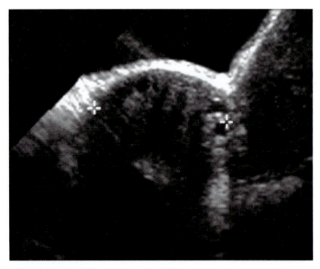

Figure 14-34. An ovarian fibroma presenting sonographically as a solid, hypoechoic mass with enhanced acoustic attenuation.

Sertoli-Leydig Cell Tumors

Sertoli-Leydig cell tumors, also called *androblastomas*, are uncommon benign tumors, accounting for less than 0.5% of all ovarian tumors. They typically present in the second to third decade of life, and about half of patients demonstrate clinical signs of androgenic hormone production such as oligomenorrhea that may proceed into amenorrhea, hirsutism, hoarseness, and breast atrophy.[28] Occasionally patients present with estrogenic manifestations, including irregular menstruation or menorrhagia in women in the reproductive age group and postmenopausal bleeding in older women. Sertoli cell tumors vary markedly in size, but most are smaller than 10 cm in diameter.[29] They tend to be solid, firm, encapsulated and lobulated masses, typically yellow or tan in color. Small cystic areas are infrequently present. They are usually unilateral but may be bilateral in phenotypic females with testicular feminization.

Sonographic Signs

There are no specific or characteristic sonographic findings that allow differentiation of Sertoli-Leydig cell tumors from other ovarian tumors.

Metastatic Tumors

About 7% of all ovarian cancers are metastatic in nature. The most common primary sites from which cancer spreads to the ovaries are the gastrointestinal tract and breast, although thyroidal and lymphatic origins occur less commonly. The routes of metastasis to the ovaries include direct invasion from tumors involving adjacent pelvic organs, from peritoneal or lymphatic fluid, and from hematogenous (blood-borne) spread.

Sonographic Signs

There are no specific or characteristic sonographic findings that allow differentiation of metastatic tumors from other ovarian tumors.

Krukenberg Tumor

A *Krukenberg tumor*, also called *carcinoma mucocellulare*, is a specific type of metastatic ovarian cancer that may produce endocrinologic abnormalities. Most commonly, these masses are spread from a primary site in the gut (stomach, intestine, or gallbladder); less commonly, from the breast, lung, or contralateral ovary. They account for nearly 50% of all metastatic ovarian lesions.[30] The endocrinologic manifestations associated with Krukenberg tumors may include vaginal bleeding, alteration in menstrual patterns, hirsutism, and virilization.

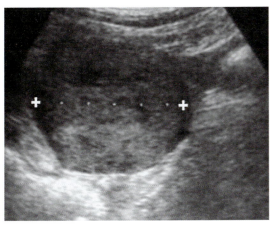

A

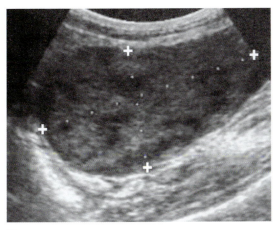

B

Figure 14-35. Krukenberg tumors: bilateral solid ovarian masses with the typical "moth-eaten" appearance. **A** Right ovary. **B** Left ovary.

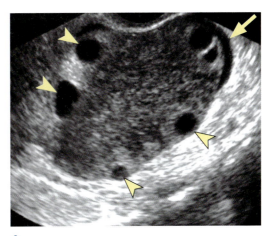

A

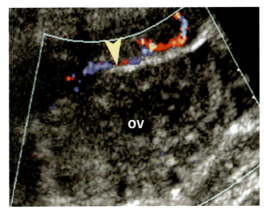

B

Figure 14-36. Ovarian torsion. **A** Endovaginal B-mode image demonstrates peripherally displaced follicles (arrowheads) and free fluid (arrow) around the ovary. **B** Doppler color imaging demonstrates absence of arterial and venous flow (arrowhead) in ovarian parenchyma (OV).

Sonographic Signs

The following are the characteristic sonographic signs of Krukenberg tumors (Figures 14-35A and B):

- Bilateral, solid ovarian masses
- Heterogeneous hyperechoic echo texture
- "Moth-eaten" appearance

OVARIAN TORSION

Ovarian torsion is the twisting of the ovary and part of the fallopian tube along the pedicle, strangulating arterial, venous, and lymphatic flow. It is a gynecologic emergency and requires urgent intervention to prevent ovarian death and necrosis. Torsion is more common in young women (15–30 years) and in postmenopausal women. Hypermobility of the ovary and adnexal masses, particularly dermoid cysts and paraovarian cysts, causes most cases of ovarian torsion.

Clinical Signs and Symptoms

Presenting signs and symptoms associated with ovarian torsion include the following:

- Severe lower abdominal pain
- Nausea and vomiting
- Leukocytosis

Sonographic Signs

The following are the characteristic sonographic signs of ovarian torsion:

- Enlarged, hypoechoic ovary
- Peripherally displaced follicles (Figure 14-36A)
- Free fluid in the pelvis (Figure 14-36A)
- Absence of arterial and venous flow in ovarian parenchyma, demonstrated by Doppler (Figure 14-36B); occasionally collateral flow

ADNEXAL PATHOLOGY

PELVIC INFLAMMATORY DISEASE

Pelvic inflammatory disease (PID) is an infectious inflammatory disease of the internal female reproductive tract that may involve the uterus, fallopian tubes, and adjacent adnexal spaces and structures. It is usually bilateral. The most common etiology of pelvic inflammatory disease is sexual transmission of infectious agents such as *Chlamydia trachomatis*, *Neisseria gonorrhoeae*, *Gardnerella vaginalis*, *Haemophilus influenzae*, and species of *Peptococcus* and *Bacteroides*. The infection begins in the vagina and cervix, ascends into the upper genital tract, and, if not diagnosed and treated successfully, spreads into the pelvic peritoneal cavity.

Clinical Signs and Symptoms

In the early stages of pelvic inflammatory disease, the patient may be asymptomatic; however, as the infection progresses, symptomatology can vary widely, from mild to acute, serious illness, including any or all of the following:

- Low-grade fever
- Pelvic discomfort
- Tubo-ovarian abscesses (TOAs) that may spread through the abdominal cavity, producing acute peritonitis and an acute perihepatitis called Fitz-Hugh–Curtis syndrome

Sonographic Signs

The sonographic presentation of pelvic inflammatory disease varies with the gross pathologic changes present in the individual patient and may include the following:

- Ill-defined uterine appearance secondary to inflammation
- Endometrial cavity thickening (endometritis) (Figure 14-37A)
- Fluid-filled fallopian tubes (hydrosalpinx or pyosalpinx) (Figure 14-37B)
- Enlarged, ill-defined ovaries (oophoritis) (Figure 14-37C)
- Free fluid in the cul-de-sac and/or peritoneal cavity (Figure 14-37D)
- With tubo-ovarian abscess, complex adnexal masses with thickened walls and cystic components (Figure 14-37E)

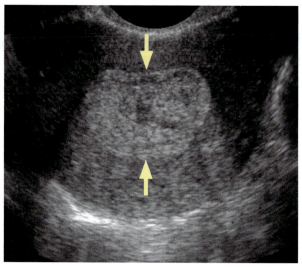

A

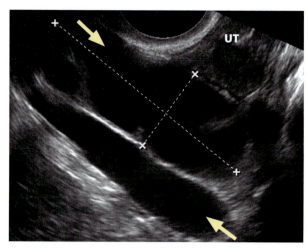

B

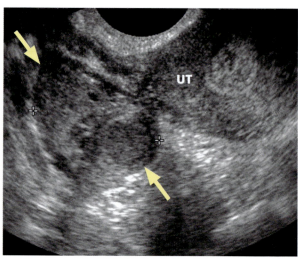

C

Figure 14-37. Pelvic inflammatory disease. **A** Endometritis—thickening of the endometrial cavity (arrows). **B** Fluid-filled fallopian tube (hydrosalpinx, arrows). UT = uterus. **C** Enlarged, ill-defined ovary (arrows). UT = uterus. (Figure continues . . .)

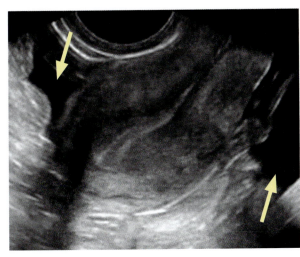

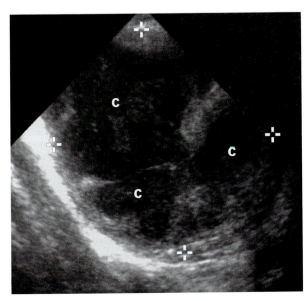

Figure 14-37, continued. D Free fluid in the anterior and posterior cul-de-sacs (arrows). **E** Complex tubo-ovarian abscess (cursors) with central cystic components (C).

ENDOMETRIOSIS

Endometriosis is the presence of normal endometrial tissue implanted anywhere outside the uterine cavity. Implants, called *endometriomas*, are most commonly located in the dependent portions of the female pelvis—i.e., the anterior and posterior cul-de-sacs, uterosacral ligament, fallopian tubes, and ovaries—although they may be found anywhere in the peritoneal cavity. As it is functional endometrial tissue, these ectopic foci respond to normal cyclic hormonal variations with proliferative and secretory responses and menstrual sloughing. The exact etiology is indeterminate in individual cases; however, general theories posit the transport of viable endometrial cells via retrograde menstruation as the most likely cause. Other etiologic possibilities include immunologic dysfunction, metaplastic conversion of endometrial cells with lymphatic or hematogenous spread, and the remains of müllerian cells in pelvic tissues.

Risk factors associated with endometriosis include:

- Family history of endometriosis
- Early menarche
- Short or long menstrual cycles
- Heavy bleeding during menses
- Parity (inverse relationship)
- Uterine or tubal defects
- Delayed childbearing

Clinical Signs and Symptoms

Many patients with endometriosis remain asymptomatic. However, when symptoms do occur they reflect the area of involvement and typically wax and wane with the hormonal cycle.[31] The classic "four D's" of endometriosis are:

- Dysmenorrhea: painful periods
- Dyspareunia: painful intercourse
- Dyschezia: painful defecation
- Dysuria: painful urination

Other symptoms include:

- Infertility
- Heavy or irregular bleeding
- Pelvic pain
- Lower abdominal or back pain
- Inguinal pain
- Pain during exercise

The diagnosis of endometriosis is accomplished with laparoscopic identification of implants and histologic confirmation of the presence of endometrial glands and stromata in a biopsy specimen. The use of sonography in evaluating patients with suspected endometriosis is limited to the identification of implants that have hemorrhaged. Blood leaks into the tissue, creating a hemorrhagic cystic mass, the so-called chocolate cyst, which is a sensitive but nonspecific finding.

Sonographic Signs

Sonography is not useful in detecting solid peritoneal implants.[32] As with other types of complex ovarian masses, sonography may reveal a wide spectrum of imaging findings:

- Well-circumscribed cystic mass with posterior acoustic enhancement.
- Lumen filled with low-level echoes (chocolate cyst) (Figure 14-38A).
- May be unilocular or multilocular.
- May contain thin or thick septations (Figure 14-38B).
- Mural nodules may be present (Figure 14-38C).

OVARIAN VEIN THROMBOSIS

Pathology in the ovarian veins is classified here under "Adnexal Pathology" (rather than ovarian) because the veins course through the ovaries toward the iliac veins and there is more venous anatomy in the adnexa than on the ovary itself. Moreover, when clot propagates, it does so outward, toward the iliacs.

Clotting of blood in the ovarian vein is a rare phenomenon but one that carries significant risk of morbidity and mortality. *Ovarian vein thrombosis* (OVT) typically arises in the presence of *Virchow's triad*: venous stasis, hypercoagulability, and venous endothelial damage. All of these hemodynamic aberrations are present in patients who are in the postpartum state, who have had recent pelvic surgery, and who have concomitant malignancies or pelvic inflammatory disease.

Computed tomographic and magnetic resonance scans are the most sensitive and specific imaging methods; however, sonography can provide a quick and inexpensive initial examination without exposing the patient to ionizing radiation or potentially nephrotoxic contrast agents. The primary limitation of ultrasound is overlying bowel gas, which frequently obscures visualization of the ovarian vasculature. As ovarian vein thrombosis is a predominantly right-sided pelvic pathology, acute appendicitis is an ever-present differential diagnostic possibility.

Clinical Signs and Symptoms

The clinical manifestations of ovarian vein thrombosis are variable, from asymptomatic or vague to potentially catastrophic (even leading to death), and include the following:[33]

- Abdominal pain
- Fever
- Pulmonary embolism

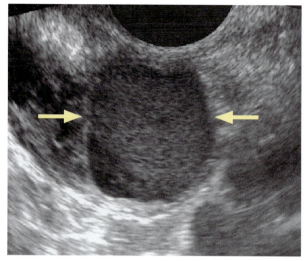

A

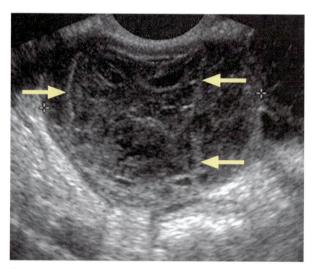

B

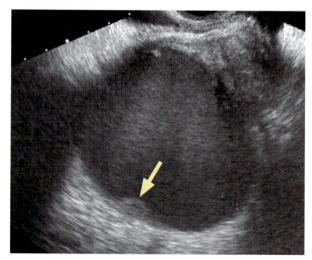

C

Figure 14-38. Endometriosis. **A** Axial endovaginal section demonstrating the lumen of a classic "chocolate cyst" (arrows) filled with low-level echoes. **B** Internal septations (arrows). **C** Presence of a mural nodule (arrow).

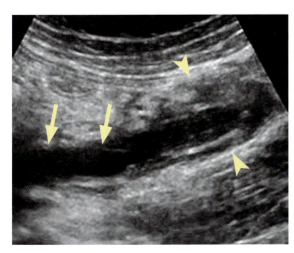

Figure 14-39. Endovaginal image demonstrating an enlarged, anechoic thrombosed ovarian vein (arrows) coursing from the ovary (arrowheads) through the adnexa.

- Sepsis
- Location on right side (80%–90% of cases), presumably due to anatomic disparities between right and left ovarian venous outflow[34]

Sonographic Signs

The following are characteristic sonographic signs of ovarian vein thrombosis:[35]

- Tubular hypoechoic or anechoic mass in adnexa (Figure 14-39)
- Tortuous tubular structure ascending from adnexa to the inferior vena cava
- Absent blood flow with Doppler interrogation

CHAPTER 14 REVIEW QUESTIONS

1. A mesonephric duct remnant that forms a cyst along the lateral or anterolateral wall of the vagina is called a:
   A. Corpus luteum cyst
   B. Paraovarian cyst
   C. Gartner's duct cyst
   D. Nabothian cyst

2. DES-related anatomic anomalies include all of the following EXCEPT:
   A. Hypoplastic uterus
   B. Constricting bands within the uterine cavity
   C. Intrauterine polyps
   D. Retroversion of the uterus

3. Congenital anatomic abnormalities resulting from the failed fusion of the paired embryonic paramesonephric ducts are referred to as:
   A. Müllerian duct anomalies
   B. Genitourinary anomalies
   C. Asherman syndrome
   D. Gartner's duct anomalies

4. The presence of a single uterine horn that may or may not communicate with the cervix is an anatomic anomaly referred to as a(n):
   A. Arcuate uterus
   B. Unicornuate uterus
   C. Bicornuate uterus
   D. Didelphic uterus

5. The anatomic anomaly consisting of two separate uterine bodies and two separate cervices, usually with the presence of a vaginal septum, is referred to as a(n):
   A. Arcuate uterus
   B. Unicornuate uterus
   C. Bicornuate uterus
   D. Didelphic uterus

6. The presence of two uterine horns contained within a single uterine body communicating with a single cervix and vagina is referred to as:
   A. Arcuate uterus
   B. Unicornuate uterus
   C. Bicornuate uterus
   D. Didelphic uterus

7. The obliteration of the endometrial cavity as a result of excessive or traumatic uterine instrumentation is called:
   A. Stein-Leventhal syndrome
   B. Beckwith-Wiedemann syndrome
   C. Adenomyosis
   D. Asherman syndrome

8. All of the following are associated with an increased prevalence of uterine fibroids EXCEPT:
   A. Obesity
   B. Hormone replacement therapy
   C. Diabetes
   D. Perimenopausal state

9. The overgrowth of endometrial tissue into the myometrium is called:
   A. Adenomyosis
   B. Asherman syndrome
   C. Choriocarcinoma
   D. Endometrial hypertrophy

10. All of the following sonographic findings are associated with adenomyosis EXCEPT:
    A. Asymmetrically enlarged uterus with focal subserosal mass
    B. Focal and diffuse bulkiness of the posterior uterine wall
    C. Heterogeneous uterine myometrial texture
    D. Focal cystic areas within the myometrium

11. Excessive proliferation of endometrial tissue without invasion of the myometrium is called:
    A. Adenomyosis
    B. Choriocarcinoma
    C. Endometrial hyperplasia
    D. Asherman syndrome

12. Endometrial hyperplasia is frequently associated with all of the following conditions EXCEPT:
    A. Polycystic ovary syndrome
    B. Gestational trophoblastic disease
    C. Late menopause
    D. Tamoxifen use

13. All of the following sonographic findings are associated with endometrial hyperplasia EXCEPT:
    A. Premenopausal endometrial thickness > 14 mm
    B. Postmenopausal endometrial thickness > 6 mm
    C. Smooth, well-defined borders
    D. Focal cystic areas in the myometrium

14. Acute inflammation of the uterine lining is called:
    A. Endometritis
    B. Parametritis
    C. Pelvic inflammatory disease
    D. Peritonitis

15. Endometrial carcinoma is more common in women aged:
    A. 20–30 years
    B. 30–40 years
    C. 40–50 years
    D. 60–70 years

16. Risk factors for endometrial carcinoma include all of the following EXCEPT:
    A. Hormone replacement therapy
    B. Late menopause
    C. Early menarche
    D. Endometritis

17. All of the following clinical signs are associated with endometrial carcinoma EXCEPT:
    A. Murphy's sign
    B. Vaginal bleeding
    C. Intermenstrual flow
    D. Lower abdominal pain

18. Masses of endometrial tissue projecting out from the surface of the endometrium and into the endometrial cavity are called:
    A. Endometrial carcinoma
    B. Endometrial polyps
    C. Fibroids
    D. Adhesions

19. All of the following are considered functional ovarian cysts EXCEPT:
    A. Cystadenomas
    B. Follicular cysts
    C. Theca-lutein cysts
    D. Corpus luteum cysts

20. Ovarian cysts that arise when the dominant follicle fails to rupture or when the fluid in an incompletely developed follicle fails to be resorbed is called a:
    A. Corpus luteum cyst
    B. Theca-lutein cyst
    C. Follicular cyst
    D. Hemorrhagic cyst

21. The functional, non-neoplastic enlargement of an ovary caused by failure of the dominant follicle to regress after ovulation is called a:
    A. Corpus luteum cyst
    B. Theca-lutein cyst
    C. Follicular cyst
    D. Hemorrhagic cyst

22. Ovarian cysts that arise in response to excessive levels of circulating gonadotropins, particularly beta-hCG, are called:
    A. Corpus luteum cysts
    B. Theca-lutein cysts
    C. Follicular cysts
    D. Hemorrhagic cysts

23. Paraovarian cysts occur in the:
    A. Omentum
    B. Cul-de-sac
    C. Round ligament
    D. Broad ligament

24. The most common histologic type of malignant ovarian neoplasm is:
    A. Brenner tumor
    B. Thecoma
    C. Dysgerminoma
    D. Cystadenocarcinoma

25. All of the following are types of sex cord stromal tumors EXCEPT:
    A. Cystadenocarcinoma
    B. Granulosa cell tumor
    C. Fibroma
    D. Sertoli-Leydig tumor

26. A metastatic type of ovarian tumor that frequently causes endocrinologic abnormalities is the:
    A. Sertoli-Leydig tumor
    B. Krukenberg tumor
    C. Granulosa cell tumor
    D. Sex cord stromal tumor

27. All of the following are considered risk factors for endometriosis EXCEPT:
    A. Late menopause
    B. Early menarche
    C. Multiparity
    D. Menorrhagia

28. All of the following are clinical symptoms reported by patients with endometriosis EXCEPT:
    A. Dysmenorrhea
    B. Dyspareunia
    C. Dyspepsia
    D. Dysuria

29. A 37-year-old woman presents with heavy menstrual periods and complains of dyspareunia. A pelvic exam reveals a symmetrically enlarged uterus with normal contours. Endovaginal sonography produces this image. The most likely diagnosis is:

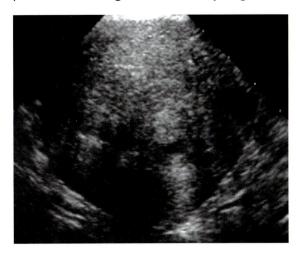

A. Adenomyosis
B. Endometrial carcinoma
C. Choriocarcinoma
D. Subserosal fibroids

30. A 65-year-old postmenopausal patient presents with sudden onset of vaginal bleeding. She is not on hormone replacement therapy and has been asymptomatic for gynecologic problems. Endovaginal sonography produces the findings seen in this image. The most likely diagnosis is:

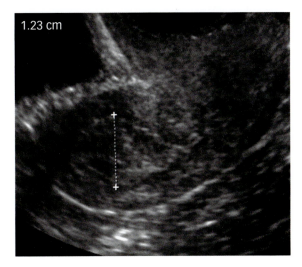

A. Degenerating fibroid
B. Early intrauterine pregnancy
C. Endometrial carcinoma
D. Adenomyosis

31. An obese patient presents with a history of infertility and hirsutism. Sonography reveals this image. The most likely diagnosis is:

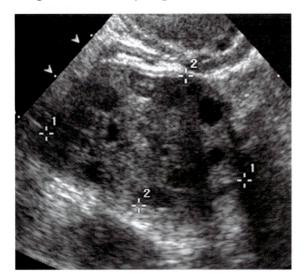

A. Polycystic ovaries
B. Ovarian torsion
C. Theca-lutein cysts
D. Anovulatory cysts

32. A 29-year-old patient presents with a history of heavy menstrual periods and an inability to conceive for the past three years. Sonography reveals this image. The most likely diagnosis is:

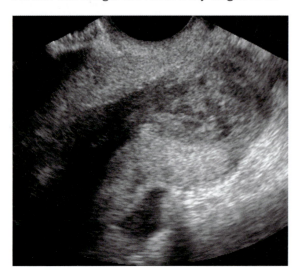

A. Uterine polyps
B. Endometrial carcinoma
C. Subserosal myoma
D. Endometritis

33. A 38-year-old patient with a history of endometriosis presents with dysuria, dyspareunia, low back pain, and heavy periods. This image most likely represents:

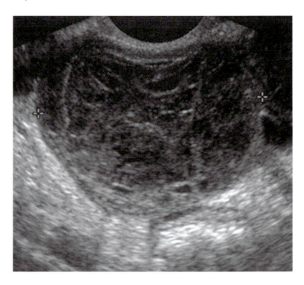

A. Hemorrhagic corpus luteum cyst
B. Endometrioma
C. Brenner tumor
D. Endometrial carcinoma

34. This image demonstrates a(n):

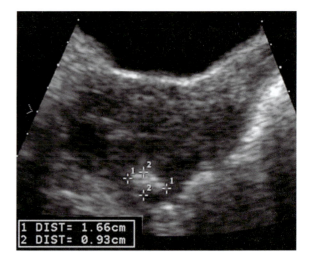

A. Cervical fibroid
B. Submucosal fibroid
C. Interstitial fibroid
D. Subserosal fibroid

35. A 42-year-old patient presents with lower abdominal pain, dyspareunia, and dysmenorrhea for several months. The uterus is firm and enlarged on pelvic exam. This image is most consistent with:

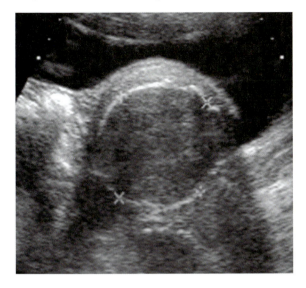

A. Calcified fibroid
B. Fetus papyraceus
C. Dysgerminoma
D. Pseudomyxoma peritonei

36. A 50-year-old woman presents complaining of generalized malaise, a full feeling in her abdomen, and an elevated CA-125 serum assay. This image is most consistent with:

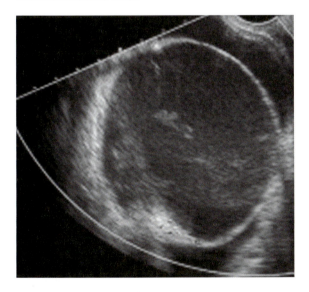

A. Hemorrhagic ovarian cyst
B. Ovarian cystadenocarcinoma
C. Dysgerminoma
D. Pelvic inflammatory disease

37. A 29-year-old patient presents with fever, elevated RBC count, and complaints of severe pain in her left lower quadrant. This image is most consistent with a diagnosis of:

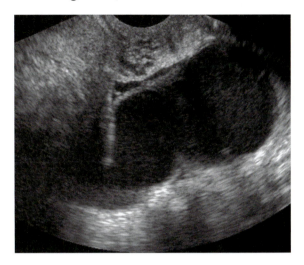

A. Ruptured ovarian cyst
B. Pelvic inflammatory disease
C. Ovarian torsion
D. Ectopic pregnancy

38. The sonographic findings in this image are most consistent with:

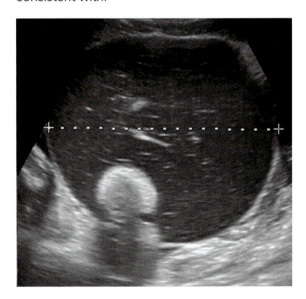

A. Sertoli-Leydig tumor
B. Cystadenocarcinoma
C. Dysgerminoma
D. Mature cystic teratoma

ANSWERS

See Appendix A on page 483 for answers.

REFERENCES

1. Dwyer PL, Rosamilia A: Congenital urogenital anomalies that are associated with the persistence of Gartner's duct: a review. Am J Obstet Gynecol 195:354–359, 2006.

2. Salle B, Sergeant P, Awada A, et al: Transvaginal ultrasound studies of vascular and morphological changes in uteri exposed to diethylstilbestrol in utero. Hum Reprod 11:2531–2536, 1996.

3. Steinkeler JA, Woodfield CA, Lazarus E, et al: Female infertility: a systematic approach to radiologic imaging and diagnosis. RadioGraphics 29:1353–1370, 2009.

4. Fedele L, Dorta M, Brioschi D, et al: Pregnancies in septate uteri: outcome in relation to site of uterine implantation as determined by sonography. Am J Roentgenol 152:781–784, 1989.

5. Hutson F: Congenital anomalies of the female genital system. In Raatz Stephenson S (ed): *Diagnostic Medical Sonography: Obstetrics and Gynecology*, 3rd edition. Philadelphia, Lippincott Williams & Wilkins, 2012, pp 31–49.

6. Schenker JG, Margalioth EJ: Intrauterine adhesions: an updated appraisal. Fertil Steril 37:593–610, 1982.

7. Munro MG: Uterine leiomyomas, current concepts: pathogenesis, impact on reproductive health, and medical, procedural, and surgical management. Obstet Gynecol Clin North Am 38:703–731, 2011.

8. Wise LA, Ruiz-Narvaez EA, Palmer JR, et al: African ancestry and genetic risk for uterine leiomyomata. Am J Epidemiol 176:1159–1168, 2012.

9. Smith SK, Riethman JL, Lomax CO Jr: Sonography of uterine leiomyosarcoma. J Diag Med Sonog 18:35–37, 2002.

10. Yeniel O, Cirpan T, Ulukus M, et al: Adenomyosis: prevalence, risk factors, symptoms and clinical findings. Clin Exp Obstet Gynecol 34:163–167, 2007.

11. Tamai K, Togashi K, Ito T, et al: MR imaging findings of adenomyosis: correlation with histopathologic features and diagnostic pitfalls. RadioGraphics 25:21–40, 2005.

12. Schneider SL, Craig M, Branning P: Improved sonographic accuracy in the presurgical diagnosis of diffuse adenomyosis: a case series and review. J Diag Med Sonog 18:71–77, 2002.

13. Atri M, Reinhold C, Mehio AR, et al: Adenomyosis: US features with histologic correlation in an in-vitro study. Radiology 215:783–790, 2000.

14. Nalaboff KM, Pellerito JS, Ben-Levi E: Imaging the endometrium: disease and normal variants. RadioGraphics 21:1409–1424, 2001.

15. Dubinsky TJ, Stroehlein K, Abu-ghazzeh Y, et al: Prediction of benign and malignant endometrial disease: hysterosonographic-pathologic correlation. Radiology 210:393–397, 1999.

16. Sorosky JI: Endometrial cancer. Obstet Gynecol 111(2 Pt 1):436–447, 2008.

17. De Muylder X, Neven P, De Somer M, et al: Endometrial lesions in patients undergoing tamoxifen therapy. Int J Gynecol Obstet 36:127–130, 1991.

18. Athey PA, Cooper NB: Sonographic features of paraovarian cysts. Am J Roentgenol 144:83–86, 1985.

19. Hart R, Hickey M, Franks S: Definitions, prevalence and symptoms of polycystic ovaries and polycystic ovary syndrome. Best Pract Res Clin Obstet Gynaecol 18:671–683, 2004.

20. Barber TM, Alvey C, Greenslade T, et al: Patterns of ovarian morphology in polycystic ovary syndrome: a study utilising magnetic resonance imaging. Eur Radiol 20:1207–1213, 2010.

21. Sassone AM, Timor-Tritsch IE, Artner A, et al: Transvaginal sonographic characterization of ovarian disease: evaluation of a new scoring system to predict ovarian malignancy. Obstet Gynecol 78:70–76, 1991.

22. Outwater EK, Siegelman ES, Hunt JL: Ovarian teratomas: tumor types and imaging characteristics. RadioGraphics 21:475–490, 2001.

23. Fibus TF: Intraperitoneal rupture of a benign cystic ovarian teratoma: findings at CT and MR imaging. Am J Roentgenol 174:261–262, 2000.

24. Sutton CL, McKinney CD, Jones JE, et al: Ovarian masses revisited: radiologic and pathologic correlation. RadioGraphics 12:853–877, 1992.

25. Van de Moortele K, Vanbeckevoort D, Hendrickx S: Struma ovarii: US and CT findings. JBR-BTR 86:209–210, 2003.

26. Jiao LZ, Xiang Y, Feng FZ, et al: Clinical analysis of 21 cases of nongestational ovarian choriocarcinoma. Int J Gynecol Cancer 20:299–302, 2010.

27. Young RH, Scully RE: Sex cord–stromal, steroid cell, and other ovarian tumors with endocrine, paracrine, and paraneoplastic manifestations. In Blaustein A, Kurman RJ (eds): *Blaustein's Pathology of the Female Genital Tract*, 5th edition. New York, Springer, 2002, p 257.

28. Lantzsch T, Stoerer S, Lawrenz K, et al: Sertoli-Leydig cell tumor. Arch Gynecol Obstet 264:206–208, 2001.

29. Oliva E, Alvarez T, Young RH: Sertoli cell tumors of the ovary: a clinicopathologic and immunohistochemical study of 54 cases. Am J Surg Pathol 29:143–156, 2005.

30. Al-Agha OM, Nicastri AD: An in-depth look at Krukenberg tumor: an overview. Arch Pathol Lab Med 130:1725–1730, 2006.

31. Buchweitz O, Poel T, Diedrich K, et al: The diagnostic dilemma of minimal and mild endometriosis under routine conditions. J Am Assoc Gynecol Laparosc 10:85–89, 2003.

32. Friedman H, Vogelzang RL, Mendelson EB, et al: Endometriosis detection by US with laparoscopic correlation. Radiology 157:217–220, 1985.

33. Salomon O, Apter S, Shaham D, et al: Risk factors associated with postpartum ovarian vein thrombosis. Thromb Haemost 82:1015–1019, 1999.

34. Savader SJ, Otero RR, Savader BL: Puerperal ovarian vein thrombosis: evaluation with CT, US, and MR imaging. Radiology 167:637–639, 1988.

35. Bilgin M, Sevket O, Yildiz S, et al: Imaging of postpartum ovarian vein thrombosis. Case Rep Obstet Gynecol 2012, Article ID #134603.

SUGGESTED READINGS

Gill KA: Gynecology. In Gill KA: *Ultrasound in Obstetrics and Gynecology: A Practitioner's Guide*. Pasadena, Davies Publishing, 2014, pp 25–88.

Goldstein C, Hagen-Ansert SL: Pathology of the uterus. In Hagen-Ansert SL (ed): *Textbook of Diagnostic Ultrasonography*, 7th edition. St. Louis, Elsevier Mosby, 2012, pp 978–1000.

Goldstein C, Hagen-Ansert SL, Vander Werff, BJ: Pathology of the adnexa. In Hagen-Ansert SL (ed): *Textbook of Diagnostic Ultrasonography*, 7th edition. St. Louis, Elsevier Mosby, 2012, pp 1028–1038.

Goldstein C, Hagen-Ansert SL, Vander Werff, BJ: Pathology of the ovaries. In Hagen-Ansert SL (ed): *Textbook of Diagnostic Ultrasonography*, 7th edition. St. Louis, Elsevier Mosby, 2012, pp 1001–1027.

Goldstein SR: Abnormal uterine bleeding: the role of ultrasound. In Callen PW (ed): *Ultrasonography in Obstetrics and Gynecology*, 5th edition. Philadelphia, Saunders Elsevier, 2008, pp 942–950.

Lerner JP, Timor-Tritsch IE, Federman A, et al: Transvaginal ultrasonographic characterization of ovarian masses with an improved, weighted scoring system. Am J Obstet Gynecol 170:81–85, 1994.

Salem S: Gynecology. In Rumack CM, Wilson SR, Charboneau JW, et al (eds): *Diagnostic Ultrasound*, 4th edition. Philadelphia, Elsevier Mosby, 2011, pp 613–638.

Schire NJ: Gestational trophoblastic neoplasia. In Callen PW (ed): *Ultrasonography in Obstetrics and Gynecology*, 5th edition. Philadelphia, Saunders Elsevier, 2008, pp 961–967.

Valentin L, Callen PW: Ultrasound evaluation of the adnexa (ovary and fallopian tubes). In Callen PW (ed): *Ultrasonography in Obstetrics and Gynecology*, 5th edition. Philadelphia, Saunders Elsevier, 2008, pp 968–985.

CHAPTER 15

Infertility

Factors Affecting Both Males and Females

Causes of Male Infertility

Causes of Female Infertility

Treatment of Infertility

Sonography in the Management of Infertility

Infertility is defined as the inability to conceive a child after 12 months of unprotected intercourse. About 14% of couples in the United States have an infertility disorder.[1] Infertility may be due to problems of female reproduction, problems with male reproduction, or factors that can affect both. Worldwide, approximately two-thirds of the cases of infertility are due to a female disorder and approximately one-third are due to a male disorder.

FACTORS AFFECTING BOTH MALES AND FEMALES

The infertility investigation begins with a detailed history and physical examination of both participants. Some causes of infertility result from factors affecting both males and females. One factor contributing to reduced fertility in many couples is postponement of childbearing. The conception rate for couples decreases with advancing age for a number of reasons. Eggs from older women ($\geq$35 years) and sperm from older men ($\geq$35 years) do not remain viable as long, so the likelihood of fertilization decreases. Additionally, older women are more likely to experience endometrial abnormalities and intraperitoneal diseases, such as endometriosis, that affect successful implantation.

Other factors that may affect the fertility of both sexes include:

- Environmental/occupational factors
- Toxic effects of drugs, including tobacco and marijuana
- Excessive exercise
- Nutritional deficiencies
- Idiopathic factors

CAUSES OF MALE INFERTILITY

Although male factors are the cause of infertility in the minority of cases, male causes of infertility are usually investigated first because the tests are less invasive and less expensive, and hence male factors are more easily ruled out.

Causes of male infertility include:[2]

- Varicoceles (40%)
- Low sperm density and motility (semen disorders)
- Abnormal sperm
- Presence of antisperm antibodies
- Cryptorchidism
- Obstruction
- Testicular failure
- Endocrine disorders
- Infections
- Genetic factors

Semen samples are studied for motility, density, morphology, signs of infection, and antisperm antibodies. If the semen analysis is normal, attention turns to the female factors.

CAUSES OF FEMALE INFERTILITY

The most common causes of female infertility are:[2]

- Ovarian/ovulatory dysfunction (40%)
- Tubal disease
- Cervical factors
- Endometriosis and other uterine factors
- Intrauterine contraceptive devices

OVULATION DISORDERS

Ovulation disorders account for approximately 25% of all infertility problems.[3] A careful history will often suggest whether or not an ovulatory problem is likely; women with normal menstrual cycles usually have normal ovulatory cycles. When ovulation disorders are suspected, a full endocrinologic workup is indicated. Even in couples in which the woman is apparently ovulatory, basal body charts and luteal phase progesterone testing may be useful. In these patients, ultrasound studies of follicular development may be helpful for diagnostic confirmation.

Three general etiologic factors are associated with anovulation:

- Failure of the hypothalamus and pituitary to produce hormones stimulating ovulation
- Failure of the follicle to rupture, as is seen in unruptured follicle syndrome or dysfunctional dominant follicle
- Polycystic ovary syndrome (PCOS)

Hypothalamic and Pituitary Causes of Anovulation

If the hypothalamus and pituitary gland cannot produce both luteinizing and follicle-stimulating hormones (Kallmann syndrome), ovulation ceases. Pharmacologic treatment consists of the administration of either gonadotropin-releasing hormone agonist (GnRH-a) or human menopausal gonadotropin (hMG) to induce ovulation. When the dominant follicle reaches 20 mm in diameter, human chorionic gonadotropin (hCG) is administered to trigger ovulation. Sonography is used to monitor follicular development and to help in determining when to add hCG to the therapeutic regimen.

Failure of Ovulation

Another cause of anovulation is *luteinized unruptured follicle* (LUF) *syndrome*. In this condition the follicle enlarges to a normal diameter but fails to rupture and release the oocyte. Sonography is useful in identifying a follicle with thickened walls and hazy, indistinct borders (Figure 15-1). The luteinized unruptured follicle gradually regresses at the time that the normal corpus luteum would regress.

Dysfunctional Follicular Development

In some women, the dominant follicle enlarges much more than a normal dominant follicle does and stays enlarged for a few days, then gradually regresses

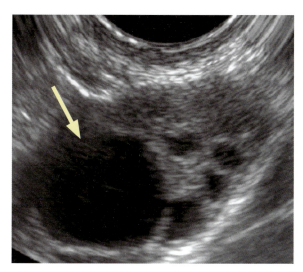

Figure 15-1. Failed ovulation: sagittal section through the ovary at day 18 demonstrating a follicle with thickened walls and hazy and indistinct borders (arrow).

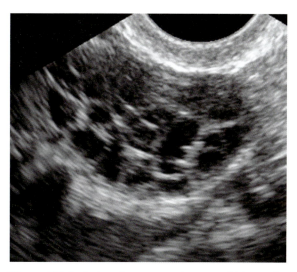

Figure 15-3. Polycystic ovary syndrome: multiple small cystic lesions replacing normal parenchyma and enlarging an ovary.

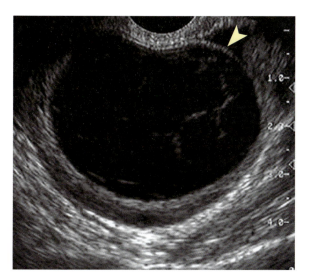

Figure 15-2. Dysfunctional dominant follicle with thin walls (arrowhead).

without follicular rupture. In this condition, the thickening of the follicle wall normally seen in luteinization does not occur. The wall appears thin with a sharp echo from the margin (Figure 15-2). The follicle then regresses in size. The menstrual cycle is not necessarily prolonged, and the degree of menses at the end of the cycle is variable.

Polycystic Ovary Syndrome

Polycystic ovary syndrome (PCOS), also known as *Stein-Leventhal syndrome*, is a common cause of infertility (see Chapter 14, page 388). In PCOS, a single dominant follicle typically does not form. Patients can be treated to induce ovulation; however, the pharmacologic agents increase the risk of inducing ovarian hyperstimulation syndrome, an undesirable sequela. Monitoring ovarian response sonographically is imperative in this patient population (Figure 15-3).

TUBAL FACTORS

Fallopian tubal factors account for approximately 35% of cases of female infertility.[4] Abnormalities of tubal transport and/or mechanical obstruction to the passage of the ovum are the primary causative mechanisms. Transport abnormalities may be caused by damage to the ciliated epithelium that normally moves the ovum through the tube and into the uterine cavity. Sources of epithelial damage include pelvic inflammatory disease, prior ectopic pregnancy, and prior tubal surgery. Transport problems may also be caused by mechanical obstruction to the passage of the ovum. Endometriosis, appendicitis, prior elective abortion, use of intrauterine contraceptive devices (IUDs), or prior tubal surgery may be the etiologic agents.

CERVICAL FACTORS

The cervix plays an important role in the transport and capacitation of sperm after intercourse. Abnormalities of cervical mucus production or the characteristics requisite for normal sperm transport can result in infertility. Factors that affect secretion of cervical mucus include hormonal changes and medications, such as the fertility drug clomiphene citrate (Clomid).

Cervical stenosis—whether congenital or acquired through surgical procedures, infections, radiation therapy, or hypoestrogenism—can cause infertility by mechanically impeding the passage of sperm from the vagina into the uterine cavity.

UTERINE FACTORS

Uterine abnormalities associated with infertility can be broadly categorized as congenital or acquired. Congenital abnormalities of the uterus include the müllerian duct anomalies of the uterus, such as septate uterus, bicornuate uterus, and didelphic uterus. Congenital abnormalities of the uterine cavity induced by diethylstilbestrol (DES) may also result in infertility.

Acquired uterine defects that have a known association with infertility are those that interfere with normal implantation of a conceptus on the endometrium. Endometritis or instrumentation of the uterine cavity may cause scarring and adhesions (Asherman syndrome) that partially or completely obliterate the endometrial lining (Figure 15-4). Uterine polyps and submucosal fibroids are common acquired defects that distort the uterine cavity and compromise blood flow to the endometrium (Figure 15-5).

Other uterine factors related to endometrial pathology include luteal phase deficiency, characterized by inadequate decidualization of the endometrium secondary to failure of the corpus luteum to produce adequate amounts of progesterone; and endometriosis, which can extrinsically compress the fallopian tube or result in internal scarring, both of which impede the normal transport of an ovum.

INTRAUTERINE CONTRACEPTIVE DEVICES

Intrauterine contraceptive devices (IUDs or IUCDs) are methods of contraception that involve the insertion of a foreign body into the central portion of the endometrial cavity. Two types of IUD are available on the American market: the nonhormonal copper device (ParaGard) and the hormone-eluting Mirena device. Nonhormonal IUDs work primarily by interfering with the normal motility and morphology of sperm cells. Copper carries spermicidal properties that prevent sperm cells from traveling through cervical mucus or kill them before they reach the fallopian tube, thus impeding fertilization. Hormonal IUDs release levonorgestrel, a type of progestogen, which thickens cervical mucus, diminishes sperm survival and ability to penetrate the ovum,

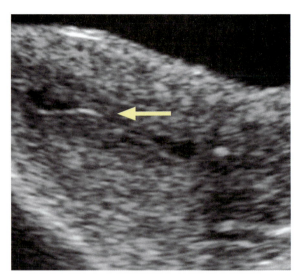

Figure 15-4. Asherman syndrome: sagittal close-up view of the uterine cavity demonstrating an endometrial synechia (arrow). Scarring and adhesions can partially or completely obliterate the endometrial lining, leading to infertility.

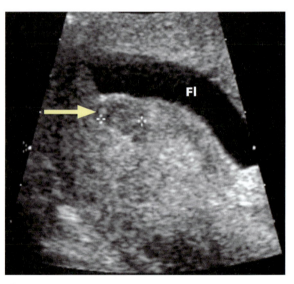

Figure 15-5. Submucosal fibroids: sagittal close-up view of the uterine cavity demonstrating instilled fluid (FI) along with a well-circumscribed fibroid located below the mucosal surface of the uterus (arrow). Fibroids can distort the uterine cavity and compromise blood flow to the endometrium, contributing to infertility.

and suppresses endometrial maturation. These combined mechanisms of action prevent fertilization.

A variety of other types of IUD that sonographers may encounter are available on the world market. Despite their individual geometric configurations, all produce a similar sonographic appearance: the presence of highly echogenic foci within the uterine cavity that cast posterior acoustic shadows and/or create ring-down and comet-tail artifacts (Figures 15-6A–C).

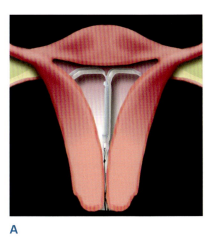
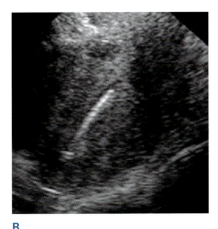
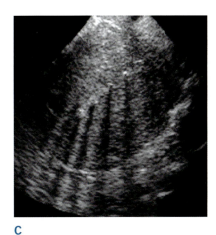

A B C

Figure 15-6. Intrauterine contraceptive devices. **A** Schematic representation of normal placement of the T-shaped ParaGard device within the uterine cavity. **B** Sonographic image of the uterine cavity containing a ParaGard device. **C** Sonogram demonstrating a Lippes loop (an early IUD widely prescribed during the 1960s and still found in some older patients). Both IUDs cast posterior acoustic shadows and/or create ring-down and comet-tail artifacts.

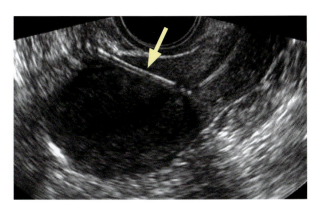

Figure 15-7. Sagittal section demonstrating an IUD (arrow) that has perforated the anterior uterine wall.

The role of sonography in evaluating a patient known to have an IUD is usually to identify its presence and proper location in the central portion of the endometrial cavity. IUDs can spontaneously pass *per vaginam* (through the vagina) or may perforate into and through the uterine wall. Any eccentric position of the device suggests uterine perforation (Figure 15-7).

TREATMENT OF INFERTILITY

A number of treatments may be used to assist infertile couples to become pregnant. Male infertility factors are usually diagnosed and treated by a urologist. Assessment and management of female factors fall within the purview of the ob/gyn practitioner and range from pharmacologic treatment of ovulatory abnormalities to surgical intervention directed at obviating mechanical causes.

PHARMACOLOGIC METHODS

A number of pharmacologic agents are available for the treatment of ovulatory dysfunction. They include clomiphene citrate, human menopausal gonadotropin (hMG), and gonadotropin-releasing hormone agonists (GnRH-a).

Clomiphene Citrate

Clomiphene citrate (sold under the names Clomid, Androxal, and Omifin) is an estrogen analog, which binds to the estrogen receptors in the hypothalamus. With clomiphene binding to the receptors, the feedback of estriol from the ovary is blocked, leading to the increased production of follicle-stimulating hormone by the pituitary gland. Under the influence of clomiphene, multiple follicles begin to form on both ovaries, increasing the likelihood that at least one will reach maturity and result in a successful ovulation.

Adverse effects include ovarian hyperstimulation syndrome (see page 414) and supernumerary pregnancy, in which multiple ova are fertilized that implant in the uterine cavity and/or in an ectopic location concomitantly. Clomiphene is usually contraindicated in patients with underlying medical disease, endometriosis, polycystic ovary syndrome, and/or uterine fibroids.

Human Menopausal Gonadotropin

Human menopausal gonadotropin (hMG) or menotropin (brand names Menopur, Pergonal, Repronex, and Humegon) contains follicle-stimulating (FSH) and

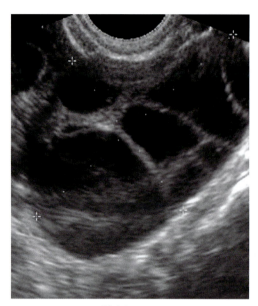
Right ovary

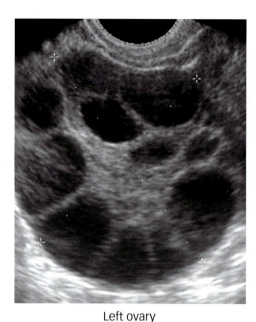
Left ovary

Figure 15-8. Ovarian hyperstimulation syndrome. Endovaginal imaging through both ovaries reveals the presence of bilateral multiple, large cystic areas.

luteinizing hormones (LH), which stimulate ovulation when a woman's ovaries can produce a follicle but hormonal stimulation is deficient. Adverse effects and contraindications are similar to those associated with clomiphene.

Gonadotropin-Releasing Hormone Agonists

Gonadotropin-releasing hormone agonists (GnRH–a) are synthetic analogs of gonadotropin-releasing hormone that stimulate the release of follicle-stimulating hormone (FSH) and luteinizing hormone (LH) by the pituitary gland. The expected response, as with the other pharmacologic treatment regimens, is the development and maturation of multiple follicles, increasing the likelihood that ovulation will occur.

Complications of Pharmacologic Methods

Ovarian hyperstimulation syndrome (OHSS) is a complication of pharmacologically induced follicular stimulation treatment. The syndrome consists of massive bilateral ovarian cystic enlargement accompanied by extravascular fluid accumulation in the peritoneal, pleural, and pericardial cavities. Risk factors for developing ovarian hyperstimulation syndrome include preexisting polycystic ovaries, low body weight, and long ovulation induction cycles.[5] Clinically the syndrome may be mild, moderate, or severe, depending on the extent or volume of fluid exudate and associated sequelae, which include hypotension, oliguria, electrolyte abnormalities, hemoconcentration, thromboembolic complications, and ovarian torsion. Rarely, ovarian hyperstimulation syndrome may occur spontaneously in response to pregnancy or as a sporadic genetic manifestation.

Sonographic Signs

The following sonographic signs are associated with ovarian hyperstimulation syndrome:

- Bilateral cystic symmetric enlargement of ovaries (Figure 15-8).
- Variably sized cysts.
- Radial arrangement of cystic areas around the ovary ("spoke-wheel" sign).
- Ascites, pleural, and/or pericardial fluid may be identified.

ASSISTED REPRODUCTIVE TECHNOLOGIES

Assisted reproductive technologies (ARTs) are methods of achieving pregnancy by artificial means, i.e., bypassing the natural method of conception through sexual intercourse. Fertilization may be induced outside the body (by means of in vitro fertilization) or inside the body (via gamete intrafallopian transfer). All methods involve the acquisition of gametes (sperm and ova) and their manipulation to achieve fertilization and implantation using microscopic technological methods.

In Vitro Fertilization

In vitro fertilization (IVF) is the method of inducing fertilization to occur outside the body (the Latin *in vitro* means "in glass"—e.g., in a test tube or Petri dish). In vitro fertilization is indicated when there are mechanical impediments to normal *in vivo* ("in the body") fertilization, such as irreversible tubal occlusion, endometriosis, fertilization defects, or male-factor infertility.

The typical IVF protocol involves stimulation of ovarian follicles with a pharmacologic agent such as Clomid or Pergonal. Endovaginal ultrasound is used to monitor the growth and development of the follicles, and when the three largest follicles reach 1.6–1.8 cm in diameter and estradiol levels are satisfactory, human chorionic gonadotropin is given to induce maturation. When mature, the oocytes can be aspirated from the follicles under direct sonographic visualization, mixed with sperm in a lab dish, and incubated until the conceptus has reached the 6- to 8-cell stage, usually three days after retrieval. Other protocols wait until the conceptus has reached the blastocyst stage, at around five days, before implanting a suitable number of embryos in the uterine cavity. Typically, two to four embryos are inserted into the uterus and placed near the fundus. If necessary, the embryos may be inserted into the uterus under direct ultrasound visualization.

Gamete Intrafallopian Transfer

In *gamete intrafallopian transfer* (GIFT), oocytes are aspirated from stimulated follicles and immediately placed into the fallopian tube along with viable sperm under laparoscopic visualization. The gametes are inserted into the fallopian tube from the abdominal approach through the fimbriated end of the tube. This procedure is used in women who have at least one functional fallopian tube and evidence of cervical disorders and in couples with unexplained infertility. In some cases, the gamete intrafallopian transfer procedure may be performed under ultrasound visualization rather than laparoscopically.

Zygote Intrafallopian Transfer

Zygote intrafallopian transfer (ZIFT) is a variant of in vitro fertilization in which the oocytes are retrieved endovaginally, fertilized in vitro, and then inserted into the fallopian tube either laparoscopically or through a transcervical tube. ZIFT implantation is performed 1 day post fertilization (rather than 3–5 days post fertilization, as is the practice in standard methods of in vitro fertilization). As with gamete intrafallopian transfer, successful zygote intrafallopian transfer requires the presence of at least one patent and functional fallopian tube.

SONOGRAPHY IN THE MANAGEMENT OF INFERTILITY

Ultrasound can aid in the diagnosis and treatment of infertility in a number of ways (see Chapter 13, "Follicular Phase," pages 364–365). Sonography can be used diagnostically to monitor the ovulatory cycle to identify abnormalities of the ovulatory process. Although hysterosalpingography with radiographic contrast is the traditional method used to evaluate tubal disease, sonography can also be used to establish tubal patency. Fluid or a contrast agent is injected into the intrauterine cavity and fallopian tubes to evaluate tubal patency. Abnormalities of endometrial maturation, uterine anomalies, and uterine fibroids can also be evaluated sonographically.

As a part of treatment for infertility, sonography can be used to follow the development of the ovarian follicles before harvesting of ova, and it can be used as a part of the procedure for inserting fertilized or unfertilized ova into the fallopian tube or uterine cavity.

Indications for sonography in infertility include:

- Follicular monitoring
- Assessment of endometrial development
- Assessment of tubal patency
- Guided follicular aspiration

FOLLICULAR MONITORING

Sonographic monitoring of ovarian follicles has become standard practice in patients undergoing infertility workup and treatment. Endovaginal B-mode imaging permits a noninvasive, quick, and accurate means of determining number, size, and position of the follicles present during each cycle and identifying clinically applicable parameters of follicular quality. Sequential studies are useful in monitoring the growth of individual follicles, and the growth patterns have a prognostic value in determining the outcome of assisted reproduction methods. Doppler methods have been studied extensively, particularly using 3D color and power Doppler measurement of flow index (FI), vascularization index (VI), and vascularization flow index (VFI) in the ovarian stromata. To date there has been poor correlation between these methods and prediction of successful oocyte retrieval or conception implantation; as a rule of thumb, however, increasing perfusion to developing follicles is an encouraging finding.[6]

Sonographic Methods

Several sonograms are obtained around the expected time of ovulation to determine which ovary will produce the dominant follicle. The dominant follicle produces the ovum for that cycle and generally measures 1.8–2.5 cm just before rupture.

Sonography may also be used to monitor follicular development when clomiphene citrate, human menopausal gonadotropin, or gonadotropin-releasing hormone agonists are being used. One of the objectives of the monitoring is to determine whether too many follicles are being stimulated and whether ovarian hyperstimulation syndrome (OHS) is developing. (See "Pharmacologic Methods" on pages 413–414.)

Transabdominal imaging of pelvic structures should be performed on the patient's first visit to identify any anatomic abnormalities or pathology that may be apparent with endovaginal scanning. Endovaginal methods are standard practice for obtaining the following information:

Baseline scan:

- Uterus: size, shape, echogenicity, presence or absence of pathology (fibroids, polyps, etc.)
- Endometrium: measurements of maximum thickness
- Ovaries: size, shape, presence or absence of pathology
- Follicles: number of antral (secondary) follicles in each ovary

Follicular monitoring:

- Endometrium: measurements of maximum thickness
- Follicles: systematic measurement of each follicle in two dimensions

Indices of Growth

Several sonographic follicular growth indices have been devised that aid in a more accurate prediction of the occurrence of ovulation:[7]

- Secondary antral follicles > 2 mm are the first follicular structures that may be visualized (Figure 15-9).
- The number of follicles present in an ovary has clinical importance in estimating ovarian age and in predicting its response to pharmacologic ovarian stimulation.
- A dominant ovulatory follicle (i.e., dominant antral follicle) can be identified between days 5 and 7 of the cycle and will continue to grow by 2 mm per day.

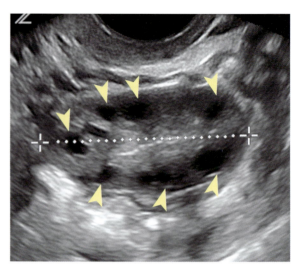

Figure 15-9. Long-axis image through an ovary (dotted line) demonstrating secondary antral follicles (arrowheads) arrayed around the periphery.

- Follicular growth patterns influence pharmacologic treatment protocols. Growth patterns are different in stimulated versus nonstimulated follicles.
- Sonographic characteristics of antral follicles include:
  - Size (largest diameter)
  - Shape (round, oval, rectangular, triangular)
  - Anechoic/hypoechoic appearance
  - Edge quality (smooth, intermediate, rough)
- *Ovulatory follicles*—those antral follicles that will eventually ovulate—are characterized by their larger size, round shape, smooth edges, and anechoic/hypoechoic appearance (Figure 15-10).
- *Nondominant* (also called *subdominant*) *follicles* are antral follicles that will not ovulate; they are characterized by smaller size, irregular shape, rough edges, and anechoic/hypoechoic appearance (Figure 15-11).

Indices of Ovulation

The greatest change in follicular appearance occurs in the last seven days preceding ovulation, caused by an increase in size and granulosa cell thickness and increased perifollicular vascularization in the thecal layer. Ovulation is further characterized by:[8]

- Sudden decrease in follicle size
- Irregularity of follicle walls (Figure 15-12)
- Free fluid in the posterior cul-de-sac (Figure 15-13)
- No difference between mean blood flow to a dominant follicle and flow to a nondominant follicle[9]

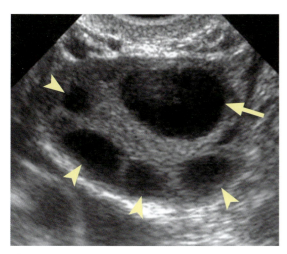

Figure 15-10. Ovulatory follicle (arrow) is characterized by its larger size in comparison with the adjacent nondominant follicles (arrowheads) that appear in this endovaginal image.

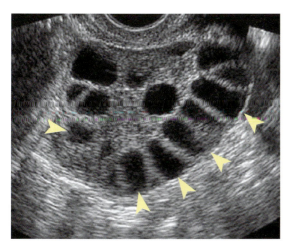

Figure 15-11. Subdominant follicles (arrowheads) are characterized by smaller size, irregular shape, rough edges, and decreased echogenicity.

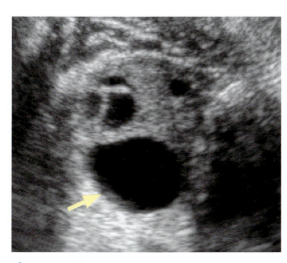

Figure 15-12. Sonographic indices of ovulation: irregularity of follicle walls (arrow).

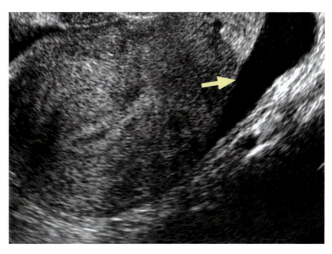

Figure 15-13. Sonographic indices of ovulation: free fluid in the posterior cul-de-sac (arrow).

Stimulated Cycles

Sonographic criteria for determining response to ovulation induction and predicting positive outcomes in patients undergoing pharmacologic treatment for ovulatory dysfunction include:

- Measurement of ovarian volume: >3 cc is associated with a higher conception rate.[10]
- Number of antral follicles present: The total number of small antral follicles in both ovaries is the most important predictive parameter of cycle outcome.[11]

ENDOMETRIAL ASSESSMENT

Normal endometrial development is critical for successful pregnancy. If the endometrium is too thin at the time of ovulation or if the endometrium does not develop in synchrony with ovulation, implantation may be impeded. Traditionally, endometrial assessment has been performed with biopsy; however, invasive methods are not acceptable in infertility patients because of the potential damage to the endometrium. Therefore, endometrial assessment should be performed prior to implantation using a noninvasive method.

Sonographic evaluation is ideally suited for this application, particularly using 3D endovaginal ultrasound methods. Several parameters have been proposed for assessing endometrial receptivity, including endometrial thickness (Figure 15-14), endometrial echotexture, endometrial and subendometrial blood flow (Figure 15-15), and endometrial volume. These parameters may identify patients with low implantation potential.

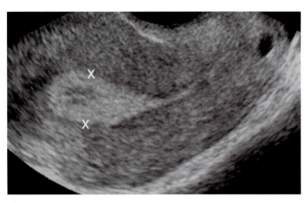

Figure 15-14. Endovaginal sonographic assessment of the endometrium, measuring its thickness (cursors). Note the hyperechoic, relatively homogeneous appearance of the endometrium.

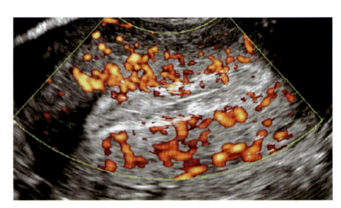

Figure 15-15. Doppler evaluation of subendometrial blood flow using, in this case, power Doppler imaging.

However, their positive predictive value is low, and there is little agreement on interpretation of absolute values obtained with sonography alone.[12,13]

Endometrial (or *uterine*) *volumetric measurements* are done using 3D volume data sets acquired with an endovaginal ultrasound probe. The endometrium is identified with traditional 2D imaging and centered within the volumetric cursor box. A data volume set is captured via an automatic sweep through the region of interest and stored in memory. Rotation and translation of the data volume set permit accurate display and measurement of the endometrium in coronal, sagittal, and axial planes. Various algorithms may be used to calculate volume from these three linear data sets (Figures 15-16A–D).

TUBAL PATENCY

Normally, the fallopian tubes are not accessible to ultrasound evaluation, unless their diameter is increased by a pathologic process, such as hydrosalpinx, pyosalpinx,

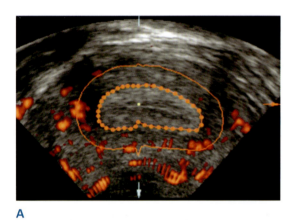

A

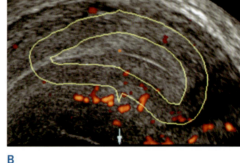

B

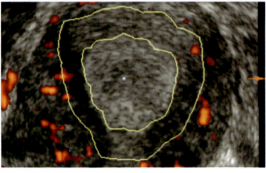

C

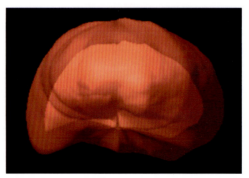

D

Figure 15-16. Endometrial volumetric measurements. Rotation and translation of the volume data set permit accurate display and measurement of the endometrium in all three sectional planes: **A** Axial. **B** Sagittal. **C** Coronal. **D** From these three data sets, various algorithms may be used to calculate endometrial volume.

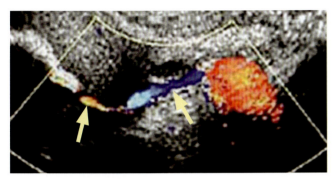

Figure 15-17. Tubal patency (arrows) is demonstrated with color Doppler imaging used in conjunction with a sonographic contrast agent instilled into the uterine cavity.

ectopic pregnancy, tubal carcinoma, or torsion. Standard diagnostic methods for assessing tubal patency include radiographic hysterosonography and laparoscopy.

A more recent addition to the diagnostic armamentarium is *hysterosalpingo contrast sonography* (HyCoSy), a procedure that involves the introduction of a fluid into the uterine cavity and the fallopian tubes. Sterile saline is used as an echo-free contrast medium for the assessment of the uterine cavity. For the examination of the fallopian tubes, color Doppler imaging in conjunction with a positive contrast medium is used, such as air-filled albumin microbubbles or galactose with micro air bubbles. Spillage of contrast into the peritoneal cavity is seen when the tubes are patent (Figure 15-17); absence of spillage suggests tubal occlusion.

GUIDED FOLLICULAR ASPIRATION

Guided follicular aspiration, also referred to as *transvaginal oocyte retrieval*, is a method of removing oocytes from the ovary for in vitro fertilization. In this procedure—usually used in conjunction with pharmacologically stimulated cycles—a needle is inserted into an ovarian follicle under ultrasound guidance (Figure 15-18). A needle guide is attached to an endovaginal transducer, the apparatus is inserted into the vagina, and the target follicle is identified. The needle is passed into the follicle and, using gentle negative pressure, the contents are aspirated. It is not unusual to retrieve multiple oocytes during a single session.

CHAPTER 15 REVIEW QUESTIONS

1. Infertility is defined as the inability to conceive a child after how many months of unprotected intercourse?
   A. 3 months
   B. 6 months
   C. 12 months
   D. 18 months

2. In an infertility patient, when can the dominant ovarian follicle be identified sonographically?
   A. Days 3–5
   B. Days 5–7
   C. Days 7–9
   D. Days 9–10

3. In an infertility patient, what is the growth rate of the dominant ovarian follicle?
   A. 2 mm/day
   B. 3 mm/day
   C. 4 mm/day
   D. 5 mm/day

4. All of the following are sonographic signs of ovarian hyperstimulation syndrome EXCEPT:
   A. Unilateral cystic enlargement of an ovary
   B. Variably sized cysts
   C. Ascites
   D. Pleural effusion

5. In an infertility patient, ovarian volume associated with a higher conception rate typically measures:
   A. > 1 cc
   B. > 2 cc
   C. > 3 cc
   D. > 4 cc

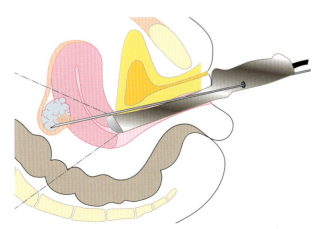

Figure 15-18. Schematic representation of ultrasound-guided follicular aspiration.

6. All of the following sonographic variables are important findings in the evaluation of an infertility patient EXCEPT:
   A. Endometrial thickness
   B. Endometrial volume
   C. Myometrial thickness
   D. Subendometrial blood flow

ANSWERS

See Appendix A on page 483 for answers.

REFERENCES

1. Data vary across time and populations. See National Survey of Family Growth, Centers for Disease Control and Prevention, 2006-2010. Available at http://www.cdc.gov/nchs/nsfg.htm.
2. Koulianos G, Gill KA: Infertility. In Gill KA: *Ultrasound in Obstetrics and Gynecology: A Practitioner's Guide*. Pasadena, Davies Publishing, 2014, p 394.
3. Mayo Clinic: Female infertility. Available at http://www.mayoclinic.org/diseases-conditions/female-infertility/basics/causes/con-20033618.
4. Yen SSC, Jaffe RB, Barbieri RL: *Reproductive Endocrinology*, 4th edition. Philadelphia, Saunders, 1999.
5. Danninger B, Brunner M, Obruca A, et al: Prediction of ovarian hyperstimulation syndrome by ultrasound volumetric assessment [corrected] of baseline ovarian volume prior to stimulation. Hum Reprod 11:1597–1599, 1996.
6. Kupesic S, Kurjak A: Uterine and ovarian perfusion during the periovulatory period assessed by transvaginal color Doppler. Fertil Steril 60:439–443, 1993.
7. Vlaisavljević V, Došen M: Clinical applications of ultrasound in assessment of follicle development and growth. Donald School J Ultrasound Obstet Gynecol 1:50–63, 2007.
8. Ecochard R, Marret H, Rabilloud M, et al: Sensitivity and specificity of ultrasound indices of ovulation in spontaneous cycles. Eur J Obstet Gynecol Reprod Biol 91:59–64, 2000.
9. Järvelä IY, Sladkevicius P, Kelly S, et al: Three-dimensional sonographic and power Doppler characterization of ovaries in late follicular phase. Ultrasound Obstet Gynecol 20:281–285, 2002.
10. Kupesic S, Kurjak A: Uterine and ovarian perfusion during the periovulatory period assessed by transvaginal color Doppler. Fertil Steril 60:439–443, 1993.
11. Vlaisavljević V, Došen M: Clinical applications of ultrasound in assessment of follicle development and growth. Donald School J Ultrasound Obstet Gynecol 1:50–63, 2007.
12. Alcázar JL: Three-dimensional ultrasound assessment of endometrial receptivity: a review. Repro Biol Endocinol 4:56, 2006.
13. Yaman C, Ebner T, Sommergruber M, et al: Three-dimensional endometrial volume estimation as a predictor of pituitary down-regulation in an IVF-embryo transfer programme. Hum Reprod 15:1698–1702, 2000.

SUGGESTED READINGS

Feigin K, Rosenblatt R, Kutcher R, et al: Sonohysterography in the evaluation of infertility. Applied Radiology 29:4–20, 2000.

Fleischer AC, Herzog J, Vasquez JM, et al: Transvaginal sonography scanning in gynecologic infertility. In Fleischer AC, Toy EC, Lee W, et al: *Sonography in Obstetrics and Gynecology: Principles and Practice*, 7th edition. New York, McGraw-Hill, 2011.

Frates MC: Infertility. In Benson CB, Arger PH, Bluth EI: *Ultrasonography in Obstetrics and Gynecology: A Practical Approach*. New York, Thieme, 2007, pp 39–49.

Koulianos G, Gill KA: Infertility. In Gill KA: *Ultrasound in Obstetrics and Gynecology: A Practitioner's Guide*. Pasadena, Davies Publishing, 2014, 393–410.

Mitchell A, Trampe B, Lebovic D: The role of ultrasound in evaluating female infertility. In Hagen-Ansert SL (ed): *Textbook of Diagnostic Sonography*, 7th edition. St. Louis, Elsevier, 2012, pp 1039–1046.

Pierson RA: Ultrasonographic imaging in infertility. In Callen PW (ed): *Ultrasonography in Obstetrics and Gynecology*, 5th edition. Philadelphia, Saunders Elsevier, 2008, pp 986–1019.

CHAPTER 16
Pediatric and Postmenopausal Gynecologic Sonography

Pediatric Sonography

Postmenopausal Sonography

Sonographic evaluation of the pediatric and postmenopausal pelvis, while pertaining to patients at disparate ends of the chronological spectrum, carries certain similarities that differentiate it from studies of women during the childbearing years. First, the internal organs of reproduction—i.e., the uterus and ovaries—are physically smaller than those found in women during the reproductively active years. Second, examination techniques are limited, in many cases, to transabdominal imaging via the full urinary bladder. The use of intracavitary probes is contraindicated in virginal pediatric patients and is frequently not well tolerated by postmenopausal patients, particularly those with vaginal atrophy. Finally, the spectrum of pathologic possibilities is lessened in these two subsets of patients, whose endocrinologic status—the dearth or complete absence of gonadotropic hormones—precludes, in all but the rarest of cases, many abnormalities almost exclusively found in women of childbearing ages.

PEDIATRIC SONOGRAPHY

ANATOMY AND PHYSIOLOGY

The anatomic appearance of the pediatric pelvis is different from that of the postmenarcheal adult pelvis, and it changes as pediatric life progresses from the neonatal period to puberty to adulthood.

The Pediatric Uterus

The *neonatal* uterus (immediately after birth), responding to in utero maternal and placental hormonal stimulation, appears more prominent and adult-like in configuration than the premenarcheal pediatric uterus. Neonatal uterine length is approximately 3.5 cm, with a typical anteroposterior (AP) diameter of approximately 1.4 cm. The endometrial lining is often echogenic, with trace amounts of fluid identified within the endometrial cavity (Figure 16-1).

As the hormonal effects dissipate within the first few months of life, the uterus assumes its more typical *premenarcheal* appearance, during which the cervix is about twice the size of the uterus, creating a fundal:cervical ratio of 1:2. The configuration of the neonatal uterus is also more tubular than the classic pear-shaped contour of a postmenarcheal uterus. The endometrium is normally not apparent; however, high-frequency transducers can demonstrate the central lining in some cases. While the uterine length at birth is about 3.5 cm, it regresses to about 3.2 cm by age 2; the AP diameter typically does not exceed 1.4 cm (Figure 16-2).

The *postmenarcheal* uterus assumes an adult configuration and relative size. Under the influence of the endocrine hormones secreted during menarche, the uterus grows to twice the size of the cervix, raising the fundal:cervical ratio to between 2:1 and 3:1 (Figure 16-3). Dimensional measurements include a length in the range of 5–9 cm, an anteroposterior diameter of approximately 3.2 cm at menarche (increasing to about 4.0 during the reproductive years), and a transverse measurement of roughly 4–5 cm. The endometrial lining is seen and varies with the phases of the menstrual cycle.[1] Approximate uterine length and AP diameter during the pediatric period are summarized in Table 16-1.

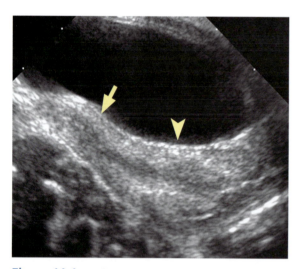

Figure 16-1. Sagittal section through a full bladder demonstrating the neonatal uterus (arrow) at approximately 4 weeks. Arrowhead = cervix.

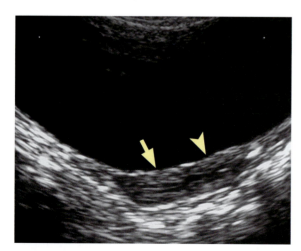

Figure 16-2. Sagittal section through a full bladder demonstrating the premenarcheal uterus (arrow) in a 6-year-old. Arrowhead = cervix. Note the tubular shape of the uterus.

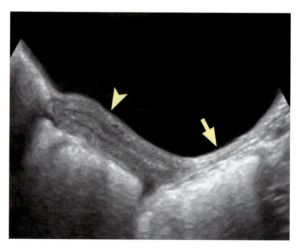

Figure 16-3. Sagittal section through a full bladder demonstrating the postmenarcheal uterus in a 12-year-old. The relational length between the cervix (arrow) and the uterine body (arrowhead) begins to assume a more adult appearance.

Pediatric Ovaries

Like the uterus, the ovaries vary in size and sonographic appearance during the pediatric period. Neonatal ovaries are slightly enlarged as a result of in utero stimulation by maternal and placental hormones, and the presence of small cysts is not an uncommon finding. From birth to approximately 1 year of age, an ovarian volume of ≥1.0 cc is expected. From 1 to 6 years, volume decreases slightly as the effects of prenatal hormone stimulation subside, typically yielding a measurement of ≤1.0 cc. From 6 years to menarche ovarian volume rises to 2–4 cc and, under the influence of pubertal hormones, reaches 8–10 cc in the postmenarcheal state. These values are summarized in Table 16-2.

Ovarian size is best assessed using volume measurements based on the traditional formula for a prolate ellipsoid (i.e., spheroid): length × width × anteroposterior diameter × 0.52. As a rule of thumb, in the prepubertal (premenarcheal) girl, uterine measurements of 4 cm length and 1.0 cm in anteroposterior diameter, along with an ovarian volume of about 4 cc, are useful benchmarks.

PEDIATRIC GYNECOLOGIC PATHOLOGY

The primary clinical indications for sonographic studies of the pediatric pelvis include:

- A palpable pelvic mass
- Amenorrhea
- Ovarian torsion
- Ambiguous genitalia
- Precocious puberty

Palpable Pelvic Masses

In the pediatric patient pelvic masses, as a rule, are rare. However, when one is present the most likely pathologic candidates include the following:

Ovarian Masses
- Physiologic cysts
- Germ cell tumors
- Ovarian torsion

Uterine Masses
- Hydrometrocolpos
- Uterine tumors (rare)

Vaginal Masses
- Sarcoma botryoides
- Vaginal rhabdomyosarcoma

Table 16-1. Mean pediatric uterine size.

Age Group	Length (cm)	AP Diameter (cm)
Neonatal	3.5	1.4
Premenarcheal	2.5–4	1.1
Postmenarcheal	5–9	3–4

Table 16-2. Mean pediatric ovarian volume.

Age Group	Volume (cc)
Neonatal	≥1.0
1–6 years	≤1.0
6 years–menarche	2–4
Postmenarcheal	8–10

Ovarian Masses

In general, solid and complex ovarian masses are not common in adolescent girls. No specific symptom or physical examination finding is pathognomonic for an ovarian mass or can distinguish a benign from a malignant one. Pregnancy should be excluded in any patient presenting with lower abdominal pain for whom there is suspicion of sexual activity. Ultrasound is the mainstay for diagnosis of an ovarian mass, with concomitant laboratory tests for those patients who display signs of androgenism or irregular menses or who appear ill.

Fortunately, most solid and complex ovarian masses in adolescents are benign; only 10% of ovarian lesions in adolescents are cancerous.[2] Many of the benign pelvic masses found in adult women also occur in the pediatric patient. The most common types of ovarian pathology identified in the pediatric patient include ovarian cysts and various types of germ cell tumors.

Ovarian Cysts

Physiologic/functional ovarian cysts (i.e., those that secrete hormones) consist of follicular, corpus luteum, and theca-lutein cysts; these cysts are quite common in adolescents. Presentation can vary, ranging from complaints of menstrual irregularity and pelvic pain to

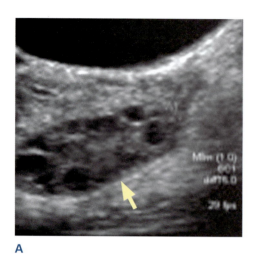
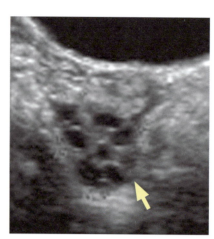

Figure 16-4. Physiologic ovarian cysts in **A** sagittal and **B** transverse sections. Arrows = enlarged ovary with multiple follicular cysts.

discovery upon palpation during a pelvic examination to an incidental finding on imaging. Compression of adjacent structures caused by a large cyst results in alteration of other organ systems and may be noted during review of systems (Figures 16-4A and B).

Germ Cell Tumors

Germ cell tumors find their origin in ectopically located embryonic cells that fail to migrate from the yolk sac to the primitive gonad. While they may arise at a wide variety of sites throughout the body, they are relatively common types of ovarian neoplasms in young girls. As a rule of thumb, cystic germ cell tumors are more likely to be benign, and solid masses tend to be malignant; however, the final diagnosis must be made histologically. Specific types of tumors include:

- *Teratomas:* These tumors contain cells from all three germ cell layers and may be benign or malignant. Mature cystic teratomas, also known as dermoid cysts, are the most common of germ cell tumors in adolescents. They account for one-third of pediatric ovarian neoplasms.[3]
- *Dysgerminomas:* Usually presenting as a solid ovarian mass, dysgerminomas are the most common malignant tumors in female patients aged 15 to 19 years.[4]
- *Endodermal sinus* or *yolk sac tumors:* These aggressive ovarian neoplasms represent the most common ovarian malignancy in children.
- *Choriocarcinomas:* These ovarian tumors are very rare but often aggressively malignant in infants. A common etiology is the spread of malignant chorionic cells from the placenta to the fetus in utero.
- *Embryonal carcinomas:* These mixed tumors contain both malignant and benign histologic components with metastatic potential.

Sonographic Signs

The sonographic signs associated with pediatric ovarian tumors vary widely, depending on the histologic nature of the mass. They may be predominantly cystic, solid, or complex in appearance.

Ovarian Torsion

Ovarian torsion is the twisting of the ovary and part of the fallopian tube along its ligamentous pedicle. Strangulation of the supporting vascular structures puts the ovary at risk of acute ischemia, creating a gynecologic surgical emergency. Unless the ovary is detorsed, ovarian loss is imminent. Ovarian torsion is an infrequent diagnosis in the pediatric age group, with an incidence of 4.9 per 100,000 girls aged 1–20 years; however, outcomes in this age group are poor, with ovarian loss reported in 60% of cases.[5] The clinical picture is nonspecific, and because children cannot always articulate their symptoms the diagnosis is often a challenge.

Sonographic Signs

The characteristic sonographic signs associated with ovarian torsion in the pediatric patient are similar to those found later in life and include:

- Enlarged, hypoechoic ovary
- Peripherally displaced follicles
- Free fluid in the pelvis
- Doppler demonstrating the absence of arterial and venous flow in ovarian parenchyma

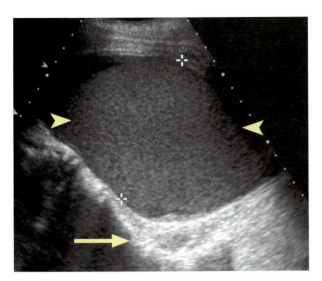

Figure 16-5. Hematometrocolpos. Arrowheads = whole blood filling the endometrial cavity. Note the pronounced posterior acoustic enhancement (arrow).

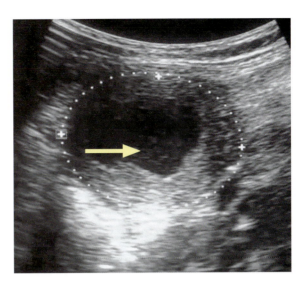

Figure 16-6. Hematometrocolpos. Arrow = thrombotic debris within a degenerating larger thrombus inside the uterine cavity.

Uterine Masses

Like their ovarian counterparts, uterine neoplastic masses are rare in the pediatric patient. The most common cause of a palpably enlarged uterus, particularly during menarche, is distention of the uterine cavity by retained menstrual products and fluid in a girl with an obstructed outflow tract.

Hematometrocolpos

Hematometrocolpos is the presence of blood in the uterine and vaginal cavities. Any type of outflow obstruction will cause blood to back up into and distend the cavities. Complete (imperforate) hymen and congenital uterovaginal obstructions such as transverse vaginal septum, cervical dysgenesis, vaginal atresia, and some müllerian duct variants may mechanically impede normal outflow.

As blood accumulates in the vaginal and uterine cavities, it assumes a range of sonographic appearances as its physical characteristics change from those of fresh whole blood to thrombus to lysed blood byproducts. Homogeneous, low-level echogenic fluid demonstrating pronounced posterior acoustic enhancement is the typical appearance of whole blood (Figure 16-5). Thrombus formation, when present, will produce focal solid areas within the larger fluid collection that metamorphose from homogeneous, soft-appearing fresh clot to heterogeneous, complex organized or degenerating clot (Figure 16-6). As blood remains confined for a period of time, it breaks down into serosanguinous

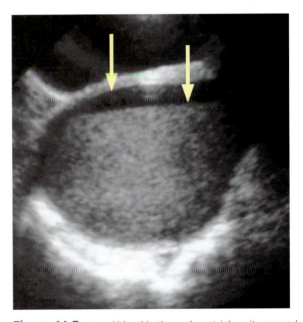

Figure 16-7. Lysed blood in the endometrial cavity secondary to hematometrocolpos. Arrows = fluid-fluid level caused by serosanguinous byproducts.

byproducts that may create the classic fluid-fluid level sonographic appearance (Figure 16-7).

Sonographic Signs

The following are the characteristic sonographic signs associated with hematometrocolpos:

- Distention of uterine and vaginal cavities with fluid
- Posterior acoustic enhancement
- Variable internal echotexture

Uterine Tumors

Neoplastic masses of the uterus are extremely rare in pediatric patients. Fibroids and diffuse myomatous changes in the myometrium have been reported in adolescents, but the incidence is exceptionally uncommon.

Vaginal Masses

Vaginal tumors are also extremely rare in the pediatric population. However, early recognition is necessary to prevent the high levels of morbidity and mortality associated with them.

Sarcoma Botryoides

Sarcoma botryoides is a type of embryonal rhabdomyosarcoma found in the walls of hollow, mucosa-lined structures such as the vagina. The term *botryoides* refers to the fact that this type of mass typically is botryoid, i.e., shaped like a bunch of grapes. The presenting symptoms may be vaginal bleeding and/or a firm, grape-like mass protruding from the vaginal introitus in girls between birth and 15 years of age (Figures 16-8A and B).

Vaginal Rhabdomyosarcoma

Similar to sarcoma botryoides, *vaginal rhabdomyosarcoma* is almost exclusively found in very young children. Sonographically, a vaginal rhabdomyosarcoma appears as a large, solid, heterogeneous or hypoechoic mass posterior to the urinary bladder.

Gartner's Duct Cysts

Gartner's duct cysts, which result from the incomplete disappearance of the mesonephric duct in female embryos, are uncommon and extremely rare findings in neonates, children, and adolescents. There is, however, a slightly increased probability of identifying such a cystic mass along the lateral or anterolateral wall of the vagina in individuals with concomitant genitourinary anatomic anomalies. The characteristic sonographic sign of a Gartner's duct cyst is a cyst located along the anterior or anterolateral wall of the vagina.

Gonadal Dysgenesis

Gonadal dysgenesis refers to a spectrum of abnormalities characterized by severely hypoplastic and dysfunctional gonads that are replaced mostly by fibrous tissue. The cause is posited to be a progressive loss of primordial germ cells on the developing embryonic gonads. The subsequent absence of gonadal hormones prevents the development of secondary sexual characteristics and results in infertility. Gonadal dysgenesis is associated with Turner and several other rare syndromes.

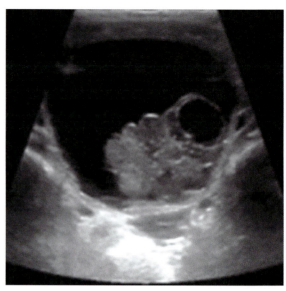

A

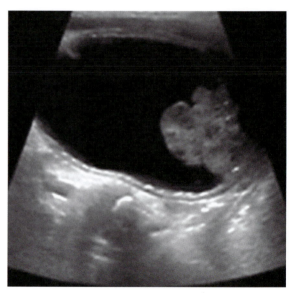

B

Figure 16-8. A rare presentation of sarcoma botryoides in **A** transverse and **B** sagittal sections, with the tumor arising from the bladder wall.

Sexual Ambiguity (Intersex State)

Sexual ambiguity, also known as *intersex state*, is characterized by chromosomal, gonadal, or genital anatomic variations that preclude the identification of an individual as distinctly male or female. There are several manifestations of intersex state, which include true hermaphroditism, ambiguous genitalia, and testicular feminization syndrome.

True Hermaphroditism

True hermaphroditism is a very rare cause of sexual ambiguity. In these individuals, there is a mosaicism, with some cells containing XX sex chromosomes and others containing XY chromosomes. These individuals often have ambiguous genitalia but with both functional ovarian and functional testicular tissue in some arrangement. On microscopic examination of the gonads, evidence of both sperm and ova production is present.

Ambiguous Genitalia

Ambiguous genitalia may be variable in appearance. In males, the scrotum may be bifid and the penis may be small or malformed. In females, the clitoris may be large and the labia may be fused. In females with a 46,XX karyotype, this condition is usually called *female pseudohermaphroditism*, and if the individual is 46,XY, the condition is labeled *male pseudohermaphroditism*. The most common cause of female pseudohermaphroditism is *congenital adrenal hyperplasia*. This condition is associated with genetic defects in the enzymes that produce the sex hormones. In females it results in male appearing genitalia. The genitalia may be ambiguous or may closely resemble normal male genitalia. In males, this condition may lead to precocious puberty. Male pseudohermaphroditism describes a condition in which a genetically determined male presents with female external genitalia and notable absence of male genitalia. Common causes include inadequate testosterone production by defective embryonic testes and androgen resistance, which blocks the action of testosterone on the developing external genitalia. A number of other steroid enzyme defects may also lead to ambiguous genitalia in both males and females.

Testicular Feminization

Testicular feminization syndrome, also known as *androgen insensitivity syndrome* (AIS), results from gonadal resistance to androgenic hormones, particularly testosterone. Affected individuals appear to be normal females externally but have 46,XY chromosomes. Internally, the vagina ends in a blind pouch without connecting to the uterus. The uterus and fallopian tubes are absent or rudimentary, and the testicles remain undescended.

Precocious Puberty

Precocious puberty is defined as complete secondary sexual development (including menarche in girls) at an early age. It differs from *early puberty* in that, while early puberty is associated with development of secondary sexual characteristics in the absence of medical anomalies, precocious puberty is usually associated with medical abnormalities that stimulate the premature release of sex hormones.

Although precocious puberty is not uncommon, a chronological definition is hard to pin down; however, a rule of thumb for medical purposes considers onset before 8 years for girls and 9 years for boys as a guide for further diagnostic evaluation. Precocious puberty is categorized as either true precocious puberty or precocious pseudopuberty.

True Precocious Puberty

The etiology of *true precocious puberty* is not fully understood, although there is a familial association and it occurs more commonly in obese children. Girls develop secondary sexual characteristics as well as changes in the uterus and ovaries normally associated with menarche as early as age 7 (range 7–13 years). Ovarian volume increases to 1 cc or greater and functional cysts may be present. The uterus enlarges to 4–5 cm in length and assumes a fundal:cervical ratio consistent with pubertal changes. Boys initially exhibit testicular enlargement with subsequent development of other secondary sexual characteristics as early as age 10 (range 10–13 years). Both genders experience the growth spurts typically associated with pubertal development, and the emotional and psychological impact on the individual can be significant.

Precocious Pseudopuberty

In *precocious pseudopuberty*, the hormones do not arise as a result of chronologically premature stimulation from the hypothalamus and pituitary gland but instead from pathologic entities that initiate activation of the hypothalamic-pituitary-gonadal axis or that secrete sex steroids independent of pituitary gonadotropin release. The condition is typically defined as the appearance of any signs of secondary sexual maturation in boys younger than 9 and in girls younger than 7. Etiologies include the following:

- Congenital adrenal hyperplasia
- Tumors of the adrenal gland, ovary, or testis
- McCune-Albright syndrome
- Exposure to exogenous sex steroid hormones

POSTMENOPAUSAL SONOGRAPHY

Menopause is the cessation of regular menstrual periods resulting from loss of ovarian sensitivity to gonadotropic hormone stimulation. Oocytes in the ovaries undergo atresia throughout a woman's life cycle, resulting in a decline in both the quantity and the quality of follicles. With fewer functional follicles present, there is a diminished response to follicle-stimulating hormone (FSH); estrogen and progesterone production tapers off, menstruation ceases, and—usually within the first five menopausal years—the uterus and ovaries begin to atrophy.

ANATOMY AND PHYSIOLOGY

The Uterus

Without the monthly stimulative effects of estrogen, the uterus shrinks until its size approaches that of the cervix (Figure 16-9). There is an inverse relationship between uterine size and the time since menopause: Uterine size and volume progressively decrease as the duration of the postmenopausal phase increases. The greatest changes occur within the first 10 years after the menopause; thereafter, change is more gradual.

A rule of thumb for normal postmenopausal uterine size is 8 × 5 × 3 cm; unlike the premenopausal uterus, the postmenopausal uterus does not significantly vary in size based on parity.[6] Atrophy and involution of the endometrium also occur in the postmenopausal state.

The normal postmenopausal endometrium should appear thin and homogeneously echogenic (Figure 16-10). There is considerable variation reported in the literature on what constitutes a normal endometrial thickness in the postmenopausal patient, particularly with regard to hormone replacement therapy. While exact measurement criteria differ, a consensus approach accepts a double-layer thickness of 5 mm or less without focal thickening as exclusive of significant disease and consistent with atrophy with or without hormone replacement therapy.[7,8]

The Ovaries

During the postmenopausal stage, the ovaries undergo anatomic changes characterized by diminution in size and volume due to the absence of physiologically active follicles. There is generally an inverse relationship between ovarian size and time since

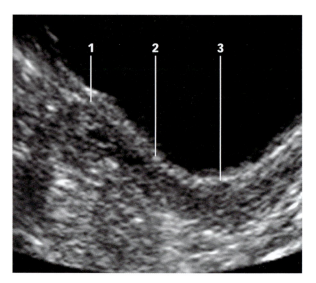

Figure 16-9. The postmenopausal uterus. 1 = fundus, 2 = body, 3 = cervix.

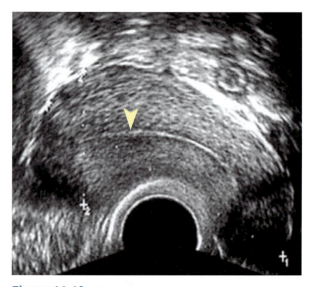

Figure 16-10. The postmenopausal endometrium. Arrowhead = thin, homogeneous endometrium.

the onset of menopause; ovarian size progressively decreases as the duration of the postmenopausal period increases.[9]

Despite their diminished size and the absence of landmark cystic follicles, both ovaries can be identified in 60% of postmenopausal women (Figure 16-11), and at least one ovary can be identified 85% of the time using an endovaginal ultrasound approach. The average size of a normal postmenopausal ovary is 2.2 × 1.2 × 1.1 cm.[10] Patients receiving hormone replacement therapy, however, may demonstrate ovaries that appear sonographically similar to those in premenopausal patients.

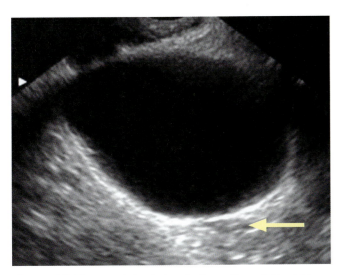

Figure 16-11. Transabdominal sagittal scan through the right adnexa demonstrating a postmenopausal ovary (arrow).

INDICATIONS FOR SONOGRAPHY

The primary indications for performing sonographic studies in postmenopausal women are the following:

- To evaluate the endometrium in a patient with vaginal bleeding
- To evaluate the endometrium in a patient on hormone replacement therapy
- To evaluate uterus and ovaries in a woman with a palpable pelvic mass
- To screen for endometrial or ovarian cancer in high-risk women

POSTMENOPAUSAL GYNECOLOGIC PATHOLOGY

Pelvic pathologies most commonly associated with the postmenopausal state are discussed below.

Postmenopausal Vaginal Bleeding

Sonographic evaluation of the pelvis in postmenopausal women experiencing vaginal bleeding has become a mandatory component of their clinical workup. Endovaginal imaging is of particular importance, as the high-resolution capabilities of the high-frequency probes used for this scan permit detailed evaluation of the various layers of the endometrium as well as the internal characteristics of the ovarian parenchyma.

The primary clinical manifestation of the postmenopausal state is the absence of menses for more than one year. The return of even a little spotting is not normal and should be investigated with tools in the diagnostic armamentarium that include clinical and sonographic evaluation, hysteroscopy, endometrial biopsy, and dilatation and curettage (D&C). The most common causes of postmenopausal vaginal bleeding include:

- Hormone replacement therapy
- Endometrial polyps
- Endometrial atrophy
- Endometrial hyperplasia
- Endometrial carcinoma

Hormone Replacement Therapy

Hormone replacement therapy (HRT), a controversial clinical topic in recent years, is a pharmacologic approach to alleviating many of the uncomfortable symptoms associated with menopause. There are two main types of hormone replacement therapy: estrogen alone and estrogen/progesterone used in combination. Both types have benefits and risks, a full discussion of which is beyond the scope of this chapter.

From a sonographic perspective, however, women on hormone replacement therapy may demonstrate sonographic findings similar to those of premenopausal women (see Table 16-3). A patient receiving unopposed estrogen may demonstrate an endometrial measurement of up to 8 mm.[11] Patients undergoing combination (estrogen/progesterone) hormone replacement therapy may demonstrate an endometrial thickness increased by 3 mm from the generally accepted measurements associated with patients not on hormone replacement therapy.

The ovaries in a postmenopausal patient on hormone replacement therapy may exhibit cyclic hemodynamic

Table 16-3. Maximum normal endometrial thickness in postmenopausal women by hormone therapy status

Hormone Therapy	Maximum Thickness (mm)
None—asymptomatic postmenopausal	≤5
Unopposed HRT	8
Combination HRT	8
Tamoxifen	10

patterns and follicular development similar to those found in a premenopausal ovulating patient.

As mentioned above, although hormone replacement therapy alleviates many of the untoward symptoms typical of menopause, pathologic complications associated with its usage have limited its application. In addition to being the most common cause of postmenopausal vaginal bleeding and the development of endometrial hyperplasia, HRT has been implicated as an etiologic factor in the development of endometrial carcinoma with estrogen-only HRT (see Chapter 15) and increased risk of breast cancer with combined estrogen and progesterone HRT.[12]

Other potential complications associated with HRT administration include an increased risk of coronary heart disease and thromboembolic sequelae such as coronary heart disease, stroke, and deep vein, mesenteric, and portal vein thrombosis.[13]

Tamoxifen

Tamoxifen is a drug most commonly administered to women who are being treated for estrogen-sensitive types of breast cancer. As an estrogen receptor antagonist, tamoxifen binds to receptor sites in breast tissue, which prevents estrogen molecules from attaching to these cells and stimulating malignant proliferation. Tamoxifen also has an estrogen-like effect on the receptors in the uterus and endometrium, causing endometrial thickening, polyps, hyperplasia, and the possibility of malignancy.[14]

The uterine sonographic findings associated with tamoxifen may include an increased endometrial thickness of up to 10 mm. As indicated above, however, any postmenopausal patient demonstrating endometrial thickening of ≥5 should prompt additional diagnostic workup. In asymptomatic postmenopausal women receiving tamoxifen, 6 mm is the optimal endometrial thickness cutoff for diagnosing endometrial abnormalities with transvaginal ultrasound. Further examination with hysterosonography can improve specificity by reducing the high false-positive rate of transvaginal ultrasound.[15] Additional sonographic findings may include an alteration in the appearance of the endometrium, particularly cystic atrophic changes. Tamoxifen is used in the management of diverse other medical conditions, including but not limited to infertility, gynecomastia, and some types of cancer.

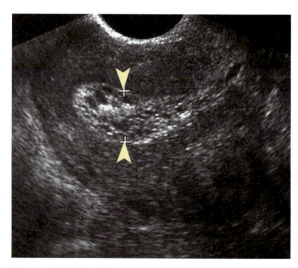

Figure 16-12. Effect of tamoxifen on the endometrium. Arrowheads = thickened, heterogeneous endometrium.

Sonographic Signs

The following are the characteristic sonographic signs associated with patients on tamoxifen:

- Increased endometrial thickness (up to 10 mm)
- Heterogeneous endometrial echo complex (Figure 16-12)
- Fluid in the endometrial cavity

Palpable Pelvic Masses

The identification of a palpable pelvic mass on gynecologic examination is another indication for pelvic sonography, just as it is in pediatric (and other premenopausal) patients. However, there are age-related differences in the types of masses found among patients in each of these groups.

In the postmenarcheal, premenopausal nonpregnant patient the most likely types of pathology presenting as a palpable pelvic mass, along with other clinical signs and symptoms, include:

Ovarian Masses

- Physiologic (follicular, corpus luteum) cysts
- Benign ovarian masses (teratomas, dermoids)
- Ovarian torsion
- Polycystic ovaries
- Some ovarian neoplasms (Sertoli-Leydig, granulosa cell tumors)

Uterine Masses

- Uterine leiomyomas (fibroids)

Adnexal Masses
- Endometriosis
- Salpingitis
- Tubo-ovarian abscesses

Gynecologic Cancer Screening

As normal cyclic hormonal levels taper off during the postmenopausal state, masses frequently encountered in younger women become less likely diagnostic possibilities. The incidence of functional cysts of the ovary diminishes (unless the patient is on cyclic hormone replacement therapy); implants of endometriosis decrease in size and symptomatology; and fibroids generally regress as estrogen levels wane. What remains are more aggressive pathologic entities with potential outcomes that generate a heightened level of concern: ovarian, uterine, and other types of pelvic malignancy.

Ovarian Cancer

The incidence of ovarian cancer increases with age. In fact, 80% of ovarian neoplasms occur in women older than 50 years of age. Recommendations for ovarian cancer screening traditionally have been organized into one of two sets of guidelines: one for women at average risk and the other for women at increased risk. Now, with the identification of gene mutations that can increase a woman's chances of developing ovarian cancer, the set of guidelines for women at increased risk has been subdivided into two groups: recommendations for women with a clear inherited risk of developing ovarian cancer due to an identified genetic mutation, and recommendations for women with a personal or family history of the disease.

Risk Factors

Risk factors associated with the occurrence of ovarian cancer can be grouped into those applicable to:

- The general population
- Patients with a family history of gynecologic cancers
- Patients with known genetic mutations associated with a heightened probability of developing cancer

Risk factors related to the *general population* include a personal history of:

- Breast cancer diagnosed at age 41 or older
- Infertility and use of assisted reproductive therapies
- Endometriosis
- Hormone replacement therapy

Increased risk factors (3–6 times that of general population) associated with *familial history* include:

- A first-degree relative (mother, sister, daughter) with ovarian cancer
- Personal history of breast cancer prior to age 40
- Personal history of breast cancer diagnosed prior to age 50, and one or more close relatives diagnosed with breast or ovarian cancer at any age
- Two or more close relatives diagnosed with breast cancer prior to age 50 or with ovarian cancer diagnosed at any age
- Ashkenazi Jewish heritage and a personal history of breast cancer prior to age 50
- Ashkenazi Jewish heritage and a first- or second-degree relative diagnosed with breast cancer prior to age 50 or with ovarian cancer at any age

Inherited risk due to known *genetic mutations* (>6 times that of the general population) include:

- Women who test positive for the presence of a BRCA1 or BRCA2 genetic mutation. BRCA1 and BRCA2 are genes involved in cell growth, division, and repair of damage to DNA that occurs naturally during one's lifetime. An altered, or mutated, BRCA1 or BRCA2 gene increases the likelihood that cancer will develop.
- Inherited mutations in other genes have also been linked to an increased risk for breast cancer. These genes include *TP53, CDH1, STK11, PTEN/MMAC1, CHEK2,* and *ATM.*

CA-125

Cancer antigen 125 (CA-125) is a tumor marker that is expressed by more than 80% of nonmucinous epithelial ovarian carcinomas and is found in most carcinomas of müllerian origin, including fallopian tube and primary serous peritoneal carcinoma.[16] Elevated CA-125 serum levels are also found in a variety of benign conditions such as fibroids, acute pelvic inflammatory disease, liver cirrhosis, nongynecologic malignancies, acute peritonitis, and normal first trimester pregnancies. While CA-125 testing has proven useful primarily in postmenopausal patients who have reached the age when many of the benign conditions

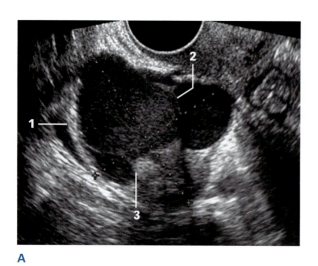 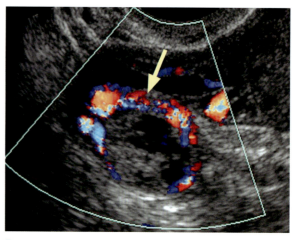

Figure 16-13. **A** A complex ovarian mass in a postmenopausal patient. 1 = thickened wall, 2 = septation, 3 = mural nodule. **B** Hypervascularity surrounding a complex ovarian mass. Arrow = low-resistance flow pattern around the periphery of the mass.

that can confound interpretation are absent, its lack of sensitivity and specificity preclude its use for screening normal risk populations for ovarian cancer.[17] In an at-risk population, CA-125 is a more useful adjunct to the clinical and sonographic evaluation in differentiating benign from malignant pelvic masses.[18]

Sonography

The American Congress of Obstetricians and Gynecologists does not recommend screening for ovarian cancer in asymptomatic women. The usual screening triad of CA-125, endovaginal sonography, and physical examination is reserved for women at increased risk as outlined above.[19]

Additionally, the American Cancer Society states that there is "no screening test proven to be effective and sufficiently accurate in the early detection of ovarian cancer. However, for women who are at high risk for ovarian cancer, the combination of a thorough pelvic examination, transvaginal ultrasonography, and a blood test for the tumor marker CA-125 may be offered."[20]

Endovaginal ultrasound is the method of choice in evaluating the ovaries in postmenopausal women identified as suitable candidates for screening. Small cystic structures may be identified within the ovaries, especially during the first 5–10 years after menopause. Even in patients on hormone replacement therapy, these simple cysts should not exceed 5–10 mm in diameter. In cysts that do exceed the upper limit of 10 mm, additional diagnostic workup is indicated, and if thick walls, septations, or nodules are noted within the cyst, surgery may be indicated on the basis of sonography alone (Figure 16-13A). Another sonographic finding that elevates suspicion of, but is not specific for, cancer is hypervascularity in or around an ovarian mass. This finding, best demonstrated with color Doppler ultrasound (Figure 16-13B) and quantified with spectral waveform analysis, has been found in association with 75% of invasive ovarian cancers.[21]

Uterine Cancer

Endometrial cancer is the most common gynecologic cancer in the United States. While endometrial cancer affects women of reproductive age as well as postmenopausal women, 75% of endometrial cancers occur in postmenopausal women, with the mean age of diagnosis at 61 years.[22] More than 90% of patients with endometrial cancer will present with abnormal vaginal bleeding, whether it is menorrhagia, metrorrhagia, or even scant postmenopausal bleeding. Approximately 10% of these patients will ultimately be diagnosed with endometrial cancer.

Risk Factors

Risk factors for uterine cancer, particularly endometrial carcinoma, include conditions that lead to increased estrogen exposure during the patient's lifetime, such as:

- Estrogen replacement therapy
- Tamoxifen administration

- Obesity
- Early menarche
- Late menopause
- Nulliparity

Sonography

Any postmenopausal woman experiencing vaginal bleeding is a candidate for endovaginal ultrasound evaluation. Particular attention is paid to the thickness and sonographic characteristic of the endometrium. As discussed above, a double-layer endometrial thickness of 5 mm or greater is an indication for additional diagnostic workup. In patients on hormone replacement therapy the maximum acceptable diameter increases.

CHAPTER 16 REVIEW QUESTIONS

1. The premenarcheal fundal-to-cervical ratio is typically:
   A. 1:2
   B. 1:3
   C. 1:4
   D. 1:5

2. The postmenarcheal fundal-to-cervical ratio is typically:
   A. 2:1–3:1
   B. 2:1–4:1
   C. 3:1–4:1
   D. 3:1–5:1

3. The normal volume measurement of a neonatal ovary is:
   A. ≥1.0 cc
   B. ≤1.0 cc
   C. 2–3 cc
   D. 3–4 cc

4. All of the following pathologic entities may be the cause of a palpable pelvic mass in the pediatric patient EXCEPT:
   A. Hydrometrocolpos
   B. Sarcoma botryoides
   C. Ovarian torsion
   D. Choriocarcinoma

5. All of the following are sonographic signs of a torsed ovary in the pediatric patient EXCEPT:
   A. Enlarged, hypoechoic ovary
   B. Peripherally displaced follicle
   C. Low-resistance Doppler flow within the ovary
   D. Free fluid in the pelvis

6. The presence of retained blood in the uterine and vaginal cavities is called:
   A. Hydrocolpos
   B. Hematometrocolpos
   C. Hydrometra
   D. Pyometrocolpos

7. A type of embryonal rhabdomyosarcoma found in the wall of the vagina more commonly in the pediatric patient is:
   A. Gartner's duct cyst
   B. Dysgerminoma
   C. Endodermal sinus tumor
   D. Sarcoma botryoides

8. All of the following are characteristics associated with true precocious puberty EXCEPT:
   A. Increase in ovarian volume
   B. Uterine enlargement
   C. Unchanged fundal:cervical ratio
   D. Appearance of secondary sexual characteristics

9. All of the following are typical etiologies of precocious pseudopuberty EXCEPT:
   A. Sarcoma botryoides
   B. Congenital adrenal hyperplasia
   C. Exposure to exogenous sex steroid hormones
   D. McCune-Albright syndrome

10. The normal postmenopausal endometrium of a patient not on hormone replacement therapy should appear:
    A. Thick and homogeneously echogenic
    B. Thin and homogeneously echogenic
    C. Hyperechoic with focal thinning
    D. Hypoechoic with focal thinning

11. A normal double-thickness measurement of the postmenopausal endometrium is generally accepted to be:
    A. <5 mm
    B. 5–7 mm
    C. 6–8 mm
    D. >5 mm

12. All of the following pathologic conditions may be responsible for postmenopausal vaginal bleeding EXCEPT:
    A. Hormone replacement therapy
    B. Endometrial polyps
    C. Postpartum state
    D. Endometrial carcinoma

13. Postmenopausal patients receiving unopposed estrogen hormone replacement therapy may exhibit a normal endometrial thickness of up to:
    A. 5 mm
    B. 6 mm
    C. 7 mm
    D. 8 mm

14. A pharmaceutical agent commonly used to treat estrogen-sensitive types of breast cancer that may alter the monographic appearance of the endometrium is:
    A. Clomid
    B. Tamoxifen
    C. Pergonal
    D. Methotrexate

15. What percentage of ovarian neoplasms occur in women over 50 years of age?
    A. 50%
    B. 60%
    C. 70%
    D. 80%

16. Elevated serum CA-125 levels may be found in all of the following pathologic conditions EXCEPT:
    A. Uterine fibroids
    B. Acute PID
    C. Ectopic pregnancy
    D. Ovarian carcinoma

17. The most common gynecologic malignancy in the United States affects the:
    A. Endometrium
    B. Ovaries
    C. Cervix
    D. Fallopian tubes

18. Factors associated with an increased risk for uterine cancer include all of the following EXCEPT:
    A. Estrogen replacement therapy
    B. Tamoxifen administration
    C. Infertility treatment
    D. Obesity

19. The term *sexual ambiguity* encompasses all of the following conditions EXCEPT:
    A. Imperforate hymen
    B. True hermaphroditism
    C. Ambiguous genitalia
    D. Testicular feminization syndrome

20. A 14-year-old girl presents with a palpable midline pelvic mass and amenorrhea. Sagittal ultrasound section through a full bladder yields the accompanying image. The diagnosis is:

    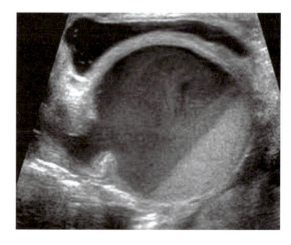

    A. Sarcoma botryoides
    B. Hydrometrocolpos
    C. Uterine tumor
    D. Vaginal rhabdomyosarcoma

21. A 65-year-old patient presents with recent onset of vaginal bleeding. The accompanying sonographic image could be consistent with all of the following diagnoses EXCEPT:

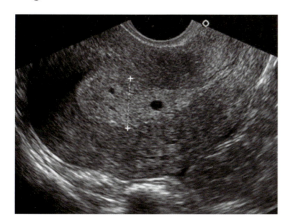

A. Endometrial carcinoma
B. Endometrial atrophy
C. Endometrial hyperplasia
D. Endometrial polyps

ANSWERS

See Appendix A on page 483 for answers.

REFERENCES

1. Garel L, Dubois J, Grignon A, et al: US of the pediatric female pelvis: a clinical perspective. RadioGraphics 21:1393–1407, 2001.

2. Kozlowski KJ: Ovarian masses. Adolesc Med 10:337–350, 1999.

3. Stepanian M, Cohn DE: Gynecologic malignancies in adolescents. Adolesc Med Clin 15:549–568, 2004.

4. Young JL Jr, Cheng Wu X, Roffers SD, et al: Ovarian cancer in children and young adults in the United States, 1992–1997. Cancer 97(Suppl 10):2694–2700, 2003.

5. Guthrie BD, Adler MD, Powell EC: Incidence and trends of pediatric ovarian torsion hospitalizations in the United States, 2000-2006. Pediatrics 125:532–538, 2010.

6. Zemlyn S: The length of the uterine cervix and its significance. J Clin Ultrasound 9:267–269, 1981.

7. Nalaboff KM, Pellerito JS, Ben-Levi E: Imaging the endometrium: disease and normal variants. RadioGraphics 21:1409–1424, 2001.

8. Smith-Bindman R, Kerlikowske K, Feldstein VA, et al: Endovaginal ultrasound to exclude endometrial cancer and other endometrial abnormalities. JAMA 280:1510–1517, 1998.

9. Flaws JA, Rhodes JC, Langenberg P, et al: Ovarian volume and menopausal status. Menopause 7:53–61, 2000.

10. Fleischer AC, McKee MS, Gordon AN, et al: Transvaginal sonography of postmenopausal ovaries with pathologic correlation. J Ultrasound Med 9:637–644, 1990.

11. Levine D, Gosink BB, Johnson LA: Change in endometrial thickness in postmenopausal women undergoing hormone replacement therapy. Radiology 197:603–608, 1995.

12. Yeh IT: Postmenopausal hormone replacement therapy: endometrial and breast effects. Adv Anat Pathol 14:17–24, 2007.

13. Gurney EP, Nachtigall MJ, Nachtigall LE, et al: The Women's Health Initiative trial and related studies: 10 years later: a clinician's view. J Steroid Biochem Mol Biol 142:4–11, 2014.

14. Kalampokas T, Sofoudis C, Anastasopoulos C, et al: Effect of tamoxifen on postmenopausal endometrium. Eur J Gynaecol Oncol 34:325–328, 2013.

15. Fong K, Kung R, Lytwyn A, et al: Endometrial evaluation with transvaginal US and hysterosonography in asymptomatic postmenopausal women with breast cancer receiving tamoxifen. Radiology 220:765–773, 2001.

16. Jacobs I, Bast RC Jr: The CA 125 tumour-associated antigen: a review of the literature. Hum Reprod 4:1–12, 1989.

17. National Comprehensive Cancer Network: *Clinical Practice Guidelines in Oncology: Ovarian Cancer*, Version 3, 2012. Available at http://www.nccn.org/professionals/physician_gls/f_guidelines.asp#site

18. Macuks R, Baidekalna I, Donina S: Comparison of different ovarian cancer detection algorithms. Eur J Gynaecol Oncol 32:408–410, 2011.

19. American College of Obstetricians and Gynecologists, Committee on Gynecologic Practice: Committee opinion no. 477: the role of the obstetrician-gynecologist in the early detection of epithelial ovarian cancer. Obstet Gynecol 117:742–746, 2011.

20. American Cancer Society: *Cancer Facts and Figures 2012*. Atlanta: American Cancer Society, 2012.

21. Barroilhet L, Vitonis A, Shipp T, et al: Sonographic predictors of ovarian malignancy. J Clin Ultrasound 41:269–274, 2013.

22. Soliman PT, Oh JC, Schmeler KM, et al: Risk factors for young premenopausal women with endometrial cancer. Obstet Gynecol 105:575–580, 2005.

SUGGESTED READINGS

Gill KA: Gynecology. In Gill KA: *Ultrasound in Obstetrics and Gynecology: A Practitioner's Guide*. Pasadena, Davies Publishing, 2014, pp 25–88.

Goldstein C, Hagen-Ansert SL: Normal anatomy and physiology of the female pelvis. In Hagen-Ansert SL (ed): *Textbook of Diagnostic Ultrasonography*, 7th edition. St. Louis, Elsevier Mosby, 2012, pp 938–954.

Goldstein C, Hagen-Ansert SL: Pathology of the uterus. In Hagen-Ansert SL (ed): *Textbook of Diagnostic Ultrasonography*, 7th edition. St. Louis, Elsevier Mosby, 2012, pp 978–1000.

Goldstein C, Hagen-Ansert SL, Vander Werff, BJ: Pathology of the adnexa. In Hagen-Ansert SL (ed): *Textbook of Diagnostic Ultrasonography*, 7th edition. St. Louis, Elsevier Mosby, 2012, pp 1028–1038.

Goldstein C, Hagen-Ansert SL, Vander Werff, BJ: Pathology of the ovaries. In Hagen-Ansert SL (ed): *Textbook of Diagnostic Ultrasonography*, 7th edition. St. Louis, Elsevier Mosby, 2012, pp 1001–1027.

Goldstein SR: Abnormal uterine bleeding: the role of ultrasound. In Callen PW (ed): *Ultrasonography in Obstetrics and Gynecology*, 5th edition. Philadelphia, Saunders Elsevier, 2008, pp 942–950.

Lerner JP, Timor-Tritsch IE, Federman A, et al: Transvaginal ultrasonographic characterization of ovarian masses with an improved, weighted scoring system. Am J Obstet Gynecol 170:81–85, 1994.

Levi CS, Lyons EA, Holt SC, et al: Normal anatomy of the female pelvis and transvaginal sonography. In Callen PW (ed): *Ultrasonography in Obstetrics and Gynecology*, 5th edition. Philadelphia, Saunders Elsevier, 2008, pp 887–918.

Rosenberg HK, Chaudhry H: Pediatric pelvic sonography. In Rumack CM, Wilson SR, Charboneau JW, et al (eds): *Diagnostic Ultrasound*, 4th edition. Philadelphia, Elsevier Mosby, 2011, pp 1925–1981.

Salem S: Gynecology. In Rumack CM, Wilson SR, Charboneau JW, et al (eds): *Diagnostic Ultrasound*, 4th edition. Philadelphia, Elsevier Mosby, 2011, pp 613–638.

Valentin L, Callen PW: Ultrasound evaluation of the adnexa (ovary and fallopian tubes). In Callen PW (ed): *Ultrasonography in Obstetrics and Gynecology*, 5th edition. Philadelphia, Saunders Elsevier, 2008, pp 968–985.

PART III
Physical Principles, Protocols, and Patient Care

Chapter 17 | Physical Principles and Instrumentation

Chapter 18 | Protocols and Patient Care

CHAPTER 17
Physical Principles and Instrumentation

Ultrasound Bioeffects

Imaging Modes

Doppler Ultrasound

Transducers

Imaging Artifacts

Alongside a mastery of the clinical knowledge and scanning skills necessary for competent practice of obstetric and gynecologic sonography lies the need for an understanding of the physical principles, instrumentation, technical components, and professional performance standards of the discipline. This chapter summarizes the basic science and instrumentation of ultrasound imaging systems and their proper application to ob/gyn studies.

ULTRASOUND BIOEFFECTS

There are two primary mechanisms of bioeffects induced by acoustic energy in human soft tissue: *thermal* and *nonthermal*.

THERMAL BIOEFFECTS

Changes in living tissue that result from temperature increases are called *thermal bioeffects*. From the perspective of an ultrasound practice, these temperature increases are caused by the absorption of acoustic energy in body tissues. If the rate of heat deposition in a particular area exceeds the body's ability to dissipate it, tissue temperatures rise, leading to hyperthermia.[1]

Hyperthermia

Several anatomic characteristics of an insonated area enhance thermal changes:

- Presence of bone: The presence of bone in the focal zone, with its associated increased attenuation levels, has been shown to induce heating in the adjacent soft tissues.[2]
- Diminished vascular perfusion: The paucity of vascular perfusion in some types of tissue (such as embryonic or ischemic tissue) diminishes the body's ability to dissipate heat via the circulatory system.
- Elevated body temperature: The elevation of the body temperature above 37° Celsius (98.6° Fahrenheit) produces an increase in attenuation and absorption of acoustic energy, presumably as the result of changes in tissue composition.[3,4]

The threshold temperature elevation for hyperthermia-induced adverse biologic effects in experimental studies is estimated to be approximately 1.5° Celsius above normal core values.[5] While this level of tissue temperature increase is unlikely to occur during routine diagnostic ultrasound examinations, achieving this level of acoustic exposure is within the capability of some modern diagnostic ultrasound devices sold both within the United States and abroad.[6]

Thermal Indices

The *thermal index* (TI) provides a method of quantifying the potential for the ultrasonic heating of human tissue.[7] Generally speaking, the thermal index is the ratio of the ultrasonic power emitted by the transducer to the ultrasonic power required to raise tissue temperature by 1° Celsius for the exposure conditions being evaluated:

$$TI = \frac{W_0}{W_{deg}}$$

where W_0 = output power of the transducer (watts), W_{deg} = power necessary to raise tissue temperature, and TI = a calculated estimate of temperature increase.

Because of the immense variety of types of tissue interfaces found in the human body, particularly when bone lies in the path of the beam, three specific types of thermal index have been devised to provide simplified averages for heating potential:

- Thermal index for soft tissue (TIs)
- Thermal index for bone (TIb)
- Thermal index for the cranium (TIc)

Each of these indices is designed to more closely approximate the energy deposition and temperature increases associated with scanning in various anatomic locations. In general obstetric imaging, the soft-tissue thermal index is most commonly used as a metric of potential tissue heating. It is generally agreed that during the course of a routine sonographic examination there is negligible risk for thermal injury to the patient and the fetus and there is no justification to limit scanning when acceptable clinical indications exist. If the thermal index does not exceed 1, currently available evidence indicates that the risk of an injury due to ultrasonic heating is negligible for the vast majority of diagnostic ultrasound examinations.[8,9] For further discussion of the bioeffects of ultrasound on patient safety, see Chapter 18, pages 472–473.

NONTHERMAL/MECHANICAL BIOEFFECTS

Nonthermal mechanisms of ultrasound bioeffects result from the mechanical interactions of an acoustic wavefront with human soft tissue. These include:

- Compression and rarefaction
- Cavitation
- Acoustic streaming

Compression/Rarefaction

The characteristic localized areas of *compression* and *rarefaction* that comprise an individual sound wave alternately push and pull on tissue particles. If the "pushing" (compression) contains enough energy, particles can be forced together with tremendous force. Conversely, the "pulling" during the rarefactory phase of wave transmission can rip particles apart with enough force to cause them to implode—a process called *cavitation*. Additionally, the transfer of energy by the loss of forward momentum of an acoustic wave can also initiate a process called *acoustic streaming*, in which flow currents are induced in the medium (i.e., human tissue).[10]

Cavitation Effects

Cavitation is the process whereby "cavities" are formed in a nonelastic medium, such as water or human tissue, as acoustic pressure waves propagate through it. When the amplitude of an ultrasound wave reaches certain threshold levels, the magnitude of the negative pressure in the areas of rarefaction becomes sufficient to tear the medium apart, causing it to fracture and allowing gases present within the medium to escape. Small "cavities" or microbubbles form and, under the continued bombardment from subsequent positive pressure waves, begin to oscillate. These microbubbles ultimately implode violently, sending shock waves into adjacent parts of the medium (Figure 17-1). These shock waves can damage adjacent cells in a variety of ways:[11]

- On the *tissue* level, studies have consistently demonstrated that cavitational effects of acoustic energy can cause hemolysis (the disintegration of blood cells), particularly when sonographic contrast agents are present.
- On the *cellular* level, cavitation bubbles have been shown to induce cell death or transient changes in the permeability of cell membranes.[12, 13]
- Cavitation can also induce changes on a *subcellular* level, causing degeneration and shrinking of a cell nucleus and clumping of the chromosomes (*pyknosis*).[14]
- Finally, on a *molecular* level, exposure to continuous insonation has been shown to cause breaks in DNA strands in rat ovary cells, presumably due to cavitational effects.[15]

Acoustic Streaming

Acoustic streaming is another nonthermal phenomenon, characterized by unidirectional flow currents in a fluid due to the introduction of acoustic energy. In human soft tissue, fluid-flowing conduits (i.e., arteries, veins, lymphatics, blood and fluid collections, and intracardiac circulation) are subject to the potential induction of acoustic streaming. When ultrasound energy propagates through a fluid collection, it applies a force to the fluid through the fluid mechanics process known as *momentum transfer*. The vibrational forces of the acoustic wavefront enhance the flow energy already present in the medium, and a streaming within the fluid results (Figure 17-2).

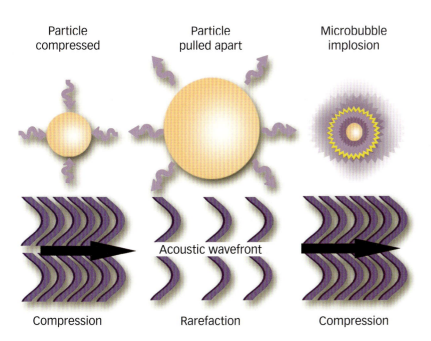

Figure 17-1. Cavitation. As a particle is compressed and pulled apart by an acoustic wavefront, microbubbles are created that implode and send shock waves into adjacent parts of the medium.

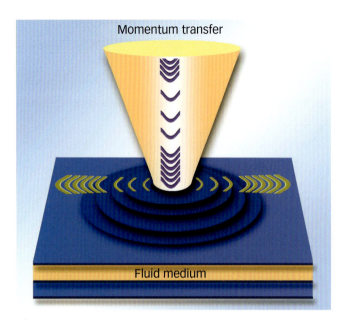

Figure 17-2. Acoustic streaming. Vibrational forces of an acoustic wavefront enhance flow energy already present in a fluid medium.

There is little evidence to support the induction of any adverse biologic effects attributable to acoustic streaming, at least from exposure to the energies employed by diagnostic ultrasound instruments. On the contrary, several studies have shown that acoustic streaming actually may reduce the temperature rise generated by ultrasound at the surface of bone. The suggestion is that the microstreams produced by momentum transfer and other acoustic physical phenomena conduct heat away from the bone, reducing the thermal effects.[16]

Mechanical Index

The *mechanical index* (MI) attempts to provide a measure of bioeffects related to the transfer of energy from acoustic waves as they propagate through human tissue.[17] The mechanical index is a measurement of the negative acoustic pressure present in the insonated area expressed as the ratio of the largest peak rarefactional (relaxation) pressure in an ultrasound beam to a constant:[18]

$$MI = \frac{P_r/f^{1/2}}{C_{MI}}$$

where P_r = peak rarefactional pressure, f = ultrasound frequency, and C_{MI} = 1 MPa/MHz. In general, MI numbers encountered in routine diagnostic ultrasound examinations are well below those necessary to induce nonthermal bioeffects.

IMAGING MODES

B-MODE

Brightness modulation, or *B-mode*, is a two-dimensional sonographic imaging method (Figure 17-3) in which a shade of gray that is proportional to the amplitude of a returning echo is assigned to each *picture element* or *pixel* to produce a single still frame. Displaying a sequential series of at least 10 single images over a short period of time (typically 1 second) creates the illusion of motion—a method known as *real time*. Two-dimensional (2D) real-time B-mode imaging is the traditional and primary ultrasound examination technique, one that permits evaluation of nearly every aspect of human anatomy.

Compounding is a B-mode method whereby several different image subframes are generated, processed, and combined into a single frame. There are several types of compounding:

- *Spatial compounding* relies on echo data obtained from several subframes, each of which has been steered into the body at slightly different angles and at slightly different times. The acoustic result is enhancement of specular reflection from tissue interfaces, yielding better spatial resolution and more reliable speckle data, which in turn improves contrast resolution.

- *Frequency compounding* employs subframes created using different fundamental transmit frequencies and/or received harmonic frequencies. Blending

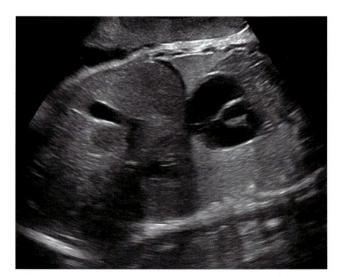

Figure 17-3. B-mode imaging: two-dimensional gray-scale representation of human anatomy, in this case a coronal section demonstrating fetal thoracoabdominal anatomy.

these fundamental and harmonic frequencies overcomes some of the limitations when each is used alone, and the compounded frame ideally enhances both near-field and far-field image quality.

- *Spatial frequency compounding* takes this technology a step further by combining both types of subframes (spatial and frequency) to create a single frame.

3D AND 4D

Three-dimensional (3D) ultrasound images (Figure 17-4) are obtained using either a mechanically or an electronically steered (matrix) transducer array. Volumetric data are acquired and stored as *volume elements* or *voxels* and can be processed and displayed in several ways.

Surface rendering yields a 3D image of the external surface of the body part being examined and is responsible for the realistic and much-in-demand "baby pictures" offered to expectant mothers. Clinical efficacy of surface rendering in obstetric scanning also includes a more accurate and useful evaluation of external anatomic abnormalities, including facial anomalies (e.g., clefting defects, facial dysmorphia, or holoprosencephaly-related anomalies) and abnormalities of the extremities (e.g., talipes equinovarus, rocker bottom foot, short limbs, amniotic banding defects, and abnormalities of the digits).

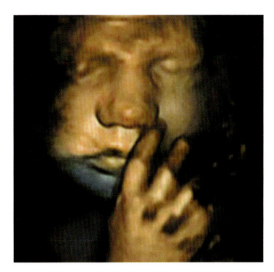

Figure 17-4. 3D surface rendering. The external surface of the imaged anatomic part is created from acquired volumetric acoustic data.

Four-dimensional (4D) imaging is simply 3D surface rendering performed in real time, yielding a video clip as opposed to a static image.

TOMOGRAPHIC SLICE

Volumetric ultrasound is a method of processing 3D ultrasound data (Figure 17-5) that permits a sequential examination of tomographic slices through a structure of interest in all three scan planes (sagittal, axial, and

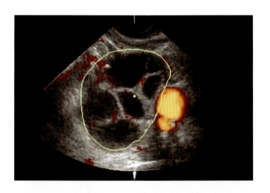
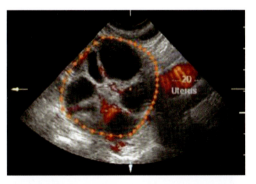
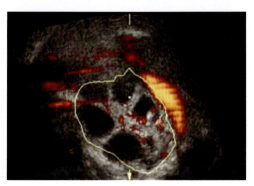
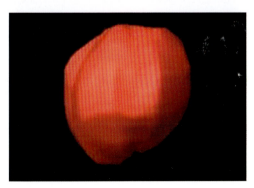

Figure 17-5. 3D tomographic slice. Three planar section images can be reconstructed from acquired volumetric acoustic data. Ovarian follicles are imaged and measured in all three planes simultaneously, resulting in the 3D image at lower right.

coronal). Much like other sectional imaging modalities (such as computed tomography and magnetic resonance imaging), volumetric ultrasound produces results that are analyzed at a viewing station after the data have been acquired and stored. In gynecologic sonography, volumetric ultrasound has proven particularly useful in evaluating and following endometrial and uterine pathology.

M-MODE

Motion mode, or *M-mode*, is a modality that displays a single B-mode line of sight along a horizontal axis as the recording medium is moved along a vertical axis (Figure 17-6). This display produces a group of lines that depict the motion of moving interfaces over time. Acoustic reflecting surfaces that remain stationary create straight lines on the display, while dynamic interfaces create lines that move up and down along the axis of the cursor line. Clinically, M-mode display is used almost exclusively in cardiac ultrasound studies. Depending on how the transducer is positioned, specific structures in the heart, particularly cardiac walls and valves, can be studied; more important, their movement can be evaluated and quantified.

DOPPLER ULTRASOUND

Doppler ultrasound applications enhance obstetric and gynecologic sonographic examinations by adding a physiologic element to the traditional 2D anatomic display. More specifically, Doppler modalities provide information about *hemodynamics*, the movement of blood in and around human soft tissue and organs. There are four primary methods of displaying Doppler information, all based on echo data created by the Doppler effect.

THE DOPPLER EFFECT

The *Doppler effect* describes changes in phase and frequency that an acoustic beam experiences as it interacts with moving structures (such as red blood cells) smaller than the incident wavelength. The Doppler-shifted echo data are detected by the transducer elements, extracted and routed by the receiver, and processed into any of the four diagnostic Doppler modes (explained below): continuous-wave (CW), pulsed-wave (PW), color Doppler imaging (CDI), or power Doppler imaging (PDI). Each has its own realm of applications and limitations in clinical obstetric and gynecologic sonography.

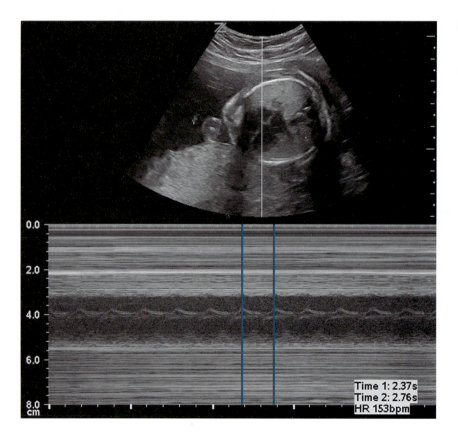

Figure 17-6. M-mode: two-dimensional display of moving interfaces, in this case fetal cardiac structures lying within a single, vertical B-mode interrogation line.

A Doppler effect occurs whenever there is relative motion between the source of an energy wave (such as sound) and the receiver of that wave. When a sound wave, for example, encounters a moving target (Figure 17-7), the frequency of the reflected portion of that wave shifts from that of the transmitted wave; this is called a *frequency shift* or *Doppler shift*. The usual example cited is a train moving toward an observer with its whistle blowing. The train's movement toward the receiver (the observer's ear) "compresses" the sound waves, resulting in the observer hearing a higher frequency than is actually being emitted from the whistle; the observer hears a higher pitch—called a *positive* frequency (or Doppler) shift. Conversely, if the train is moving away from the receiver/hearer, the sound waves are "stretched apart" relative to the receiver, and the perceived frequency (pitch) is lower than the transmitted frequency—called a *negative* frequency shift.

In Doppler imaging applications, structures moving toward the ultrasound probe create a positive Doppler shift, while those moving away create a negative shift. If both the sound's source and the person hearing the sound (the receiver) are moving at the same speed in the same direction (as would be the case for the engineer located *on* the train), there is no perceived frequency shift.

Mathematically, the Doppler effect can be defined as the difference between the frequencies of a transmitted, or incident, ultrasound beam and those of the returning, or reflected, echoes:

$$F_d = F_r - F_i$$

where F_d = Doppler frequency, F_i = incident frequency, and F_r = reflected frequency.

Example: If the central incident frequency is 5 MHz, and the receiver detects a 4.5 MHz returning frequency, the Doppler shift is -0.5 MHz. If it detects a 5.5 MHz returning frequency, the Doppler shift is $+0.5$ MHz. Conveniently, in medical applications Doppler frequencies fall within the range of human hearing (20–20,000 Hz). This makes fetal monitoring devices and Doppler stethoscopes, which produce a simple audio output, easy to design and use.

The more complete expression of the Doppler formula and the one that is relative to medical imaging applications describes the Doppler frequency (F_d) as a function not only of the incident frequency (F_i) but also of velocity of the insonated medium (V), the cosine of the angle of incidence (cos θ), and the constant velocity of sound (C) in the medium:

$$F_d = \frac{2F_i V}{C} \times \cos \theta$$

Two of these variables—incident frequency and angle of incidence—are operator selectable and are important criteria in optimizing Doppler display information.

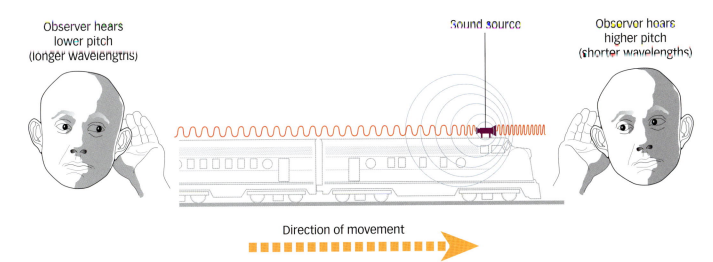

Figure 17-7. The Doppler effect: An observer (receiver) hearing the sound waves as they approach will hear "compressed" (resulting in higher) frequencies and thus a higher pitch, called a *positive* Doppler shift. Conversely, if the train is moving away from the receiver, the sounds waves are "stretched apart" (resulting in lower frequencies) relative to the receiver, who will hear a lower pitch, called a *negative* Doppler shift.

As an ultrasound beam propagates through the human body, it encounters a variety of interfaces, each of which will alter the course and transmission of the acoustic wavefront. (An interface is the apposition of any two substances of disparate acoustic impedance.) Interfaces that are dimensionally larger than the wavelength of the sound beam and are struck at close to 90° will produce the specular reflections that generate the borders and margins displayed in anatomic structures. Immobile interfaces smaller than the incident wavelength create speckle data, which forms the basis of the smooth textural appearance seen in solid parenchymal organs. Equally small or smaller moving interfaces (red blood cells) generate phase-shifted Rayleigh scattering, which provides the raw data used to generate all of the Doppler display modalities available on contemporary ultrasound imaging systems.

The returning Doppler data contain frequency, phase, and amplitude information about the Rayleigh scattering that occurred in the area being interrogated. Software-driven mathematical restatement of the Doppler equation converts frequency-shifted information into velocity information about the moving scatterers; phase change correlates with directionality of flow (toward or away from the transducer); and amplitude data yield information about the quantity of red blood cells (RBCs) moving through the insonated area. When these three echo data parameters are processed in various ways, any or all of the Doppler display modalities can be generated.

DOPPLER MODALITIES

The primary Doppler display modalities used in clinical hemodynamic evaluation are:

- Continuous-wave Doppler
- Color Doppler imaging
- Power Doppler imaging
- Spectral (pulsed-wave) Doppler

Continuous-Wave Doppler

Continuous-wave (CW) *Doppler* is the simplest and technologically least complicated method of displaying blood flow information. CW Doppler devices have two transducer crystals (Figure 17-8A), one continuously emitting and one continuously receiving acoustic information.

Continuous-wave Doppler is used in fetal monitoring devices and Doppler stethoscopes (Figure 17-8B) and provides a quick, sensitive, and inexpensive tool for detecting blood flow anywhere within the sensitivity zone of the transducer.

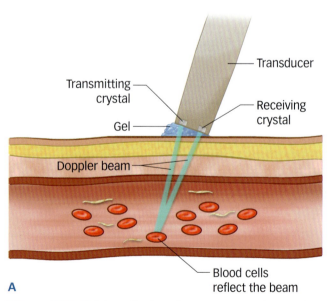
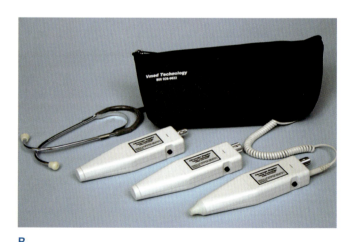

Figure 17-8. A Schematic of continuous-wave Doppler transducer, showing how transmitting crystals will continuously transmit a signal at a particular frequency while receiving crystals receive the reflected signal, which will be Doppler-shifted if the reflectors (here, red blood cells) are moving. **B** Handheld continuous-wave Doppler devices. CW Doppler instruments are used in a variety of clinical applications: vascular stethoscopes (top) and obstetric fetal heart transducer (bottom).

Because true continuous-wave Doppler is not based on pulse-echo imaging technology, it cannot be "gated," or directed to obtain depth-specific Doppler signals, as can spectral Doppler, nor can it be used for any imaging applications.

Color Doppler Imaging

Color Doppler imaging (CDI) integrates a global hemodynamic map on a two-dimensional real-time anatomic image (Figure 17-9). Using pulse-echo imaging technology, CDI extracts Doppler signals from the returning echo data set and sends them along separate processing channels to create a pixel-by-pixel map of blood flow. This hemodynamic information is either overlaid by or interwoven with a simultaneous gray-scale image of the corresponding anatomy. Each CDI pixel encodes blood flow characteristics typical of Doppler displays, i.e., presence, direction, relative velocity, and amplitude.

The primary utility of color Doppler imaging is in quickly, sensitively, and accurately displaying all hemodynamic activity within a selected field of view. Advantages of this mode include instantaneous differentiation of vascular from nonvascular structures (presuming they are normal and patent), real-time observation of flow patterns into and out of vascular beds, identification of abnormal hemodynamic patterns created by significant vascular stenoses or occlusions, and guidance in accurate range-gate placement for spectral Doppler interrogation of specific sites within a blood vessel.

The primary limitation of color Doppler imaging is that it cannot yield the quantitative data about blood flow (such as peak systolic and end-diastolic velocity values) that are requisite bits of information in the ratios and indices used as diagnostic criteria in many Doppler examination protocols.

Power Doppler Imaging

Power Doppler imaging (PDI) operates on the same engineering principles as color Doppler imaging: A color-coded image is presented simultaneously with a two-dimensional gray-scale image to provide a global hemodynamic picture of the area being examined (Figure 17-10A). The difference is that color pixels in power Doppler imaging display only presence and relative amplitude of flow, not flow directionality.

The primary advantage of power Doppler imaging is its increased sensitivity to very low-flow states, permitting the detection of blood flow even in very small vascular beds under very slow and sluggish conditions. Like color Doppler imaging, it is useful as a guide for accurate range-gate placement for subsequent spectral Doppler interrogation.

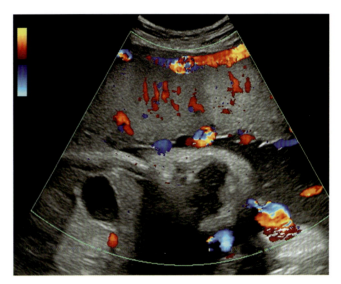

Figure 17-9. Color Doppler velocity imaging: a global hemodynamic map demonstrating the presence, direction, and relative velocity of blood flow within the selected field of view.

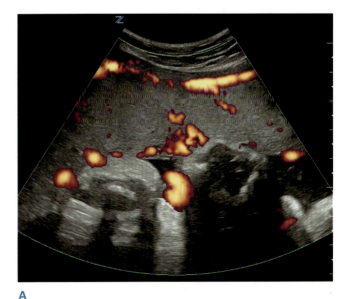

A

Figure 17-10. A Power Doppler imaging: a global hemodynamic map demonstrating the presence and relative amplitudes of blood flow within the selected field of view. (Figure continues . . .)

The primary limitations of power Doppler imaging include its inability to display flow directionality—toward or away from the transducer—and its inability to provide quantitative measurements. *Directional power Doppler imaging* (dPDI) is a hybrid display that adds positive/negative phase-shifted information extracted from CDI to the amplitude data used in PDI (Figure 17-10B). The result is a hemodynamic display modality that maintains sensitivity to low-flow states but adds the directionality information associated with CDI and spectral Doppler.

Spectral Doppler

Also called *pulsed* or *pulsed-wave* (PW) *Doppler*, *spectral Doppler* (Figure 17-11) is the only Doppler modality that can provide numeric values associated with blood flow: the quantitative information that is necessary in rendering a clinical interpretation of hemodynamic states. As pulsed-wave information is obtained using pulse-echo imaging methods, Doppler data can be obtained at a specific, operator-selected location from within a field of view. Using color Doppler imaging or power Doppler imaging to guide the placement of the pulsed-wave cursor assists in the more rapid and accurate use of this range gate. When activated, the gate captures an echo data set from its specific location, which is then processed into a graph-like spectral display. The same information displayed with other Doppler modes is present on a frequency spectrum: presence, direction, amplitude, and velocity.

Unique to spectral Doppler is its ability to demonstrate absolute, measurable velocity values—as opposed to the relative values displayed with color Doppler imaging. Quantifiable hemodynamic parameters that can be obtained from an arterial spectral Doppler waveform include peak systolic velocity (PSV), end-diastolic velocity (EDV), acceleration time (AT), and time-averaged mean velocity (TAMV). Incorporating these data points into a plethora of hemodynamic formulas yields the diagnostic criteria employed in many clinical Doppler examination protocols. Examples include the systolic/diastolic (S/D) ratio, the resistivity index (RI), the pulsatility index (PI), the acceleration index (AI), and volume flow measurements.

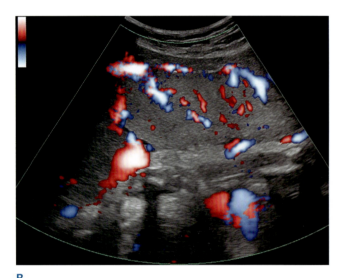

Figure 17-10, continued. B Directional power Doppler imaging: a global hemodynamic map demonstrating blood flow within the selected field of view that combines the sensitivity of power Doppler imaging and the directionality of color Doppler imaging.

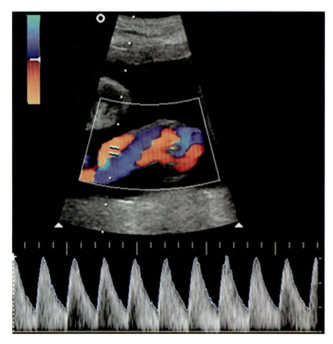

Figure 17-11. Spectral Doppler imaging. Blood flow presence, direction, and amplitude are displayed on a frequency spectral waveform in a duplex ultrasound image.

TRANSDUCERS

Transducers are the heart of every ultrasound imaging system, and their proper selection, use, and care form a core component of sonographic practice. Each probe—which is a collection of small piezoelectric transducer elements acting in unison—produces the acoustic wavefront that insonates the anatomy being examined and receives the returning echo data that constitute the basis of each sonographic image. Contemporary imaging probes are highly sophisticated medical instruments capable of producing very high spatial and contrast resolution (at the submillimeter level) in color Doppler and B modes as well as accurate spatial and temporal resolution of hemodynamic states in spectral and color Doppler modes. Several probe characteristics are pertinent to obstetric and gynecologic imaging: frequency range, array configuration, field of view, and footprint. (These parameters are discussed in the description of each probe type listed in "Array Configuration" on page 450.)

FREQUENCY RANGE

The traditional rule of thumb in sonographic imaging posits that higher-frequency probes produce images with higher spatial resolution but lack the ability to penetrate deep into the human body. *Spatial resolution* is the ability to distinguish between two point reflectors in close proximity within a single imaging frame. Lower frequencies, on the other hand, penetrate to deeper depths but generally yield images with diminished spatial resolution. It follows, therefore, that the first challenge in selecting the appropriate probe for a given exam type is to identify the highest frequency that can penetrate to the depth required for adequately imaging the areas of interest. Transabdominal imaging in the second and third trimesters, for example, will require lower-frequency probes (typically 3–7 MHz) than endovaginal imaging in first trimester or gynecologic examinations (typically 5–12 MHz).

Most of today's ultrasound probes operate within a frequency range that is somewhat operator selectable. For example, a convex 6–3 MHz probe permits adequate imaging of deeper structures when the 3 MHz end of the frequency bandwidth is employed, while allowing improved imaging of more superficial structures when the 6 MHz end is used. Operator selection of imaging frequencies from the control console eliminates the need to change probes physically during a single examination in which structures both near and far need to be examined. While an operator-selected single frequency is displayed on the monitor, it is important to remember that virtually all ultrasound probes actually utilize a bandwidth of frequencies in creating images; the displayed frequency typically represents either the highest or the mean value within the full bandwidth.

Today's ultrasound systems also allow the user to select fundamental, harmonic, or both frequency types to enhance penetration and contrast resolution of images. *Contrast resolution* is the ability to distinguish between subtle textural differences within a single soft tissue structure.

Fundamental frequencies are those generated by the piezoelectric elements in the probe and are a function of the physical properties of the ceramic crystals and of the way the system transmitter is programmed to perform. By integrating crystals with broad bandwidth capabilities and pulsing them in complex patterns, the operator can—to some degree—change the fundamental frequency of the transmitted acoustic wave. Using the example given above, a 6–3 MHz convex probe can be instructed by the operator to transmit a higher frequency (6 MHz) for optimal near-field imaging or a lower frequency (3 MHz) for better far-field penetration. The primary clinical advantage of fundamental frequency imaging is better near-field spatial resolution and a wider B-mode bandwidth, which produces softer textures within solid parenchymal organs.

Harmonic frequencies, on the other hand, are generated within the soft tissue being insonated. As an acoustic beam propagates through a tissue medium, shifts in amplitude, frequency, and phase occur—the reflected component of which is received by the transducer and used to create all the sonographic display modes.

By use of sophisticated electronic filters and mode-specific digital signal-processing channels, the system receiver is capable of extricating these individual echo data parameters. Changes in amplitude permit the construction of a B-mode image; changes in phase yield the various Doppler display modes; and changes in frequency provide the harmonic waves useful in enhancing two-dimensional gray-scale imaging. The clinical advantages of harmonic imaging are increased penetration without sacrificing spatial resolution and a "cleaner" image devoid of much of the noise and clutter created when a fundamental wavefront strikes the skin surface and body wall. This increased signal-to-noise ratio results in enhanced contrast resolution.

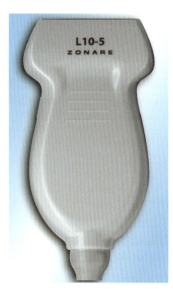

Figure 17-12. Linear array probe. Transducer elements are arranged along a straight line: wide footprint, rectangular field of view.

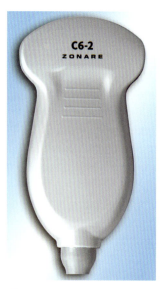

Figure 17-13. Convex array probe. Transducer elements are arranged along a curved line: wide footprint, wedge-shaped field of view with wide near field.

ARRAY CONFIGURATION

Ultrasound probes are available with different array configurations to address the broad diversity of imaging needs in obstetric and gynecologic practice. *Array* refers to the number of piezoelectric crystal elements present in a particular probe and the geometric pattern in which they are arranged. The number of elements integrated into a given probe varies widely by manufacturer and is constrained by the physical size of the probe footprint and the number of processing channels the system receiver employs.

Obviously, probes with a small footprint—an endovaginal instrument, for example—accommodate fewer individual crystal elements than probes with a large footprint, e.g., a wide-aperture convex transabdominal probe. Imaging systems that employ larger numbers of individual processing channels—1024 compared with 128, for example—typically integrate an equal number of individual crystal elements into their probes. While image quality in traditional beamformer-based sonographic imaging systems is directly related to the number of crystal elements and processing channels on board, image quality in more recent zone sonography imaging methods is not. Rather, they rely on high-capacity, high-speed digital signal-processing components and advanced software algorithms to produce images of equal or better spatial, contrast, and temporal resolution.

Traditional types of ultrasound probes include the linear array, convex array, phased array, matrix array, and endovaginal. Each has a signature *footprint*, which is the physical dimensionality that comes in contact with the human body, and *field of view*, which is the displayed image geometry.

Linear Array Probes

In a *linear array* probe (Figure 17-12), the piezoelectric transducer elements are arranged along a straight line. They can be fired sequentially or in complex group patterns that allow the acoustic beam to be focused and steered. Images produced by linear array probes are rectangular. Imaging advantages of linear arrays include better spatial resolution and a wider field of view in the near field. Disadvantages include a large footprint that can render them impractical for use with tight anatomic windows, such as the intercostal spaces in the abdomen and suprapubic transvesicular scanning in the pelvis.

Convex Array Probes

Convex array probes (Figure 17-13), also called *curved linear* or *curvilinear* probes, combine the near-field advantages of linear array and the far-field advantages of phased sector probes. The piezoelectric elements are arranged along a single convex line, which creates a wider, higher-resolution image in the near field while maintaining image width and quality in the far

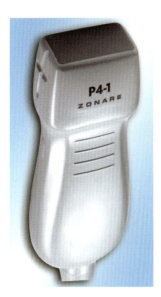

Figure 17-14. Phased array probe. Transducer elements are arranged in a short, compact line: narrow footprint, wedge-shaped field of view with narrow near field.

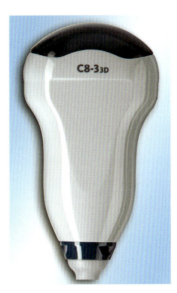

Figure 17-15. Matrix array probe. Transducer elements are arranged in several parallel lines for acquiring volumetric data sets used in 3D application: narrow footprint, wedge-shaped field of view.

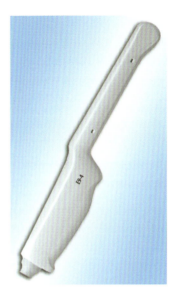

Figure 17-16. Endovaginal probe. Transducer elements are compactly arranged at the tip of the probe for intracavitary imaging. Tight, narrow footprint; wedge-shaped image with narrow near field.

field. Convex array footprints can vary considerably in width and are best suited for soft tissue windows rather than windows narrowed by adjacent bony or gas-containing structures. The field of view produced by convex array probes is wedge-shaped with a wide near field.

Phased Array Probes

Phased array probes (Figure 17-14) are constructed with the piezoelectric elements arranged in a short, compact, linear configuration; however, they are fired using timing delays to create a wedge-shaped, or sector, image. The advantages of these probes include a smaller footprint that is ideal for tight anatomic windows and a wide far field of view. Disadvantages affect primarily the near field and include a narrow field of view and diminished spatial resolution. Phased array probes can be designed for extracorporeal or intracavitary use. Most endovaginal transducers are phased array.

Matrix Array Probes

The piezoelectric elements in a *matrix array* transducer (Figure 17-15) are arranged in several parallel lines that permit acquisition of two orthogonal planes of echo data simultaneously. The acoustic wavefront can be steered through the anatomic structures of interest either mechanically or electronically. On-board computers register the locations of the returning echo and create voxels (volume elements) that can be processed to create 3D and 4D images. The footprint of a matrix array probe is large and the field of view varies with the volumetric imaging mode selected.

ENDOVAGINAL PROBES

Endovaginal probes (Figure 17-16) utilize a convex or phased array configuration of piezoelectric elements placed directly at the tip of the probe (*end fire*) or angled slightly toward the area of interest (*offset*). Offset probes are by far the most commonly available type on contemporary sonographic imaging systems. They require less "torquing" of the device in the vagina and are therefore better tolerated by the patient. The widely divergent wedge-shaped field of view obtained via a small footprint is ideally suited for panning through the entire female pelvis with minimal transducer manipulation.

IMAGING ARTIFACTS

A sonographic imaging artifact can be defined as a structure or feature not really present but visible as the result of a breakdown in the way an ultrasound system constructs an image. The pulse-echo imaging method forming the core of all sonographic systems relies on several assumptions about acoustic energy and its interaction with human soft tissue. Key among these assumptions are the following:

- that ultrasound travels at 1540 m/sec in human soft tissue
- that an echo received by a particular element originated from that element
- that an ultrasound beam is two-dimensional, i.e., it has no thickness

If there is any deviation from these suppositions, which happens every time human anatomy is insonated, errors in the placement of echo data information in the appropriate corresponding image pixels occur. These are called *artifacts*. Some artifacts are characterized by the appearance of excess echoes in the image where none should be seen, some by the absence of echoes where they should appear, and others by the incorrect placement of echoes in the image itself.

The entire realm of sonographic image artifacts is broad and complex, and a complete discussion of them is beyond the scope of this chapter. Several artifacts pertinent to a review of obstetric and gynecologic sonography are discussed below. These include:

- posterior acoustic shadowing
- posterior acoustic enhancement
- reverberation artifacts
- refraction artifacts
- section-thickness artifacts
- mirror-image artifacts
- secondary lobe artifacts

POSTERIOR ACOUSTIC SHADOWING

Posterior acoustic shadowing (Figure 17-17) is the reduction in amplitude of echoes lying beyond, or deep to, a highly reflective interface. This reduction in amplitude is the result of near total attenuation of acoustic energy as it encounters a surface interface of substantially different acoustic impedance from that of the medium through which it has been traveling. Since a large proportion of the incident beam is reflected and/or absorbed at this interface surface, little energy remains to travel deeper into tissue and continue creating echo information. Reduction in beam intensity deep to a high-level attenuator appears as a shadow on the image.

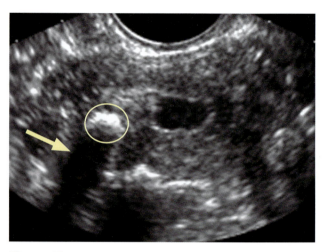

Figure 17-17. Posterior acoustic shadowing (arrow) behind a focally calcified uterine fibroid (circled).

POSTERIOR ACOUSTIC ENHANCEMENT

Posterior acoustic enhancement is the opposite of shadowing. As an acoustic beam of given intensity encounters a structure that is less attenuating than adjacent soft tissue, it continues to propagate through the structure unimpeded. As the beam exits the structure, the beam intensity remains strong enough to produce high-amplitude echoes as it encounters interfaces deep to the structure. As a result, the echogenicity of the area behind the structure appears increased compared to that of adjacent tissue areas. This appearance of increased echogenicity in tissue relative to that adjacent to it is also called *posterior acoustic enhancement* or *enhanced through-transmission*.

Posterior acoustic enhancement is strong evidence of the presence of a fluid-filled structure and is normally seen, for example, behind the full urinary bladder or behind an ovarian cyst (Figures 17-18A and B). The presence of enhancement behind other complex or echo-filled masses is evidence that the mass has a definite fluid component or high water content. Other common examples of structures that appear with posterior acoustic enhancement include normal ovaries, hematomas, and abscesses (Figures 17-18C and D).

REVERBERATION ARTIFACTS

Reverberation artifacts are observed as equally spaced, bright linear echoes resulting from repeated reflections from specular-type interfaces. They are commonly seen in the near field of a sonographic image when the transmitted acoustic wave strikes the interface

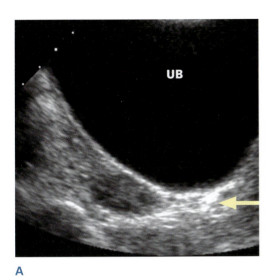
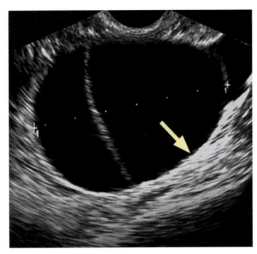
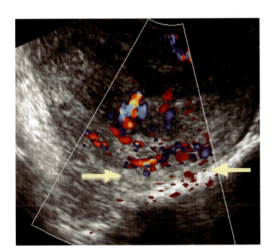
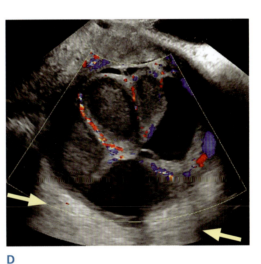

Figure 17-18. Posterior acoustic enhancement (arrows) demonstrated behind **A** a full urinary bladder (UB), **B** an ovarian cystic mass, **C** intrauterine retained products of conception with hematoma, and **D** a tubo-ovarian abscess.

between the transducer face and the body wall. The large magnitude of difference in acoustic impedance between transducer face and body wall creates a high-amplitude reflection that then returns back to the transducer face, reflects off it, and is once again sent back toward the body wall. This back-and-forth "ringing" of the acoustic pulse continues until all the acoustic energies are attenuated. Since the ultrasound machine is registering echoes as a function of time, each successive line of echoes returning to the transducer will be registered at a greater distance from the probe face with diminishing amplitude (Figure 17-19A).

Reverberation artifacts are also commonly seen behind anechoic fluid collections, such as amniotic fluid and simple or complex ovarian cysts (Figures 17-19B and C) as the acoustic wavefront bounces back and forth between the posterior wall of the fluid collection and specular reflectors behind it.

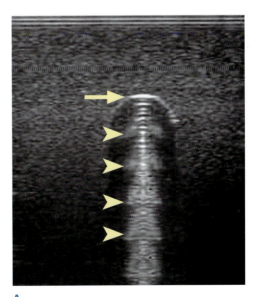

Figure 17-19. Reverberation. **A** Test phantom imaging demonstrates the initial reflector (arrow) and equally spaced reverberatory reflections (arrowheads). (Figure continues . . .)

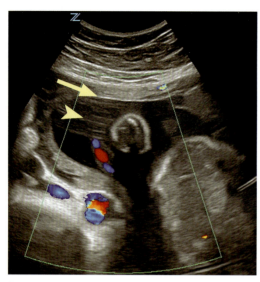

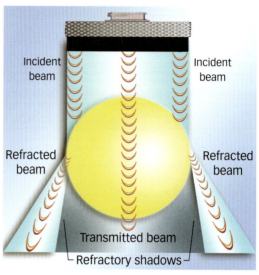

B

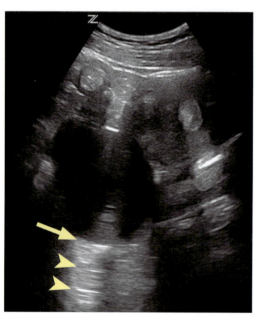

C

Figure 17-19, continued. B Sonographic demonstration of reverberation seen in amniotic fluid emanating from the specular interface (arrow) at the chorioamniotic membrane interface (arrowhead). **C** Sonographic demonstration of reverberation seen behind the back wall (arrow) of a bright specular ovarian cyst (arrowheads).

REFRACTION ARTIFACTS

A *refraction artifact* is observed as a triangular area of echo dropout adjacent to a curved structure whose acoustic impedance differs significantly from that of surrounding tissue (Figure 17-20A). The two physical conditions that must be met for acoustic refraction to occur are oblique incidence of the sound beam and a change in velocity through the medium. *Oblique incidence* happens when the acoustic wave strikes

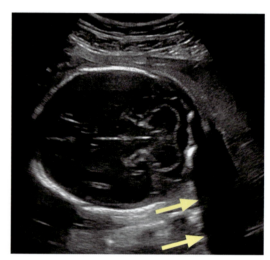

B

Figure 17-20. Refraction artifacts. **A** Schematic illustration of areas of acoustic shadowing produced by sound beam refraction. **B** Sonographic demonstration of refractory shadow (arrows) emanating from the highly reflective, curved surface of the fetal occipital bone. (Figure continues . . .)

a convex surface; *velocity changes* occur when the sound beam encounters an anatomic structure with significantly different acoustic impedance. The net effect of these two physical phenomena is a redirecting of a portion of the sound beam away from its incident path and a loss of echo data information.

Refraction artifacts, or *refractory shadows* as they are sometimes called, are frequently seen arising from the lateral aspect of the fetal head in axial section (Figure 17-20B), from the edges of cysts (Figure 17-20C), and from the edges of uterine fibroids (Figure 17-20D), to mention a few examples.

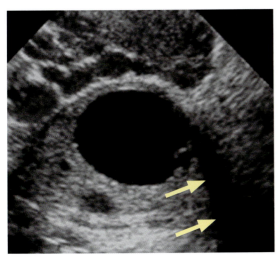

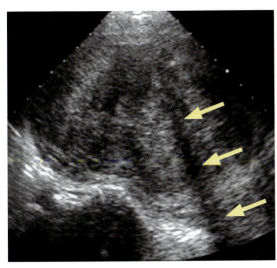

Figure 17-20, continued. C Sonographic demonstration of refractory shadow (arrows) from the lateral surface of an ovary containing a mature ovarian follicle. **D** Sonographic demonstration of refractory shadow (arrows) from the curved surface of an intramural uterine fibroid.

SECTION-THICKNESS ARTIFACTS

Theoretically, a two-dimensional sectional image should be produced by a two-dimensional ultrasound beam, or one of infinite "thinness." In reality, however, the ultrasound beam is three-dimensional and possesses a thickness that varies at different distances from the transducer face. Because of this disparity in beam thickness, some echoes received from the sides of the wider portion of the beam are recorded and displayed as if they came from the thinnest part of the beam, the beam axis (Figure 17-21A). Because of the assumption that all echoes originate along the axis of

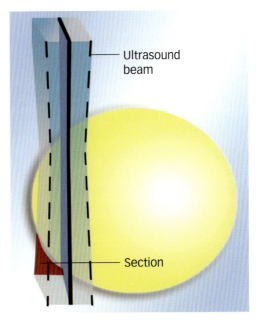

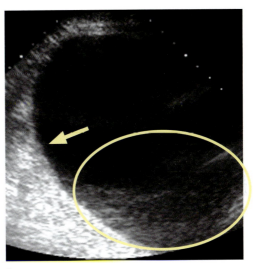

Figure 17-21. Section-thickness artifact. **A** Schematic shows echoes generated by tissue (section) that is out of the acquisition plane of the transducer (broken black lines) and will be displayed on the image as low-level clutter. **B** Echoes generated by tissue that is out of the acquisition plane of the transducer are displayed and circled as misregistered echoes from the curvature of the lateral bladder wall (arrow).

the transducer, the result is a misregistration artifact in which low-level echoes are erroneously placed on the image. These are called *section-thickness* or *slice-thickness artifacts*.

A typical example of this type of artifact is the low-level echoes that may be seen near the inner lateral walls of the fluid-filled urinary bladder (Figure 17-21B).

MIRROR-IMAGE ARTIFACTS

A *mirror-image artifact* is a type of multipath artifact in which a structure is anomalously placed on the display due to redirection of the sound beam as it interacts with strong reflectors. This phenomenon occurs when an object is located in front of a highly reflective surface at which near total reflection takes place. The accompanying image, using a tissue-equivalent test phantom, demonstrates duplication of the true object (in the case of Figure 17-22A, embedded in liver-mimicking phantom material). During its initial pass through the real material, the acoustic beam produces imaging data that are appropriately displayed above the mirror plane. As the beam continues its forward path, it strikes the mirror plane, ricochets off it, and sends a duplicate imaging data set back to the transducer. As this data set is received later in time, it is displayed as a duplicate structure deeper in the image.

In clinical practice, mirror-image artifacts are most commonly seen in the abdomen, near the strongly reflective liver/diaphragm interface (Figure 17-22B), and in the pelvis, arising from the posterior uterine wall/bowel interface (Figure 17-22C).

SECONDARY LOBE ARTIFACTS

By nature of their geometric configuration, electronic transducer arrays form "puddles" of acoustic energy both between and at the edges of the piezoelectric crystals (Figure 17-23A). One of the assumptions used by ultrasound imaging systems is that the ultrasound beam is infinitely thin—lacking a z-axis (width). In reality, however, diffraction prevents this from being realized. These *secondary lobes* radiate outward at various angles to the main beam, interact with near-field soft tissue, and generate image artifacts due to error in the positioning of the returning echoes. When echo data received at the surface of an individual transducer element are actually transmitted by a different element and at asynchronous moments in firing time, they are registered in the scan convertor erroneously. There are two types of secondary lobes: side lobes and grating lobes.

Side lobes are typically low in intensity compared with the main beam. Because the energy present in side lobes is typically very low, they generally do not create noticeable imaging degradation. However, if these lobes encounter a strong specular reflector, the

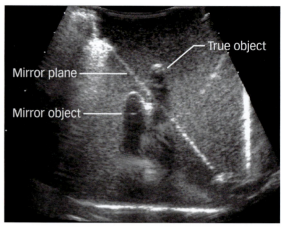

A

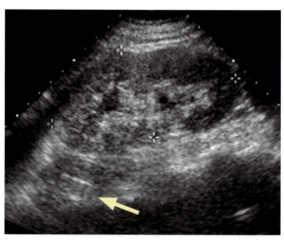

B

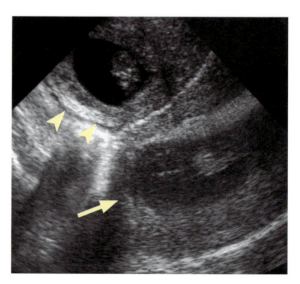

C

Figure 17-22. Mirror-image artifact. **A** Test phantom image demonstrating a mirror image of tissue-equivalent material with an embedded focal true object. **B** Sagittal sonogram demonstrating a mirror image (arrow) of the kidney. **C** Mirror image of a first trimester gravid uterus (arrow) emanating from the specular interface between the posterior uterine wall and gas-filled bowel (arrowheads).

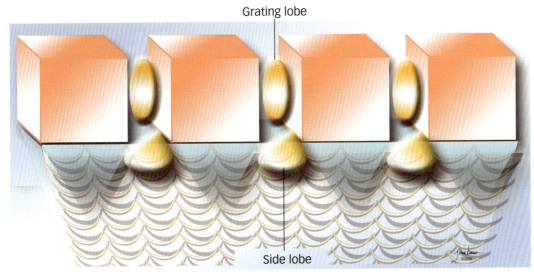

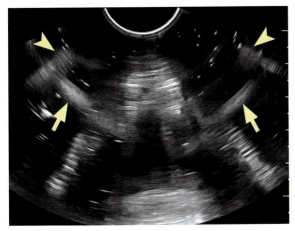

Figure 17-23. Secondary lobe artifacts. **A** Schematic representation of the origins of grating lobe and side-lobe artifacts. **B** Water path scanning, demonstrating "cloud-like" grating (arrowheads) and crescent-shaped side-lobe artifacts (arrows).

reflected energy will be added to the energy from the main beam that is used to create the image and will appear as a crescent-shaped band of spurious echoes within the image (Figure 17-23B).

Grating lobes are the result of the summation of side lobes from individual crystals. Low-intensity side lobes, when added together, create significant secondary lobes of energy when multiple crystals are pulsed simultaneously and appear as swatches of spurious echoes usually in the central portion of the image. Grating lobes assume a more "cloud-like" appearance than their side-lobe counterparts (Figure 17-23B).

CHAPTER 17 REVIEW QUESTIONS

1. All of the following indices are measures of potential tissue heating by acoustic energy EXCEPT:
   A. MI
   B. TIs
   C. TIb
   D. TIc

2. The bioeffect that results from compression and rarefaction of a medium as an acoustic wave travels through it is called:
   A. Cavitation
   B. Acoustic streaming
   C. Hyperthermia
   D. Insonation

3. Which of the following is NOT subject to the potential induction of acoustic streaming?
   A. Arteries
   B. Veins
   C. Ovaries
   D. Lymphatics

4. The mechanical index measures:
   A. Thermal changes in soft tissue
   B. Positive acoustic pressure present in a medium
   C. Negative acoustic pressure present in a medium
   D. Cavitational changes

5. The two-dimensional sonographic method of displaying the amplitude of a returning echo as a shade of gray on the display is called:
   A. Real time
   B. Static scanning
   C. M-mode
   D. B-mode

6. The sonographic display modality that displays a single B-mode line of site along a horizontal axis is called:
   A. M-mode
   B. B-mode
   C. PW Doppler
   D. Continuous-wave Doppler

7. The simplest mathematical expression of the Doppler effect is stated as:
   A. $F_d = F_r - F_i$
   B. $F_r = F_d - F_i$
   C. $F_r = F_i - F_d$
   D. $F_d = F_i - F_r$

8. Doppler information is obtained from analyzing and displaying:
   A. Specular reflectors
   B. Nonspecular reflectors
   C. Rayleigh scatter
   D. Transmitted energy

9. Doppler data received by the transducer include all of these signal parameters EXCEPT:
   A. Frequency
   B. Depth
   C. Amplitude
   D. Phase

10. The simplest and technologically least complicated method of displaying blood flow information is:
    A. Color Doppler imaging
    B. Power Doppler imaging
    C. Continuous-wave Doppler
    D. Spectral Doppler

11. The two-dimensional sonographic imaging modality that provides a global display of the presence, direction, and relative velocities present in a hemodynamic state is:
    A. Color Doppler imaging
    B. Power Doppler imaging
    C. Continuous-wave Doppler
    D. Spectral Doppler

12. The only Doppler ultrasound modality that permits the quantification of flow states is:
    A. Color Doppler imaging
    B. Power Doppler imaging
    C. Continuous-wave Doppler
    D. Spectral Doppler

13. Higher-frequency ultrasound probes, compared with lower-frequency probes, are associated with:
    A. Better penetration and better spatial resolution
    B. Less penetration and better spatial resolution
    C. Less penetration and less spatial resolution
    D. Better penetration and less spatial resolution

14. Ultrasound frequencies returning to the transducer that are generated by shifts in phase and frequency within the tissue itself are called:
    A. Fundamental
    B. Secondary
    C. Harmonic
    D. Tertiary

15. The B-mode method of generating, processing, and combining several image subframes into a single frame is called:
    A. Compounding
    B. Harmonics
    C. Enhancement
    D. Digital signal processing

16. Ultrasound probes constructed with the piezoelectric elements arranged in a short, compact, linear configuration and fired using timing delays to create a wedge-shaped, or sector, image are called:
    A. Linear arrays
    B. Matrix arrays

C. Convex arrays

D. Phased arrays

17. What is the name of an ultrasound probe constructed with the piezoelectric elements arranged in several parallel lines, permitting acquisition of two orthogonal planes of echo data simultaneously and used in 3D and 4D imaging?

    A. Linear arrays
    B. Matrix arrays
    C. Convex arrays
    D. Phased arrays

18. The reduction in amplitude of echoes lying beyond, or deep to, a highly reflective interface is an artifact called:

    A. Posterior acoustic enhancement
    B. Posterior acoustic shadowing
    C. Section-thickness artifact
    D. Mirror-image artifact

19. What is the name of the sonographic imaging artifact that appears as equally spaced, bright linear echoes resulting from repeated reflections from specular-type interfaces?

    A. Reverberation
    B. Refractions
    C. Section thickness
    D. Side lobes

ANSWERS

See Appendix A on page 484 for answers.

REFERENCES

1. American Institute of Ultrasound in Medicine: *Medical Ultrasound Safety*. Laurel, American Institute of Ultrasound in Medicine, 2014, p 7.

2. Myers MR: Transient temperature rise due to ultrasound absorption at a bone/soft-tissue interface. J Acoust Soc Am 115:2887–2891, 2004.

3. Damianou CA, Sanghvi NT, Fry FJ, et al: Dependence of ultrasonic attenuation and absorption in dog soft tissues on temperature and thermal dose. J Acoust Soc Am 102:628–634, 1997.

4. Arthur RM, Straube WL, Trobaugh JW, et al: Noninvasive estimation of hyperthermia temperatures with ultrasound. Int J Hyperthermia 21:589–600, 2005.

5. Bacon DR, Carstensen EL: Measurement of enhanced heating due to ultrasound absorption in the presence of nonlinear propagation. Proc 1989 IEEE Ultrasonics Symposium, 1989, pp 1057–1060.

6. Miller MW, Nyborg WL, Dewey WC, et al: Hyperthermic teratogenicity, thermal dose and diagnostic ultrasound during pregnancy: implications of new standards on tissue heating. Int J Hyperthermia 18:361–384, 2002.

7. Lubbers J, Hekkenberg RT, Bezemer RA: Time to threshold (TT), a safety parameter for heating by diagnostic ultrasound. Ultrasound Med Biol 29:755–764, 2003.

8. Health Canada. *Guidelines for the Safe Use of Diagnostic Ultrasound*. Ottawa, Health Canada, 2001. Available at http://www.hc-sc.gc.ca/ewh-semt/pubs/radiation/01hecs-secs255/index-eng.php.

9. Miller MW, Nyborg WL, Dewey WC, et al: Hyperthermic teratogenicity, thermal dose and diagnostic ultrasound during pregnancy: implications of new standards on tissue heating. Int J Hyperthermia 18:361–384, 2002.

10. Dyson M: Non-thermal cellular effects of ultrasound. Br J Cancer Suppl 45:165–171, 1982.

11. Miller MW, Miller DL, Brayman AA: A review of in vitro bioeffects of inertial ultrasonic cavitation from a mechanistic perspective. Ultrasound Med Biol 22:1131–1154, 1996.

12. Liu Y, Yang H, Sakanishi A: Ultrasound: mechanical gene transfer into plant cells by sonoporation. Biotechnol Adv 24:1–16, 2006.

13. Guzmán HR, Nguyen DX, Khan S, et al: Ultrasound-mediated disruption of cell membranes, II: heterogeneous effects on cells. J Acoust Soc Am 110:597–606, 2001.

14. Prat F, Chapelon JY, Chauffert B, et al: Cytotoxic effects of acoustic cavitation on HT-29 cells and a rat peritoneal carcinomatosis in vitro. Cancer Res 51:3024–3029, 1991.

15. Miller DL, Thomas RM, Frazier ME: Single strand breaks in CHO cell DNA induced by ultrasonic cavitation in vitro. Ultrasound Med Biol 17:401–406, 1991.

16. Wu J, Winkler AJ, O'Neill TP: Effect of acoustic streaming on ultrasonic heating. Ultrasound Med Biol 20:195–201, 1994.

17. Carstensen EL, Dalecki D, Gracewski SM, et al: Nonlinear propagation and the output indices. J Ultrasound Med 18:69–80, 1999.

18. Apfel RE, Holland CK: Gauging the likelihood of cavitation from short-pulse, low-duty cycle diagnostic ultrasound. Ultrasound Med Biol 17:179–185, 1991.

SUGGESTED READINGS

Fowlkes JB, Holland CK: Biologic effects and safety. In Rumack CM, Wilson SR, Charboneau JW, et al (eds): *Diagnostic Ultrasound*, 4th edition. Philadelphia, Elsevier Mosby, 2011, pp 34–52.

Hagen-Ansert SL, Craig M, Coffin C, et al: Foundations of sonography. In Hagen-Ansert SL (ed): *Textbook of Diagnostic Ultrasonography*, 7th edition. St. Louis, Elsevier Mosby, 2012, pp 2–116.

Hedrick WR, Hykes DL, Starchman DE: *Ultrasound Physics and Instrumentation*, 4th edition. St. Louis, Elsevier Mosby, 2005.

Kremkau FW: *Sonography: Principles and Instruments*, 9th edition. St. Louis, Elsevier Saunders, 2016.

Merritt CRB: The physics of ultrasound. In Rumack CM, Wilson SR, Charboneau JW, et al (eds): *Diagnostic Ultrasound*, 4th edition. Philadelphia, Elsevier Mosby, 2011, pp 2–33.

Owen CA, Zagzebski JA: *Ultrasound Physics Review: A Review for the ARDMS SPI Exam*. Pasadena, Davies Publishing, 2012.

CHAPTER 18

Protocols and Patient Care

Examination Protocols

Preparing for the Exam

Endovaginal and Transperineal Imaging

Sonographic Approaches

Measurement Techniques

Integration of Data

Reporting Results

The Sonographer's Role in Invasive Procedures

Patient Safety

Quality Assurance

EXAMINATION PROTOCOLS

Examination protocols are standardized methods of conducting sonographic studies aimed at ensuring consistent quality by establishing conventional performance criteria for each type of exam. Examinations should always be performed in accordance with clear and specific protocols, and the requisite images and clips should be obtained, labeled, and stored for subsequent physician review and interpretation. (See Appendix C, "AIUM Practice Guidelines," published by the American Institute of Ultrasound in Medicine, on the performance of pelvic ultrasound examinations, obstetric ultrasound examinations, and ultrasonography in reproductive medicine.)

Generally speaking, examination protocols encompass the following preliminary tasks:

- Gathering clinical information
- Selecting the proper instrumentation (transducers) and sonographic approach (transabdominal, endovaginal, transperineal, etc.)
- Selecting appropriate exam-specific technical parameters (frequency, post-processing parameters, consideration of ALARA principles)
- Obtaining and documenting an established and comprehensive series of images utilizing appropriate imaging modes (B-mode, color Doppler, spectral Doppler, and/or M-mode)

The exact content and location of images contained within these series vary widely from practice to practice; however, standards have been established by several national professional associations. Examples of imaging standards for each type of obstetric and gynecologic ultrasound examination are included in Appendix C, "AIUM Practice Guidelines."

Examination protocols are intended to be a roadmap to the performance of a particular type of sonographic examination—whether directed (targeted), limited, or complete in scope.

CLINICAL STANDARDS AND GUIDELINES

As valued members of the healthcare team, sonographers are expected to adopt and adhere to established professional performance standards. The Society of Diagnostic Medical Sonography publishes *Diagnostic Ultrasound Clinical Practice Standards*,[1] which outlines minimum practice standards, including the following:

- Patient education and communication
- Analysis and determination of the proper method of implementing and conducting a diagnostic ultrasound examination
- Documentation and evaluation of the examination results
- Implementation and conduct of quality assurance performance standards
- Maintaining quality of patient care in the ultrasound laboratory
- Participation in self-assessment and continuing educational activities
- Ongoing collaboration with all members of the healthcare team
- Adherence to an established code of medical ethics

PREPARING FOR THE EXAM

SONOGRAPHER PREPARATION

Prior to the start of any obstetric or gynecologic sonographic examination, the sonographer should obtain and record pertinent clinical information about the patient. It is imperative that the patient be properly identified and that orders for the appropriate examination have been generated. If a chart is available, relevant medical history, physical findings, and laboratory results should be gleaned and recorded on the sonography worksheet or in the electronic medical record, according to the protocols and requirements of the institution under whose auspices the examination is being performed. Both the reports and images of prior ultrasound studies should be reviewed when these are available. Care should be taken to enter correct and complete data into the patient identification page of the ultrasound system software, and the appropriate examination preset that is proprietary to each manufacturer should be selected prior to the start of the examination.

PATIENT PREPARATION

When the patient arrives in the examination room, the sonographer should introduce him- or herself and explain to the patient, in understandable language, what examination is to be performed and what the patient can expect during the procedure. A brief interview with the patient is useful in obtaining additional medical information about indications for the exam, pertinent medical history and symptomatology, and prior testing and/or imaging studies that have been performed.

Gynecologic Exams

Preparation for a sonographic examination of the female reproductive tract traditionally involves the patient's filling her urinary bladder. A full urinary bladder displaces loops of small intestine upward and out of the false pelvis, providing a wide-open acoustic window for viewing the uterus, cervix, vagina, ovaries, adnexa, and potential spaces deep within the pelvic cavity. The typical instruction to the patient for filling the bladder is to remain well hydrated for 24 hours prior to the scheduled appointment and, one hour before the examination, to drink four 8-ounce glasses of water, refraining from emptying the bladder until the exam is completed. While filling the bladder and holding it for up to an hour is uncomfortable and may be unnecessary for limited studies that can be performed using a transvaginal (endovaginal) approach alone, the full bladder remains requisite when a complete examination of the true pelvis is required.

In volumetric terms an adequately full urinary bladder requires, in most patients, approximately 500 cc of retained urine. From an imaging perspective, the bladder is considered adequately full when the dome of the bladder extends cephalad to the fundus of the uterus (Figure 18-1A). This level of filling permits complete visualization of not only the uterine fundus but also any focal lesions, particularly fibroids that may be extending exophytically from the fundus. If the dome of the bladder extends only to the level of the fundus, refractory artifacts from the curved surfaces of both the uterus and the bladder preclude an adequate anatomic evaluation (Figure 18-1B).

Obstetric Exams

The requirement of a full urinary bladder for obstetric ultrasound examination varies from practice to practice. During the first trimester, an endovaginal approach is usually adequate for visualizing intrauterine contents, permitting biometric measurements of the embryo(s) when present, establishing viability, and examining the adnexa and the anterior and posterior cul-de-sac for any concomitant pathology. A full bladder may be necessary to evaluate any uterine pathology, particularly fibroids, extending beyond the endovaginal field of view or transducer frequency limitations.

During the second and third trimesters, a full bladder is necessary for a transabdominal evaluation of the lower uterine segment and to establish the position of the lower edge of the placenta relative to the cervix.

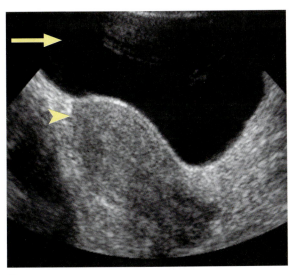

A

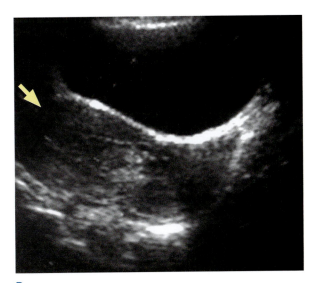

B

Figure 18-1. **A** Adequate bladder filling. Sagittal section through the uterus demonstrating the dome (arrow) of the urinary bladder extending cephalad to the uterine fundus (arrowhead).
B Inadequate bladder filling. Refraction from the curved anatomic surfaces anterior to the uterus casts an acoustic shadow (arrow).

However, an overly full urinary bladder may result in a false-positive diagnosis of placenta previa as the bladder compresses the lower uterine segment and the intrauterine contents. Repeat post-void imaging will decompress the pelvic anatomy and permit a more accurate determination of the relationship between the placenta and the cervix. In some practices, patient discomfort and the time necessary for patients to fill their bladders along with this potential for false-positive findings have been obviated by the routine use of translabial and/or endovaginal imaging of the lower uterine segment and cervix. Patients who have had a prior sonogram that has ruled out lower uterine segment abnormalities and placenta previa may also be spared the discomfort and inconvenience of a full urinary bladder.

ENDOVAGINAL AND TRANSPERINEAL IMAGING

Endovaginal (or transvaginal) and transperineal (translabial) imaging require direct contact of the ultrasound transducer with the patient's external genitalia; the endovaginal approach requires the instrumentation of the vagina itself. Both should be performed after clearly communicating with the patient why these approaches are necessary and how they will be conducted. If the patient has been holding on to a full bladder, it usually comes as a great relief when she is allowed to void prior to the next stage of the examination.

Upon returning to the exam room and undressing as she would for a pelvic exam, the patient is shown the probe, covered with a sterile sheath or condom, and invited to ask questions. (Nonlatex probe covers should be available for those patients with a latex allergy.) For endovaginal imaging, a generous amount of lubricant is applied to the probe and the patient is offered the option of inserting the probe herself or having the sonographer do it. In either case, the patient's modesty is maintained throughout the examination with a covering sheet. For translabial imaging, the contact must be made by the sonographer. Adequate scanning gel is applied to the probe and gentle contact with the labia is maintained throughout the procedure.

When either an endovaginal or a translabial examination is performed by a male sonographer, it is advisable (and in many facilities and practices mandatory) to have a female staff member present in the exam room to serve as a chaperone during this portion of the sonographic examination. It is always the patient's prerogative to undergo or forgo either of these imaging approaches.

Patients for whom an endovaginal or translabial examination is not advisable and generally not performed include the following:

- Patients who are confused, unable to cooperate, or in any way *non compos mentis* (of unsound mind)
- Patients who are virginal
- Patients who have received pelvic radiation for cervical carcinoma, in whom the vagina will be scarred and the endovaginal approach is likely to be painful and unsuccessful

SONOGRAPHIC APPROACHES

EXTRACORPOREAL APPROACH

An extracorporeal sonographic approach relies on the utilization of externally accessible anatomic windows through which the acoustic wavefront can be directed. Depending on the body part being examined and the application selected, these acoustic windows are referred to variously as:

- *Transabdominal*: through the anterior abdominal wall
- *Transvesicular*: through the full urinary bladder
- *Transperineal*: across the perineum
- *Intercostal*: through a rib interspace
- *Subcostal*: from beneath the costal margin
- *Substernal*: from beneath the sternum
- *Suprasternal*: from above the sternal notch

In obstetric and gynecologic sonography, the most commonly utilized extracorporeal windows are the transvesicular and transperineal approaches. Using a full urinary bladder as the acoustic window, the transvesicular approach is the standard initial examination method for evaluation of the entire pelvis in gynecologic applications. In first trimester obstetric applications, it is useful for assessing the uterus, its contents, the adnexa, and parauterine spaces. In second and third trimester obstetric applications, the transabdominal approach (Figure 18-2A) permits visualization of the lower uterine segment, cervix, and vagina.

A potential difficulty in scanning a patient with a gravid uterus, particularly in the late second and third trimesters, is *supine hypovolemic syndrome* (also known as *supine hypotensive syndrome*). During the scan the patient is lying on her back, and the weight of the uterus compresses the inferior vena cava and reduces the volume of venous return to the right heart, decreasing cardiac output. The patient typically complains of feeling lightheaded, dizzy, faint, and bradycardic. Management is simple and consists of having the patient turn onto her left side, into a left lateral decubitus position.

The transperineal approach (Figure 18-2B) directs the acoustic beam through the soft tissue structures that form the external genitalia and pelvic floor. This method generates uncompromised imaging of the vagina, cervix, and inferior-most portion of the lower uterine segment. It is ideally suited to evaluating the relationship between the placenta and internal cervical os, especially in patients with a suspected placenta previa.

INTRACAVITARY APPROACH

Intracavitary approaches utilize imaging probes that are inserted into a body cavity. Again, depending on the anatomy being examined and the application selected, intracavitary windows include:

- *Transrectal*: through the rectum, primarily for prostate and rectal wall imaging
- *Transesophageal*: through the esophagus, for echocardiographic imaging
- *Transvaginal (endovaginal)*: through the vaginal vault, for ovarian, adnexal, uterine, and obstetric imaging (Figure 18-2C)

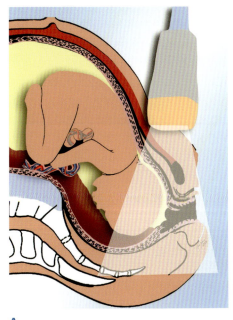

A

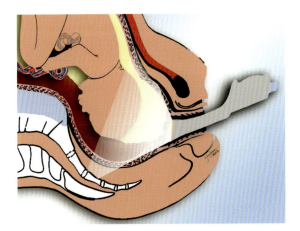

B

C

Figure 18-2. A Transabdominal approach to imaging. A phased sector or tight-footprint convex extracorporeal probe is placed in long axis on the anterior abdominal wall just above the symphysis pubis for visualization of the vagina, cervix, and lower uterine segment. **B** Transperineal approach. A phased sector or small-footprint extracorporeal probe is placed in long axis externally on the labia, providing a sagittal sectional view through the vagina, cervix, and lower uterine segment. **C** Transvaginal (endovaginal) approach. An intracavitary phased sector probe is inserted into the vagina and can be manipulated to obtain sagittal or coronal sectional views of the cervix, lower uterine segment, both adnexa, and parauterine spaces.

In obstetric and gynecologic imaging applications, transvaginal/endovaginal ultrasound is ideally suited to high-resolution imaging of pelvic structures close to the face of the probe. The proximity of these structures to the source of the acoustic wavefront minimizes the effects of attenuation and permits the use of higher frequencies, which yield higher spatial and contrast resolution. Endovaginal imaging has become the sonographic gold standard in many ob/gyn applications. These include:

- Ovarian/adnexal imaging:
  - Monitoring follicular development
  - Identifying and characterizing ovarian pathology
  - Evaluating normal and pathologic ovaries using Doppler imaging
  - Identifying and characterizing tubal pathology
  - Identifying and characterizing pathology in the parauterine spaces
- Uterine imaging:
  - Evaluating the endometrium
  - Identifying and characterizing subtle myometrial pathology
  - Evaluating the cervix
- Obstetric imaging:
  - First trimester
    - Assessing intrauterine contents
    - Determining embryonic viability
    - Evaluating normal and pathologic gestations using Doppler imaging
    - Identifying concomitant ovarian findings
    - Evaluating parauterine spaces in patients with suspected ectopic pregnancy
  - Second/third trimesters
    - Evaluating the cervix
    - Assessing internal cervical os/placenta relationship

Prior to insertion of the probe it should be disinfected in compliance with institutional infection control standards, using either a submersion method or an aerosol method, and covered with a gel-filled sheath. (See Appendix C, "Guidelines for Cleaning and Preparing Endocavitary Ultrasound Transducers between Patients," pages 510–512). Lubricant applied to the sheath prior to vaginal insertion may be a commercially available vaginal lubricant, ultrasound gel, or simply sterile water.

MEASUREMENT TECHNIQUES

Contemporary real-time ultrasound imaging systems are capable of providing B-mode measurements at the submillimeter level. Correct placement of measurement calipers in an appropriately obtained sectional image is critical to accurate and reproducible results. See Tables 18-1 and 18-2 as well as the figures cited in those tables.

(Text continues on page 470 . . .)

Table 18-1. Cursor placement for common gynecologic measurements.

Figure	Gyn Part	Sectional Image	Cursor Placement
18-3A	Cervix	Longitudinal (long axis)	Internal cervical os to external cervical os
18-3B	Uterus	Longitudinal (long axis)	Serosal surface of fundus to external cervical os
18-3C	Uterus	Transverse (broadest portion)	Serosal surfaces, both lateral aspects
18-3D	Endometrium	Endovaginal (long axis)	Basalis layer anterior and posterior at 90° to long axis
18-3E	Ovary	Longitudinal (anteroposterior)	Outer surface, both longitudinal endpoints
18-3F	Ovary	Transverse (axial axis)	Outer surface, both axial endpoints
18-3G	Follicles	Longest axis	Inner surface, each axis
18-3H	Pathology	Longitudinal (long axis)	Outer surface, both longitudinal endpoints
18-3I	Pathology	Transverse (axial axis)	Outer surface, both axial endpoints

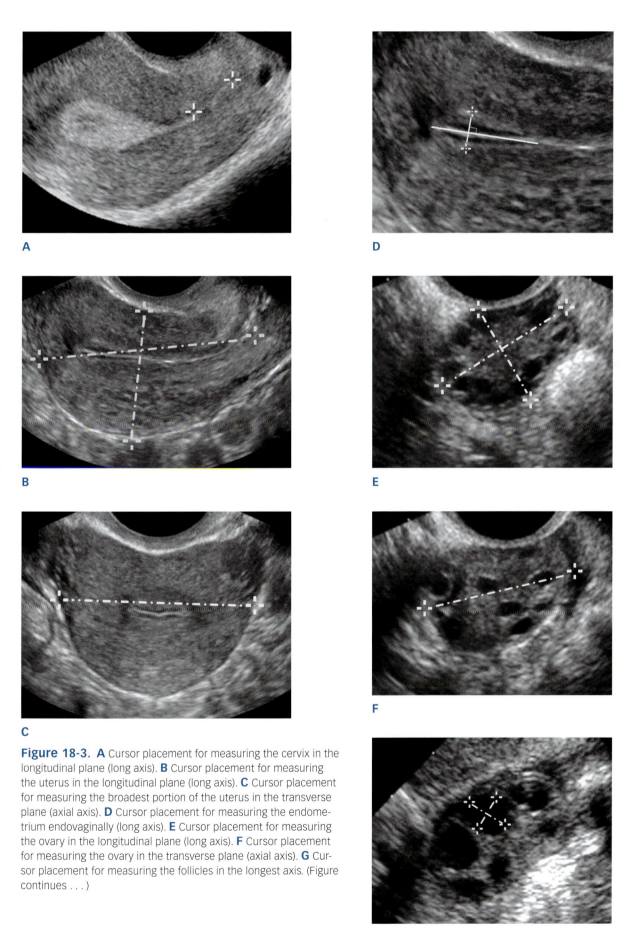

Figure 18-3. A Cursor placement for measuring the cervix in the longitudinal plane (long axis). **B** Cursor placement for measuring the uterus in the longitudinal plane (long axis). **C** Cursor placement for measuring the broadest portion of the uterus in the transverse plane (axial axis). **D** Cursor placement for measuring the endometrium endovaginally (long axis). **E** Cursor placement for measuring the ovary in the longitudinal plane (long axis). **F** Cursor placement for measuring the ovary in the transverse plane (axial axis). **G** Cursor placement for measuring the follicles in the longest axis. (Figure continues . . .)

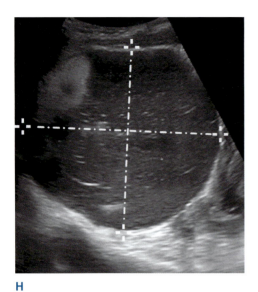
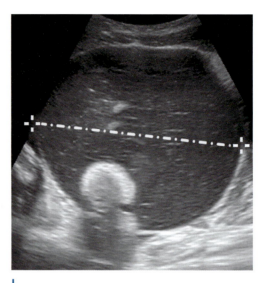

**Figure 18-3, continued.
H** Cursor placement for measuring a pathologic mass in the longitudinal plane (long axis).
I Cursor placement for measuring a pathologic mass in the transverse plane (axial axis).

H

I

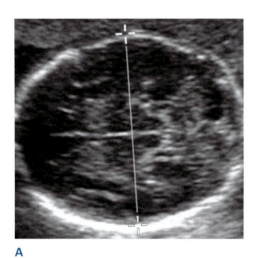
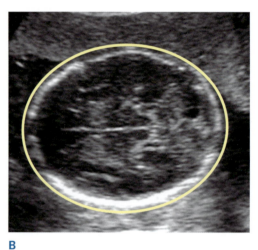

A

B

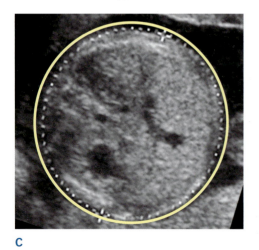
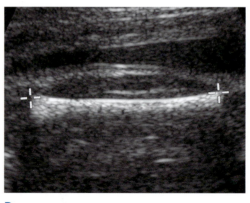

C

D

Figure 18-4. A Biparietal diameter measurement in axial section at the level of the thalamus and cavum septi pellucidi. **B** Cursor placement for measuring head circumference in axial section at the level of the thalamus and cavum septi pellucidi. **C** Cursor placement for measuring abdominal circumference in axial section at the level of the portal sinus and stomach.
D Cursor placement for measuring femur length in long axis through the ossified diaphysis. (Figure continues . . .)

Table 18-2. Cursor placement for common fetal measurements.

Figure	Fetal Measurement	Sectional Image	Cursor Placement
18-4A	Biparietal diameter	Axial at level of thalamus and cavum septi pellucidi	Outer-edge upper parietal bone, inner-edge lower parietal bone
18-4B	Head circumference	Axial at level of thalamus and cavum septi pellucidi	Ellipse to include all scalp echoes
18-4C	Abdominal circumference	Axial at level of portal sinus and stomach	Ellipse to include skin line
18-4D	Femur length	Long axis through ossified diaphysis	Both ends of ossified diaphysis
18-4E	Lateral ventricle	Axial at level of thalamus and cavum septi pellucidi	Inner edges of atrium
18-4F	Cisterna magna	Axial oblique through posterior fossa	Inner edges at midline
18-4G	Fetal heart rate	M-mode tracing	Any similar points on the cardiac cycle

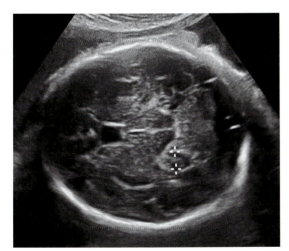

E

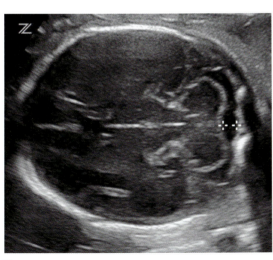

F

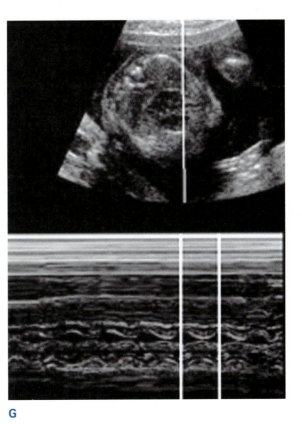

G

Figure 18-4, continued. E Cursor placement for measuring the lateral ventricle in axial section at the level of the thalamus and cavum septi pellucidi. **F** Cursor placement for measuring the cisterna magna in axial oblique section through the posterior fossa. **G** M-mode tracing measuring fetal heart rate.

INTEGRATION OF DATA

An essential component of any sonographic examination is the integration of appropriate clinical data with the images obtained during the course of the study. While many diagnoses, particularly those with characteristic anatomic or structural aberrations, can be made on the basis of the sonographic images alone, others require interpretation of the images in the context of the broader clinical picture. Useful correlative clinical information includes laboratory data and the results of prior sonograms and/or other imaging studies such as radiography, computed tomography, magnetic resonance imaging, and nuclear imaging scans.

Prior sonographic studies can direct attention to a particular area of interest and, in some cases, may limit the scope of the study to answer a specific question about changes in a previously identified abnormality. Similarly, ancillary imaging studies may have revealed an abnormality that requires additional sonographic information to help hone the specificity of a diagnosis. Acoustic characteristics of a lesion can often provide valuable information about its gross pathologic nature—for example, whether it is a cystic or solid mass—which other imaging modalities cannot do with the same level of reliability.

Serial ultrasound exams offer a method of following clinical scenarios noninvasively and without the repetitive expense and exposure to ionizing radiation that alternative imaging modalities may entail. Monitoring uterine fibroids, assessing ovarian size in ovarian hyperstimulation syndrome, and checking for the resolution of an ovarian cyst are but a few examples of the efficacious way serial sonography can be used in gynecologic practice. In obstetrics, serial studies are requisite in monitoring changes in fetal size, and the integration of biometric data from earlier studies is essential in plotting growth curves. Serial sonographic imaging is also a practical way of following physiologic abnormalities associated with pregnancy, such as fetal pyelectasis and ventriculomegaly, changes associated with hydrops fetalis, variations in amniotic fluid volume, and placental maturity.

Lab results provide another level of information that can augment and direct the cognitive (critical thinking) component of sonographic diagnosis. While a complete overview of biochemical tissue and serum analysis is beyond the scope of this book, results of the commonly ordered serum lab values are included in Tables 18-3, 18-4, and 18-5. The values included here are representative normal values; each testing laboratory typically includes its own range of normal values on the report.

Table 18-3. Normal reference values for complete blood count (CBC).

	Units	Values
Without differential		
WBC	$10^6/mm^3$	4.0–10.5
RBC	$10^6/mm^3$	4.14–5.8
Hemoglobin	g/Dl	13–18
Hematocrit	%	37–51
MCV	fL	80–100
MCH	pg	27–30
MCHC	g/Dl	31–36
RDW	%	10%
Platelets	$10^6/mm^3$	140–415
With differential		
Neutrophils	$10^9/mm^3$	2–7
Lymphocytes	$10^9/mm^3$	1–3
Monocytes	$10^9/mm^3$	0.2–1.0
Eosinophils	$10^9/mm^3$	0.02–0.5
Basophils	$10^9/mm^3$	0.02–0.1

Notes: WBC = white blood cell count; RBC = red blood cell count; MCV = mean corpuscular volume; MCH = mean corpuscular hemoglobin; MCHC = mean corpuscular hemoglobin concentration; RDW = red cell distribution width (mean corpuscular hemoglobin concentration).

Source: Data from Jacobs DS, DeMott WR, Oxley DK: *Jacobs & DeMott Laboratory Test Handbook with Key Word Index*, 5th edition. Cleveland, Lexi-Comp, 2001.

REPORTING RESULTS

It falls within the scope of practice of the diagnostic medical sonographer to communicate the preliminary results of an ultrasound examination to the managing clinician. In fact, it is a responsibility incumbent upon the sonographer as a key member of the patient care team to get this information to the referring practitioner, particularly when the referring practitioner indicates that "immediate medical attention is necessary."[2] Results communicated by the sonographer are frequently categorized as "preliminary results,"

Table 18-4. Normal reference values for beta-hCG serum levels (1st IRP).

Weeks since LMP	mIU/mL
3	5–50
4	5–426
5	18–7340
6	1080–56,500
7–8	7650–229,000
9–12	25,700–288,000
13–16	13,300–254,000
17–24	4060–165,400
25–40	3640–117,000
Nonpregnant females	<5.0
Postmenopausal females	<9.5

Source: Data from Jacobs DS, DeMott WR, Oxley DK: *Jacobs & DeMott Laboratory Test Handbook with Key Word Index*, 5th edition. Cleveland, Lexi-Comp, 2001.

Table 18-5. Normal reference values for chromosomal and neoplastic markers.

	Units	Values
Chromosomal markers		
MSAFP	MoM	0.4–2.5
PAPP-A	MoM	>0.4
Beta-hCG—free	MoM	<2
µE3	MoM	>0.5
Inhibin A	MoM	>2.5
Neoplastic markers		
CA-125	U/mL	<35
Beta-hCG—GTD	% rise*	10%
Beta-hCG—GTD	mIU/L**	40,000
Beta-hCG—ovarian tumor	mIU/L**	>50,000
AFP	ng/mL	>1000
Inhibin A***	pg/mL	<5

Notes: MSAFP = maternal serum alpha-fetoprotein; PAPP-A = pregnancy-associated plasma protein A; beta-hCG = beta subunit of human chorionic gonadotropin; µE3 = estriol; GTD = gestational trophoblastic disease; AFP = alpha-fetoprotein; MoM = multiple of the median.

*Over 3 weekly titers

**4–5 months post uterine evacuation

***Postmenopausal

Source: Data from Jacobs DS, DeMott WR, Oxley DK: *Jacobs & DeMott Laboratory Test Handbook with Key Word Index*, 5th edition. Cleveland, Lexi-Comp, 2001.

"sonographer's impression," or "technical findings" to obviate the concern of overstepping boundaries and rendering a diagnosis—a task reserved for those licensed to do so. Whatever semantic approach is adopted by a particular ultrasound lab, the critical task is to communicate this information to the managing clinician in an accurate and timely manner.

THE SONOGRAPHER'S ROLE IN INVASIVE PROCEDURES

A sonographer is often called upon to participate in the performance of invasive procedures conducted under ultrasound guidance. Ultrasound provides an accurate, quick, and inexpensive method of directing a needle, or needle-directed catheter, into the body for a plethora of clinical indications both diagnostic and therapeutic. Its primary usage is in the identification of an entry site that is safely away from critical fetal and maternal anatomic and pathologic structures that, if inadvertently pierced by a needle, could cause significant complications and sequelae. Ultrasound guidance also provides visual guidance for the exact placement of a needle device into small and otherwise inaccessible locations within the human body, such as mature ovarian follicles for ova retrieval.

The sonographer's role in assisting in invasive procedures begins with preparing the patient for the procedure, assisting the physician in acquiring signed informed consent documentation, and preparing laboratory orders and specimen containers. A pre-procedural sonographic examination of the area is conducted and, depending on the procedure being contemplated, may encompass a complete diagnostic protocol or may be limited to directed imaging of the area of interest. Immediately prior to the start of the invasive procedure, a "time out" is called in which all members of the procedural team are required to participate. This protocol, which is mandated by healthcare regulatory agencies, verifies that the correct procedure will be performed on the correct site, on the correct patient.

The procedure then begins. In some practices and in some procedures, the physician scans with one hand while directing the needle with the other. In others, the sonographer scans while the physician directs the needle. Upon completion of the invasive procedure, specimens, when obtained, are sent to the lab and the sonographer may be asked to reexamine the needle site to identify any post-procedural bleeding or other sequelae.

Common types of ultrasound-directed invasive procedures performed within the purview of obstetrics and gynecology include:

- *Oocyte retrieval*: Under endovaginal ultrasound guidance, a needle is inserted into an ovarian follicle and its contents are aspirated. Ova that are retrieved are used for in vitro fertilization methods.
- *Sonohysterography*: Sterile saline is introduced into the uterine cavity to permit a more detailed endovaginal sonographic evaluation of the endometrial lining.
- *Fetal interventional techniques* (amnioreduction, shunt placement): Under transabdominal ultrasound guidance, a needle or a catheter is advanced into a polyhydramniotic cavity to reduce the amount of fluid and improve fetal outcomes.
- *Amniocentesis*: Amniotic fluid is withdrawn from the uterine cavity between 15 and 20 weeks' gestation to be tested for genetic karyotype information about the fetus. When amniocentesis is performed closer to term, the fluid is useful in assessing fetal lung maturity. (See Chapter 11, pages 275–276.) The sonographer's role in transabdominal amniocentesis includes performing a pre-procedure imaging protocol and, in some cases, assisting with transabdominal transducer placement for needle guidance.
- *Chorionic villus sampling*: Chorionic villi are obtained by either endovaginal or transabdominal needle sampling. The specimens are analyzed to provide genetic karyotype information about the fetus. (See Chapter 11, pages 274–275.) The sonographer's role in chorionic villus sampling includes performing a pre-procedure imaging protocol and, in some cases, assisting with either the transabdominal or endovaginal transducer placement for needle guidance.
- *Amnioreduction*: Excess amniotic fluid is therapeutically removed in pregnancies complicated by severe polyhydramnios.
- *Amnioinfusion*: Normal saline is therapeutically introduced into the uterine cavity in pregnancies complicated by severe oligohydramnios.
- *Fetal blood sampling*: Also called *cordocentesis* or *percutaneous umbilical blood sampling* (PUBS), this invasive needle procedure collects blood samples useful in assessing fetal complications such as anemia, intrauterine infection, and alloimmune diseases. (See Chapter 12, pages 336–337.)
- *Intrauterine fetal transfusion*: Donor blood is introduced into the cord vessels for treatment of fetal anemia.
- *Contrast procedures*: Hysterosalpingo-contrast sonography is a procedure that uses endovaginal imaging in conjunction with the introduction of an ultrasound contrast agent into the uterine cavity and fallopian tubes. It is useful in assessing tubal patency and endometrial defects.
- *Assisted reproductive techniques*: A variety of methods employed to achieve pregnancy by artificial means that include:
  - *In vitro fertilization*, whereby oocytes are retrieved from stimulated follicles under endovaginal ultrasound guidance, combined with viable sperm in a Petri dish, and, after 3–5 days, placed in the endometrial cavity via a small transcervical tube.
  - *Gamete intrafallopian transfer*, whereby oocytes are aspirated from stimulated follicles and immediately placed under laparoscopic visualization in the fallopian tube with viable sperm.
  - *Zygote intrafallopian transfer*, a variant of in vitro fertilization whereby oocytes are retrieved transvaginally, fertilized in vitro, and then inserted into the fallopian tube under laparoscopic guidance or through a transcervical tube.

PATIENT SAFETY

BIOEFFECTS AND FETAL SAFETY

Ultrasound is used widely in medicine as both a diagnostic and a therapeutic tool. Through several physical mechanisms (see Chapter 17), acoustic energy produces a variety of biologic effects in human tissues both *in vitro* (in the laboratory) and *in vivo* (in the living organism).[3] Usually these mechanisms are viewed as the potentially negative aspect associated with insonating the human body, and certainly some tissue changes have been reported in laboratory-controlled experiments following exposures at intensities within the diagnostic range.[4,5] However, since the 1970s numerous clinical studies have been performed to evaluate for possible bioeffects on the fetus of routine ultrasound imaging during pregnancy.[6] These studies have shown no evidence of significant biologic effects on fetuses of pregnant women undergoing routine diagnostic sonography and no long-term somatic effects even twenty years later.

Nevertheless, as sonographic imaging systems become more complex and increasingly capable of simultaneous multimodal interrogation, the exposure rates associated with standard-of-care examination protocols have increased.[7] It therefore remains imperative, particularly in embryonic and fetal ultrasound examinations, that sonographers be cognizant of this and incorporate the ALARA principle, elucidated below, into every examination that they perform.

ALARA PRINCIPLE

While the routine use of ultrasound imaging in obstetrics has been deemed safe by professional associations tasked with safeguarding patients' health and safety, levels of exposure to acoustic energy should always be kept to a minimum. This, of course, is true for all sonographic clinical applications, not just obstetric ones. To achieve this goal of minimum exposure, the ALARA principle prescribes that exposure to ultrasound waves should be "as low as reasonably achievable" during all sonographic imaging protocols. This principle is based on two primary practice guidelines:

- Reduce exposure (*dwell time*) by maintaining transducer contact with the patient's body only when actively imaging.
- Adjust system controls that affect acoustic output to the lowest setting that still permits acquisition of necessary diagnostic information.

The American Institute of Ultrasound in Medicine (AIUM) provides additional specific guidelines for fetal safety:

> A thermal index for soft tissue (TIs) should be used at earlier than 10 menstrual weeks' gestation, and a thermal index for bone (TIb) should be used at 10 weeks' gestation or later when bone ossification is evident. In keeping with the ALARA principle, M-mode imaging should be used instead of spectral Doppler imaging to document embryonic/fetal heart rate.[8]

The use of pulsed and color Doppler imaging modalities requires the introduction of, in some instances, several hundred additional focused pulse/wave cycles

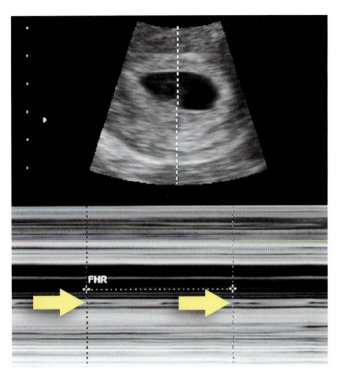

Figure 18-5. M-mode tracing of an embryonic heart at 6 weeks.

to produce the desired information. M-mode, on the other hand, relies on the same number of cycles as B-mode imaging, keeping the exposure levels to a minimum. For routine documentation of embryonic and fetal cardiac activity, M-mode (Figure 18-5) is the method of choice; pulsed and color Doppler assessment should be used only when clinical concerns warrant it.

QUALITY ASSURANCE

The goals of a quality assurance (QA) program in a diagnostic ultrasound laboratory are to prevent mistakes in diagnosis and/or injury to the patient or sonographer. Organizations that accredit ultrasound facilities, such as the Intersocietal Accreditation Commission (IAC), the American College of Radiology (ACR), and the American Institute of Ultrasound in Medicine (AIUM), all include some level of quality assurance measures in their essentials and guidelines, making QA programs a requirement for successful accreditation.

Components of a routine QA program should focus on patient and sonographer safety, cleanliness, and basic performance testing. With the exception of a daily inspection of an ultrasound system for cleanliness, breakage, or operator control malfunction, most technical and engineering parameters are assessed by a commercial field service technician during routine preventative maintenance testing. A comprehensive ultrasound QA program should assure the following:

- Electrical and mechanical safety
- Sterility and cleanliness
- Proper transducer and system performance
- Distance measurement accuracy
- Proper workstation image display

ASSURANCE OF ELECTRICAL AND MECHANICAL SAFETY

The ultrasound systems should be examined on a daily basis for:

- Transducer cracks, delaminations, and discolorations
- Frayed transducer or power cables
- Breakage of buttons, knobs, or switches on the user interface

ASSURANCE OF STERILITY AND CLEANLINESS

The ultrasound systems should be examined on a daily basis for:

- Air filter cleanliness
- User interface and monitor cleanliness
- Transducer cleanliness
- Proper working condition of user interface lights and indicators
- Proper working condition and stability of wheels and wheel locks

TRANSDUCER AND SYSTEM PERFORMANCE

On an annual basis transducer performance should be evaluated for:

- Dead elements
- Maximum depth of visualization (for each frequency setting)
- Target resolution performance

DISTANCE MEASUREMENT ACCURACY

On an annual basis the measurement accuracy of an ultrasound system should be assessed in both vertical and horizontal planes.

WORKSTATION IMAGE DISPLAY

The monitor at each workstation should be set to display the same gray-scale and echo levels as the monitor on the machine. All gray bar transitions should be visible. This check can be done visually or using a test pattern, available on most ultrasound imaging systems, that displays a gray bar pattern (from 0% to 100%) and squares for detecting geometric distortion of the monitor.

CHAPTER 18 REVIEW QUESTIONS

1. In volumetric terms, an adequately full urinary bladder for transabdominal sonography requires approximately how much retained urine?
   A. 200 cc
   B. 300 cc
   C. 400 cc
   D. 500 cc

2. Prior to the beginning of any obstetric or gynecologic ultrasound examination, the following information should be obtained:
   A. Results of prior imaging studies
   B. Pertinent laboratory results
   C. Relevant medical history
   D. All of the above

3. Serial ultrasound examinations are useful for assessing all of the following clinical conditions EXCEPT:
   A. Fetal pyelectasis
   B. Malignant ovarian carcinoma
   C. Fetal growth
   D. Ovarian hyperstimulation syndrome

4. In reporting the results of a sonographic examination to a referring practitioner, the most important consideration is:
   A. Making it clear that it is only a preliminary report
   B. Categorizing the report as "technical findings only"
   C. Providing the information in an accurate and timely manner
   D. Obtaining interpreting physician approval first

5. Which of the following is NOT a routine part of performing an endovaginal ultrasound?
   A. Asking the patient to continue to maintain a full bladder
   B. Clearly explaining the nature and importance of the procedure to the patient
   C. Applying a protective sheath to the probe
   D. Applying generous amounts of lubricant to the probe

6. All of the following are considered extracorporeal approaches to ultrasound imaging EXCEPT:
   A. Transvesicular
   B. Transvaginal
   C. Transperineal
   D. Transabdominal

7. All of the following are considered intracavitary approaches to ultrasound imaging EXCEPT:
   A. Transrectal
   B. Transperineal
   C. Transesophageal
   D. Transvaginal

8. Proper cursor placement for measurement of the long axis of the cervix is from:
   A. Uterine isthmus to internal os
   B. Uterine isthmus to external os
   C. Vaginal introitus to external os
   D. Internal os to external os

9. Proper cursor placement for measuring the long axis of the uterus is from:
   A. Serosal surface of the fundus to the external cervical os
   B. Serosal surface of the fundus to the internal cervical os
   C. Cornu of the uterus to the isthmus
   D. Cornu of the uterus to the external cervical os

10. The goals of a quality assurance program in diagnostic medical sonography include all of the following EXCEPT:
    A. Preventing mistakes in diagnosis
    B. Avoiding injury to patient or operator
    C. Reducing nosocomial infections
    D. Standardizing imaging protocols

11. All of the following technical parameters are important ALARA considerations EXCEPT:
    A. Dwell time
    B. Acoustic output
    C. Thermal index
    D. Transducer configuration

12. All of the following are components of a quality assurance program in diagnostic medical sonography EXCEPT:
    A. Assurance of electrical and mechanical safety
    B. Assurance of sterility and cleanliness
    C. Assurance of appropriate examination methods
    D. Assurance of distance measurement accuracy

ANSWERS

See Appendix A on page 484 for answers.

REFERENCES

1. Society of Diagnostic Medical Sonography: *Diagnostic Ultrasound Clinical Practice Standards*. Dallas, Society of Diagnostic Medical Sonography, 1993–2000. Available at https://www.sdms.org/positions/clinicalpractice.asp.

2. Society of Diagnostic Medical Sonography: *Diagnostic Ultrasound Clinical Practice Standards*. Dallas, Society of Diagnostic Medical Sonography, 1994, 1.5.5.

3. Dalecki D: Mechanical bioeffects of ultrasound. Ann Rev Biomed Eng 6:229–248, 2004.

4. Barnett SB, Ziskin MC, Ter Haar GR, et al: International recommendations and guidelines for the safe use of diagnostic ultrasound in medicine. Ultrasound Med Biol 26:355–366, 2000.

5. Miller DL: Safety assurance in obstetrical ultrasound. Semin Ultrasound CT MR 29:156–164, 2008.

6. Fowlkes JB, Bioeffects Committee of the American Institute of Ultrasound in Medicine: American Institute of Ultrasound in Medicine consensus report on potential bioeffects of diagnostic ultrasound: executive summary. J Ultrasound Med 27:503–515, 2008.

7. Cibull SL, Harris GR, Nell DM: Trends in diagnostic ultrasound acoustic output from data reported to the US Food and Drug Administration for device indications that include fetal applications. J Ultrasound Med 32:1921–1932, 2013.

8. American Institute of Ultrasound in Medicine: *AIUM Practice Guideline for the Performance of Obstetric Ultrasound Examinations*. Laurel, American Institute of Ultrasound in Medicine, 2013, p 12.

SUGGESTED READINGS

American Institute of Ultrasound in Medicine: *AIUM Practice Guideline for the Performance of Obstetric Ultrasound Examinations*. Laurel, American Institute of Ultrasound in Medicine, 2013.

Wax J, Minkoff H, Johnson A, et al: Consensus report on the detailed fetal anatomic ultrasound examination: indications, components, and qualifications. J Ultrasound Med 33:189–195, 2014.

APPENDIX A

Answers to Chapter Review Questions

CHAPTER 1

1. C. Luteinizing hormone.
2. A. Trophoblastic tissue.
3. C. Twice the 1st IRP level.
4. C. Blastocyst.
5. C. During gastrulation.
6. A. Decidual thickening.
7. D. Conceptual age is 14 days less than menstrual age.
8. A. 4.5–5.0 menstrual weeks.
9. B. 1.0 mm per day.
10. C. Intradecidual sign.
11. B. Irregular, echogenic borders.
12. B. Double bleb sign.
13. B. Double decidual sac sign.
14. C. 5.5–6.0 weeks.
15. C. 5–6 weeks.
16. C. 5.0 mm.
17. D. ≥8.0 mm.

18. B. 2–4 mm.
19. C. 8 menstrual weeks.
20. B. 12 menstrual weeks.
21. C. Embryonic rhombencephalon.
22. A. Mean sac diameter < 8 mm without a yolk sac.
23. B. Double sac sign.
24. C. Spontaneous abortion.
25. A. Complex echogenic material in the uterine cavity.
26. D. Empty uterus with "clean" endometrial stripe.
27. B. Anembryonic pregnancy.
28. A. Ectopic pregnancy.
29. C. Ampullary portion of the fallopian tube.
30. B. Identification of an extrauterine gestational sac with live embryo.
31. B. Heterotopic pregnancy.
32. C. Identification of an extrauterine gestational sac with yolk sac.
33. A. Beta-hCG levels less than expected for dates.
34. D. Theca-lutein cysts.
35. A. Hydatidiform mole.
36. A. Chorioadenoma destruens.
37. C. Ectopic pregnancy.
38. A. Interstitial ectopic pregnancy.
39. B. Incomplete abortion.
40. A. Complete hydatidiform mole.
41. B. Normal embryonic midgut herniation.
42. C. Interstitial ectopic pregnancy.
43. C. Recurrent trophoblastic disease.

CHAPTER 2

1. C. Syncytiotrophoblast.
2. B. Villi.
3. B. Intrauterine growth restriction (IUGR).
4. B. 4 cm.
5. D. Grade III.
6. A. Circumvallate.
7. C. Succenturiate.
8. D. Annular.
9. B. Partial previa.
10. D. Vasa previa.
11. C. Placental abruption.
12. B. Placenta increta.
13. C. Placenta percreta.
14. C. Complete placenta previa.
15. C. Placenta increta.

CHAPTER 3

1. B. Two arteries and one vein.
2. A. Oxygenated blood from the placenta to the fetus.
3. B. 8.
4. C. Iliac arteries.
5. B. Polyhydramnios.
6. A. Single umbilical artery (SUA).
7. B. Umbilical cord cysts.
8. D. Cord entanglement.
9. A. Battledore placenta and velamentous insertion.
10. A. Placenta previa.
11. D. Monochorionic/monoamniotic pregnancies.
12. A. Umbilical vein thrombosis.
13. A. Cord stricture.
14. C. Secondary atrophy of a previously normal vessel.

CHAPTER 4

1. C. 4.5 weeks.
2. B. Mean sac diameter.
3. A. 1 mm per day.
4. A. < 5 mm.

5. A. Cavum septi pellucidi, falx cerebri, and thalamic nuclei.
6. B. Head circumference.
7. C. Normal somatic growth of the fetus.
8. D. Abdominal circumference.
9. B. 33 weeks.
10. A. Fetal femur length.
11. D. 8.
12. A. >2 cm.

CHAPTER 5

1. C. 6 menstrual weeks.
2. C. 6–7 menstrual weeks.
3. B. Secondary palate.
4. B. Maxilla.
5. C. Orbital rim.
6. B. Complete cleft palate.
7. A. Cleft lip and palate.
8. A. Micrognathia.
9. B. Cleft lip.
10. B. Polyhydramnios.
11. C. Hypertelorism.
12. D. Cyclopia.
13. D. Alobar holoprosencephaly.
14. A. Trisomy 21.
15. D. Anophthalmia.
16. C. Anophthalmia.
17. D. Cyclopia.
18. B. Micrognathia.
19. A. Macroglossia.
20. A. Hypotelorism.
21. B. Epignathus.
22. D. All of the above.
23. C. Teratoma.

24. C. Thyroglossal duct cysts.
25. A. Cystic hygroma.
26. C. Turner syndrome.
27. A. Cystic hygroma.

CHAPTER 6

1. B. Cavum septi pellucidi.
2. D. Choroid plexus.
3. B. Atrium.
4. B. Third ventricle.
5. A. Falx cerebri.
6. C. Cisterna magna.
7. A. Circle of Willis.
8. C. Cerebellar hemispheres.
9. A. Choroid plexus.
10. D. Cavum septi pellucidi.
11. B. Spinous process.
12. D. A normal spine.
13. D. Ventriculomegaly.
14. A. Enlargement of the ventricular system with concomitant compression atrophy of adjacent cerebral parenchyma.
15. B. Enlargement of the ventricular system without concomitant compression atrophy of adjacent cerebral parenchyma.
16. A. Hydrocephalus.
17. B. Hydranencephaly.
18. B. Hydranencephaly.
19. A. Holoprosencephaly.
20. A. Holoprosencephaly.
21. C. Alobar.
22. B. Lobar holoprosencephaly.
23. D. Holoprosencephaly.
24. D. Dandy-Walker malformation.
25. B. Cyclopia.

26. A. Dandy-Walker malformation.
27. C. Agenesis of the corpus callosum.
28. A. Agenesis of the corpus callosum.
29. A. Epignathus.
30. B. Microcephaly.
31. D. Neural tube defects.
32. D. Holoprosencephaly.
33. B. Spina bifida.
34. D. Anencephaly.
35. B. Anencephaly.
36. A. Encephalocele.
37. C. Encephalocele.
38. D. Iniencephaly.
39. A. Spina bifida aperta.
40. B. Meningomyelocele.

CHAPTER 7

1. D. Abdominal visceral situs.
2. D. All of the above.
3. C. 40%.
4. A. Transposition of the great vessels.
5. C. Pulmonary artery.
6. C. Pulmonary hypoplasia.
7. D. Cystic adenomatoid malformation.
8. B. Ventricular septal defect.
9. D. Tricuspid atresia.
10. D. Transposition of the great vessels.
11. D. Hypoplastic left heart syndrome.
12. A. Coarctation of the aorta.
13. B. Ectopia cordis.
14. A. Tricuspid valve displaced inferiorly in the right ventricle.
15. D. Single great artery arising from truncal root.
16. A. Endocardial cushion defect.
17. C. Pulmonary sequestration.
18. A. Hydrothorax.
19. B. Left ventricle.
20. C. Right atrium.
21. D. Aortic root.
22. B. Left atrium.
23. A. Aortic coarctation.
24. C. Cystic adenomatoid malformation of the lung.
25. B. Pulmonary stenosis.
26. C. Cystic adenomatoid malformation of the lung.
27. B. Pulmonary sequestration.
28. A. Diaphragmatic hernia.

CHAPTER 8

1. A. Long bones.
2. A. Normal ossified metaphysis.
3. C. Micromelia.
4. A. Rhizomelia.
5. C. Polydactyly.
6. B. Osteochondrodysplasia.
7. C. Osteogenesis imperfecta.
8. D. Severe bowing of the long bones.
9. A. Hypophosphatasia.
10. B. Hypomineralization of bone.
11. D. Talipes equinovarus.
12. C. Rocker bottom foot.
13. A. Dysostosis.
14. A. Achondrogenesis.
15. D. Thanatophoric dysplasia.
16. A. Talipes equinovarus.
17. B. Rocker bottom foot.
18. B. Achondroplasia.
19. C. Achondrogenesis.

20. D. Soft tissue or bony fusion of digits.
21. A. Homozygous dominant achondroplasia.
22. D. Cloverleaf skull.
23. A. Hypophosphatasia.
24. D. Osteogenesis imperfecta.
25. B. Thanatophoric dysplasia.

CHAPTER 9

1. B. Right portal vein.
2. C. Umbilical arteries.
3. B. Stomach.
4. B. It is less echogenic than bone and more echogenic than liver.
5. A. Omphalocele.
6. B. Gastroschisis.
7. A. Omphalocele.
8. D. Limb–body wall complex.
9. B. Gastrointestinal atresia.
10. B. Double bubble.
11. D. Hepatosplenomegaly.
12. A. Abdominal circumference measurements less than expected for dates.
13. D. Duodenal atresia.
14. C. Gonorrhea.
15. C. External sacrococcygeal teratoma.
16. D. Presacral teratoma.
17. C. Sacrococcygeal teratoma.
18. A. Duodenal atresia.
19. C. Hepatosplenic calcifications.
20. A. Bladder exstrophy.

CHAPTER 10

1. B. Beginning of the 6th menstrual week.
2. A. Pronephroi.
3. C. Mesonephroi.
4. D. 12–14 menstrual weeks.
5. A. 1 mm per week of gestation.
6. C. 30–45.
7. C. 12 menstrual weeks.
8. A. Renal agenesis.
9. B. Potter sequence.
10. B. Hydrops fetalis.
11. A. Severe oligohydramnios.
12. D. Bladder exstrophy.
13. B. Normal amount of amniotic fluid.
14. C. Renal ectopia.
15. A. Multiple large cysts replacing renal parenchyma.
16. B. Large hyperechoic kidneys bilaterally.
17. D. Renal agenesis.
18. B. Obstructive uropathy.
19. C. Ureteropelvic junction obstruction.
20. A. Congenital primary megaureter.
21. A. Hydronephrosis.
22. C. Ureteropelvic junction obstruction.
23. C. Multicystic dysplastic kidney disease.
24. D. Posterior urethral valves.

CHAPTER 11

1. A. Maternal age > 30 years.
2. D. Serial serum beta-hCG titers.
3. D. Luteinizing hormone.
4. B. Multicystic dysplastic renal disease.
5. D. 14 weeks' gestation.
6. A. Trisomy 21.
7. B. Human chorionic gonadotropin.
8. D. Hypotelorism.
9. B. Talipes equinovarus.
10. C. 40–80 mm.
11. A. <2.5 mm.

12. D. ≥6 mm.
13. D. 15 and 20 weeks.
14. C. <6 mm.
15. A. Spina bifida.
16. D. Autosomal recessive.
17. A. 23 pairs of chromosomes.
18. A. Trisomy.
19. D. Demineralized bone.
20. C. Edwards syndrome.
21. D. Echogenic bowel.
22. A. Turner syndrome.
23. B. Syndrome.
24. B. Hydrocephalus.
25. A. Anencephaly.
26. D. Macroglossia.
27. A. Holoprosencephaly.
28. D. Amniotic band syndrome.
29. A. Trisomy 18.
30. D. Beckwith-Wiedemann.
31. C. Meckel-Gruber.
32. B. Pentalogy of Cantrell.
33. B. VACTERL association.

CHAPTER 12

1. C. Hydrops fetalis.
2. D. Turner syndrome.
3. B. Nonimmue hydrops.
4. D. Abnormally small and mature placenta.
5. A. Intrauterine growth restriction.
6. B. Symmetric intrauterine growth restriction.
7. A. AC measuring > 2 weeks behind HC.
8. D. Intrauterine growth restriction (IUGR).
9. A. A single amnion and a single chorion.
10. C. Dizygotic.
11. C. Twin-twin transfusion syndrome.
12. C. Double placentation.
13. A. Oligohydramnios.
14. C. Hydrops fetalis.
15. B. Craniopagus.
16. A. Omphalopagus.
17. D. Monochorionic/monoamniotic twinning.
18. B. Rh isoimmunization.
19. A. Twin-to-twin transfusion syndrome.
20. C. Conjoined twins.
21. A. Monoamniotic/monochorionic.

CHAPTER 13

1. B. Rectus abdominis.
2. C. Linea terminalis.
3. A. Mesovarium ligament.
4. A. Round ligament.
5. D. Cardinal ligament.
6. B. Broad ligament.
7. C. Fundus.
8. C. Corpus.
9. B. 2–3 cm.
10. A. Serosa.
11. B. Basalis layer.
12. B. Retroverted.
13. C. Retroflexed.
14. A. Fornix.
15. B. Space of Retzius.
16. C. Pouch of Douglas.
17. D. Interstitial portion.
18. A. Isthmic portion.
19. B. Cortex.

20. D. Tunica albuginea.
21. C. Abdominal aorta.
22. A. Internal iliac artery.
23. A. Laterally, superior to the cervix.
24. B. Low resistance.
25. B. Menarche.
26. D. Corpus luteum.
27. A. Follicular phase.
28. B. 2–3 mm/day.
29. B. Presence of a cumulus oophorus.
30. C. 14 days.
31. B. Levator ani muscle group.
32. A. Ovulation will occur within 36 hours.

CHAPTER 14

1. C. Gartner's duct cyst.
2. D. Retroversion of the uterus.
3. A. Müllerian duct anomalies.
4. B. Unicornuate uterus.
5. D. Didelphic uterus.
6. C. Bicornuate uterus.
7. D. Asherman syndrome.
8. B. Hormone replacement therapy.
9. A. Adenomyosis.
10. A. Asymmetrically enlarged uterus with focal subserosal mass.
11. C. Endometrial hyperplasia.
12. B. Gestational trophoblastic disease.
13. D. Focal cystic areas in the myometrium.
14. A. Endometritis.
15. D. 60–70 years.
16. D. Endometritis.
17. A. Murphy's sign.
18. B. Endometrial polyps.
19. A. Cystadenomas.
20. C. Follicular cyst.
21. A. Corpus luteum cyst.
22. B. Theca-lutein cysts.
23. D. Broad ligament.
24. D. Cystadenocarcinoma.
25. A. Cystadenocarcinoma.
26. B. Krukenberg tumor.
27. C. Multiparity.
28. C. Dyspepsia.
29. A. Adenomyosis.
30. C. Endometrial carcinoma.
31. A. Polycystic ovaries.
32. A. Uterine polyps.
33. B. Endometrioma.
34. D. Subserosal fibroid.
35. A. Calcified fibroid.
36. B. Ovarian cystadenocarcinoma.
37. B. Pelvic inflammatory disease.
38. D. Mature cystic teratoma.

CHAPTER 15

1. C. 12 months.
2. B. Days 5–7.
3. A. 2 mm/day.
4. A. Unilateral cystic enlargement of an ovary.
5. C. > 3 cc.
6. C. Myometrial thickness.

CHAPTER 16

1. A. 1:2.
2. A. 2:1–3:1.
3. A. ≥1.0 cc.
4. D. Choriocarcinoma.

5. C. Low-resistance Doppler flow within the ovary.
6. B. Hematometrocolpos.
7. D. Sarcoma botryoides.
8. C. Unchanged fundal:cervical ratio.
9. A. Sarcoma botryoides.
10. B. Thin and homogeneously echogenic.
11. A. <5 mm.
12. C. Postpartum state.
13. D. 8 mm.
14. B. Tamoxifen.
15. D. 80%.
16. C. Ectopic pregnancy.
17. A. Endometrium.
18. C. Infertility treatment.
19. A. Imperforate hymen.
20. B. Hydrometrocolpos.
21. B. Endometrial atrophy.

CHAPTER 17

1. A. MI.
2. A. Cavitation.
3. C. Ovaries.
4. C. Negative acoustic pressure present in a medium.
5. D. B-mode.
6. A. M-mode.
7. A. $F_d = F_r - F_i$
8. C. Rayleigh scatter.
9. B. Depth.
10. C. Continuous-wave Doppler.
11. A. Color Doppler imaging.
12. D. Spectral Doppler.
13. B. Less penetration and better spatial resolution.
14. C. Harmonic.
15. A. Compounding.
16. D. Phased arrays.
17. B. Matrix arrays.
18. B. Posterior acoustic shadowing.
19. A. Reverberation.

CHAPTER 18

1. D. 500 cc.
2. D. All of the above.
3. B. Malignant ovarian carcinoma.
4. C. Providing the information in an accurate and timely manner.
5. A. Asking the patient to continue to maintain a full bladder.
6. B. Transvaginal.
7. B. Transperineal.
8. D. Internal os to external os.
9. A. Serosal surface of the fundus to the external cervical os.
10. D. Standardizing imaging protocols.
11. D. Transducer configuration.
12. C. Assurance of appropriate examination methods.

APPENDIX B

Chapters Cross-Referenced to the ARDMS Exam Content Outline

Publisher's note: *Ob/Gyn Sonography: An Illustrated Review* is a comprehensive text review that will continue to prepare candidates for the ob/gyn specialty exam even as ARDMS makes incremental changes to and rearrangements of its exam outline. Both publisher and author have carefully surveyed prior and current exam outlines, best practices, and essential knowledge needed to pass the ARDMS exam. For the convenience of registrants for the ARDMS ob/gyn specialty examination, below we cross-reference the book's contents to the 2016 ARDMS ob/gyn exam content outline.

It is important to note that the latest exam outlines from ARDMS provide a *generalized* categorical overview within which *very specific* (but not always exhaustive) clinical tasks are arranged. These ARDMS tasks do not, in and of themselves, constitute all the key intermediate topics you must know to pass your exam. In *Ob/Gyn Sonography: An Illustrated Review*, you get it all—the book itself is a full review of ob/gyn sonography, while this index identifies where specific ARDMS tasks are discussed within the more comprehensive coverage of the book. Remember: The ARDMS exam content outlines change periodically, so for the latest exam updates be sure to visit www.ardms.org.

ARDMS EXAM CONTENT CATEGORY/TASK	CHAPTER
ANATOMY AND PHYSIOLOGY (25%)	
Normal Anatomy and Physiology	
GYN	
Assess both adnexa (i.e., ovaries, fallopian tubes)	1, 12, 13, 14, 16
Assess the endometrium	13, 14, 15
Assess the uterus (i.e., position, orientation, contour)	13
Assess the cervix	12, 13, 14, 15
Assess the cul-de-sacs	1, 13, 14
Assess patients of reproductive age	1–15, 18
Assess postmenopausal patients	16
Assess premenarcheal patients	16
OB	
Identify structures in the first trimester obstetrical exam at less than 10 weeks (i.e., decidual reaction, gestational sac, yolk sac, embryo)	1
Identify fetal anatomy in the first trimester obstetrical exam at 10–14 weeks (i.e., calvaria, stomach, cord insertion, extremities)	1
Identify multiple gestations (i.e., fetal number, chorionicity/amnionicity)	12
Assess the placenta (i.e., size, location)	2
Assess the umbilical cord (i.e., insertion into placenta, vessel number)	3
Assess amniotic fluid volume	7
Assess fetal lie and presentation	12
Assess the fetal heart (i.e., axis, chambers, outflow tracts)	7
Assess the neck	5
Assess intracranial structures	6
Assess the facial anatomy (i.e., nose, lips, nasal bones, orbits, profile)	5
Assess the diaphragm	7
Assess the thorax (i.e., thymus, lungs)	7
Assess the abdomen (i.e., gallbladder, stomach, liver)	9
Assess the skeletal system (e.g., cranial contour, long bones evaluation, ribs, vertebrae, skull, spine)	8
Assess the ankles and feet	8
Assess the hands/fingers	8
Assess the genitalia	10

ARDMS EXAM CONTENT CATEGORY/TASK	CHAPTER
PATHOLOGY (41%)	
Abnormal Physiology and Perfusion	
GYN	
Identify adnexal pathology other than ovarian	14
Identify ovarian pathology	14
Identify endometrial pathology (i.e., polyps, hyperplasia)	14
Identify uterine masses (e.g., leiomyomas, sarcomas)	14
Identify müllerian duct developmental anomalies (e.g., septated, subseptate, bicornuate, unicornis uterus)	14
Identify adenomyosis	14
Identify cervical pathology (e.g., polyps)	12, 13, 14
Identify free fluid in the pelvis	1, 13, 14, 15
Identify vaginal pathology (e.g., imperforate hymen)	14
OB	
Identify maternal pelvic pathology	12, 14
Congenital Anomalies	
Assess multiple gestations (e.g., conjoined twins, acardiac twin, twin-to-twin transfusion syndrome, discordance)	12
Identify abnormal multiple gestations	12
Identify molar degeneration	1
Identify ectopic pregnancy	1
Identify embryonic/fetal demise	1, 12
Identify anembryonic pregnancy	1
Identify abnormal trisomy (e.g., 13, 18, 21)	11
Identify abnormal congenital anomalies	5–12
Identify abnormal amniotic fluid volume	4, 7, 10
Identify abnormal fetal growth	2, 4, 8, 12
Identify abnormal yolk sac	1, 2, 12
Identify abnormal central nervous system anomaly (e.g., anencephaly, acrania, hydranencephaly, Dandy-Walker malformation, encephalocele)	6
Identify abnormal intracranial structures (e.g., choroid plexus cyst)	6
Identify a thickened nuchal translucency	1, 11
Identify abnormal face (i.e., nose/ lips, orbits, profile)	4, 5
Identify abnormal neck (e.g., goiter, cystic hygroma)	5

ARDMS EXAM CONTENT CATEGORY/TASK	CHAPTER
Congenital Anomalies (continued)	
Identify abnormal fetal heart (e.g., axis, chambers, outflow tracts)	7
Identify abnormal diaphragm	7
Identify abnormal thorax	7
Identify abnormal abdomen (e.g., gallbladder, stomach, liver)	9
Identify abnormal abdominal wall defect (e.g., omphalocele, gastroschisis)	9
Identify abnormal umbilical cord (e.g., insertion, vessels)	3
Identify abnormal gastrointestinal system (e.g., echogenic bowel, duodenal atresia, bowel obstruction, esophageal atresia, cysts)	9
Identify abnormal genitourinary system (e.g., hydronephrosis, cystic renal dysplasia, hydroureter, renal agenesis, bladder outlet obstruction, ureterocele, abnormal genitalia, ovarian cyst)	10
Identify abnormal genitalia	10
Identify abnormal skeletal system (e.g., skull, spine)	8
Identify abnormal ankles and feet (e.g., clubfeet, polydactyly)	8
Identify abnormal hands/fingers	8
Placental Abnormalities	
Identify previa	2, 18
Identify vasa previa	2, 3
Identify subchorionic hemorrhage	1, 2
Identify abruption	2, 14
Identify accreta, increta, percreta	2
Identify infarction	2
Identify abnormal membrane/insertion shape (i.e., circumvallate)	2
Identify accessory lobe	2
Identify masses (e.g., chorioangioma)	2
PROTOCOLS (25%)	
Clinical Standards and Guidelines	
Obtain pertinent clinical history as a part of the exam	1, 15, 16, 18
Correlate previous exams	18 and throughout
Review lab results as a part of the exam (e.g., hCG levels, CA-125)	1, 2, 11, 14, 15, 18
Perform quality assurance checks on the equipment	18

ARDMS EXAM CONTENT CATEGORY/TASK	CHAPTER
Perform transabdominal technique	17, 18
Perform transvaginal/endovaginal technique	18
Perform translabial/transperineal technique	18
Measurement Techniques	
GYN	
Measure endometrium thickness	13–16, 18
Measure ovarian dimensions	13–16, 18
Measure uterine dimensions	13–16, 18
Measure cervical length	13–16, 18
OB	
Perform biophysical profiles	4
Measure amniotic fluid (i.e., amniotic fluid index, deepest pocket)	4, 7, 12
Measure crown-rump length	1, 4, 11
Measure mean sac diameter	1, 4
Measure the yolk sac	1
Measure biparietal diameter	4, 18
Measure biparietal diameter corrected	4
Measure head circumference	4, 6, 18
Measure cisterna magna	6, 18
Measure cerebellum	4, 6
Measure transverse cerebellar diameter	4, 12
Measure cerebral lateral ventricle	6, 18
Measure cephalic index	4
Measure nuchal translucency in first trimester	1, 11
Measure nuchal fold between 15 and 20 weeks' gestation	11
Measure orbital, intraorbital, and outer orbital diameters	4, 5
Measure nasal bone	4, 11
Measure abdominal circumference	4, 9, 18
Measure humerus length	4, 8
Measure femur length	4, 8, 18
Measure other long bones (e.g., radius, ulna, tibia)	4, 8

ARDMS EXAM CONTENT CATEGORY/TASK	CHAPTER
PHYSICS AND INSTRUMENTATION (8%)	
Hemodynamics	
GYN	
Assess ovarian vasculature with Doppler	13, 17
Assess the uterine arteries with Doppler	13, 17
Assess arteriovenous malformations using Doppler	6, 17
OB	
Assess embryonic and/or fetal heart rate and rhythm with M-mode	1, 7, 17
Assess the middle cerebral artery with Doppler	6
Assess the ductus venosus	7, 9
Assess fetal heart rate using Doppler	1, 7
Assess the umbilical cord vessels with Doppler	2, 3, 9
Imaging Instruments	
Apply M-mode	1, 7, 17, 18
Apply color flow imaging	17, 18
Apply power (angio, amplitude) Doppler	1, 2, 3, 10, 15, 17
Apply pulsed spectral Doppler	17
Apply harmonics	17, 18
Perform 3D imaging	5, 6, 8, 9, 11, 15, 17
Apply knowledge of artifacts	15, 17
TREATMENT (1%)	
Sonographer Role in Procedures	
Provide guidance for sonohysterography	18
Provide guidance for amniocentesis after 15 weeks	7, 11, 18
Provide guidance for chorionic villus sampling	11, 18

APPENDIX C

AIUM Practice Guidelines

Publisher's note: *These AIUM practice guidelines are reprinted with the kind permission of the American Institute of Ultrasound in Medicine (AIUM). These standards are the most current as of press time. Because standards are periodically updated, you should visit www.aium.org for the most recent versions of practice guidelines in specialties related to obstetrics and gynecology, where acknowledgments and references also appear. Practice Guidelines may be downloaded for free from the AIUM website by both members and nonmembers.*

- Obstetric Ultrasound Examinations   491
- Pelvic Ultrasound Examinations   498
- Sonohysterography   501
- Ultrasonography in Reproductive Medicine   504
- A Focused Reproductive Endocrinology and Infertility Scan   512
- Fetal Echocardiography   515

AIUM PRACTICE GUIDELINE FOR THE PERFORMANCE OF OBSTETRIC ULTRASOUND EXAMINATIONS

Guideline developed in conjunction with the American College of Radiology (ACR), the American College of Obstetricians and Gynecologists (ACOG), and the Society of Radiologists in Ultrasound (SRU)

I. INTRODUCTION

The clinical aspects contained in specific sections of this guideline (Introduction, Classification of Fetal Sonographic Examinations, Specifications of the Examination, Equipment Specifications, and Fetal Safety) were revised collaboratively by the American Institute of Ultrasound in Medicine (AIUM), the American College of Radiology (ACR), the American College of Obstetricians and Gynecologists (ACOG), and the Society of Radiologists in Ultrasound (SRU). Recommendations for personnel qualifications, written request for the examination, procedure documentation, and quality control vary among the organizations and are addressed by each separately.

This guideline has been developed for use by practitioners performing obstetric sonographic studies. Fetal ultrasound[a] should be performed only when there is a valid medical reason, and the lowest possible ultrasonic exposure settings should be used to gain the necessary diagnostic information. A limited examination may be performed in clinical emergencies or for a limited purpose such as evaluation of fetal or embryonic cardiac activity, fetal position, or amniotic fluid volume. A limited follow-up examination may be appropriate for reevaluation of fetal size or interval growth or to reevaluate abnormalities previously noted if a complete prior examination is on record.

While this guideline describes the key elements of standard sonographic examinations in the first trimester and second and third trimesters, a more detailed anatomic examination of the fetus may be necessary in some cases, such as when an abnormality is found or suspected on the standard examination or in pregnancies at high risk for fetal anomalies. In some cases, other specialized examinations may be necessary as well.

While it is not possible to detect all structural congenital anomalies with diagnostic ultrasound, adherence to the following guidelines will maximize the possibility of detecting many fetal abnormalities.

II. CLASSIFICATION OF FETAL SONOGRAPHIC EXAMINATIONS

A. First-Trimester Examination

A standard obstetric sonogram in the first trimester includes evaluation of the presence, size, location, and number of gestational sac(s). The gestational sac is examined for the presence of a yolk sac and embryo/fetus. When an embryo/fetus is detected, it should be measured and cardiac activity recorded by a 2-dimensional video clip or M-mode imaging. Use of spectral Doppler imaging is discouraged. The uterus, cervix, adnexa, and cul-de-sac region should be examined.

B. Standard Second- or Third-Trimester Examination

A standard obstetric sonogram in the second or third trimester includes an evaluation of fetal presentation, amniotic fluid volume, cardiac activity, placental position, fetal biometry, and fetal number, plus an anatomic survey. The maternal cervix and adnexa should be examined as clinically appropriate when technically feasible.

C. Limited Examination

A limited examination is performed when a specific question requires investigation. For example, in most routine nonemergency cases, a limited examination could be performed to confirm fetal heart activity in a bleeding patient or to verify fetal presentation in a laboring patient. In most cases, limited sonographic examinations are appropriate only when a prior complete examination is on record.

D. Specialized Examinations

A detailed anatomic examination is performed when an anomaly is suspected on the basis of the history, biochemical abnormalities, or the results of either the limited or standard scan. Other specialized examinations might include fetal Doppler ultrasound, a biophysical profile, a fetal echocardiogram, and additional biometric measurements.

III. QUALIFICATIONS AND RESPONSIBILITIES OF PERSONNEL

See the AIUM Official Statement *Training Guidelines for Physicians Who Evaluate and Interpret Diagnostic Abdominal, Obstetric, and/or Gynecologic Ultrasound Examinations* and the AIUM *Standards and Guidelines for the Accreditation of Ultrasound Practices*.

IV. WRITTEN REQUEST FOR THE EXAMINATION

The written or electronic request for an ultrasound examination should provide sufficient information to allow for the appropriate performance and interpretation of the examination.

---

[a] The consensus of the committee was that the use of the terms *ultrasound* and *sonography* is at the discretion of each organization.

The request for the examination must be originated by a physician or other appropriately licensed health care provider or under the provider's direction. The accompanying clinical information should be provided by a physician or other appropriate health care provider familiar with the patient's clinical situation and should be consistent with relevant legal and local health care facility requirements.

V. SPECIFICATIONS OF THE EXAMINATION

A. First-Trimester Ultrasound Examination

1. **Indications**

   Indications for first-trimester[b] sonography include but are not limited to:

   a. Confirmation of the presence of an intrauterine pregnancy;

   b. Evaluation of a suspected ectopic pregnancy;

   c. Defining the cause of vaginal bleeding;

   d. Evaluation of pelvic pain;

   e. Estimation of gestational (menstrual)[c] age;

   f. Diagnosis or evaluation of multiple gestations;

   g. Confirmation of cardiac activity;

   h. Imaging as an adjunct to chorionic villus sampling, embryo transfer, and localization and removal of an intrauterine device;

   i. Assessing for certain fetal anomalies, such as anencephaly, in high-risk patients;

   j. Evaluation of maternal pelvic masses and/or uterine abnormalities;

   k. Measuring the nuchal translucency (NT) when part of a screening program for fetal aneuploidy; and

   l. Evaluation of a suspected hydatidiform mole.

   Comment
   A limited examination may be performed to evaluate interval growth, estimate amniotic fluid volume, evaluate the cervix, and assess the presence of cardiac activity.

2. **Imaging Parameters**

   Comment
   Scanning in the first trimester may be performed either transabdominally or transvaginally. If a transabdominal examination is not definitive, a transvaginal scan or transperineal scan should be performed whenever possible.

   a. The uterus (including the cervix) and adnexa should be evaluated for the presence of a gestational sac. If a gestational sac is seen, its location should be documented. The gestational sac should be evaluated for the presence or absence of a yolk sac or embryo, and the crown-rump length should be recorded when possible.

   Comment
   A definitive diagnosis of intrauterine pregnancy can be made when an intrauterine gestational sac containing a yolk sac or embryo/fetus with cardiac activity is visualized. A small, eccentric intrauterine fluid collection with an echogenic rim can be seen before the yolk sac and embryo are detectable in a very early intrauterine pregnancy. In the absence of sonographic signs of ectopic pregnancy, the fluid collection is highly likely to represent an intrauterine gestational sac. In this circumstance, the intradecidual sign may be helpful. Follow-up sonography and/or serial determination of maternal serum human chorionic gonadotropin levels are/is appropriate in pregnancies of undetermined location to avoid inappropriate intervention in a potentially viable early pregnancy.

   The crown-rump length is a more accurate indicator of gestational (menstrual) age than is the mean gestational sac diameter. However, the mean gestational sac diameter may be recorded when an embryo is not identified.

   Caution should be used in making the presumptive diagnosis of a gestational sac in the absence of a definite embryo or yolk sac. Without these findings, an intrauterine fluid collection could represent a pseudo–gestational sac associated with an ectopic pregnancy.

   b. The presence or absence of cardiac activity should be documented with a 2-dimensional video clip or M-mode imaging.

---

[b] For the purpose of this document, first trimester represents 1 week to 13 weeks 6 days.

[c] For the purpose of this document, the terms *gestational age* and *menstrual age* are considered equivalent.

Comment
With transvaginal scans, while cardiac motion is usually observed when the embryo is 2 mm or greater in length, if an embryo less than 7 mm in length is seen without cardiac activity, a subsequent scan in 1 week is recommended to ensure that the pregnancy is nonviable.

c. Fetal number should be documented.

Comment
Amnionicity and chorionicity should be documented for all multiple gestations when possible.

d. Embryonic/fetal anatomy appropriate for the first trimester should be assessed.

e. The nuchal region should be imaged, and abnormalities such as cystic hygroma should be documented.

Comment
For those patients desiring to assess their individual risk of fetal aneuploidy, a very specific measurement of the NT during a specific age interval is necessary (as determined by the laboratory used). See the guidelines for this measurement below.

NT measurements should be used (in conjunction with serum biochemistry) to determine the risk of having a fetus with aneuploidy or other anatomic abnormalities such as heart defects.

In this setting, it is important that the practitioner measure the NT according to established guidelines for measurement. A quality assessment program is recommended to ensure that false-positive and false-negative results are kept to a minimum.

f. The uterus including the cervix, adnexal structures, and cul-de-sac should be evaluated. Abnormalities should be imaged and documented.

Comment
The presence, location, appearance, and size of adnexal masses should be documented. The presence and number of leiomyomata should be documented. The measurements of the largest or any potentially clinically significant leiomyomata should be documented. The cul-de-sac should be evaluated for the presence or absence of fluid. Uterine anomalies should be documented.

Guidelines for NT Measurement:

i. The margins of the NT edges must be clear enough for proper placement of the calipers.

ii. The fetus must be in the midsagittal plane.

iii. The image must be magnified so that it is filled by the fetal head, neck, and upper thorax.

iv. The fetal neck must be in a neutral position, not flexed and not hyperextended.

v. The amnion must be seen as separate from the NT line.

vi. The + calipers on the ultrasound must be used to perform the NT measurement.

vii. Electronic calipers must be placed on the inner borders of the nuchal line space with none of the horizontal crossbar itself protruding into the space.

viii. The calipers must be placed perpendicular to the long axis of the fetus.

ix. The measurement must be obtained at the widest space of the NT.

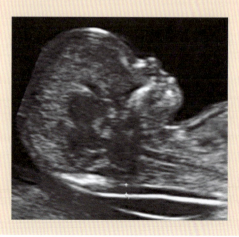

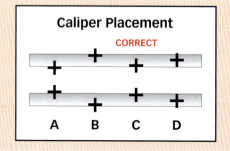

B. Second- and Third-Trimester Ultrasound Examination

1. Indications

Indications for second- and third-trimester sonography include but are not limited to:

a. Screening for fetal anomalies;
b. Evaluation of fetal anatomy;
c. Estimation of gestational (menstrual) age;
d. Evaluation of fetal growth;
e. Evaluation of vaginal bleeding;
f. Evaluation of abdominal or pelvic pain;
g. Evaluation of cervical insufficiency;
h. Determination of fetal presentation;
i. Evaluation of suspected multiple gestation;
j. Adjunct to amniocentesis or other procedure;
k. Evaluation of a significant discrepancy between uterine size and clinical dates;
l. Evaluation of a pelvic mass;
m. Evaluation of a suspected hydatidiform mole;
n. Adjunct to cervical cerclage placement;
o. Suspected ectopic pregnancy;
p. Suspected fetal death;
q. Suspected uterine abnormalities;
r. Evaluation of fetal well-being;
s. Suspected amniotic fluid abnormalities;
t. Suspected placental abruption;
u. Adjunct to external cephalic version;
v. Evaluation of premature rupture of membranes and/or premature labor;
w. Evaluation of abnormal biochemical markers;
x. Follow-up evaluation of a fetal anomaly;
y. Follow-up evaluation of placental location for suspected placenta previa;
z. History of previous congenital anomaly;
aa. Evaluation of the fetal condition in late registrants for prenatal care; and
bb. Assessment for findings that may increase the risk for aneuploidy.

Comment
In certain clinical circumstances, a more detailed examination of fetal anatomy may be indicated.

2. Imaging Parameters for a Standard Fetal Examination

a. Fetal cardiac activity, fetal number, and presentation should be documented.

Comment
An abnormal heart rate and/or rhythm should be documented.

Multiple gestations require the documentation of additional information: chorionicity, amnionicity, comparison of fetal sizes, estimation of amniotic fluid volume (increased, decreased, or normal) in each gestational sac, and fetal genitalia (when visualized).

b. A qualitative or semiquantitative estimate of amniotic fluid volume should be documented.

Comment
Although it is acceptable for experienced examiners to qualitatively estimate amniotic fluid volume, semiquantitative methods have also been described for this purpose (e.g., amniotic fluid index, single deepest pocket, and 2-diameter pocket).

c. The placental location, appearance, and relationship to the internal cervical os should be documented. The umbilical cord should be imaged and the number of vessels in the cord documented. The placental cord insertion site should be documented when technically possible.

Comment
It is recognized that the apparent placental position early in pregnancy may not correlate well with its location at the time of delivery.

Transabdominal, transperineal, or transvaginal views may be helpful in visualizing the internal cervical os and its relationship to the placenta.

Transvaginal or transperineal ultrasound may be considered if the cervix appears shortened or cannot be adequately visualized during the transabdominal sonogram.

A velamentous (also called membranous) placental cord insertion that crosses the internal os of the cervix is vasa previa, a condition that has a high risk of fetal mortality if not diagnosed before labor.

d. Gestational (menstrual) age assessment.

First-trimester crown-rump measurement is the most accurate means for sonographic dating of pregnancy. Beyond this period, a variety of sonographic parameters such as biparietal diameter, abdominal circumference, and femoral diaphysis length can be used to estimate gestational (menstrual) age. The variability of gestational (menstrual) age estimation, however, increases with advancing pregnancy. Significant discrepancies between gestational (menstrual) age and fetal measurements may suggest the possibility of a fetal growth abnormality, intrauterine growth restriction, or macrosomia.

Comment

The pregnancy should not be redated after an accurate earlier scan has been performed and is available for comparison.

i. The biparietal diameter is measured at the level of the thalami and cavum septi pellucidi or columns of the fornix. The cerebellar hemispheres should not be visible in this scanning plane. The measurement is taken from the outer edge of the proximal skull to the inner edge of the distal skull.

Comment

The head shape may be flattened (dolichocephaly) or rounded (brachycephaly) as a normal variant. Under these circumstances, certain variants of normal fetal head development may make measurement of the head circumference more reliable than biparietal diameter for estimating gestational (menstrual) age.

ii. The head circumference is measured at the same level as the biparietal diameter, around the outer perimeter of the calvarium. This measurement is not affected by head shape.

iii. The femoral diaphysis length can be reliably used after 14 weeks' gestational (menstrual) age. The long axis of the femoral shaft is most accurately measured with the beam of insonation being perpendicular to the shaft, excluding the distal femoral epiphysis.

iv. The abdominal circumference or average abdominal diameter should be determined at the skin line on a true transverse view at the level of the junction of the umbilical vein, portal sinus, and fetal stomach when visible.

Comment

The abdominal circumference or average abdominal diameter measurement is used with other biometric parameters to estimate fetal weight and may allow detection of intrauterine growth restriction or macrosomia.

e. Fetal weight estimation.

Fetal weight can be estimated by obtaining measurements such as the biparietal diameter, head circumference, abdominal circumference or average abdominal diameter, and femoral diaphysis length. Results from various prediction models can be compared to fetal weight percentiles from published nomograms.

Comment

If previous studies have been performed, appropriateness of growth should also be documented. Scans for growth evaluation can typically be performed at least 2 to 4 weeks apart. A shorter scan interval may result in confusion as to whether measurement changes are truly due to growth as opposed to variations in the technique itself.

Currently, even the best fetal weight prediction methods can yield errors as high as ±15%. This variability can be influenced by factors such as the nature of the patient population, the number and types of anatomic parameters being measured, technical factors that affect the resolution of ultrasound images, and the weight range being studied.

f. Maternal anatomy.

Evaluation of the uterus, adnexal structures, and cervix should be performed when appropriate. If the cervix cannot be visualized, a transperineal or transvaginal scan may be considered when evaluation of the cervix is needed.

Comment

This will allow recognition of incidental findings of potential clinical significance. The presence, location, and size of adnexal masses and the presence of at least the largest and potentially clinically significant leiomyomata should be documented. It is not always possible to image the normal maternal ovaries during the second and third trimesters.

g. Fetal anatomic survey.

Fetal anatomy, as described in this document, may be adequately assessed by ultrasound after approximately 18 weeks' gestational (menstrual) age. It may be possible to document normal structures before this time, although some structures can be difficult to visualize due to fetal size, position, movement, abdominal scars, and increased maternal abdominal wall thickness. A second- or third-trimester scan may pose technical limitations for an anatomic evaluation due to imaging artifacts from acoustic shadowing. When this occurs, the report of the sonographic examination should document the nature of this technical limitation. A follow-up examination may be helpful.

The following areas of assessment represent the minimal elements of a standard examination of fetal anatomy. A more detailed fetal anatomic examination may be necessary if an abnormality or suspected abnormality is found on the standard examination.

i. Head, face, and neck:
   Lateral cerebral ventricles;
   Choroid plexus;
   Midline falx;
   Cavum septi pellucidi;
   Cerebellum;
   Cistern magna; and
   Upper lip.

Comment

A measurement of the nuchal fold may be helpful during a specific age interval to assess the risk of aneuploidy.

ii. Chest:
   Heart:
   Four-chamber view;
   Left ventricular outflow tract; and
   Right ventricular outflow tract.

iii. Abdomen:
   Stomach (presence, size, and situs);
   Kidneys;
   Urinary bladder;
   Umbilical cord insertion site into the fetal abdomen; and
   Umbilical cord vessel number.

iv. Spine:
   Cervical, thoracic, lumbar, and sacral spine.

v. Extremities:
   Legs and arms.

vi. Sex:
   In multiple gestations and when medically indicated.

VI. DOCUMENTATION

Adequate documentation is essential for high-quality patient care. There should be a permanent record of the ultrasound examination and its interpretation. Images of all appropriate areas, both normal and abnormal, should be recorded. Variations from normal size should be accompanied by measurements. Images should be labeled with the patient identification, facility identification, examination date, and side (right or left) of the anatomic site imaged. An official interpretation (final report) of the ultrasound findings should be included in the patient's medical record. Retention of the ultrasound examination should be consistent both with clinical needs and with relevant legal and local health care facility requirements.

Reporting should be in accordance with the AIUM *Practice Guideline for Documentation of an Ultrasound Examination*.

VII. EQUIPMENT SPECIFICATIONS

These studies should be conducted with real-time scanners, using a transabdominal and/or transvaginal approach. A transducer of appropriate frequency should be used. Real-time sonography is necessary to confirm the presence of fetal life through observation of cardiac activity and active movement.

The choice of transducer frequency is a trade-off between beam penetration and resolution. With modern equipment, 3- to 5-MHz abdominal transducers allow sufficient penetration in most patients while providing adequate resolution. A lower-frequency transducer may be needed to provide adequate penetration for abdominal imaging in an obese patient. During early pregnancy, a 5-MHz abdominal transducer or a 5- to 10-MHz or greater vaginal transducer may provide superior resolution while still allowing adequate penetration.

VIII. FETAL SAFETY

Diagnostic ultrasound studies of the fetus are generally considered safe during pregnancy. This diagnostic procedure should be performed only when there is a valid medical indication, and the lowest possible ultrasonic exposure setting should be used to gain the necessary diagnostic information under the ALARA (as low as reasonably achievable) principle.

A thermal index for soft tissue (Tis) should be used at earlier than 10 weeks' gestation, and a thermal index for bone (Tib) should be used at 10 weeks' gestation or later when bone ossification is evident. In keeping with the ALARA principle, M-mode imaging should be used instead of spectral Doppler imaging to document embryonic/fetal heart rate.

The promotion, selling, or leasing of ultrasound equipment for making "keepsake fetal videos" is considered by the US Food and Drug Administration to be an unapproved use of a medical device. Use of a diagnostic ultrasound system for these purposes, without a physician's order, may be in violation of state laws or regulations.

IX. QUALITY CONTROL AND IMPROVEMENT, SAFETY, INFECTION CONTROL, AND PATIENT EDUCATION

Policies and procedures related to quality control, patient education, infection control, and safety should be developed and implemented in accordance with the AIUM *Standards and Guidelines for the Accreditation of Ultrasound Practices*.

Equipment performance monitoring should be in accordance with the AIUM *Standards and Guidelines for the Accreditation of Ultrasound Practices*.

X. ALARA PRINCIPLE

The potential benefits and risks of each examination should be considered. The ALARA principle should be observed when adjusting controls that affect the acoustic output and by considering transducer dwell times. Further details on ALARA may be found in the AIUM publication *Medical Ultrasound Safety*, Third Edition.

AIUM PRACTICE GUIDELINE FOR THE PERFORMANCE OF ULTRASOUND OF THE FEMALE PELVIS

Guideline developed in collaboration with the American College of Radiology (ACR), the American College of Obstetricians and Gynecologists (ACOG), the Society for Pediatric Radiology (SPR), and the Society of Radiologists in Ultrasound (SRU).

I. INTRODUCTION

The clinical aspects contained in specific sections of this guideline (Introduction, Indications, Specifications of the Examination, and Equipment Specifications) were developed collaboratively by the American Institute of Ultrasound in Medicine (AIUM), the American College of Radiology (ACR), the American College of Obstetricians and Gynecologists (ACOG), the Society for Pediatric Radiology (SPR), and the Society of Radiologists in Ultrasound (SRU). Recommendations for physician requirements, written request for the examination, documentation, and quality control vary among the organizations and are addressed by each separately.

This guideline has been developed to assist physicians performing sonographic studies of the female pelvis. Ultrasound examinations of the female pelvis should be performed only when there is a valid medical reason, and the lowest possible ultrasonic exposure settings should be used to gain the necessary diagnostic information. In some cases, additional or specialized examinations may be necessary. Although it is not possible to detect every abnormality, adherence to the following guideline will maximize the probability of detecting most abnormalities. For ultrasound examinations of the urinary bladder, see the AIUM *Practice Guideline for the Performance of an Ultrasound Examination of the Abdomen and/or Retroperitoneum*.

II. INDICATIONS

Indications for pelvic sonography include but are not limited to:

1. Evaluation of pelvic pain;
2. Evaluation of pelvic masses;
3. Evaluation of endocrine abnormalities, including polycystic ovaries;
4. Evaluation of dysmenorrhea (painful menses);
5. Evaluation of amenorrhea;
6. Evaluation of abnormal bleeding;
7. Evaluation of delayed menses;
8. Follow-up of a previously detected abnormality;
9. Evaluation, monitoring, and/or treatment of infertility patients;
10. Evaluation in the presence of a limited clinical examination of the pelvis;
11. Evaluation for signs or symptoms of pelvic infection;
12. Further characterization of a pelvic abnormality noted on another imaging study;
13. Evaluation of congenital uterine and lower genital tract anomalies;
14. Evaluation of excessive bleeding, pain, or signs of infection after pelvic surgery, delivery, or abortion;
15. Localization of an intrauterine contraceptive device;
16. Screening for malignancy in high-risk patients;
17. Evaluation of incontinence or pelvic organ prolapse;
18. Guidance for interventional or surgical procedures; and
19. Preoperative and postoperative evaluation of pelvic structures.

III. QUALIFICATIONS OF PERSONNEL

See the AIUM Official Statement *Training Guidelines for Physicians Who Evaluate and Interpret Diagnostic Ultrasound Examinations* and the AIUM *Standards and Guidelines for the Accreditation of Ultrasound Practices*.

IV. WRITTEN REQUEST FOR THE EXAMINATION

The written or electronic request for an ultrasound examination should provide sufficient information to allow for the appropriate performance and interpretation of the examination.

The request for the examination must be originated by a physician or other appropriately licensed health care provider or under the provider's direction. The accompanying clinical information should be provided by a physician or other appropriate health care provider familiar with the patient's clinical situation and should be consistent with relevant legal and local health care facility requirements.

V. SPECIFICATIONS OF THE EXAMINATION

The following sections detail the examination to be performed for each organ and anatomic region in the female pelvis. All relevant structures should be identified by the transabdominal and/or transvaginal approach. A transrectal or transperineal approach may be useful in patients who are not candidates for introduction of a vaginal probe and in assessing the patient with pelvic organ prolapse. More than 1 approach may be necessary.

A. General Pelvic Preparation

For a complete transabdominal pelvic sonogram, the patient's bladder can be distended if necessary to displace the small bowel from the field of view. Occasionally, overdistention of the bladder may compromise the evaluation. When this occurs, imaging may be repeated after partial bladder emptying. If an abnormality of the urinary bladder is detected, it should be documented and reported.

For a transvaginal sonogram, the urinary bladder is preferably empty. The patient, the sonographer, or the physician may introduce the vaginal transducer, preferably under real-time monitoring. Consideration of having a chaperone present should be in accordance with local policy.

B. Uterus

The vagina and uterus provide anatomic landmarks that can be used as reference points for the other pelvic structures, whether normal or abnormal. In examining the uterus, the following should be evaluated: (1) the uterine size, shape, and orientation; (2) the endometrium; (3) the myometrium; and (4) the cervix. The vagina may be imaged as a landmark for the cervix. The overall uterine length is evaluated in a sagittal view from the fundus to the cervix (to the external os, if it can be identified). The depth of the uterus (anteroposterior dimension) is measured in the same sagittal view from its anterior to posterior walls, perpendicular to the length. The maximum width is measured in the transverse or coronal view. If volume measurements of the uterine corpus are performed, the cervical component should be excluded from the uterine length measurement.

Abnormalities of the uterus should be documented. The myometrium and cervix should be evaluated for contour changes, echogenicity, masses, and cysts. Masses that may require followup or intervention should be measured in at least 2 dimensions, acknowledging that it is not usually necessary to measure all uterine fibroids. The size and location of clinically relevant fibroids should be documented.

The endometrium should be analyzed for thickness, focal abnormalities, echogenicity, and the presence of fluid or masses in the cavity. The thickest part of the endometrium should be measured perpendicular to its longitudinal plane in the anteroposterior diameter from echogenic to echogenic border (Figure 1). The adjacent hypoechoic myometrium and fluid in the cavity should be excluded (Figure 2). Assessment of the endometrium should allow for variations expected with phases of the menstrual cycle and with hormonal supplementation. It should be reported if the endometrium is not adequately seen in its entirety or is poorly defined. Sonohysterography may be a useful adjunct to evaluate the patient with abnormal uterine bleeding or to further clarify an abnormally thickened endometrium. (See the AIUM *Practice Guideline for the Performance of Sonohysterography*.) If the patient has an intrauterine contraceptive device, its location should be documented.

The addition of 3-dimensional to 2-dimensional ultrasound (transabdominal, transvaginal, transperineal, and/or transrectal) can be helpful in many circumstances, including but not limited to evaluating the relationship of masses with the endometrial

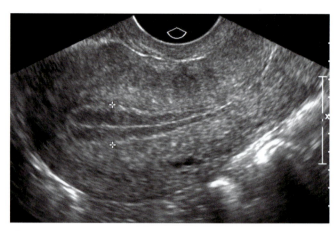

Figure 1. Measurement of endometrial thickness. The endometrial thickness is measured in its thickest portion from echogenic to echogenic border (calipers) perpendicular to the midline longitudinal plane of the uterus.

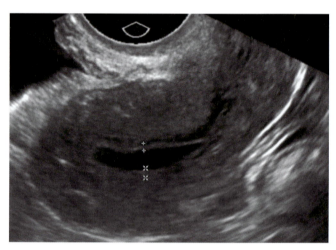

Figure 2. Measurement of endometrium with fluid in the cavity. In the presence of endometrial fluid, measurements of the 2 separate layers of the endometrium (calipers), excluding the fluid, are added to determine the endometrial thickness.

cavity, identifying uterine congenital anomalies and a thickened and/or heterogeneous endometrium, and evaluating the location of an intrauterine device and the integrity of the pelvic floor.

C. Adnexa, Including Ovaries and Fallopian Tubes

When evaluating the adnexa, an attempt should be made to identify the ovaries first, since they can serve as a major point of reference for assessing the presence of adnexal pathology. The ovarian size may be determined by measuring the ovary in 3 dimensions (width, length, and depth) on views obtained in 2 orthogonal planes. Any ovarian abnormalities should be documented.

The ovaries may not be identifiable in some patients. This occurs most frequently before puberty, after menopause, or in the presence of a large leiomyomatous uterus. The adnexal region should be surveyed for abnormalities, particularly masses and dilated tubular structures.

If an adnexal abnormality is noted, its relationship with the ovaries and uterus should be assessed. The size and sonographic characteristics of adnexal masses should be documented.

Spectral, color, and/or power Doppler ultrasound may be useful to evaluate the vascular characteristics of pelvic lesions.

D. Cul-de-Sac

The cul-de-sac and bowel posterior to the uterus may not be clearly defined. This area should be evaluated for the presence of free fluid or a mass. If a mass is detected, its size, position, shape, sonographic characteristics, and relationship to the ovaries and uterus should be documented. Differentiation of normal loops of bowel from a mass may be difficult if only a transabdominal examination is performed. A transvaginal examination may be helpful to distinguish a suspected mass from fluid and feces within the normal rectosigmoid colon.

VI. DOCUMENTATION

Adequate documentation is essential for high-quality patient care. There should be a permanent record of the ultrasound examination and its interpretation. Images of all appropriate areas, both normal and abnormal, should be recorded. Variations from normal size should be accompanied by measurements. Images should be labeled with the patient identification, facility identification, examination date, and side (right or left) of the anatomic site imaged. An official interpretation (final report) of the ultrasound findings should be included in the patient's medical record. Retention of the ultrasound examination should be consistent both with clinical needs and with relevant legal and local health care facility requirements.

Reporting should be in accordance with the AIUM *Practice Guideline for Documentation of an Ultrasound Examination*.

VII. EQUIPMENT SPECIFICATIONS

A sonographic examination of the female pelvis should be conducted with a real-time scanner, preferably using sector, curved linear, and/or endovaginal transducers. The transducer or scanner should be adjusted to operate at the highest clinically appropriate frequency, realizing that there is a trade-off between resolution and beam penetration.

VIII. QUALITY CONTROL AND IMPROVEMENT, SAFETY, INFECTION CONTROL, AND PATIENT EDUCATION

Policies and procedures related to quality control, patient education, infection control, and safety should be developed and implemented in accordance with the AIUM *Standards and Guidelines for the Accreditation of Ultrasound Practices*. Equipment performance monitoring should be in accordance with the AIUM *Standards and Guidelines for the Accreditation of Ultrasound Practices*.

IX. ALARA PRINCIPLE

The potential benefits and risks of each examination should be considered. The ALARA (as low as reasonably achievable) principle should be observed when adjusting controls that affect the acoustic output and by considering transducer dwell times. Further details on ALARA may be found in the AIUM publication *Medical Ultrasound Safety*, Third Edition.

AIUM PRACTICE GUIDELINE FOR THE PERFORMANCE OF SONOHYSTEROGRAPHY

Guideline developed in collaboration with the American College of Radiology, the American College of Obstetricians and Gynecologists, and the Society of Radiologists in Ultrasound

I. INTRODUCTION

The clinical aspects contained in specific sections of this guideline (Introduction, Indications and Contraindications, Specifications for Individual Examinations, and Equipment Specifications) were developed collaboratively by the American Institute of Ultrasound in Medicine (AIUM), the American College of Radiology (ACR), the American College of Obstetricians and

Gynecologists (ACOG), and the Society of Radiologists in Ultrasound (SRU). Recommendations for physician qualifications, written request for the examination, procedure documentation, and quality control may vary among the 4 organizations and are addressed by each separately.

This guideline has been developed to assist qualified physicians performing sonohysterography. Properly performed sonohysterography can provide information about the uterus, endometrium, and fallopian tubes. Additional studies may be necessary for complete diagnosis. Adherence to the following guideline will maximize the diagnostic benefit of sonohysterography.

Sonohysterography is the evaluation of the endometrial cavity using the transcervical injection of sterile fluid. Various terms such as saline infusion sonohysterography and simply sonohysterography have been used to describe this technique. The primary goal of sonohysterography is to visualize the endometrial cavity in more detail than is possible with routine endovaginal sonography. Sonohysterography can also be used to assess tubal patency. An increase in the amount of free pelvic fluid at the end of the procedure indicates that at least one tube is patent.

II. INDICATIONS AND CONTRAINDICATIONS

A. Indications

Indications include but are not limited to evaluation of:

1. Abnormal uterine bleeding;
2. Uterine cavity, especially with regard to uterine myomas, polyps, and synechiae;
3. Abnormalities detected on endovaginal sonography, including focal or diffuse endometrial or intracavitary abnormalities;
4. Congenital or acquired abnormalities of the uterus;
5. Infertility;
6. Recurrent pregnancy loss; and
7. Suboptimal visualization of the endometrium on endovaginal ultrasound.

B. Contraindications

Sonohysterography should not be performed in a woman who is pregnant or who could be pregnant. This is usually avoided by scheduling the examination in the follicular phase of the menstrual cycle, after menstrual flow has essentially ceased but before the patient has ovulated. In a patient with regular cycles, sonohysterography should not in most cases be performed later than the 10th day of the menstrual cycle. Sonohysterography should not be performed in patients with a pelvic infection or unexplained pelvic tenderness, which could be due to pelvic inflammatory disease. Active vaginal bleeding is not a contraindication to the procedure but may make the interpretation more challenging.

III. QUALIFICATIONS AND RESPONSIBILITIES OF THE PHYSICIAN

See www.aium.org for AIUM Official Statements including *Standards and Guidelines for the Accreditation of Ultrasound Practices* and relevant Physician Training Guidelines.

IV. WRITTEN REQUEST FOR THE EXAMINATION

The written or electronic request for an ultrasound examination should provide sufficient information to allow for the appropriate performance and interpretation of the examination.

The request for the examination must be originated by a physician or other appropriately licensed health care provider or under the provider's direction. The accompanying clinical information should be provided by a physician or other appropriate health care provider familiar with the patient's clinical situation and should be consistent with relevant legal and local health care facility requirements.

V. SPECIFICATIONS FOR INDIVIDUAL EXAMINATIONS

A. Patient Preparation

Pelvic organ tenderness should be assessed during the preliminary endovaginal sonogram. If the patient's history or physical exam is concerning for active pelvic inflammatory disease, the examination should be deferred until an appropriate course of treatment has been completed. In the presence of nontender hydrosalpinges, consideration may be given to administering antibiotics at the time of the examination; in this case, it is prudent to discuss the antibiotic regimen with the referring physician. A pregnancy test is advised when clinically indicated. Patients should be questioned about a latex allergy or a reaction to betadine or other topical antiseptic before use of these products. A sonohysterogram should be performed in the early follicular phase, as close to the end of the menstrual period as possible.

B. Procedure

A previous endovaginal sonogram is useful for measurement of the endometrium and evaluation of the uterus, ovaries, and pelvic free fluid. A speculum is used to allow visualization of the cervix. The presence of unusual pain, lesions, or purulent vaginal or cervical discharge may require rescheduling the procedure pending further evaluation. Before insertion, the catheter should be flushed with sterile fluid to avoid introducing air during the study. After cleansing the external os, the cervical canal and/or uterine cavity should be catheterized using aseptic technique, and appropriate sterile fluid should be instilled slowly by means of manual injection under real-time sonographic imaging. Imaging should include real-time scanning of the endometrial and cervical canal. Imaging may include evaluation of fallopian tube patency if indicated.

C. Contrast Agent

Appropriate sterile fluid such as normal saline or water should be used for sonohysterography. If the requesting physician is interested in tubal patency, then a sonosalpingogram can be offered using agitated saline.

D. Images

Precatheterization images should be obtained and recorded, in at least 2 planes, to show normal and abnormal findings. These images should include the thickest bilayer endometrial measurement, which includes the anterior and posterior endometrial thicknesses, obtained in a sagittal view.

Once the uterine cavity is filled with fluid, a complete survey of the uterine cavity should be performed and representative images obtained to document normal and abnormal findings. If a balloon catheter filled with saline is used for the examination, images should be obtained at the end of the procedure with the balloon deflated to fully evaluate the endometrial cavity, particularly the cervical canal and lower portion of the endometrial cavity.

Color Doppler sonography may be helpful in evaluating the vascularity of an intrauterine abnormality and tubal patency.

Three-dimensional imaging, in particular reconstructed coronal plane imaging, is useful in the assessment of Müllerian duct anomalies and for preoperative mapping of myomas.

E. Postprocedure Care

The imaging or referring physician should discuss the sonohysterogram findings with the patient. The patient should be instructed to contact her physician if she develops fever, persistent pain, or unusual bleeding following the procedure. The patient should be told to expect leaking of fluid after the procedure that may be blood-tinged or may have a similar color as the cleaning solution.

VI. DOCUMENTATION

Adequate documentation is essential for high-quality patient care. There should be a permanent record of the ultrasound examination and its interpretation. Images of all appropriate areas, both normal and abnormal, should be recorded. Variations from normal size should be accompanied by measurements. Images should be labeled with the patient identification, facility identification, examination date, and side (right or left) of the anatomic site imaged. An official interpretation (final report) of the ultrasound findings should be included in the patient's medical record. Retention of the ultrasound examination should be consistent both with clinical needs and with relevant legal and local health care facility requirements.

Reporting should be in accordance with the AIUM *Practice Guideline for Documentation of an Ultrasound Examination*.

VII. EQUIPMENT SPECIFICATIONS

Sonohysterography is usually conducted with a high-frequency endovaginal transducer. In cases of an enlarged uterus, additional transabdominal images during infusion may be required to fully evaluate the endometrium. The transducer should be adjusted to operate at the highest clinically appropriate frequency under the ALARA (as low as reasonably achievable) principle.

VIII. QUALITY CONTROL AND IMPROVEMENT, SAFETY, INFECTION CONTROL, AND PATIENT EDUCATION

Policies and procedures related to quality control, patient education, infection control, and safety should be developed and implemented in accordance with the AIUM *Standards and Guidelines for the Accreditation of Ultrasound Practices*.

Equipment performance monitoring should be in accordance with the AIUM *Standards and Guidelines for the Accreditation of Ultrasound Practices*.

IX. ALARA PRINCIPLE

The potential benefits and risks of each examination should be considered. The ALARA (as low as reasonably achievable) principle should be observed when adjusting controls that affect the acoustic output and by considering transducer dwell times. Further details on ALARA may be found in the AIUM publication *Medical Ultrasound Safety*, Third Edition.

AIUM PRACTICE GUIDELINE FOR THE PERFORMANCE OF ULTRASONOGRAPHY IN REPRODUCTIVE MEDICINE

Prepared in collaboration with the American Institute of Ultrasound in Medicine (AIUM) and the Society for Reproductive Endocrinology and Infertility (SREI), an affiliate of the American Society of Reproductive Medicine (ASRM)

ULTRASOUND EXAMINATION OF THE FEMALE PELVIS FOR INFERTILITY AND REPRODUCTIVE MEDICINE

The following are proposed guidelines for ultrasound evaluation of the female pelvis. The document consists of 2 parts:

Part I: Equipment and Documentation Guidelines

Part II: Guidelines for Performance of the Ultrasound Examination of the Female Pelvis for Infertility and Reproductive Medicine

This guideline has been developed to provide assistance to practitioners performing ultrasound studies of the female pelvis. In some cases, additional and/or specialized examinations may be necessary. While it is not possible to detect every abnormality, adherence to the following will maximize the probability of detecting most of the abnormalities that occur.

This guideline includes excerpts from various previously published guidelines of the AIUM. The latest versions of all AIUM guidelines are available at www.aium.org.

Part I: Equipment and Documentation Guidelines

Equipment

The sonographic examination of the female pelvis should be conducted with a real-time scanner, with the availability of multiple types of transducers. The transducer or scanner should be adjusted to operate at the highest clinically appropriate frequency, realizing that there is a trade-off between resolution and beam penetration. With modern equipment, studies performed from the anterior abdominal wall can usually use frequencies of 3.5 MHz or higher, while scans performed from the vagina should use frequencies of 5 MHz or higher.

Care of the Equipment

All probes should be cleaned after each patient examination. Transvaginal probes should be covered by a protective sheath prior to insertion. Patients should be questioned about latex allergy prior to use of a latex sheath. Following each examination, the sheath should be disposed, and the probe washed, dried, and appropriately disinfected (see section below: "Guidelines for Cleaning and Preparing Endocavitary Ultrasound Transducers Between Patients"). The type of antimicrobial solution and the methodology for disinfection depend on manufacturer and infectious disease recommendations.

Documentation

Adequate documentation is essential for high-quality patient care. A permanent record of the ultrasound examination and its interpretation should be kept by the facility performing the study. Images of all appropriate areas, both normal and abnormal, should be recorded. Variations from normal size should be accompanied by measurements. Images are to be appropriately labeled with the examination date, facility name, patient identification, and image orientation and/or organ imaged when appropriate. A report of the ultrasound findings should be included in the patient's medical record. Urgent or clinically important unexpected results should be communicated verbally to any referring and/or treating physician and this communication documented in the report. Retention of the permanent record of the ultrasound examination should be consistent both with clinical needs and with the relevant legal and local health care facility requirements.

Part II: Guidelines for Performance of the Ultrasound Examination of the Female Pelvis for Infertility and Reproductive Medicine

The following guidelines describe the examination to be performed for each organ and anatomic region in the female pelvis. Whenever possible, all relevant structures should be identified by the vaginal approach. When a transvaginal scan fails to image all areas needed for diagnosis, a transabdominal scan should be performed. In some cases, both a transabdominal and a transvaginal scan may be needed.

General Pelvic Preparation

For a pelvic sonogram performed transabdominally, the patient's urinary bladder should, in general, be distended adequately to displace the small bowel and its contained gas from the field of view. Occasionally, overdistension of the bladder may compromise evaluation. When this occurs, imaging may be repeated after the patient partially empties her bladder.

For a transvaginal sonogram, the urinary bladder is preferably empty. The patient, the sonographer, or the physician may introduce the transvaginal transducer, preferably under real-time monitoring. Transvaginal sonography is a specialized form of a pelvic examination. Therefore, policies applied locally regarding chaperone or patient privacy issues during a pelvic examination should also be applied during a transvaginal ultrasound examination.

Uterus

The vagina and the uterus provide anatomic landmarks that can be used as reference points when evaluating the pelvic structures. In evaluating the uterus, the following should be documented: (1) uterine size, shape, and orientation; (2) the endometrium; (3) the myometrium; and (4) the cervix. The vagina may be imaged as a landmark for the cervix and lower uterine segment. Uterine length is evaluated on a long-axis view as the distance from the fundus to the cervix. The anteroposterior (AP) diameter of the uterus is measured in the same long-axis view from its anterior to posterior walls, perpendicular to its long axis. The transverse diameter is measured from the transaxial or coronal view, perpendicular to the long axis of the uterus. If volume measurements of the uterine corpus are performed, the cervical component should be excluded from the uterine measurement.

Abnormalities of the uterus should be documented. The endometrium should be analyzed for thickness, focal abnormalities, and the presence of fluid or masses in the endometrial cavity. Assessment of the endometrium should allow for variations expected with phases of the menstrual cycle and with hormonal supplementation. The endometrial thickness measurement should include both layers, measured anterior to posterior, in the sagittal plane. Any fluid within the endometrial cavity should be excluded from this measurement. If the endometrial echo is difficult to image or ill-defined, a comment should be added to the report.

The myometrium and cervix should be evaluated for contour changes, echogenicity, and masses. Masses, if identified, should be measured in at least 2 dimensions and their locations recorded.

Adnexa (Ovaries and Fallopian Tubes)

When evaluating the adnexa, an attempt should be made to identify the ovaries first since they can serve as a major point of reference for assessing the presence of adnexal pathology. Although their location is variable, the ovaries are most often situated anterior to the internal iliac (hypogastric) vessels, lateral to the uterus, and superficial to the obturator internus muscle. The ovaries should be measured, and ovarian abnormalities should be documented. Ovarian size can be determined by measuring the ovary in 3 dimensions on views obtained in 2 orthogonal planes. It is recognized that the ovaries may not be identifiable in some women. This occurs most frequently after menopause or in patients with a large leiomyomatous uterus.

The normal fallopian tubes are not commonly identified. This region should be surveyed for abnormalities, particularly dilated tubular structures.

If an adnexal mass is noted, its relationship to the uterus and the ovaries, if separately visualized, should be documented. Its size, echogenicity, and internal characteristics (cystic, solid, or complex) should be determined. Doppler ultrasound may be useful in select cases to identify the vascular nature of pelvic structures.

Cul-de-sac

The cul-de-sac and bowel posterior to the uterus may not be clearly defined. This area should be evaluated for the presence of free fluid or masses. When free fluid is detected, its echogenicity should be assessed. If a mass is detected, its size, position, shape, echogenicity, internal characteristics (cystic, solid, or complex), and relationship to the ovaries and uterus should be documented. Identification of peristalsis can be helpful in distinguishing a loop of bowel from a pelvic mass. In the absence of peristalsis, differentiation of normal loops of bowel from a mass may be difficult. A transvaginal examination may be helpful to distinguish a suspected mass from fluid and feces within the normal rectosigmoid. An ultrasound water enema study or a repeat examination after a cleansing enema may also help to distinguish a suspected mass from bowel.

Limited Examination

In some circumstances, a limited pelvic ultrasound examination is appropriate, especially when monitoring ovarian stimulation (e.g., an ovarian folliculogram study or determining endometrial qualities prior to cryopreserved embryo transfer). A comprehensive exam should have previously been performed in the preceding 4 to 6 months to rule out other gynecologic pathology. The limited exam can be restricted to the organ or measurements of interest. In the case of an ovarian folliculogram, the following should be documented: ovarian follicle number in each ovary, endometrial thickness, and endometrial morphologic appearance. In addition, follicular diameters in 2 dimensions for each follicle above 10 mm should be recorded. A single recorded value representing the mean of 2 diameter measurements performed at right angles is also acceptable. Given that these patients will have had a full pelvic exam at the appropriate interval prior to initiating therapy, for infertility patients undergoing limited folliculogram studies, permanent recorded images should be obtained as indicated. Pertinent clinical information should be recorded in the patient record.

Ultrasound-Guided Procedures

A. **Follicle Puncture:** Ultrasound-assisted (transvaginal or transabdominal) follicle puncture for retrieving eggs for in vitro fertilization (IVF) is appropriate in the following circumstances:

1. The patient has undergone comprehensive sonographic evaluation of the pelvis within 4 to 6 months prior to the start of hormonal stimulation of the ovaries.

2. Real-time continuous guidance is available, and the image demonstrates a safe approach for the needle path.

3. The ovaries can be brought in close proximity to the ultrasound transducer, thus avoiding the puncture of vital structures (e.g., bowel and blood vessels).

B. **Cyst Aspiration:** Ultrasound-assisted (transvaginal or transabdominal) ovarian cyst puncture and aspiration is appropriate in patients who have been diagnosed with a persistent ovarian cyst and who meet the following criteria:

1. Failed resolution of the cyst following observation and/or hormonal manipulation.

2. The cyst is unilocular and thin-walled without internal excrescences or septations.

3. Real-time continuous guidance is available, and the image demonstrates a safe approach for the needle path.

4. The cyst can be brought in close proximity to the ultrasound transducer, thus avoiding the puncture of vital structures (e.g., bowel and blood vessels).

C. **Embryo Transfer:** Ultrasound-assisted embryo transfer is appropriate in patients undergoing a "fresh" IVF cycle or following embryo cryopreservation or embryo/egg donation. If an abdominal ultrasound examination is performed, the bladder should be full to facilitate visualization of the endometrium and the transfer catheter.

Qualifications and Responsibilities of the Physician

Physicians who perform or supervise ultrasound-guided follicular aspiration or embryo transfer should be skilled in pelvic ultrasonography and appropriate placement of catheters and ultrasound-guided needle placement. They should understand the indications, limitations, and possible complications of the procedure. Physicians should have training, experience, and demonstrated competence in gynecologic ultrasonography and treatment procedures. Physicians are responsible for the documentation of the examination, quality control, and patient safety. Urgent or clinically important unexpected results should be communicated verbally to any referring and/or treating physician and this communication documented in the report.

ULTRASOUND EXAMINATION OF THE FEMALE PELVIS IN THE FIRST 10 WEEKS (EMBRYONIC PERIOD) OF PREGNANCY

Introduction

This portion of the guideline has been developed for use by practitioners performing sonographic studies only during the first 10 menstrual weeks of pregnancy. Such sonography should be performed only when there is a valid medical reason, and the lowest possible ultrasonic exposure settings should be used to gain the necessary diagnostic information. A limited examination may be performed in clinical emergencies or in specific clinical scenarios, such as evaluation of fetal or embryonic cardiac activity. A limited follow-up examination may be appropriate if a complete prior examination is on record. While this guideline describes the key elements of standard sonographic examinations in the first 10 weeks of pregnancy, in some cases, other specialized examinations may be necessary as well.

Specifications of the Examination

1. **Indications**

    A sonographic examination can be of benefit in many circumstances in the embryonic period of pregnancy, including but not limited to the following indications:

    a. To confirm the presence of an intrauterine pregnancy.

    b. To evaluate a suspected ectopic pregnancy.

    c. To define the cause of vaginal bleeding.

    d. To evaluate pelvic pain.

    e. To date the pregnancy.

    f. To diagnose or evaluate multiple gestations.

    g. To confirm cardiac activity.

    h. To evaluate maternal pelvic masses and/or uterine abnormalities.

    i. To evaluate a suspected hydatidiform mole.

    Comment

    A limited examination may be performed to assess the presence of cardiac activity.

2. **Imaging Parameters**

    Overall Comment

    Scanning in the first 10 weeks of pregnancy may be performed either transabdominally or transvaginally, although transvaginal scanning is preferred. Patients should be questioned about latex allergy prior to use of a latex sheath.

    a. The uterus, including the cervix, and adnexa should be evaluated for the presence of a gestational sac. If a gestational sac is seen, its location should be documented. The gestational sac should be evaluated for the presence or absence of a yolk sac or embryo, and the embryonic size should be measured and recorded, when possible.

    Comment

    Embryonic size is a more accurate indicator of gestational (menstrual) age than is mean gestational sac diameter. However, the mean gestational sac diameter may be measured and recorded when an embryo is not identified. Caution should be used in making the presumptive diagnosis of a gestational sac in the absence of a definite embryo or yolk sac. Without these findings, an intrauterine fluid collection could represent a pseudo–gestational sac associated with an ectopic pregnancy.

    b. Presence or absence of cardiac activity should be reported.

    Comment

    With transvaginal scans, cardiac motion is usually observed when the embryo is 5 mm or greater in length. If an embryo less than 5 mm in length is seen without cardiac activity, a subsequent scan at a later time may be needed to document cardiac activity. If possible, the M-mode function of the scanner should be used to document cardiac activity.

    c. Embryonic number should be reported.

    Comment

    Amnionicity and chorionicity should be documented for all multiple pregnancies when possible.

    d. Evaluation of the uterus, adnexal structures, and cul-de-sac should be performed.

    Comment

    The presence, location, and size of adnexal masses should be recorded. The presence of leiomyomata should be recorded, and measurements of the largest or any potentially clinically significant leiomyomata should be recorded. The cul-de-sac should be scanned for the presence or absence of fluid.

3. **Equipment Specifications**

   These studies should be conducted with real-time scanners, using a transabdominal and/or a Transvaginal approach. A transducer of appropriate frequency should be used.

   Comment

   Real-time sonography is necessary to confirm the presence of cardiac activity. A transvaginal scanning approach is preferred for this indication.

4. **Fetal Safety**

   Diagnostic ultrasound studies of the fetus are generally considered to be safe during pregnancy. This diagnostic procedure should be performed only when there is a valid medical indication, and the lowest possible ultrasonic exposure setting should be used to gain the necessary diagnostic information under the as low as reasonably achievable (ALARA) principle.

   The promotion, selling, or leasing of ultrasound equipment for making "keepsake fetal videos" is considered by the US Food and Drug Administration (FDA) to be an unapproved use of a medical device. Use of a diagnostic ultrasound system for these purposes, without a physician's order, may be in violation of state laws or regulations.

SONOHYSTEROGRAPHY IN REPRODUCTIVE MEDICINE AND INFERTILITY

Introduction

This portion of the guideline has been developed to provide assistance to qualified physicians performing sonohysterography. Properly performed sonohysterography can provide information about the uterus and the endometrium. Additional studies may be necessary for complete diagnosis. However, adherence to the following standard will maximize the diagnostic benefit of sonohysterography.

Definition

Sonohysterography consists of sonographic imaging of the uterus and uterocervical cavity, using real-time sonography during injection of sterile fluid (saline or water) into the uterine cavity.

Goal

The goal of sonohysterography is to visualize the endometrial cavity in more detail than is possible with routine transvaginal sonography.

Indications and Contraindications

The most common indication for sonohysterography is abnormal uterine bleeding in both premenopausal and postmenopausal women. Other indications include but are not limited to:

A. Indications

1. Infertility and habitual abortion.
2. Congenital abnormalities and/or anatomic variants of the uterine cavity.
3. Preoperative and postoperative evaluation of the uterine cavity, especially with regard to uterine myomas, polyps, and cysts.
4. Suspected uterine cavity synechiae.
5. Further evaluation of suspected abnormalities seen on transvaginal sonography, including focal or diffuse endometrial thickening or debris.
6. Inadequate imaging of the endometrium by transvaginal sonography.
7. Screening evaluation of the uterine cavity prior to fertility treatment(s) using assisted reproductive technologies.

B. Contraindications

Sonohysterography should not be performed in a woman who is pregnant or who could be pregnant. This is usually avoided by scheduling the examination in the follicular phase of the menstrual cycle, after menstrual flow has essentially ceased, but before the patient has ovulated. In a patient with regular cycles, sonohysterography should not in most cases be performed later than the 10th day of the menstrual cycle. Sonohysterography should not be performed in patients with a pelvic infection or unexplained pelvic tenderness, which may be due to chronic pelvic inflammatory disease. Pelvic organ tenderness should be assessed during the preliminary transvaginal sonogram. Active vaginal bleeding is not a contraindication to the procedure but may make the interpretation more challenging.

Qualifications and Responsibilities of the Physician

Physicians who perform or supervise diagnostic sonohysterography should be skilled in pelvic ultrasonography and appropriate placement of catheters. They should understand the indications, limitations, and possible complications of the procedure. Physicians should have training, experience, and demonstrated competence in gynecologic ultrasonography and sonohysterography. Physicians are responsible for the documentation of the examination, quality control, and patient safety. Urgent or clinically important unexpected results should be communicated verbally to any referring and/or treating physician and this communication documented in the report.

Specifications of the Examination

A. Patient Preparation

The referring physician may elect to prescribe prophylactic antibiotics if patients routinely take these for other invasive procedures. If painful, dilated, and/or obstructed fallopian tubes are found prior to fluid infusion, and the patient is not taking prophylactic antibiotics, the examination should be delayed until treatment can be administered. In the presence of nontender hydrosalpinges, consideration may be given to administering antibiotics at the time of the examination. A pregnancy test is advised when clinically indicated. Patients should be questioned about latex allergy prior to use of a latex sheath.

B. Procedure

Preliminary routine transvaginal sonography with measurements of the endometrium and evaluation of the uterus and the ovaries should be performed prior to sonohysterography. A speculum is used to allow visualization of the cervix. The presence of unusual pain, lesions, or purulent vaginal or cervical discharge may require rescheduling the procedure pending further evaluation. After cleansing the external os, the cervical canal and/or uterine cavity should be catheterized using aseptic technique, and appropriate sterile fluid should be instilled slowly by means of manual injection under real-time sonographic imaging. Imaging should include real-time scanning of the endometrial and cervical canals.

For infertility patients, tubal patency may be determined during sonohysterography by using the following methods: During the preliminary sonogram, the posterior cul-de-sac and pelvis should be evaluated for the presence of free fluid. If none is present before injection of fluid and it is present after fluid injection, then one can state that at least 1 tube is patent. Additionally, contrast material or a small amount of air injected with the fluid may be used with concurrent real-time sonographic imaging of the cornua, adnexae, and cul-de-sac to assess tubal patency. This can facilitate assessing patency of each fallopian tube.

C. Distension Media

Appropriate sterile fluid such as normal saline or water should be used for sonohysterography.

D. Images

Appropriate images, in at least 2 planes, using a high-frequency transvaginal ultrasound probe, should be produced and recorded to demonstrate normal and abnormal findings. Precatheterization images should be obtained, including the thickest bilayer endometrial measurement on a sagittal image.

Once the uterine cavity is filled with fluid, representative images with a complete survey of the uterine cavity are obtained as necessary for diagnostic evaluation. If a balloon catheter is used for the examination, images should be obtained at the end of the procedure with the balloon deflated to fully evaluate the endometrial cavity and particularly the cervical canal and the lower uterine segment.

E. Equipment Specifications

Sonohysterography is usually conducted with a transvaginal transducer. In cases of an enlarged uterus, additional transabdominal images during infusion may be required to fully evaluate the endometrium. The transducer should be adjusted to operate at the highest clinically appropriate frequency under the ALARA principle.

TRAINING GUIDELINES FOR PHYSICIANS WHO EVALUATE AND INTERPRET DIAGNOSTIC ULTRASOUND EXAMINATIONS

Adapted from the AIUM Official Statement *Training Guidelines for Physicians Who Evaluate and Interpret Diagnostic Ultrasound Examinations*, ©2008 by the American Institute of Ultrasound in Medicine.

Physicians who evaluate and interpret diagnostic ultrasound examinations should be licensed medical practitioners who have a thorough understanding of the indication[s] and guidelines for ultrasound examinations as well as familiarity with the basic physical principles and limitations of the technology of ultrasound imaging. They should be familiar with alternative and complementary imaging and diagnostic procedures and should be capable of correlating the results of these other procedures with the ultrasound examination findings. They should have an understanding of ultrasound technology and instrumentation, ultrasound power output, equipment calibration, and safety. Physicians responsible for ultrasound examinations should be able to demonstrate familiarity with the anatomy, physiology, and pathophysiology of those organs or anatomic areas that are being examined. These physicians should provide evidence of training and requisite competence needed to successfully perform and interpret diagnostic ultrasound examinations in the area(s) they practice. The training should include methods of documentation and reporting of ultrasound studies. Physicians performing diagnostic ultrasound examinations should meet at least one of the following:

1. Completion of an approved residency program, fellowship, or postgraduate training that includes the equivalent of at least 3 months of diagnostic ultrasound training in the area(s) they practice under the supervision of a qualified physician(s),* during which the trainees will have evidence of being involved with the performance, evaluation, and interpretation of at least 300** sonograms.

2. In the absence of formal fellowship or postgraduate training or residency training, documentation of clinical experience could be acceptable providing the following could be demonstrated:

   a. Evidence of 100 *AMA PRA Category 1 Credits*™ dedicated to diagnostic ultrasound in the area(s) they practice, and

   b. Evidence of being involved with the performance, evaluation, and interpretation of the images of at least 300** sonograms within a 3-year period. It is expected that in most circumstances, examinations will be under the supervision of a qualified physician(s).* These sonograms should be in the area(s) they are practicing.

Cases presented as preselected, limited image sets, such as in lectures, case conferences, and teaching files, are excluded. The ability to analyze a full image set, determining its completeness and the adequacy of image quality, and performing the diagnostic process, distinguishing normal from abnormal, is considered a primary goal of the training experience.

GUIDELINES FOR CLEANING AND PREPARING ENDOCAVITARY ULTRASOUND TRANSDUCERS BETWEEN PATIENTS

Adapted from the AIUM Official Statement *Guidelines for Cleaning and Preparing Endocavitary Ultrasound Transducers Between Patients*, ©2003 by the American Institute of Ultrasound in Medicine.

The purpose of this document is to provide guidance regarding the cleaning and disinfection of transvaginal ultrasound probes.

All sterilization/disinfection represents a statistical reduction in the number of microbes present on a surface. Meticulous cleaning of the instrument is the essential key to an initial reduction of the microbial/organic load by at least 99%. This cleaning is followed by a disinfecting procedure to ensure a high degree of protection from infectious disease transmission, even if a disposable barrier covers the instrument during use.

Medical instruments fall into different categories with respect to potential for infection transmission. The most critical level of instruments is that which is intended to penetrate skin or mucous membranes. These require sterilization. Less critical instruments (often called "semicritical" instruments) that simply come into contact with mucous membranes such as fiber-optic endoscopes require high-level disinfection rather than sterilization.

Although endocavitary ultrasound probes might be considered even less critical instruments because they are routinely protected by single-use disposable probe

---

*A qualified physician is one who, at minimum, meets the criteria defined above in this document.

**Three hundred cases were selected as a minimum number needed to gain experience and proficiency with ultrasonography as a diagnostic modality. This is necessary to develop technical skills, to appreciate the practical applications of basic physics as it affects image quality and artifact formation, and to acquire an experience base for understanding the range of normal and recognizing deviations from normal.

covers, leakage rates of 0.9% to 2% for condoms and 8% to 81% for commercial probe covers have been observed in recent studies. For maximum safety, one should therefore perform high-level disinfection of the probe between each use and use a probe cover or condom as an aid to keeping the probe clean.

There are 4 generally recognized categories of disinfection and sterilization. Sterilization is the complete elimination of all forms or microbial life, including spores and viruses. Disinfection, the selective removal of microbial life, is divided into 3 classes:

- High-Level Disinfection: Destruction/removal of all microorganisms except bacterial spores.
- Mid-Level Disinfection: Inactivation of *Mycobacterium tuberculosis*, bacteria, most viruses, and most fungi and some bacterial spores.
- Low-Level Disinfection: Destruction of most bacteria, some viruses, and some fungi. Low-level disinfection will not necessarily inactivate *M. tuberculosis* or bacterial spores.

The following specific recommendations are made for the use of endocavitary ultrasound transducers. Users should also review the Centers for Disease Control and Prevention (CDC) document on sterilization and disinfection of medical devices to be certain that their procedures conform to the CDC principles for disinfection of patient care equipment.

1. **Cleaning:** After removal of the probe cover, use running water to remove any residual gel or debris from the probe. Use a damp gauze pad or other soft cloth and a small amount of mild nonabrasive liquid soap (household dishwashing liquid is ideal) to thoroughly cleanse the transducer. Consider the use of a small brush especially for crevices and areas of angulation depending on the design of your particular transducer. Rinse the transducer thoroughly with running water, and then dry the transducer with a soft cloth or paper towel.

2. **Disinfection:** Cleaning with a detergent/water solution as described above is important as the first step in proper disinfection since chemical disinfectants act more rapidly on clean surfaces. However, the additional use of a high-level liquid disinfectant will ensure further statistical reduction in the microbial load. Because of the potential disruption of the barrier sheath, additional high-level disinfection with chemical agents is necessary.

Examples of such high-level disinfectants include but are not limited to

a. 2.4% to 3.2% glutaraldehyde products (a variety of available proprietary products, including Cidex, Metricide, and Procide).

b. Non-glutaraldehyde agents, including Cidex OPA (*o*-phthalaldehyde) and Cidex PA (hydrogen peroxide and peroxyacetic acid).

c. 7.5% hydrogen peroxide solution.

d. Common household bleach (5.25% sodium hypochlorite) diluted to yield 500 parts per million chlorine (10 cc in 1 L of tap water). This agent is effective but generally not recommended by probe manufacturers because it can damage metal and plastic parts.

Other agents such as quaternary ammonium compounds are not considered high-level disinfectants and should not be used. Isopropanol is not a high-level disinfectant when used as a wipe, and probe manufacturers generally do not recommend soaking probes in the liquid.

The FDA has published a list of approved sterilants and high-level disinfectants for reprocessing reusable medical and dental devices. That list can be consulted to identify agents that may be useful for probe disinfection.

Practitioners should consult the labels of proprietary products for specific instructions. They should also consult instrument manufacturers regarding compatibility of these agents with probes. Many of the chemical disinfectants are potentially toxic, and many require adequate precautions such as proper ventilation, personal protective devices (gloves, face/eye protection, etc) and thorough rinsing before reuse of the probe.

3. **Probe Covers:** The transducer should be covered with a barrier. If the barriers used are condoms, these should be nonlubricated and nonmedicated. Practitioners should be aware that condoms have been shown to be less prone to leakage than commercial probe covers and have a 6-fold enhanced acceptable quality level (AQL) when compared to standard examination gloves. They have an AQL equal to that of surgical gloves. Users should be aware of latex sensitivity issues and have available non–latex-containing barriers.

4. **Aseptic Technique:** For the protection of the patient and the health care worker, all endocavitary examinations should be performed with the operator properly gloved throughout the procedure. Gloves should be used to remove the condom or other barrier from the transducer and to wash the transducer as outlined above. As the barrier (condom) is removed, care should be taken not to contaminate the probe with secretions from the patient. At the completion of the procedure, hands should be thoroughly washed with soap and water.

   Note: An obvious disruption in condom integrity does not require modification of this protocol. These guidelines take into account possible probe contamination due to a disruption in the barrier sheath.

In summary, routine high-level disinfection of the endocavitary probe between patients plus the use of a probe cover or condom during each examination is required to properly protect patients from infection during endocavitary examinations. For all chemical disinfectants, precautions must be taken to protect workers and patients from the toxicity of the disinfectant.

AIUM PRACTICE GUIDELINE FOR THE PERFORMANCE OF A FOCUSED REPRODUCTIVE ENDOCRINOLOGY AND INFERTILITY SCAN

Guideline developed in conjunction the American College of Nurse-Midwives (ACNM), the American College of Obstetricians and Gynecologists (ACOG), the American College of Osteopathic Obstetricians and Gynecologists (ACOOG), the American Society for Reproductive Medicine–Society for Reproductive Endocrinology and Infertility (ASRM-SREI), and the Association of Women's Health, Obstetric and Neonatal Nurses (AWHONN).

I. INTRODUCTION

The clinical aspects contained in specific sections of this guideline (Introduction, Indications, Specifications of the Examination, and Equipment Specifications) were developed collaboratively by the American Institute of Ultrasound in Medicine (AIUM), the American College of Nurse-Midwives (ACNM), the American College of Obstetricians and Gynecologists (ACOG), the American College of Osteopathic Obstetricians and Gynecologists (ACOOG), the American Society for Reproductive Medicine–Society for Reproductive Endocrinology and Infertility (ASRM-SREI), and the Association of Women's Health, Obstetric and Neonatal Nurses (AWHONN). Recommendations for practitioner requirements, written request for the examination, procedure documentation, and quality control vary among the organizations and are addressed by each separately.

This guideline has been developed to provide assistance to practitioners performing focused ultrasound studies of the female pelvis in the practice of reproductive medicine and infertility. In some cases, additional and/or specialized examinations may be necessary. While it is not possible to detect every abnormality, adherence to the following will maximize the probability of detecting most of the abnormalities that occur.

II. INDICATIONS

Indications for an ultrasound examination for a focused reproductive endocrinology and infertility scan include, but are not limited to, monitoring of ovulation induction and ovarian stimulation.

III. QUALIFICATIONS AND RESPONSIBILITIES OF THE PHYSICIAN

See www.aium.org for AIUM Official Statements including *Standards and Guidelines for the Accreditation of Ultrasound Practices* and relevant Physician Training Guidelines.

IV. WRITTEN REQUEST FOR THE EXAMINATION

The written or electronic request for an ultrasound examination should provide sufficient information to allow for the appropriate performance and interpretation of the examination. When an ultrasound examination is performed within a practice as part of established patient care, the indication for the examination should be documented, but a formal request is not needed.

A request for an ultrasound examination must be originated by a physician or other appropriately licensed health care provider or under the provider's direction. The accompanying clinical information should be provided by a physician or other appropriate health care provider familiar with the patient's clinical situation and should be consistent with relevant legal and local health care facility requirements.

V. SPECIFICATIONS OF THE EXAMINATION

The following guidelines describe the examination to be performed for each organ and anatomic region in the female pelvis. Whenever possible, all relevant structures should be identified by the vaginal approach. When a transvaginal scan fails to image all areas needed for diagnosis, a transabdominal scan should be performed. In some cases, both a transabdominal and a transvaginal scan may be needed.

General Pelvic Preparation

For a pelvic ultrasound examination performed transabdominally, the patient's urinary bladder should, in general, be distended adequately to displace the small bowel and its contained gas from the field of view. Occasionally, overdistension of the bladder may compromise evaluation. When this occurs, imaging may be repeated after the patient partially empties her bladder.

For a transvaginal sonogram, the urinary bladder is preferably empty. The patient, the sonographer, or the practitioner may introduce the transvaginal transducer, preferably under real-time monitoring. Transvaginal sonography is a specialized form of a pelvic examination. Therefore, policies applied locally regarding chaperone or patient privacy issues during a pelvic examination should also be applied during a transvaginal ultrasound examination.

Focused Reproductive Endocrinology and Infertility Examination

A focused pelvic ultrasound examination is appropriate when monitoring ovarian stimulation (e.g., an ovarian folliculogram study or determining endometrial qualities before embryo transfer). A comprehensive examination should have previously been performed in the preceding 4 to 6 months to rule out other gynecologic pathology. The limited examination can be restricted to the organ or measurements of interest. In the case of an ovarian folliculogram, the following should be documented: ovarian follicle number in each ovary, endometrial thickness, and endometrial morphologic appearance. Endometrial thickness is measured from outside to outside in an anterior-posterior view at the widest point. In addition, follicular diameters in 2 dimensions for each follicle larger than 10 mm should be recorded. A single recorded value representing the mean of 2 diameter measurements performed at right angles is also acceptable. Permanent recorded images should be obtained and stored in accordance with local, state, and federal regulations. Pertinent clinical information should be recorded in the patient record.

VI. DOCUMENTATION

Adequate documentation is essential for high-quality patient care. A permanent record of the ultrasound examination and its interpretation should be kept by the facility performing the study. Images of all appropriate areas, both normal and abnormal, should be recorded. Variations from normal size should be accompanied by measurements. Images are to be appropriately labeled with the examination date, facility name, and, when appropriate, organ imaged. A report of the ultrasound findings should be included in the patient's medical record. Urgent or clinically important unexpected results should be communicated verbally to any referring and/or treating provider and this communication documented in the report. Retention of the permanent record of the ultrasound examination should be consistent both with clinical needs and with the relevant legal and local health care facility requirements.

VII. EQUIPMENT SPECIFICATIONS

Equipment

An ultrasound examination of the female pelvis should be conducted with a real-time scanner, with the appropriate transabdominal and transvaginal transducers. The transducer or scanner should be adjusted to operate at the highest clinically appropriate frequency, realizing that there is a trade-off between resolution and beam penetration. With modern equipment, studies performed from the anterior abdominal wall can usually use frequencies of 3.5 MHz or higher, while scans performed from the vagina should use frequencies of 5 MHz or higher.

Care of the Equipment

All probes should be cleaned after each patient examination. Transvaginal probes should be covered by a protective sheath before insertion. Patients should be questioned about a latex allergy before use of a latex sheath. After each examination, the sheath should be discarded, and the probe should be washed, dried, and appropriately disinfected (see "Guidelines for Cleaning and Preparing Endocavitary Ultrasound Transducers Between Patients"). The type of antimicrobial solution and the methods for disinfection depend on manufacturer and infectious disease recommendations.

VIII. QUALITY CONTROL AND IMPROVEMENT, SAFETY, INFECTION CONTROL, AND PATIENT EDUCATION

Policies and procedures related to quality control, patient education, infection control, and safety should be developed and implemented in accordance with the *AIUM Standards and Guidelines for the Accreditation of Ultrasound Practices*.

Equipment performance monitoring should be in accordance with the AIUM Standards and Guidelines for the Accreditation of Ultrasound Practices.

IX. ALARA PRINCIPLE

The potential benefits and risks of each examination should be considered. The ALARA (as low as reasonably achievable) principle should be observed when adjusting controls that affect the acoustic output and by considering transducer dwell times. Further details on ALARA may be found in the AIUM publication *Medical Ultrasound Safety*, Third Edition.

GUIDELINES FOR CLEANING AND PREPARING ENDOCAVITARY ULTRASOUND TRANSDUCERS BETWEEN PATIENTS

Previously published by the AIUM

The purpose of this document is to provide guidance regarding the cleaning and disinfection of transvaginal ultrasound probes.

All sterilization/disinfection represents a statistical reduction in the number of microbes present on a surface. Meticulous cleaning of the instrument is the essential key to an initial reduction of the microbial/organic load by at least 99%. This cleaning is followed by a disinfecting procedure to ensure a high degree of protection from infectious disease transmission, even if a disposable barrier covers the instrument during use.

Medical instruments fall into different categories with respect to potential for infection transmission. The most critical level of instruments is that which is intended to penetrate skin or mucous membranes. These require sterilization. Less critical instruments (often called "semicritical" instruments) that simply come into contact with mucous membranes such as fiber-optic endoscopes require high-level disinfection rather than sterilization.

Although endocavitary ultrasound probes might be considered even less critical instruments because they are routinely protected by single-use disposable probe covers, leakage rates of 0.9% to 2% for condoms and 8% to 81% for commercial probe covers have been observed in recent studies. For maximum safety, one should therefore perform high-level disinfection of the probe between each use and use a probe cover or condom as an aid to keeping the probe clean.

There are 4 generally recognized categories of disinfection and sterilization. Sterilization is the complete elimination of all forms or microbial life, including spores and viruses. Disinfection, the selective removal of microbial life, is divided into 3 classes:

- High-Level Disinfection—Destruction/removal of all microorganisms except bacterial spores.
- Mid-Level Disinfection—Inactivation of *Mycobacterium tuberculosis*, bacteria, most viruses, and most fungi and some bacterial spores.
- Low-Level Disinfection—Destruction of most bacteria, some viruses, and some fungi. Low-level disinfection will not necessarily inactivate *M. tuberculosis* or bacterial spores.

The following specific recommendations are made for the use of endocavitary ultrasound transducers. Users should also review the Centers for Disease Control and Prevention document on sterilization and disinfection of medical devices to be certain that their procedures conform to the Centers for Disease Control and Prevention principles for disinfection of patient care equipment.

1. **Cleaning:** After removal of the probe cover, use running water to remove any residual gel or debris from the probe. Use a damp gauze pad or other soft cloth and a small amount of mild nonabrasive liquid soap (household dishwashing liquid is ideal) to thoroughly cleanse the transducer. Consider the use of a small brush especially for crevices and areas of angulation depending on the design of your particular transducer. Rinse the transducer thoroughly with running water, and then dry the transducer with a soft cloth or paper towel.

2. **Disinfection:** Cleaning with a detergent/water solution as described above is important as the first step in proper disinfection because chemical disinfectants act more rapidly on clean surfaces. However, the additional use of a high-level liquid

disinfectant will ensure further statistical reduction in the microbial load. Because of the potential disruption of the barrier sheath, additional high-level disinfection with chemical agents is necessary. Examples of such high-level disinfectants include but are not limited to:

a. 2.4% to 3.2% glutaraldehyde products (a variety of available proprietary products, including Cidex, Metricide, and Procide);

b. Nonglutaraldehyde agents, including Cidex OPA (o-phthalaldehyde) and Cidex PA (hydrogen peroxide and peroxyacetic acid);

c. 7.5% hydrogen peroxide solution; and

d. Common household bleach (5.25% sodium hypochlorite) diluted to yield 500 parts per million chlorine (10 mL in 1 L of tap water). This agent is effective but generally not recommended by probe manufacturers because it can damage metal and plastic parts.

Other agents such as quaternary ammonium compounds are not considered high-level disinfectants and should not be used. Isopropanol is not a high-level disinfectant when used as a wipe, and probe manufacturers generally do not recommend soaking probes in the liquid.

The US Food and Drug Administration has published a list of approved sterilants and high-level disinfectants for reprocessing reusable medical and dental devices. That list can be consulted to identify agents that may be useful for probe disinfection.

Practitioners should consult the labels of proprietary products for specific instructions. They should also consult instrument manufacturers regarding compatibility of these agents with probes. Many of the chemical disinfectants are potentially toxic, and many require adequate precautions such as proper ventilation, personal protective devices (e.g., gloves and face/eye protection) and thorough rinsing before reuse of the probe.

3. **Probe Covers:** The transducer should be covered with a barrier. If the barriers used are condoms, these should be nonlubricated and nonmedicated. Practitioners should be aware that condoms have been shown to be less prone to leakage than commercial probe covers and have a 6-fold enhanced acceptable quality level when compared to standard examination gloves. They have an acceptable quality level equal to that of surgical gloves. Users should be aware of latex sensitivity issues and have non–latex-containing barriers available.

4. **Aseptic Technique:** For the protection of the patient and the health care worker, all endocavitary examinations should be performed with the operator properly gloved throughout the procedure. Gloves should be used to remove the condom or other barrier from the transducer and to wash the transducer as outlined above. As the barrier (condom) is removed, care should be taken not to contaminate the probe with secretions from the patient. At the completion of the procedure, hands should be thoroughly washed with soap and water.

Note: Obvious disruption in condom integrity does not require modification of this protocol. These guidelines take into account possible probe contamination due to a disruption in the barrier sheath.

In summary, routine high-level disinfection of the endocavitary probe between patients, plus the use of a probe cover or condom during each examination, is required to properly protect patients from infection during endocavitary examinations. For all chemical disinfectants, precautions must be taken to protect workers and patients from the toxicity of the disinfectant.

AIUM PRACTICE GUIDELINE FOR THE PERFORMANCE OF FETAL ECHOCARDIOGRAPHY

Guideline developed in conjunction with the American College of Obstetricians and Gynecologists (ACOG), the Society for Maternal-Fetal Medicine (SMFM), and the American Society of Echocardiography (ASE), and endorsed by the American College of Radiology (ACR).

I. INTRODUCTION

Congenital heart disease is a leading cause of infant morbidity and mortality from birth defects with an estimated incidence of 6 per 1000 live births for moderate to severe forms. Accurate prenatal diagnosis offers potential clinical benefit with regard to infant outcome, especially in those cases that are likely to require prostaglandin infusion to maintain patency of the ductus arteriosus. Fetal echocardiography is broadly defined as a detailed sonographic evaluation that is used to identify and characterize fetal heart anomalies before delivery. This specialized diagnostic procedure is an extension of the "basic" and "extended basic" fetal cardiac screening guidelines that have been previously described for the 4-chamber view and outflow tracts. It should be performed only when there is a valid medical reason, and the lowest possible ultrasonic exposure settings should be used to gain the necessary diagnostic information. While it is not possible to detect every abnormality, adherence to the following guideline will maximize the probability of detecting most cases of clinically significant congenital heart disease.

II. QUALIFICATIONS AND RESPONSIBILITIES OF PERSONNEL

Performance and interpretation of fetal echocardiography require a unique set of advanced skills and knowledge. Specific training requirements and maintenance of competency guidelines have been developed by the AIUM as well as the ASE in conjunction with the American Heart Association, the American College of Cardiology, and the American Academy of Pediatrics. Appropriately trained obstetricians, maternal-fetal medicine specialists, pediatric cardiologists, and radiologists with special expertise in fetal imaging who have acquired the appropriate knowledge base and skills as outlined in these statements may perform fetal echocardiography.

III. INDICATIONS

Indications for fetal echocardiography are often based on a variety of parental and fetal risk factors for congenital heart disease. However, most cases are not associated with known risk factors. Common indications for a detailed scan of the fetal heart include but are not limited to the following:

A. Maternal Indications
- Autoimmune antibodies, anti-Ro (SSA)/anti-La (SSB);
- Familial inherited disorders (e.g., 22q11.2 deletion syndrome);
- In vitro fertilization;
- Metabolic disease (e.g., diabetes mellitus and phenylketonuria); and
- Teratogen exposure (e.g., retinoids and lithium).

B. Fetal Indications
- Abnormal cardiac screening examination;
- First-degree relative of a fetus with congenital heart disease;
- Abnormal heart rate or rhythm;
- Fetal chromosomal anomaly;
- Extracardiac anomaly;
- Hydrops;
- Increased nuchal translucency; and
- Monochorionic twins.

IV. WRITTEN REQUEST FOR THE EXAMINATION

The written or electronic request for an ultrasound examination should provide sufficient information to allow for the appropriate performance and interpretation of the examination.

A request for the examination must be originated by a physician or other appropriately licensed health care provider or under the provider's direction. The accompanying clinical information should be provided by a physician or other appropriate health care provider familiar with the patient's clinical situation and should be consistent with relevant legal and local health care facility requirements.

V. SPECIFICATIONS OF THE EXAMINATION

The following section describes required and optional elements for fetal echocardiography.

A. General Considerations

Fetal echocardiography is commonly performed between 18 and 22 weeks' gestational age. Some forms of congenital heart disease may even be recognized during earlier stages of pregnancy. Optimal views of the heart are usually obtained when the cardiac apex is directed toward the anterior maternal wall. Technical limitations (e.g., maternal obesity, prone fetal position, and late gestation) can make a detailed heart evaluation very difficult due to acoustic shadowing, especially during the third trimester. It may be necessary to examine the patient at a different time if the heart is poorly visualized. The examiner can optimize sonograms by appropriate adjustment of technical settings, such as acoustic focus, frequency selection, signal gain, image magnification, temporal resolution, harmonic imaging, and Doppler-related parameters (e.g., velocity scale, frequency wall filter, and frame rate). Because the heart is a dynamic structure, a complete evaluation can only be made if real-time imaging with acquisition of analog recordings or digital video clips is used as a standard part of every fetal echocardiogram.

B. Cardiac Imaging Parameters: Basic Approach

The fetal echocardiogram is a detailed evaluation of cardiac structure and function. This method typically involves a sequential segmental analysis of 3 basic areas that include the atria, ventricles, and great arteries and their connections. A segmental analysis includes an initial assessment of fetal right/left orientation, followed by an assessment of the following segments and their relationships:

- Visceral/abdominal situs:
  - Stomach position; and
  - Cardiac apex position;
- Atria:
  - Situs;
  - Systemic and pulmonary venous connections;
  - Venous anatomy; and
  - Atrial anatomy (including septum);
- Ventricles:
  - Position;
  - Atrial connections;
  - Ventricular anatomy (including septum);
  - Relative and absolute size;
  - Function; and
  - Pericardium; and
- Great arteries (aorta, main and branch pulmonary arteries, and ductus arteriosus):
  - Position relative to the trachea;
  - Ventricular connections; and
  - Vessel size, patency, and flow (both velocity and direction).

In addition to a segmental analysis, the following connections should be evaluated:

- Atrioventricular junction: anatomy, size, and function of atrioventricular (e.g., mitral and tricuspid) valves; and
- Ventriculoarterial junction: anatomy, size, and function of semilunar (e.g., aortic and pulmonary) valves, including assessment of both the subpulmonary and subaortic regions.

C. Grayscale Imaging (Required)

Key scanning planes can provide useful diagnostic information about the fetal heart (Figures 3–5). Evaluation should include the following criteria, noting abnormalities of the heart and pericardium:

- Four-chamber view;
- Left ventricular outflow tract;
- Right ventricular outflow tract;
- Three-vessel and trachea view;
- Short-axis views ("low" for ventricles, "high" for outflow tracts);
- Long-axis view;
- Aortic arch view;
- Ductal arch view; and
- Superior and inferior vena cava views.

D. Color Doppler Sonography (Required)

Color Doppler sonography should be used to evaluate the following structures for potential flow disturbances:

- Systemic veins (including superior and inferior venae cavae and ductus venosus);
- Pulmonary veins;
- Foramen ovale;
- Atrioventricular valves;
- Atrial and ventricular septa;
- Semilunar valves;
- Ductal arch;
- Aortic arch; and
- Umbilical vein and artery (optional).

In addition, pulsed Doppler sonography should be used as an adjunct to evaluate the following:

- Atrioventricular valves;
- Semilunar valves;
- Ductus venosus;
- Umbilical vein and artery (optional);
- Cardiac rhythm disturbance; and
- Any structure in which an abnormality on color Doppler sonography is noted.

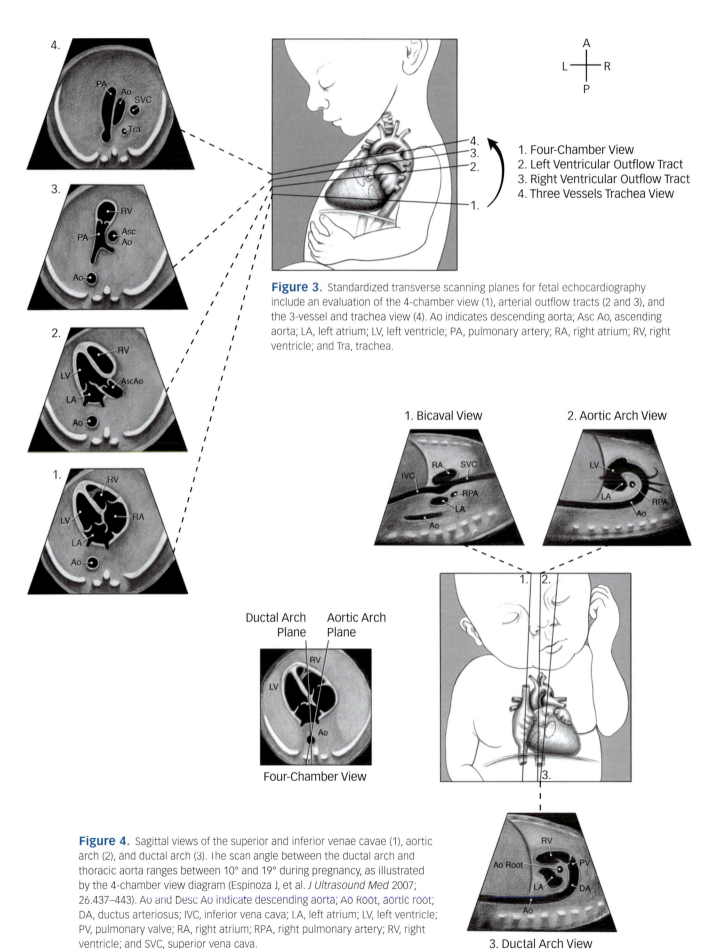

Figure 3. Standardized transverse scanning planes for fetal echocardiography include an evaluation of the 4-chamber view (1), arterial outflow tracts (2 and 3), and the 3-vessel and trachea view (4). Ao indicates descending aorta; Asc Ao, ascending aorta; LA, left atrium; LV, left ventricle; PA, pulmonary artery; RA, right atrium; RV, right ventricle; and Tra, trachea.

Figure 4. Sagittal views of the superior and inferior venae cavae (1), aortic arch (2), and ductal arch (3). The scan angle between the ductal arch and thoracic aorta ranges between 10° and 19° during pregnancy, as illustrated by the 4-chamber view diagram (Espinoza J, et al. *J Ultrasound Med* 2007; 26.437–443). Ao and Desc Ao indicate descending aorta; Ao Root, aortic root; DA, ductus arteriosus; IVC, inferior vena cava; LA, left atrium; LV, left ventricle; PV, pulmonary valve; RA, right atrium; RPA, right pulmonary artery; RV, right ventricle; and SVC, superior vena cava.

E. Heart Rate and Rhythm Assessment

Documentation of the heart rate and rhythm should be made by cardiac cycle length measurements obtained by the Doppler technique or M-mode interrogation. A normal fetal heart rate at mid-gestation is 120 to 180 beats per minute. If bradycardia or tachycardia is documented, or if the rhythm is noted to be irregular, simultaneous assessment of atrial and ventricular contraction should be performed using either simultaneous Doppler sonography of the mitral inflow–aortic outflow or superior vena cava–ascending aorta or by M-mode sonography of the atrium and ventricle to determine the underlying mechanism. An alternative approach using tissue Doppler sonography of the atrium and ventricle has also been described.

F. Cardiac Biometry

(Optional But Should Be Considered for Suspected Structural or Functional Anomalies)

Normal ranges for fetal cardiac measurements have been published as percentiles and z scores that are based on gestational age or fetal biometry. Individual measurements can be determined from 2-dimensional images or M-mode images in some situations and may include the following parameters:

- Aortic and pulmonary valve annulus in systole and tricuspid and mitral valve annulus in diastole (absolute size with comparison of left- to right-sided valves; left-sided valves measure equal or slightly smaller than right-sided valves);
- Right and left ventricular length (should measure equal);
- Aortic arch and isthmus diameter measurements;
- Main pulmonary artery and ductus arteriosus measurements;
- End-diastolic ventricular diameter just inferior to the atrioventricular valve leaflets;
- Thickness of the ventricular free walls and interventricular septum just inferior to the atrioventricular valves;
- Cardiothoracic ratio; and
- Additional measurements if warranted, including:
  ▸ Systolic dimensions of the ventricles;
  ▸ Transverse dimensions of the atria; and
  ▸ Diameters of branch pulmonary arteries.

G. Cardiac Function Assessment

(Optional But Should Be Considered for Suspected Structural or Functional Cardiac Anomalies)

Right and left heart function should be qualitatively assessed in all studies. Signs of cardiomegaly, atrioventricular valve regurgitation, and hydrops fetalis should be noted. If abnormal ventricular function is suspected, quantitative assessment of heart function should be considered and can include measures such as fractional shortening, ventricular strain, and the myocardial performance index.

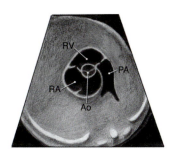

1. High Short-Axis View: Great Arteries

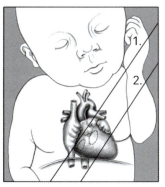

Fetal Heart: Coronal View

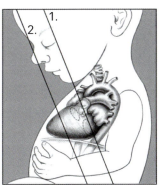

Fetal Heart: Sagittal View

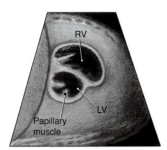

2. Low Short-Axis View: Ventricles

Figure 5. Low and high short-axis views of the fetal heart. Ao indicates aortic valve; LV, left ventricle; PA, pulmonary artery; RA, right atrium; and RV, right ventricle.

H. Complementary Imaging Strategies (Optional)

Other adjunctive imaging modalities, such as 3- and 4-dimensional sonography, have been used to evaluate anatomic defects and to quantify fetal hemodynamic parameters, such as cardiac output. Adjunctive Doppler modalities that have been used include tissue and continuous wave Doppler.

VI. REPORTING AND DOCUMENTATION

Adequate documentation is essential for high-quality patient care. There should be a permanent record of the fetal echocardiographic examination and its interpretation. Motion video clips, in conjunction with still images, are an essential part of the documentation of a fetal echocardiogram. Motion analog recordings or digital video clips, in conjunction with still images, are an essential part of the documentation of a fetal echocardiogram. Digital video clips should include at least the 4-chamber view, left and right ventricular outflow tracts, 3-vessel and trachea view, and sagittal aortic and ductal arches using both real-time grayscale and color Doppler techniques. Variations from normal size should be accompanied by measurements. Images should be labeled with the patient identification, facility identification, examination date, and side (right or left) of the anatomic site imaged. An official interpretation (final report) of the diagnostic findings should be included in the patient's medical record. Retention of the sonographic examination should be consistent both with clinical need and with relevant legal and local health care facility requirements. Reporting should be in accordance with recognized practice guidelines for documentation and communication of diagnostic ultrasound findings.

VII. EQUIPMENT SPECIFICATIONS

A sonographic examination of the fetal heart should be conducted using a real-time scanner. Sector, curvilinear, and endovaginal transducers are used for this purpose. The transducer or scanner should be adjusted to operate at the highest clinically appropriate frequency, realizing that there is a trade-off between resolution and beam penetration. With modern equipment, fetal imaging studies performed from the anterior abdominal wall can usually use frequencies of 5.0 MHz or higher, whereas scans performed from the vagina should be performed using frequencies of 7 MHz or higher. Acoustic shadowing and maternal body habitus may limit the ability of higher-frequency transducers from providing greater anatomic detail for the fetal heart.

VIII. QUALITY CONTROL AND IMPROVEMENT, SAFETY, INFECTION CONTROL, AND PATIENT EDUCATION

Policies and procedures related to quality control, patient education, infection control, and safety should be developed and implemented in accordance with the AIUM *Standards and Guidelines for the Accreditation of Ultrasound Practices*. The potential benefits and risks of each examination should be considered. The ALARA (as low as reasonably achievable) principle should be observed when adjusting controls that affect the acoustic output and by considering transducer dwell times. Further details on ALARA may be found in the AIUM publication *Medical Ultrasound Safety*, Third Edition. Equipment performance monitoring should be in accordance with the AIUM *Standards and Guidelines for the Accreditation of Ultrasound Practices*.

APPENDIX D

Application for CME Credit

OB/GYN SONOGRAPHY: AN ILLUSTRATED REVIEW
2nd Edition

Introduction

Who May Apply for CME Credit

Objectives of This Activity

How to Obtain CME Credit

Applicant Information

Evaluate This CME Activity—You Grade Us!

Answer Sheet

CME Quiz

INTRODUCTION

Ob/Gyn Sonography: An Illustrated Review, 2nd Edition is a continuing medical educational (CME) activity approved for 15 hours of credit by the Society of Diagnostic Medical Sonography and may be used by more than one person (see *Note* on page 523).

WHO MAY APPLY FOR CME CREDIT

This credit may be applied as follows:

- Sonographers and technologists may apply these hours toward the CME requirements of the ARDMS and ARRT, as well as to the CME requirements of most facility-accrediting organizations. CCI also accepts SDMS-approved CME credits but stipulates that 30 of the triennial requirement of 36 CME credits be related to the cardiovasculature; the remaining 6 CME credits can be related to any topic.

- SDMS-approved credit is not applicable toward the AMA Physician's Recognition Award but may be applicable to the CME requirements for physicians associated with accredited ultrasound facilities. Be sure to confirm requirements with the pertinent organizations.

If you have any questions whatsoever about CME requirements that affect you, please contact the responsible organization directly for current information. CME requirements can and sometimes do change.

OBJECTIVES OF THIS ACTIVITY

Upon completion of this educational activity, you will be able to:

1. Describe and identify normal and abnormal fetal and female pelvic anatomy and physiology.
2. Describe how, when, and why ultrasonography is applied in the practice of obstetrics and gynecology.
3. Differentiate normal from abnormal obstetric and gynecologic sonographic findings and explain the correlations between these findings and pertinent laboratory and imaging studies.
4. Describe how, when, and why fetal and gynecologic measurements are made.
5. Explain the role of medical genetics in the practice of obstetrics and gynecology.
6. Describe the diseases, complications, and coexisting disorders of the female reproductive system, pregnancy, and antepartum and postpartum fetus.
7. Explain how to prepare for and perform the techniques of sonographic examination in the practice of obstetrics and gynecology.

HOW TO OBTAIN CME CREDIT

To apply for credit, please do all of the following:

1. Read and study the book and complete the interactive exercises it contains.
2. Make copies of the applicant information page, evaluation questionnaire (you grade us!), and answer sheet.
3. Complete these forms, make copies for your records, and send the completed forms together with payment (paper check or full credit card information) to the following address:

   Davies Publishing, Inc.
   Attn: CME Coordinator
   32 South Raymond Avenue, Suite 4
   Pasadena, California 91105-1961

   You may also fax us the applicable pages and pay by credit card. Our fax number is 626-792-5308. You may call us with your credit card, expiration date, and 3- or 4-digit security code or include it with the fax. We grade quizzes within 24 business hours of receipt and will email your certificate. Questions? Please call us at 626-792-3046 or (toll-free within the continental U.S.) 877-792-0005.

4. If more than one person will be applying for credit, be sure to photocopy the original (uncompleted) applicant information form, evaluation form, and CME answer sheet so that you always have the original on hand for use.

APPLICANT INFORMATION

Ob/Gyn Sonography: An Illustrated Review, 2nd Edition

Name _____ Date of birth _____

Current credentials _____

Home address _____

City/State/ZIP (City/Country/Postal Code) _____

Telephone _____ Email address _____

ARDMS # _____ ARRT # _____ SDMS # _____

CCI # _____ Sonography Canada (CARDUP) # _____

Check enclosed ❑ _____

Credit Card # _____ Expiration date _____ Security code _____

❑ The name and address given above apply to BOTH credit card billing and mailing.

❑ The name on the credit card and/or the billing address is different; for billing, please use this:

Name on credit card _____

Billing address _____

City/State/ZIP (City/Country/Postal Code) _____

❑ I purchased this book myself (new, not used).   ❑ I borrowed the book or purchased it used.

Signature certifying your completion of the activity _____

NOTE

The original purchaser of this CME activity is entitled to submit this CME application for an administrative fee of $39.50. Please enclose a check payable to Davies Publishing, Inc., with your application. Others may also submit applications for CME credit by completing the activity as explained above and enclosing an administrative fee of $49.50. The CME administrative fee helps to defray the cost of processing, evaluating, and maintaining a record of your application and the credit you earn. Fees may change without notice. For the current fee, call us at 626-792-3046, email us at cme@daviespublishing.com, or write to us at the aforementioned address. We will be happy to help!

EVALUATE THIS CME ACTIVITY—YOU GRADE US!

Ob/Gyn Sonography: An Illustrated Review, 2nd Edition

Please let us know what you think of this book. Participating in this quality survey is a requirement for CME applicants, and it benefits future readers by ensuring that current readers are satisfied and, if not, that their comments and opinions are heard and taken into account.

1. Why did you purchase this book? (Check your primary reason.)
   - ❏ Registry review
   - ❏ Course text
   - ❏ Clinical reference
   - ❏ CME activity

2. Have you used the book for other reasons, too? (Check all that apply.)
   - ❏ Registry review
   - ❏ Course text
   - ❏ Clinical reference
   - ❏ CME activity

3. To what extent did this book meet its stated objectives and your needs? (Check one.)
   - ❏ Greatly
   - ❏ Moderately
   - ❏ Minimally
   - ❏ Insignificantly

4. The content of this book was (check one):
   - ❏ Just right
   - ❏ Too basic
   - ❏ Too advanced

5. The quality of the exercises, illustrations, and case examples was mainly (check one):
   - ❏ Excellent
   - ❏ Good
   - ❏ Fair
   - ❏ Poor

6. The manner in which the book presents the material is mainly (check one):
   - ❏ Excellent
   - ❏ Good
   - ❏ Fair
   - ❏ Poor

7. If you used this book to prepare for the registry exam, did you also use other materials or take any exam-preparation courses?
   - ❏ No
   - ❏ Yes (please specify what materials and courses)

   _____
   _____
   _____

8. If you used this book for a course, please cite the course, the instructor's name, the name of the school or program, and any other textbooks you may have used:

   Course/Instructor/School or program

   _____
   _____
   _____

   Other textbooks

   _____
   _____
   _____

9. What did you like best about this book?

   _____
   _____
   _____

10. What did you like least about this book?

    _____
    _____
    _____

11. If you used this book to prepare for your registry exam in ob/gyn sonography, did you pass?
    - ❏ Yes
    - ❏ No
    - ❏ Haven't yet taken it

12. May we quote any of your comments in our catalogs or promotional material?
    - ❏ Yes
    - ❏ No
    - ❏ Further comment . . .

    _____
    _____
    _____
    _____
    _____
    _____

ANSWER SHEET

Ob/Gyn Sonography: An Illustrated Review, 2nd Edition

Circle the correct answer below and return this sheet to Davies Publishing Inc.
Passing criterion is 70%. Applicant may not have more than 3 attempts to pass.

1. A B C D	31. A B C D	61. A B C D	91. A B C D	121. A B C D
2. A B C D	32. A B C D	62. A B C D	92. A B C D	122. A B C D
3. A B C D	33. A B C D	63. A B C D	93. A B C D	123. A B C D
4. A B C D	34. A B C D	64. A B C D	94. A B C D	124. A B C D
5. A B C D	35. A B C D	65. A B C D	95. A B C D	125. A B C D
6. A B C D	36. A B C D	66. A B C D	96. A B C D	126. A B C D
7. A B C D	37. A B C D	67. A B C D	97. A B C D	127. A B C D
8. A B C D	38. A B C D	68. A B C D	98. A B C D	128. A B C D
9. A B C D	39. A B C D	69. A B C D	99. A B C D	129. A B C D
10. A B C D	40. A B C D	70. A B C D	100. A B C D	130. A B C D
11. A B C D	41. A B C D	71. A B C D	101. A B C D	131. A B C D
12. A B C D	42. A B C D	72. A B C D	102. A B C D	132. A B C D
13. A B C D	43. A B C D	73. A B C D	103. A B C D	133. A B C D
14. A B C D	44. A B C D	74. A B C D	104. A B C D	134. A B C D
15. A B C D	45. A B C D	75. A B C D	105. A B C D	135. A B C D
16. A B C D	46. A B C D	76. A B C D	106. A B C D	136. A B C D
17. A B C D	47. A B C D	77. A B C D	107. A B C D	137. A B C D
18. A B C D	48. A B C D	78. A B C D	108. A B C D	138. A B C D
19. A B C D	49. A B C D	79. A B C D	109. A B C D	139. A B C D
20. A B C D	50. A B C D	80. A B C D	110. A B C D	140. A B C D
21. A B C D	51. A B C D	81. A B C D	111. A B C D	141. A B C D
22. A B C D	52. A B C D	82. A B C D	112. A B C D	142. A B C D
23. A B C D	53. A B C D	83. A B C D	113. A B C D	143. A B C D
24. A B C D	54. A B C D	84. A B C D	114. A B C D	144. A B C D
25. A B C D	55. A B C D	85. A B C D	115. A B C D	145. A B C D
26. A B C D	56. A B C D	86. A B C D	116. A B C D	146. A B C D
27. A B C D	57. A B C D	87. A B C D	117. A B C D	147. A B C D
28. A B C D	58. A B C D	88. A B C D	118. A B C D	148. A B C D
29. A B C D	59. A B C D	89. A B C D	119. A B C D	149. A B C D
30. A B C D	60. A B C D	90. A B C D	120. A B C D	150. A B C D

CME QUIZ

Please answer the following questions after you have completed the CME activity. There is one *best* answer for each question. Circle it on the answer sheet above. Be sure to make a copy of this quiz and uncompleted forms if more than one person will be taking it.

1. Which sonographic finding is NOT associated with adenomyosis?
   A. Focal and diffuse bulkiness of the posterior uterine wall
   B. Asymmetrically enlarged uterus with focal subserosal mass
   C. Heterogeneous uterine myometrial texture
   D. Focal cystic areas within the myometrium

2. What is the name for a fetal head measuring more than 3 standard deviations below mean for gestational age?
   A. Macrocephaly
   B. Anencephaly
   C. Microcephaly
   D. Schizencephaly

3. When can the dominant ovarian follicle be identified sonographically in an infertility patient?
   A. Days 3–5
   B. Days 5–7
   C. Days 7–9
   D. Days 9–11

4. Which is the potential space between the anterior abdominal wall and anterior bladder surface?
   A. Fornix
   B. Pouch of Douglas
   C. Space of Retzius
   D. Cul-de-sac

5. Which of these congenital metabolic disorders results in demineralization of fetal bone?
   A. Hypophosphatasia
   B. Radial ray anomaly
   C. Talipes equinovarus
   D. Meckel-Gruber syndrome

6. Which sonographic finding is NOT associated with endometrial hyperplasia?
   A. Focal cystic areas in the myometrium
   B. Premenopausal endometrial thickness greater than 14 mm
   C. Postmenopausal endometrial thickness greater than 6 mm
   D. Smooth, well-defined borders

7. What is the most common gynecologic malignancy in the United States?
   A. Ovarian cancer
   B. Cervical cancer
   C. Endometrial cancer
   D. Fallopian tube cancer

8. Which is the most common histologic type of malignant ovarian neoplasm?
   A. Brenner tumor
   B. Cystadenocarcinoma
   C. Thecoma
   D. Dysgerminoma

9. DES-related anatomic anomalies include all of the following EXCEPT:
   A. Hypoplastic uterus
   B. Constricting bands within the uterine cavity
   C. Intrauterine polyps
   D. Retroversion of the uterus

10. Which Doppler ultrasound modality permits the quantification of flow states?
    A. Spectral Doppler
    B. Color Doppler imaging
    C. Power Doppler imaging
    D. Continuous-wave Doppler

11. The earliest sonographic sign of an intrauterine pregnancy is:
    A. Double bleb sign
    B. Decidual thickening
    C. Double sac sign
    D. Yolk sac

12. Which of the following congenital abnormalities is NOT associated with Dandy-Walker malformation?
    A. Cleft palate
    B. Hydrocephalus
    C. Cyclopia
    D. Agenesis of the corpus callosum

13. Which of these terms refers to congenital skeletal syndromes of abnormal bony formation that result in shortening of the long bones?
    A. Osteochondrodysplasia
    B. Achondrogenesis
    C. Osteogenesis imperfecta
    D. Hypophosphatasia

14. Which of these pathologies would you expect to see in a patient with a hydatidiform mole?
    A. Corpus luteum cysts
    B. Follicular cysts
    C. Theca-lutein cysts
    D. Paraovarian cysts

15. Which of the following is NOT considered an extracorporeal approach to ultrasound imaging?
    A. Transvesicular
    B. Transperineal
    C. Transvaginal
    D. Transabdominal

16. What is the name of the highly vascularized structure lying along the floor of both lateral ventricles and extending along the roof of the third ventricle?
    A. Choroid plexus
    B. Cavum septi pellucidi
    C. Falx cerebri
    D. Corpus callosum

17. Which of these chromosomal anomalies is most commonly associated with cystic hygroma?
    A. Trisomy 13
    B. Trisomy 21
    C. Treacher Collins syndrome
    D. Turner syndrome

18. The anteroposterior (AP) diameter of a placenta at term should not exceed:
    A. 6 cm
    B. 5 cm
    C. 4 cm
    D. 3 cm

19. What is the name of the space lying between the frontal horns and bodies of the two lateral ventricles?
    A. Cavum vergae
    B. Foramen of Monro
    C. Cavum septi pellucidi
    D. Falx cerebri

20. What is the term for a placenta with a loose chorionic membrane that folds back upon itself and encircles the surface of the fetus?
    A. Circummarginate
    B. Circumvallate
    C. Succenturiate
    D. Annular

21. A maternal serum triple test involves all EXCEPT which of the following?
    A. Maternal serum AFP
    B. Luteinizing hormone
    C. Serum beta-hCG
    D. Estriol

22. Which of the following is NOT a typical etiology of precocious pseudopuberty?
    A. Sarcoma botryoides
    B. Congenital adrenal hyperplasia
    C. Exposure to exogenous sex steroid hormones
    D. McCune-Albright syndrome

23. Which factor is NOT associated with an increased risk for uterine cancer?
    A. Estrogen replacement therapy
    B. Tamoxifen administration
    C. Obesity
    D. Infertility treatment

24. Which condition is associated with facial anomalies such as cyclopia and proboscis?
    A. Holoprosencephaly
    B. Hydranencephaly
    C. Hydrocephalus
    D. Median facial cleft

25. How do conceptual age and menstrual age differ?
    A. Conceptual age is 7 days greater than menstrual age.
    B. Conceptual age is 14 days greater than menstrual age.
    C. Conceptual age is 7 days less than menstrual age.
    D. Conceptual age is 14 days less than menstrual age.

26. What does the mechanical index measure?
    A. Thermal changes in soft tissue
    B. Negative acoustic pressure present in a medium
    C. Positive acoustic pressure present in a medium
    D. Cavitational changes

27. Which of these ovarian tumors is a metastatic type that frequently causes endocrinologic abnormalities?
    A. Sertoli-Leydig tumor
    B. Granulosa cell tumor
    C. Krukenberg tumor
    D. Sex cord stromal tumor

28. Which is the most common congenital cardiac anomaly?
    A. Tetralogy of Fallot
    B. Atrial septal defect
    C. Ventricular septal defect
    D. Aortic coarctation

29. What is the name for abnormal congenital hypomineralization of fetal bony structure?
    A. Achondrogenesis
    B. Osteogenesis imperfecta
    C. Osteochondrodysplasia
    D. Campomelic dysplasia

30. Which of the following would be an indication for fetal echocardiography?
    A. Dextrocardia
    B. Two-vessel umbilical cord
    C. Increased diameter of nuchal translucency
    D. All of the above

31. What is the normal double-thickness measurement of the postmenopausal endometrium?
    A. <5 mm
    B. >5 mm
    C. 5–7 mm
    D. 6–8 mm

32. What is the mean sac diameter at the earliest point that the normal yolk sac becomes visible?
    A. 4.0 mm
    B. 4.5 mm
    C. 5.0 mm
    D. 5.5 mm

33. Which of the following is a uniformly lethal defect characterized by an absent umbilical cord and exteriorization of abdominal contents that attach directly to the placental surface?
    A. Limb–body wall complex
    B. Gastroschisis
    C. Cloacal exstrophy
    D. Abdominoschisis

34. What rate of growth is typical for a dominant ovarian follicle?
    A. 1–2 mm/day
    B. 2–3 mm/day
    C. 3–4 mm/day
    D. 4–5 mm/day

35. Which of the following is NOT associated with an increased prevalence of uterine fibroids?
    A. Obesity
    B. Diabetes
    C. Perimenopausal state
    D. Hormone replacement therapy

36. Which of these congenital anomalies is NOT associated with VACTERL?
    A. Spina bifida
    B. Holoprosencephaly
    C. Cleft lip
    D. Polydactyly

37. When can you first visualize the fluid-filled gestational sac?
    A. 4.5–5.0 menstrual weeks
    B. 5.0–5.5 menstrual weeks
    C. 5.5–6.0 menstrual weeks
    D. 6.0–6.5 menstrual weeks

38. What is the name for the congenital narrowing of the aortic lumen?
    A. Tetralogy of Fallot
    B. Coarctation of the aorta
    C. Ebstein's anomaly
    D. Aortic stenosis

39. Which of the following is NOT a major component of the diagnostic triad in a prenatal genetic testing program?
    A. Serial serum beta-hCG titers
    B. Maternal serum testing
    C. Amniocentesis
    D. Sonographic fetal anatomic survey

40. Which of the following is a congenital anomaly characterized by incomplete development of the structures comprising the left side of the fetal heart?
    A. Tetralogy of Fallot
    B. Conotruncal abnormality
    C. Hypoplastic left heart syndrome
    D. Persistent truncus arteriosus

41. What is the term for the congenital absence of an eyeball?
    A. Hypertelorism
    B. Hypotelorism
    C. Anophthalmia
    D. Microphthalmia

42. Which pathology may result from disruption of the normal outflow of the urinary tract?
    A. Renal agenesis
    B. Renal ectopia
    C. Obstructive uropathy
    D. Polycystic renal disease

43. Which of the following values indicates an increased risk of spontaneous abortion?
    A. MSD − CRL < 5 mm
    B. MSD − CRL < 7 mm
    C. MSD − CRL < 10 mm
    D. MSD − CRL < 12 mm

44. What is the name for retained blood in the uterine and vaginal cavities?
    A. Hydrocolpos
    B. Hydrometra
    C. Hematometrocolpos
    D. Pyometrocolpos

45. Which of the following is NOT associated with echogenic fetal bowel?
    A. Trisomy 13
    B. Duodenal atresia
    C. Cytomegalovirus infection
    D. Cystic fibrosis

46. Which of the following is NOT a parameter assessed in a fetal biophysical profile?
    A. Fetal breathing
    B. Fetal femur length
    C. Amniotic fluid volume
    D. Fetal tone

47. Once the conceptus is implanted in the uterine lining, it is called the:
    A. Blastocyst
    B. Zygote
    C. Morula
    D. Yolk sac

48. Which of these sonographic signs is NOT associated with ovarian hyperstimulation syndrome?
    A. Variably sized cysts
    B. Unilateral cystic enlargement of an ovary
    C. Ascites
    D. Pleural effusion

49. Which type of facial clefting is most prevalent?
    A. Cleft lip alone
    B. Cleft lip and palate
    C. Cleft palate alone
    D. Median facial clefting

50. How much urine must a patient retain in her bladder during transabdominal sonography?
    A. 200 cc
    B. 300 cc
    C. 400 cc
    D. 500 cc

51. Which of the following umbilical cord conditions may cause fetal death?
    A. Cord stricture
    B. Excessive Wharton's jelly
    C. Short cord
    D. Long cord

52. What is the primary characteristic of Ebstein's anomaly?
    A. Mitral valve displaced inferiorly in the left ventricle
    B. Tricuspid valve displaced inferiorly in the right ventricle
    C. Overriding aorta
    D. All or part of heart located outside the thoracic cavity

53. Which of the following conditions is NOT associated with orbital hypertelorism?
    A. Trisomy 21
    B. Trisomy 13
    C. Alobar holoprosencephaly
    D. Turner syndrome

54. What is the term for the incomplete covering of the internal cervical os by the lower edge of the placenta?
    A. Complete previa
    B. Marginal previa
    C. Partial previa
    D. Low-lying placenta

55. Which of these germ cell layers contributes to the tissue components of a teratoma?
    A. Endoderm
    B. Ectoderm
    C. Mesoderm
    D. All of the above

56. Using Grannum's scale, what grade would you assign to a placenta with the appearance of scattered echogenic calcifications and focal cystic spaces?
    A. Grade 0
    B. Grade I
    C. Grade II
    D. Grade III

57. Which of these sonographic findings is NOT found in a fetus with sirenomelia?
    A. Absent feet
    B. Macroglossia
    C. Oligohydramnios
    D. Single umbilical artery

58. Which nuchal thickness is considered normal?
    A. <6 mm
    B. <8 mm
    C. <4 mm
    D. <2 mm

59. The fetal skeletal abnormality characterized by a cloverleaf skull and a bell-shaped chest is:
    A. Short rib–polydactyly syndrome
    B. Thanatophoric dysplasia
    C. Campomelic dysplasia
    D. Chondrodysplasia punctata

60. How should the normal postmenopausal endometrium appear?
    A. Thick and homogeneously echogenic
    B. Hyperechoic with focal thinning
    C. Hypoechoic with focal thinning
    D. Thin and homogeneously echogenic

61. To get the best estimation of the gestational age of a dolichocephalic fetus, use the:
    A. Head circumference
    B. Biparietal diameter
    C. Cephalic index
    D. BPD/AC ratio

62. The term for dorsal and lateral dislocation of the talonavicular joint with a prominent calcaneus is:
    A. Talipes equinovarus
    B. Clubfoot
    C. Syndactyly
    D. Rocker bottom foot

63. Which of these anomalies is NOT associated with Beckwith-Wiedemann syndrome?
    A. Omphalocele
    B. Macroglossia
    C. Hydrocephalus
    D. Hepatosplenomegaly

64. Which is the most severe form of holoprosencephaly?
    A. Lobar
    B. Alobar
    C. Semilobar
    D. Nonlobar

65. What is the name of the anomalous condition characterized by an accessory fragment of lung that has no connection to the tracheobronchial tree and maintains a separate arterial circulation?
    A. Cystic adenomatoid malformation
    B. Diaphragmatic hernia
    C. Diaphragmatic eventration
    D. Pulmonary sequestration

66. A defect in the abdominal wall lateral to the cord insertion through which intra-abdominal content herniates into the amniotic cavity is known as:
    A. Omphalocele
    B. Umbilical hernia
    C. Gastroschisis
    D. Rachischisis

67. Absent ossification of the vertebral bodies is the primary characteristic of:
    A. Thanatophoric dysplasia
    B. Achondroplasia
    C. Diastrophic dysplasia
    D. Achondrogenesis

68. What is the name for the spectrum of congenital anatomic abnormalities resulting from the failed fusion of the paired embryonic paramesonephric ducts?
    A. Müllerian duct anomalies
    B. Genitourinary anomalies
    C. Asherman syndrome
    D. Gartner's duct anomalies

69. What is the classic sonographic sign of duodenal atresia?
    A. Short umbilical cord
    B. Echogenic bowel
    C. Double bubble
    D. Tip of the iceberg

70. Which of the following cardiac anomalies is NOT detected on the four-chamber view of the fetal heart?
    A. Single ventricle
    B. Transposition of the great vessels
    C. Ebstein's anomaly
    D. Ventricular hypoplasia

71. The most common abnormality of the umbilical cord is:
    A. Four-vessel cord
    B. Single umbilical artery (SUA)
    C. Cord cyst
    D. Short cord

72. Which of these cardiac segments is NOT assessed during a routine sonographic examination of the fetal heart?
    A. Abdominal visceral situs
    B. Visceroatrial situs
    C. Ventricular loop
    D. Truncus arteriosus

73. Which of these sonographic findings is inconsistent with asymmetric intrauterine growth restriction?
    A. AC measuring > 2 weeks behind HC
    B. HC measuring > 2 weeks behind AC
    C. Normal femur length measurement
    D. Early grade III placenta

74. In twin reversed arterial perfusion (TRAP) sequence, the recipient twin may demonstrate all of the following sonographic findings EXCEPT:
    A. Acardiacus
    B. Hydrops fetalis
    C. Cystic hygroma
    D. Absent upper body

75. In twin-twin transfusion syndrome, the recipient twin may demonstrate all of the following sonographic findings EXCEPT:
    A. Hydropic changes
    B. Oligohydramnios
    C. Hepatosplenomegaly
    D. Ascites

76. In postmenopausal patients receiving unopposed estrogen hormone replacement therapy, how thick can the endometrium be and still be within normal limits?
    A. 5 mm
    B. 6 mm
    C. 7 mm
    D. 8 mm

77. Which of these soft sonographic markers is NOT associated with trisomy 18?
    A. Choroid plexus cysts
    B. Single umbilical artery
    C. Echogenic bowel
    D. Brachycephaly

78. The condition in which the placenta has prematurely separated from the myometrium is known as:
    A. Placenta previa
    B. Placenta percreta
    C. Placenta accreta
    D. Placental abruption

79. Fetuses affected by campomelic dysplasia exhibit which hallmark sonographic finding?
    A. Bell-shaped chest
    B. Severe demineralization of long bones
    C. Severe bowing of the long bones
    D. Absent vertebral ossification

80. Which sonographic finding is NOT associated with meconium peritonitis?
    A. Hepatosplenomegaly
    B. Ascites
    C. Intraperitoneal calcifications
    D. Polyhydramnios

81. What is the term for an accessory cotyledon located away from the main placental body?
    A. Circumvallate
    B. Succenturiate
    C. Circummarginate
    D. Annular

82. Which of the following identifies a monochorionic/monoamniotic twin pregnancy?
    A. Two amnions and a single chorion
    B. A single amnion and a single chorion
    C. A single amnion and two chorions
    D. Two amnions and two chorions

83. Which two-dimensional sonographic imaging modality provides a global display of the presence, direction, and relative velocities in a hemodynamic state?
    A. Color Doppler imaging
    B. Power Doppler imaging

C. Continuous-wave Doppler

D. Spectral Doppler

84. Which of the following best describes hydrocephalus?

    A. Enlargement of the ventricular system without concomitant compression atrophy of adjacent cerebral parenchyma

    B. Enlarged, single midline ventricle surrounded by a mantle of cerebral tissue

    C. Enlargement of the ventricular system with concomitant compression atrophy of adjacent cerebral parenchyma

    D. Cystic dilatation of the cisterna magna with compression atrophy of the cerebellum

85. What is the term for the obliteration of the endometrial cavity through excessive or traumatic uterine instrumentation?

    A. Asherman syndrome

    B. Stein-Leventhal syndrome

    C. Beckwith-Wiedemann syndrome

    D. Adenomyosis

86. Which sonographic finding does NOT characterize campomelic dysplasia?

    A. Hydrocephalus

    B. Cloverleaf skull

    C. Micrognathia

    D. Narrowed thorax

87. In a nonpregnant patient, when should regression of the corpus luteum be complete?

    A. 28 days

    B. 14 days

    C. 7 days

    D. 24 hours

88. What would you call a uterus whose body is directed toward the hollow of the sacrum without a marked bend in the endometrial stripe?

    A. Anteverted

    B. Retroflexed

    C. Involuted

    D. Retroverted

89. Which of the following is NOT considered a functional ovarian cyst?

    A. Follicular cyst

    B. Theca-lutein cyst

    C. Corpus luteum cyst

    D. Cystadenoma

90. Which of these is the LEAST reliable indicator of gestational age?

    A. Crown-rump length

    B. Biparietal diameter

    C. Abdominal circumference

    D. Mean sac diameter

91. What is the name of the ligament formed by the double fold of peritoneum that arises from the lateral aspect of the uterus and divides the true pelvis into anterior and posterior compartments?

    A. Round ligament

    B. Uterosacral ligament

    C. Broad ligament

    D. Cardinal ligament

92. The protrusion of intracranial contents through a defect in the bony calvarium is known as:

    A. Encephalocele

    B. Anencephaly

    C. Schizencephaly

    D. Holoprosencephaly

93. Which of these pathologic entities does NOT cause a palpable pelvic mass in the pediatric patient?

    A. Choriocarcinoma

    B. Hydrometrocolpos

    C. Sarcoma botryoides

    D. Ovarian torsion

94. Fetal bowel echogenicity is:

    A. Less echogenic than bone and more echogenic than liver

    B. More echogenic than bone and less echogenic than liver

    C. More echogenic than liver and less echogenic than spleen

    D. More echogenic than spleen and isoechoic with liver

95. When is the double decidual sac sign typically demonstrated sonographically?
    A. 4.5–5.0 weeks
    B. 5.0–5.5 weeks
    C. 5.5–6.0 weeks
    D. 6.0–6.5 weeks

96. Which nuchal translucency measurement is considered abnormal?
    A. ≥1 mm
    B. ≥2 mm
    C. ≥4 mm
    D. ≥6 mm

97. Which of the following is a fetal condition characterized by all biometric parameters measuring less than expected for a given gestational age?
    A. Trisomy 21
    B. Beckwith-Wiedemann syndrome
    C. Asymmetric intrauterine growth restriction
    D. Symmetric intrauterine growth restriction

98. Which anatomic anomaly consists of two separate uterine bodies and two separate cervices, usually with the presence of a vaginal septum?
    A. Arcuate uterus
    B. Didelphic uterus
    C. Unicornuate uterus
    D. Bicornuate uterus

99. In the pediatric patient, which of the following is NOT associated with a torsed ovary?
    hypoechoic ovary
    A. Low-resistance Doppler flow within the ovary
    B. A peripherally displaced follicle
    C. An enlarged, hypoechoic ovary
    D. Free fluid in the pelvis

100. Which of these clinical signs is NOT associated with endometrial carcinoma?
    A. Murphy's sign
    B. Vaginal bleeding
    C. Intermenstrual flow
    D. Lower abdominal pain

101. Doppler findings in the ovarian artery supplying the dominant ovary typically demonstrate:
    A. High resistance
    B. High pulsatility
    C. Low resistance
    D. A dicrotic notch

102. Anatomic landmarks identified at a proper plane of section for head circumference include:
    A. Cavum septi pellucidi, cerebellar hemispheres, and thalamic nuclei
    B. Falx cerebri, interhemispheric fissure, and thalamic nuclei
    C. Cavum septi pellucidi, falx cerebri, and thalamic nuclei
    D. Falx cerebri, Sylvian fissure, and cerebellar hemispheres

103. When you see the upward and outward displacement of both lateral ventricles on the sonogram, you should suspect:
    A. Holoprosencephaly
    B. Hydranencephaly
    C. Hydrocephalus
    D. Agenesis of the corpus callosum

104. Acute inflammation of the uterine lining is known as:
    A. Parametritis
    B. Peritonitis
    C. Endometritis
    D. Pelvic inflammatory disease

105. Which of the following clinical signs is NOT associated with gestational trophoblastic disease?
    A. Beta-hCG levels greater than expected for dates
    B. Beta-hCG levels less than expected for dates
    C. First trimester vaginal bleeding
    D. Hyperemesis gravidarum

106. The midgut herniation normally regresses back into the fetal abdominal cavity by:
    A. 11 menstrual weeks
    B. 12 menstrual weeks

C. 14 menstrual weeks
D. 16 menstrual weeks

107. Which of these sonographic findings is NOT consistent with a spontaneous complete abortion?
    A. Empty uterus with "clean" endometrial stripe
    B. Complex echogenic material in the uterine cavity
    C. Moderate to bright endometrial echoes
    D. Uterine enlargement

108. How do higher-frequency ultrasound probes compare with lower-frequency probes?
    A. They provide less penetration and better spatial resolution.
    B. They provide better penetration and better spatial resolution.
    C. They provide less penetration and less spatial resolution.
    D. They provide better penetration and less spatial resolution.

109. What is the term for the artifact caused by a reduction in amplitude of echoes lying deep to a highly reflective interface?
    A. Posterior acoustic enhancement
    B. Section-thickness artifact
    C. Posterior acoustic shadowing
    D. Mirror-image artifact

110. When does the umbilical cord become sonographically visible?
    A. 4 menstrual weeks
    B. 6 menstrual weeks
    C. 8 menstrual weeks
    D. 10 menstrual weeks

111. What is the most common neural tube defect affecting the spinal column?
    A. Spina bifida
    B. Encephalocele
    C. Iniencepaly
    D. Anencephaly

112. Deep invasion of placental villi into the myometrium but not the serosal layer is known as:
    A. Placenta accreta
    B. Chorioangioma
    C. Placental abruption
    D. Placenta increta

113. How early can the fetal external genitalia be differentiated sonographically?
    A. 8 menstrual weeks
    B. 10 menstrual weeks
    C. 12 menstrual weeks
    D. 14 menstrual weeks

114. The earliest measure of sonographically demonstrable gestational age is:
    A. Mean sac diameter
    B. Biparietal diameter
    C. Yolk sac size
    D. Crown rump length

115. Which type of pregnancy is most likely to encounter cord entanglement?
    A. Diamniotic/monozygotic pregnancy
    B. Monoamniotic/dizygotic pregnancy
    C. Monochorionic/monoamniotic pregnancy
    D. Singleton pregnancy

116. A fetus visualized in "stargazer" posture suggests the presence of which neural tube defect?
    A. Iniencephaly
    B. Anencephaly
    C. Spina bifida
    D. Encephalocele

117. What term refers to masses of endometrial tissue projecting out from the surface of the endometrium and into the endometrial cavity?
    A. Endometrial carcinoma
    B. Fibroids
    C. Adhesions
    D. Endometrial polyps

118. Abnormalities of the ureter (as opposed to distal obstructive pathology) can result in a chronic dilatation of the ureter known as:
    A. Ectopic ureterocele
    B. Congenital primary megaureter
    C. Hydronephrosis
    D. Hydroureter

119. The rounded, superior aspect of the uterus located above the insertion of the fallopian tubes is known as the:
    A. Fundus
    B. Corpus
    C. Body
    D. Cornu

120. What is the term for the congenital chest anomaly in which all or part of the heart is located outside of the thoracic cavity?
    A. Ebstein's anomaly
    B. Diaphragmatic hernia
    C. Ectopia cordis
    D. Omphalocele

121. Potter type II (multicystic renal dysplasia) is NOT characterized by:
    A. Multiple large cysts replacing renal parenchyma
    B. Echogenic renal parenchyma
    C. Large hyperechoic kidneys bilaterally
    D. Lobulated renal contour

122. What is the primary anatomic abnormality associated with persistent truncus arteriosus?
    A. Single great artery arising from truncal root
    B. Aorta arising from the right ventricle
    C. Pulmonary artery arising from the left ventricle
    D. Pulmonary hypoplasia

123. Which sonographic finding is NOT associated with unilateral renal agenesis?
    A. Normal amount of amniotic fluid
    B. Down syndrome
    C. Potter sequence
    D. Obstructive uropathies

124. Which congenital abdominal wall defect is associated with Beckwith-Wiedemann syndrome?
    A. Gastroschisis
    B. Omphalocele
    C. Umbilical hernia
    D. Rachischisis

125. Which of the following findings is diagnostic for an ectopic pregnancy?
    A. Empty uterus in a patient with a positive pregnancy test
    B. Free fluid in the cul-de-sac
    C. Identification of an extrauterine gestational sac with live embryo
    D. Complex adnexal mass in a patient with a positive pregnancy test

126. What is the normal cervical length in a nulliparous woman?
    A. 1–2 mm
    B. 2–3 mm
    C. 1–2 cm
    D. 2–3 cm

127. Which of the following anomalies is associated with both Beckwith-Wiedemann syndrome and trisomy 21?
    A. Branchial cleft cyst
    B. Macroglossia
    C. Cyclopia
    D. Epignathus

128. When should you be able to detect a normal yolk sac using ultrasound?
    A. 4.5 weeks
    B. 4.0 weeks
    C. 5.0 weeks
    D. 5.5 weeks

129. Which of the following fetal vessels will help identify the umbilical cord?
    A. Umbilical arteries
    B. Iliac arteries
    C. Umbilical vein
    D. Hepatic vein

130. Which of the following is a congenital anomaly characterized by incomplete development of the fetal lungs?
    A. Diaphragmatic hernia
    B. Pulmonary sequestration
    C. Congenital cystic adenomatoid malformation
    D. Pulmonary hypoplasia

131. Potter type I (infantile polycystic renal disease) is NOT characterized by:
    A. Large echogenic kidneys
    B. Multiple large cysts replacing renal parenchyma
    C. Nonfilling of the urinary bladder
    D. Loss of corticomedullary differentiation

132. Which of these fetal anomalies is NOT associated with caudal regression syndrome?
    A. Hydronephrosis
    B. Pulmonary hypoplasia
    C. Myelomeningocele
    D. Anencephaly

133. Which of these soft sonographic markers is NOT associated with trisomy 21?
    A. Nuchal thickening
    B. Echogenic bowel
    C. Pyelectasis
    D. Demineralized bone

134. Which of the following is NOT a histopathologic type of intracranial tumor?
    A. Epignathus
    B. Glioblastoma
    C. Craniopharyngioma
    D. Sarcoma

135. Which of the following anomalies is suggested by an abnormal decrease in maternal serum alpha-fetoprotein?
    A. Spina bifida
    B. Trisomy 21
    C. Omphalocele
    D. Multiple gestations

136. Which is the ONLY type of twinning that can result in conjoined twins?
    A. Monochorionic/monoamniotic twinning
    B. Monochorionic/diamniotic twinning
    C. Dichorionic/diamniotic twinning
    D. Dizygotic twinning

137. What is the name for congenital limb shortening that affects only the proximal segment of an extremity?
    A. Mesomelia
    B. Rhizomelia
    C. Micromelia
    D. Amelia

138. What should the maximum vertical pocket of amniotic fluid measure in order to be considered normal in a fetal biophysical profile?
    A. >2 cm
    B. >4 cm
    C. >6 cm
    D. >8 cm

139. What is the name of the clinically serious condition in which velamentously inserted cord vessels precede the fetal presenting part?
    A. Vasa previa
    B. Prolapsed cord
    C. Complete previa
    D. Partial previa

140. Which of these anatomic structures is NOT identified on the left ventricular outflow tract (LVOT) view?
    A. Left atrium
    B. Aortic root
    C. Ventricular septum
    D. Pulmonary artery

141. When measuring the long axis of the uterus, where should you place the cursors?
    A. Serosal surface of the fundus to the internal cervical os
    B. Serosal surface of the fundus to the external cervical os
    C. Cornu of the uterus to the isthmus
    D. Cornu of the uterus to the external cervical os

142. How does the Second International Standard (2IS) compare to the International Reference Preparation (1st IRP) in measuring serum levels of beta-hCG?
    A. The 2IS level is equal to the 1st IRP level.
    B. The 2IS level is half the 1st IRP level.
    C. The 2IS level is twice the 1st IRP level.
    D. The 2IS level is three times greater than the 1st IRP level.

143. What is the typical crown-rump length when embryonic cardiac activity can first be visualized?
    A. 1–3 mm
    B. 2–4 mm
    C. 3–5 mm
    D. 4–6 mm

144. What is the term for a mesonephric duct remnant that forms a cyst along the lateral or anterolateral wall of the vagina?
    A. Gartner's duct cyst
    B. Corpus luteum cyst
    C. Paraovarian cyst
    D. Nabothian cyst

145. An intraorbital distance that measures above the 95th percentile is termed:
    A. Anophthalmia
    B. Hypotelorism
    C. Cyclopia
    D. Hypertelorism

146. Which of these fetal conditions does NOT result in immune hydrops fetalis?
    A. Fetal anemia
    B. Hemolytic diseases
    C. Rh isoimmunization
    D. Turner syndrome

147. How often does the fetal urinary bladder empty and refill?
    A. Every 10–25 minutes
    B. Every 20–30 minutes
    C. Every 30–45 minutes
    D. Every 45–60 minutes

148. How early can the fetal kidneys be identified?
    A. 6–8 menstrual weeks
    B. 8–10 menstrual weeks
    C. 10–12 menstrual weeks
    D. 12–14 menstrual weeks

149. What anomaly can result if complete canalization of the renal pelvis and proximal ureter fails at about 10–12 weeks' gestation?
    A. Renal agenesis
    B. Ureteropelvic junction obstruction
    C. Bladder exstrophy
    D. Multicystic dysplastic kidney

150. When should you measure nuchal translucency?
    A. When CRL is approximately 20–40 mm
    B. When CRL is approximately 40–50 mm
    C. When CRL is approximately 40–80 mm
    D. When CRL is approximately 80–120 mm

Subject Index

Publisher's note: *Entries on anatomy and pathologies refer to the fetus unless otherwise indicated. The letter "f" following a page number denotes an image or illustration; the letter "t" refers to a table.*

A

Abdomen, 219–241. *See also* Gastrointestinal tract
    abnormalities, 221–241, 226t
    embryology, 219–221
    vasculature, 222f, 224f

Abdominal circumference (AC), 72t, 75–76, 76f, 77t, 468–469, 468f, 469t

Abdominal wall (fetal), 220, 220f

Abdominal wall defects (fetal), 226–230

Abdominoschisis. *See* Gastroschisis

Abortion. *See also* Fetal demise
    complete, 15
    elective, x
    incomplete, 15, 15f
    spontaneous, 15–17, 310
    subchorionic hemorrhage, 17
    threatened, 16–17

Abruption. *See* Placental abruption

Abscesses
    postpartum, 334f
    puerperal, 333–334
    tubo-ovarian, 398–399, 399f, 453f

AC. *See* Abdominal circumference
ACC. *See* Agenesis of the corpus callosum
Accessory placental variants, 39–40
Acetylcholinesterase, 275
Achondrogenesis, 203–204, 203f
Achondroplasia, 204–205
Acoustic streaming, 441–442
Activity. *See* Fetal activity
Adenocarcinoma, 381, 382, 390. *See also* Cystadenocarcinoma
Adenomyosis, 379, 379f
Adherence abnormalities, placental
 accreta, 47–48, 47f
 increta, 47–48, 47f, 49
 percreta, 47–48, 47f, 49
Adnexal pathologies, 398–400. *See also* Ovarian pathologies; Uterine pathologies
 endometriosis, 399–400
 mass in ectopic pregnancy, 18–19
 ovarian venous thrombosis, 400–401
 pelvic inflammatory disease, 398
ADPKD. *See* Autosomal dominant polycystic kidney disease
Adrenal glands (fetal), 249, 250f
Adrenal hyperplasia, 427
Adrenal neuroblastomas, 265f
Adult polycystic kidney disease (APKD), 256
AFI. *See* Amniotic fluid index
AFP. *See* Alpha-fetoprotein
Agenesis of the corpus callosum, 132–133, 132f, 133f
AIS. *See* Androgen insensitivity syndrome
AIUM. *See* American Institute of Ultrasound in Medicine
ALARA principle, 11, 307, 473, 498
Allantoic cysts, 62, 63f
Alobar holoprosencephaly, 126, 126f, 127, 128f
Alpha-fetoprotein (AFP)
 in amniotic fluid, 273
 in maternal serum, 273–274, 471t
Alveolar phase of lung development, 151–153, 152f
Alveolar ridge, 95f
Ambiguous genitalia, 427

Amelia, 201
American Institute of Ultrasound in Medicine, 462, 473
 fetal echocardiography practice guidelines, 515–520
 focused reproductive endocrinology and infertility scan practice guidelines, 512–515
 obstetric ultrasound practice guidelines, 491–498
 pelvic ultrasound practice guidelines, 498–504
 reproductive medicine ultrasound practice guidelines, 504–512
 sonohysterography practice guidelines, 501–504
Amniocentesis
 biochemical assays, 275, 275f
 chromosomal analysis, 275–276
 indications, 276
 procedure, 275–276, 472
 pulmonic maturity studies, 155–156
 risks/complications, 276
 sonographer's role, 472
Amnioinfusion, 472
Amnion, 6–7, 7f, 9, 10f, 13, 13f, 33
Amnioreduction, 472
Amniotic band syndrome, 287–288, 288f
Amniotic cavity, 6, 32f
Amniotic fluid, 153–156. *See also* Oligohydramnios; Polyhydramnios
 abnormal, 154–155, 154f, 155f
 in biophysical profile, 83t
 echogenicity, 155
 and gestational age, 154t
 normal, 155f
 volume estimation, 153–155
Amniotic fluid index (AFI), 83, 153–155, 154t. *See also* Oligohydramnios; Polyhydramnios
Amniotic sac, 7, 9, 13
Ampulla (fallopian tube), 356
Anasarca, 303f
Anatomy and physiology. *See* Pelvic anatomy
Androblastomas. *See* Sertoli-Leydig cell tumors
Androgen insensitivity syndrome (AIS), 427
Androxal. *See* Clomiphene citrate
Anembryonic pregnancy, 15f, 16

Anemia (fetal), 309
Anencephaly, 137–138, 138f
Aneuploidy, 282
Aneurysms. See also Varices
    umbilical artery, 63
    vein of Galen, 130–131, 130f
Angiogenesis, 7
Anhydramnios, 155
Annular placenta, 40, 40f
Anophthalmia, 96, 100–101, 101f
Anteflexion, uterine, 352–353, 352f, 353f
Antepartum/postpartum risks, 330–335
Anterior cerebral arteries, 119
Anterior cul-de-sac, 355, 355f
Anteverted/anteflexed uterus, 352f, 353f
Antral follicles, 416–417, 416f
Aorta (fetal)
    abdominal, 224, 224f
    anatomy, 161f
    ascending, 157f, 160–161, 161f, 163, 164, 178, 181
    coarctation of, 184–185
    descending, 158f, 160–161
    in double-inlet left ventricle, 182
    in double-outlet right ventricle, 179–180
    embryology, 156–157, 157f
    in hypoplastic heart syndrome, 180–181
    in persistent truncus arteriosus, 178–179
    in pulmonary sequestration, 167–168
    in tetralogy of Fallot, 176
    in transposition of the great vessels, 177
Aortic arch, 157f, 158, 161, 161f, 178, 181, 184, 185f
Aorticopulmonary septum, 157f
Apical five-chamber view of fetal heart, 165f
APKD. See Autosomal dominant polycystic kidney disease
Appendicular skeleton, 198
Aqueduct of Sylvius, 116, 117f
Arachnoid mater, 117
Arcuate uterus, 373, 373f, 374f
ARPKD. See Autosomal recessive polycystic kidney disease

ART. See Assisted reproductive technologies
Artifacts (imaging), 451–457
    grating lobes, 457, 457f
    mirror-image, 456, 456f
    posterior acoustic enhancement, 452, 453f
    posterior acoustic shadowing, 452, 452f
    refractory shadows, 454–455, 454f, 455f
    reverberation, 452–454, 453f
    secondary lobe, 456, 457f
    section-thickness, 455, 455f
    side lobes, 456, 457f
"As low as reasonably achievable." See ALARA principle
Ascites, 50f, 105, 124, 234, 234f, 236f, 238, 302, 303f, 316, 316f, 317, 326, 327, 336, 355f, 391, 391f, 396, 414
ASD. See Atrial septal defect
Asherman syndrome, 375, 375f, 412, 412f
Asphyxiating thoracic dystrophy, 208–209
Assisted reproductive technologies (ART)
    gamete intrafallopian transfer, 415, 472
    in vitro fertilization, 414–415, 472
    and multiple gestations, 311
    zygote intrafallopian transfer, 415, 472
Associations. See also Sequences; Syndromes
    CHARGE, 293–294
    defined, 287
    VACTERL, 293
Asymmetric intrauterine growth restriction, 306–307
At-risk pregnancies, 301–337
    antepartum/postpartum risks, 330–335
    fetal complications, 302–311, 302t
    fetal therapy, 335–337
    maternal complications, 302t, 311, 321–330
    multiple gestations, 311–321
Atria (fetal brain), 115–116, 116f, 117f
Atria (fetal heart), 156–159, 161–165, 173–190
Atrial flutter, 190, 190f
Atrial septal defect (ASD), 163, 173, 174–175, 176, 178, 179f, 181, 181f, 183
Atrial septations, 157
Atrioventricular block, 191, 191f, 193

Atrioventricular septal defect (AVSD), 173–176, 175f, 176f
Autosomal dominant disorders (defined), 282
Autosomal dominant polycystic kidney disease (ADPKD), 254t, 256, 256f
Autosomal recessive disorders (defined), 282
Autosomal recessive polycystic kidney disease (ARPKD), 253–255, 254t
AV block. *See* Atrioventricular block
AVSD. *See* Atrioventricular septal defect
Axial skeleton, 197

B

B-mode imaging, 442–443, 442f
Banana sign, 142–143, 143f
Basal plate, 33f
    infarction, 41
    lesions, 41–42, 42f
Battledore placenta, 60–61, 61f
Beckwith-Wiedemann syndrome, 288, 288f, 289f
Bell-shaped chest, 206f
beta-hCG. *See* Human chorionic gonadotropin, beta subunit
Bicaval view of fetal heart, 518f
Bicornuate uterus, 330f, 373, 373f, 374f
Bifid renal collecting system, 262
Bilaminar embryonic disc, 6–7, 7f, 9
Bilateral renal agenesis, 252, 253f
Bilirubin, 275
Binocular distance (BOD), 80, 80t, 81f, 92f, 96f, 97t
Bioeffects of ultrasound
    mechanical, 440–442
        acoustic streaming, 441–442
        cavitation, 441
        compression, 440–441
        rarefaction, 440–441
    thermal, 440
        hyperthermia, 440
        thermal indices, 440
Biometry. *See* Fetal biometry

Biophysical profile (BPP)
    management recommendations, 83, 83t
    scoring, 83, 83t
Biparietal diameter (BPD), 72–73, 72t, 73f, 468–469, 468f, 469t
Bipartite placenta, 39, 39f, 40
Bladder outlet obstruction, 262
Bladder. *See* Urinary bladder
Blastocyst, 6–7, 6f
Bleeding, 4, 7, 13, 15–16, 18
    implantation, 4, 13
    per vaginam, 7, 13, 15–16, 18, 20
Blighted ovum. *See* Anembryonic pregnancy
Blood flow (fetal), 157–159. *See also* Cardiovascular system; Doppler sonography; Fetoplacental circulation; Great vessels; Pulsatility indices; Resistivity indices
    with coarctation of the aorta, 184
    with cord anomalies, 58, 61–62, 61f, 62f, 319–320, 320f
    in the embryo, 8
    in the endometrium, 412, 417, 418, 418f
    in the fetal heart, 159
    as a factor in infertility, 412
    mass assessment, 390–391, 391f
    during the menstrual cycle, 358–359
    with ovarian torsion, 377
    in pelvic vessels, 358–360
    in the placenta, 33–34, 48f
    renal, 253
    shunting of, 158–159, 173f, 175f, 181
    with twin reversed arterial perfusion sequence, 317
    umbilical vessels, 222f, 306–307
    with venous thrombosis, 335, 335f, 401
Bochdalek hernia, 168, 168f
BOD. *See* Binocular distance
Body stalk anomaly. *See* Limb–body wall complex
Bone measurements (fetal). *See* Femur length; Nasal bone length
Bony thorax, 159f

Bowel (fetal), 223, 278–279
    echogenicity, 225, 225f, 235f, 279f
    hyperechogenic, 278–279
    large (colon), 225
    obstruction of, 233f
    small, 224–225
BPD. See Biparietal diameter
BPP. See Biophysical profile
Brachiocephalic artery, 161
Bradycardia, embryonic, 1, 11, 11t, 14
Brain. See also Central nervous system; entries under Intracranial
    blood supply, 118–119
    brain stem, 117–118
    embryonic, 12
    fetal, 73f, 113–119f
    measuring BPD, 72–73
Brain sparing, 305, 308f
Breathing motion. See Fetal breathing motion
Breech presentation, 330
Brenner tumor, 392f. See also Transitional cell tumors
Brightness modulation. See B-mode imaging
Broad ligament, 349
Bulbus cordis, 156–157, 157f, 178

C

CA-125 tumor marker, 431–432, 471t
Calcaneus, 200, 200f, 213
Calcifications
    with cytomegalovirus, 327
    facial bones, 88
    hepatic, 238–239, 238f, 239f
    intracranial, 135, 309–310, 310f, 325
    with meconium peritonitis, 234, 234f
    with ovarian masses, 390–391
    placental, 37, 37f, 40, 40f, 305f
    with teratomas, 103, 104f, 392, 393, 394f
Caliectasis, 258f, 259, 259f, 260f
Calvaria, 72, 73, 75, 75f, 114, 138–140, 139f, 140f, 210, 211f

Campomelic dysplasia, 207–208, 208f
Canalicular phase of lung development, 152, 152f
Cancer antigen 125. See CA-125 tumor marker
Cancer. See Malignant masses; specific types
Caput membranaceum, 203, 204f
Cardiac activity, embryonic, 11f. See also Heart
Cardiac myxomas, 187
Cardiac positional abnormalities
    ectopia cordis, 186, 186f
    situs abnormalities, 184–186
Cardiac tumors, 187–188, 189f, 190
Cardiac wall abnormalities
    cardiac tumors, 187–190
    cardiomyopathy, 187
    pericardial effusion, 188–189
Cardinal ligament, 349
Cardiomegaly, 160, 160f, 187
Cardiomyopathy, 187, 188f
Cardiothoracic (C/T) circumference, 187
Cardiovascular system. See also Fetoplacental circulation; Heart
    abnormalities, 166t, 172–191
    anatomy, 156–159
    circulation, 156, 157–159
    embryology, 6–8, 11, 156–157, 156f
    sonographic anatomy, 159–165
    tube formation, 156
Carotid arteries (fetal), 118, 119, 119f, 161, 161f
Caudal neurophore, 112, 112f
Caudal regression syndrome, 289, 289f, 290f
Cavitation, 441, 441f
Cavum septi pellucidi, 114–115, 114f, 117f
Cavum vergae, 114–115, 114f
CBC. See Complete blood count
CDH. See Congenital diaphragmatic hernia
CDI. See Color Doppler imaging
Cebocephaly, 127
Central nervous system (fetal). See also Brain; entries under Intracranial; Neural
    abnormalities, 121–142, 122t

Central nervous system (fetal) *(continued)*
    brain development, 113–119
    embryology, 111–113
    spinal development, 119–120
Cephalic index (CI), 75
Cephalic presentation, 330
Cephalocele, 139–140
Cerclage procedures, 322, 323f
Cerebellar vermis, 114, 118, 129, 129f
Cerebellomedullary cistern. *See* Cisterna magna
Cerebellum, 73f, 81f, 82t, 114, 116f, 117–118, 117f, 118f, 119, 125f, 131f
Cerebral aqueduct, 116
Cerebral arteries, 118–119
Cerebral cortex, 116, 126, 128f
Cerebral hemispheres, 116–117
Cerebral peduncles, 117, 117f
Cervical anomalies (gynecologic)
    atresia (stenosis), 372
    DES-related, 372–373
    fibroids, 377
    nabothian cysts, 372
Cervical cerclage, 322, 323f
Cervical os (internal and external), 350–351, 354
Cervix
    anatomy, 350, 352–354, 354f
    anomalies, 372–373, 377
    cerclage procedures, 322, 323f
    incompetent, 321–322, 322f
    and infertility, 411–412
    measurement of, 467f
    os (internal and external), 350, 354, 354f
Cesarean section, 334, 334f
Chamber partitioning (fetal heart), 156–157
CHARGE association, 293–294, 294f
Chest (fetal), 151–172
    abnormalities, 151–152, 165–191, 166t
    bell-shaped, 206f
    circumference, 160
    embryology, 152f, 156–157
    masses, 166, 166t, 172–173, 172f

Chiari II malformation, 142–143
Chin abnormalities, 92, 101–105
Chocolate cysts, 400f
Choledochal cysts, 237, 237f
Chondroectodermal dysplasia. *See* Ellis–van Creveld syndrome
Chorioadenoma destruens, 23
Chorioangioma, 35, 49, 49f
Choriocarcinoma
    ovarian (gynecologic), 395, 395f
    uterine (gestational), 23–24, 24f
Chorion, 10f, 32f, 33
Chorion frondosum, 17, 32, 32f
Chorion laeve. *See* Chorion
Chorionic cavity, 7, 13
Chorionic plate, 33, 34, 34f, 37, 38, 41
Chorionic sac, 69–70
Chorionic villi, 7f, 33
Chorionic villus sampling (CVS), 274–275, 274f, 472
Choroid plexus, 113–116, 115f, 116f, 123
    cysts, 131, 131f, 207f, 280, 280f
    dangling, 123, 124f
Chromosomal analysis. *See also* Genetic testing
    amniocentesis, 275–276
    chromosomal markers, 471, 471t
Chronic retroplacental submembranous hematoma, 45, 46
CI. *See* Cephalic index
Circle of Willis, 118, 119f
Circulatory system. *See* Fetoplacental circulation; Heart
Circummarginate placenta, 38, 38f
Circumvallate placenta, 38, 38f
Cisterna magna, 117f, 118, 118f, 120f, 123f
    measurement of, 469, 469f, 469t
Clear cell carcinoma, 390
Clefting anomalies
    anterior, 92–94
    lip, 92–95, 93f, 95f
    median cleft facial syndrome, 93–94
    palate, 92–95, 93f, 95f

posterior, 92–93
prevalence, 94
Clinical standards and guidelines, 462, 491–520. *See also* Examinations
Cloacal exstrophy, 230–231, 230f, 231f
Clomid. *See* Clomiphene citrate
Clomiphene citrate, 413
Cloverleaf skull, 206f
Clubfoot. *See* Talipes equinovarus
CMN. *See* Congenital mesoblastic nephroma
CMV. *See* Cytomegalovirus
CNS. *See* Central nervous system
Coarctation of the aorta, 173, 180, 182, 184, 184f, 185f
Coccyx, 347f
Colon. *See* Bowel
Color Doppler imaging (CDI). *See also specific anatomy and pathologies*
    contraindications, 3, 11, 473
    umbilical imaging, 319–320, 320f
    pelvic vasculature, 358–361
    velocity imaging, 447f
Communicating hydrocephalus, 122
Complete abortion, 15
Complete blood count, 470, 470t
Complete hydatidiform mole, 20–21
Complete previa, 42–43, 43f
Compounding, 442–443
Compression, 440–441
Concealed abruption, 45–46, 46f
Conceptual age, 4–5, 5t. *See also* Gestational age; Menstrual age
Conceptus period, 6–7
Congenital adrenal hyperplasia, 427
Congenital cardiac abnormalities. *See also* Cardiac positional abnormalities; Cardiac wall abnormalities; Conotruncal anomalies; Fetal heart rate; Septal defects; Single ventricle anomalies; Ventricular septal size
    cardiac wall abnormalities, 173, 187–189
    conotruncal anomalies, 172, 176–180, 182
    disproportionate ventricular size, 183–184
    heart rate/rhythm abnormalities, 173, 189–191
    septal defects, 163, 173–176
    single ventricle anomalies, 163, 173, 180–182
Congenital diaphragmatic hernia (CDH), 167, 168–169, 186
Congenital mesoblastic nephroma (CMN), 265
Congenital primary megaureter, 260–261, 261f
Congenital pulmonary airway malformation. *See* Cystic adenomatoid malformation of the lung
Congenital rubella syndrome, 326–327
Conjoined twins, 312, 320–321, 321f
Conotruncal anomalies
    double-inlet left ventricle, 182
    double-outlet right ventricle, 164, 173, 176, 179–180
    persistent truncus arteriosus, 173, 176, 178–179
    tetralogy of Fallot, 164, 173, 176–177, 184
    transposition of the great vessels, 164, 176, 177–178, 182, 184, 186
Continuous wave (CW) Doppler, 446–447
Contrast procedures, 472
Conus medullaris, 120
Convex array transducers, 450f
Convex/curvilinear array transducers, 450–451
Cord. *See* Umbilical cord
Cord prolapse. *See* Prolapse
Cordocentesis, 336, 336f, 472
Coronal view of fetal heart, 519f
Corpora quadrigemina, 117
Corpus (uterine), 346, 350, 352, 352f, 353f
Corpus callosum, 114, 114f, 115
    agenesis of, 132f, 133f
Corpus luteum, 15, 16, 361, 364, 366, 366f
Corpus luteum cysts
    pathologic, 329, 385, 385f, 386f
    of pregnancy, 16, 386
Cortex (ovarian), 346–357, 357f
Cotyledons (placenta), 34, 40f, 41
CP cysts. *See* Choroid plexus
CPAM (cystic adenomatoid malformation of the lung). *See* Cystic adenomatoid malformation of the lung

CPCs. *See* Choroid plexus
Cranial fossae, 198f
Craniopagus twinning, 320
Craniopharyngiomas, 133
Crista dividens, 159
CRL. *See* Crown-rump length
Crown-rump length (CRL), 10, 14, 68, 69, 70–71, 71f
CRS. *See* Congenital rubella syndrome
C/T circumference. *See* Cardiothoracic (C/T) circumference
Cul-de-sacs, pelvic
    anterior, 355
    free fluid in, 19f
    posterior, 355
Cumulus oophorus, 364–365
Curvilinear (curved linear) transducers. *See* Convex/curvilinear array transducers
CVS. *See* Chorionic villus sampling
CW Doppler. *See* Continuous-wave (CW) Doppler
Cyclocephaly. *See* Cyclopia
Cyclopia, 96, 99–100, 100f
    with holoprosencephaly, 127, 127f
Cystadenocarcinoma, 389
    ovarian, 391f
Cystadenoma, 329, 329f, 390, 390f
Cystic adenomatoid malformation of the lung (CAML), 166, 169, 170, 170f, 171f
Cystic chest masses, 172
Cystic hepatic masses, 237f
Cystic hygroma, 101, 105, 105f
Cystic ovarian masses, 329–330
Cystic placental lesions, 40–42
    basal plate, 41–42
    mid-placental, 40, 41
    subchorionic, 40–41
Cystic/solid chest masses, 172
Cystic teratomas, 329
Cysts. *See also* entries under Cystic; Masses; Solid masses; *specific pathologies*
    chin and neck, 101, 103
    corpus luteum, 385f, 386f
    decidual, 9, 20
    follicular, 385f
    hemorrhagic (ovarian), 387f
    neck, 103, 103f
    ovarian (fetal), 240f, 329–330
    periventricular, 326f
    placental, 37, 40–41
    splenic, 240f
    subchorionic, 41f
Cytomegalovirus, 235f, 327, 327f
Cytotrophoblast, 7f, 32

D

Dandy-Walker malformation, 12, 129, 129f, 130f
Dangling choroid, 123, 124f
Data integration, 470
DD gestation. *See* Dichorionic/diamniotic gestations
Decidua basalis. *See* Decidual layers
Decidua capsularis. *See* Decidual layers
Decidua parietalis. *See* Decidual layers
Decidua reflexa. *See* Decidual layers
Decidua serotina. *See* Decidual layers
Decidua vera. *See* Decidual layers
Decidual cyst, 9, 20
Decidual layers 32, 32f, 34f, 36f
    decidua basalis (serotina), 9f, 10f, 16f, 17, 32–33, 32f, 34, 35, 47
    decidua capsularis (reflexa), 9f, 10f, 16f, 32, 32f
    decidua parietalis (vera), 9f, 10f, 16f, 32, 32f
Decidual thickening, 8
Demineralized cranial bones, 211f
Demise (fetal), 310–311. *See also* Abortion
DES-related anomalies. *See* Diethylstilbestrol
Diabetes (maternal)
    fetal effects, 323–324
    gestational, 323
    maternal effects, 323–324
    mellitus type I, 323
    mellitus type II, 323
    sonographic management, 324

Diagnostic Ultrasound Clinical Practice Standards (SDMS), 462
Diaphragm (fetal), 151, 159, 160, 160f, 166, 167, 169, 225
    hernia, 160, 166, 167, 168–169, 168f, 169f, 184, 186
Dichorionic/diamniotic gestations, 313, 313f, 314f
Didelphic uterus, 373, 373f, 374f
Diencephalon, 112, 113f, 116, 117f
Diethylstilbestrol, 372
Disomy, 282, 286–287
Disproportionate ventricular size, 183–184
    coarctation of the aorta, 180, 182, 184
    Ebstein's anomaly, 183, 190
Distance measurement accuracy, 474
Dizygotic gestations, 313
Dome of urinary bladder, 349
Dominant follicle, 359, 364–366, 365f–366f, 417f
    dysfunctional, 411f
Doppler effect, 444–446, 445f
Doppler shift, 445
Doppler sonography. *See also* Color Doppler imaging; Continuous-wave (CW) Doppler; Power Doppler imaging; Pulsatility indices; Pulsed-wave (PW) Doppler sonography; Resistivity indices; Spectral Doppler sonography; *specific clinical applications*
    color Doppler imaging, 447
    continuous-wave Doppler, 446–447
    contraindications, 3, 11, 307, 473
    power Doppler, 447–448
    spectral Doppler, 448
DORV. *See* Double-outlet right ventricle
Double bleb sign, 7, 9, 9f
    notochord, 7–8
Double bubble sign, 232
Double decidual sac sign, 10, 10f
Double-inlet left ventricle, 182, 182f, 183f, 184
Double-outlet right ventricle (DORV), 164, 173, 176, 179–180, 180f
Double sac sign, 9–10, 19–20, 32
Douglas, pouch of, 355
Down syndrome. *See* Trisomy 21

DUB. *See* Dysfunctional uterine bleeding
Ductal arch view of fetal heart, 518f
Ductus arteriosus, 158–159, 160–161, 176, 177, 181, 184
Ductus venosus, 158–159, 158f, 222, 222f
Duodenal atresia, 232, 232f
Duplex renal collecting system, 262
Dura mater, 117
Dural landmarks, 117
Dwell time, 473
Dysfunctional dominant follicle, 410–411
Dysfunctional uterine bleeding, 380–381
Dysgerminoma, 394, 395f
Dysostoses, 212–214
    radial ray anomaly, 212
    rocker bottom foot, 214
    talipes equinovarus, 212–213
Dystocia, 377
    fibroid-related, 377

E

Eagle-Barrett syndrome. *See* Prune belly syndrome
Ear (fetal), 91f
Early pregnancy factor (EPF), 4
Ebstein's anomaly, 163, 183, 183f, 190
Echocardiography (fetal), 165
Echogenic fetal bowel (EFB), 235
Echogenic intracardiac focus (EIF), 279–280, 280f
Ectopia cordis, 184, 186, 186f
Ectopic pregnancy, 17–20
    adnexal mass, 18–19
    decidual cyst, 9, 20
    diagnostic criteria, 18
    etiologies, 17
    free fluid, 18–19, 19f
    heterotopic, 14, 18–19, 19f
    implantation sites, 18, 18t
    incidence, 18, 18t
    presentation, 18
    progesterone levels, 4
    pseudogestational sac, 9, 19–20

Ectopic pregnancy *(continued)*
    ring of fire sign, 19, 19f
    risk factors, 17
    sonographic signs, 14, 18–20
Ectopic ureterocele, 260, 260f, 261f
EDC. *See* Estimated date of confinement
Edema, scalp, 303f
Edwards syndrome. *See* Trisomy 18
EFB. *See* Echogenic fetal bowel
EIF. *See* Echogenic intracardiac focus
Electrical/mechanical performance, 474
Ellis–van Creveld syndrome, 290–291, 291f
Embryology, 6–13
    anatomy, 10
    cardiovascular system, 6–8, 11, 11f, 156–157, 156f
    central nervous system, 111–113
    chest, 152f, 156–157
    conceptus period, 6–7
    embryonic period, 8
    face, 88–92
    gastrointestinal tract, 6–8, 219–221, 220f
    genitalia, 6–8
    genitourinary system, 6–8, 247–248
    heart, 6–8, 11f, 156–157
    lungs, 151–152, 152f
    measurements, 69–71
    musculoskeletal system, 8, 201–214
    neck, 89–92
    placenta, 31–50
    time line, 5t, 6–8
    umbilical cord, 53
Embryonic buds, 11f
Embryonic demise, 14f. *See also* Abortion; Fetal demise
Embryonic disc
    bilaminar, 6–7, 7f, 9
    trilaminar, 7
Embryonic gut, 220f
Embryonic membranes
    amniotic, 33, 33f
    chorionic, 33, 33f, 35, 35f, 38, 41f
    formation of, 33
    umbilical cord formation, 53
Embryonic period, 8
    cardiac activity, 10–11, 18
Embryonic phase of lung development, 151–152
Encephalocele, 98, 101, 139–140
    frontal, 96
    occipital 139f, 140f, 141f
Encephalomalacia, 134
Endocardial cushions, 156–157, 157f, 163, 175–176
Endometrial assessment (infertility treatment), 417–418
Endometrial carcinoma, 382f
Endometrial epithelium, 7f
Endometrial hyperplasia, 380, 380f
Endometrial pathologies
    carcinoma, 381
    dysfunctional uterine bleeding, 380–381
    endometritis, 381
    hyperplasia, 380
    polyps, 383
Endometrial polyps, 383f, 384f
Endometrioid carcinoma, 390
Endometriomas, 399
Endometriosis, 399–400, 400f
Endometritis, 381, 381f, 398f
Endometrium, 350–352, 351f, 352f
    assessment in infertility, 418f
    measurement technique, 467f
    measurements, 352t
    postmenopausal, 428f
    thickness, 352t, 429t, 500f
Endovaginal and transperineal imaging, 464, 465, 465f
    contraindications, 464
    first trimester, 9, 10, 11, 13
    patient preparation, 464
    transducers, 451, 451f
Enhanced through-transmission. *See* Posterior acoustic enhancement
EPF. *See* Early pregnancy factor
Epignathus, 102, 103, 104, 104f

Epiphyses, 198
    appearance, 77f, 79–80, 79f, 79t
Epithelial ovarian tumors, 390–391
Erythroblastosis fetalis, 302
Esophageal atresia, 231, 231f
Estimated due date, 69
Estimated date of confinement (EDC), 69
Estradiol, 361
    levels during menstrual cycle, 362f
Estriol (μE3), 273t, 274, 471t
Ethmocephaly, 127, 127f
Examinations. *See also* Clinical standards and guidelines
    preparation, 462–464
    protocols, 462–474
Exencephaly (acrania), 137f, 138–139, 139f
Exophytic fibroids, 377
Expected date of delivery, 69
External abruption, 45, 46, 46f
Extrachorial placental variants, 35, 38–39, 38f
Extrauterine pregnancy. *See* Ectopic pregnancy

F

Face (fetal), 87–105
    abnormalities, 92–105, 92t
    anatomy, 88f, 89f, 90f, 91f, 92f
    embryology, 88–92
    skeletal anatomy, 198f
Failed pregnancy, 13–23
    diagnostic criteria, 4–5, 14, 18–20
    progesterone levels, 4
    sonographic signs, 5, 10, 14–23, 24f
Fallopian tubes, 356
    anatomy, 356f
    and infertility, 411
    tissue layers, 356
    tubal transit, 6f
Fallot, tetralogy of, 176f
False-negative results, 273
False pelvis, 347, 347f, 348f
False-positive results, 272–273
Falx cerebri, 117, 117f
FBS. *See* Cordocentesis
Feet, 200f
Female infertility. *See* Infertility
Femur, 199f, 210f, 211f
Femur length (FL), 72t, 76–77, 77f, 77t, 79f 468–469, 468f, 469t
Fertilization, 4, 5, 6, 6f, 12
Fetal activity, 83
Fetal anemia, 309
Fetal biometry, 67–85
    first trimester, 67–71
    multiple gestations, 68
    parameters, 68, 71, 72t, 80, 83
    second/third trimesters, 72–82
Fetal biophysical profile. *See* Biophysical profile
Fetal blood sampling. *See* Cordocentesis
Fetal breathing motion, 83, 83t
Fetal circulation. *See* Fetoplacental circulation
Fetal complications, 302–311, 302t
    anemia, 309
    demise, 310–311
    diabetes-related, 323–324
    hydrops fetalis, 302–304
    intracranial calcifications, 309–310
    intrauterine growth restriction, 304–308
    with multiple gestations, 311
    therapies, 335–337
Fetal demise, 310–311. *See also* Abortion
Fetal echocardiography, 165
    indications for, 165
    practice guidelines, 515–520
    scanning planes, 518f
Fetal growth parameters, 67–83. *See also* Abdominal circumference; Biparietal diameter; Crown-rump length; Femur length; Head circumference; Mean sac diameter; Orbits; Transcerebellar diameter
Fetal heart rate, 11, 11t, 83, 189–191, 190f, 469, 469f, 469t, 473

Fetal lie. *See* Fetal position
Fetal pericardial effusion, 183, 186, 188–189
Fetal position
    lie, 330–331, 331f
    presentation, 330–331, 331f
Fetal presentation. *See* Fetal position
Fetal supraventricular tachycardia, 189–190
Fetal therapy, 335–337
Fetal tone, 83, 83t
Fetal weight percentile chart, 309f
Fetoplacental circulation, 33f, 34f, 54f, 157–159, 158f
Fetus papyraceus, 318–319, 319f
FHR. *See* Fetal heart rate
Fibroids, 329f
    leiomyomas, 376
    myomas, 376
    submucosal, 412f
    uterine, 376f, 377f, 378f
Fibromas
    cardiac, 187
    ovarian, 396, 396f
Fibula, 200f
Filly's rule, 123, 123f
Fimbria, 356
Fingers, 199f, 202f
First International Reference Preparation (1st IRP), 5, 5t
First trimester, 3–29. *See also* Embryology
    abnormal, 13–24
    examination protocols, 3–4, 463, 464, 466
    normal, 4–13
    time line, 5t, 6–8
FL. *See* Femur length
Focused reproductive endocrinology and infertility scan practice guidelines, 512–515
Follicle-stimulating hormone (FSH), 361
    levels during menstrual cycle, 362f
Follicles, 356–357, 357f, 359, 361, 363–366
    antral, 416f
    aspiration, 419, 419f
    cysts, 385f
    dominant, 365f, 366f
    measurement of, 467f
    monitoring (infertility treatment), 415–417
    subdominant, 417f
Follicular phase of menstrual cycle, 359f, 364, 365f
Foramen of Magendie, 116
Foramen ovale, 156–157, 158f, 159, 162–163, 174–175, 178, 180, 181
Foramina of Luschka, 116, 118, 122
Foramina of Monro, 115, 116
Forebrain, 112, 116–117
    diverticulation, 126
Fornix of cerebrum, 114
Four-chamber view of fetal heart, 162f, 175f, 176f, 518f
    tricuspid regurgitation, 184f
Four-dimensional (4D) ultrasound, 443
Four-quadrant amniotic fluid index. *See* Amniotic fluid index
Fraternal twins. *See* Dizygotic gestations
Free fluid
    in cul-de-sacs, 18, 19, 19f, 399f, 417f
    in paracolic gutters, 19
Frequencies (transducers), 449
    fundamental, 449
    harmonic, 449
Frequency compounding, 442–443
Frequency shift, 445
    negative, 445
Frontonasal dysplasia sequence. *See* Median cleft facial syndrome
Frontonasal prominence, 88, 88f
FSH. *See* Follicle-stimulating hormone
Functional ovarian cysts, 384–388
Fundus, uterine, 350, 350f, 353f

G

Gallbladder (fetal), 224, 224f
    abnormalities, 238f, 239
Gamete intrafallopian transfer (GIFT), 415, 472
Gamma-glutamyl transpeptidase (GGTP), 275
Gartner's duct cysts, 372f, 426
Gastrointestinal atresia, 231–232

Gastrointestinal tract (fetal), 8, 13. *See also* Abdomen (fetal)
    abnormalities, 219–241
    embryology, 6–8, 219–221, 220f
Gastroschisis, 226, 227–229, 228f
Genetic sonographic fetal anatomic survey, 276–281
Genetic testing (prenatal), 271–294
    abnormalities, 282–287
    anatomic survey, 276–281
    associations, 287, 293–294
    chromosomal analysis, 278–276
    indications, 272
    invasive procedures, 274–276
    maternal serum testing, 272–273, 273t
    sequences, 287
    syndromes, 287–293
Genital system (fetal). *See* Genitourinary system
Genitalia (fetal), 250–251
    ambiguous, 427
    embryology, 6–8
    female, 250, 250f
    male, 250–251, 250f
Genitourinary neoplasms, 264–266, 266f
Genitourinary system (fetal), 247–266
    abnormalities, 251–266, 252t
    anatomy, 248–251
    embryology, 6–8, 247–248
Germ cell tumors, 392–395
    ovarian, 392–395
German measles, 326–327
Germinal epithelium (ovarian), 356
Gestational age, 5, 68–69, 70–83, 72t. *See also* Conceptual age; Fetal growth parameters; Menstrual age
    conceptual age, 4, 5, 5t, 68–69
    determining, 68–69
    menstrual age, 4, 5, 5t, 6, 68–69
Gestational diabetes, 323
Gestational hypertension, 324–325
Gestational sac, 5, 7–20, 9f, 14f, 69–71
    measurement, 70f

    pseudogestational, 9, 19–20
    sonographic signs, 9–10
Gestational trophoblastic disease (GTD), 20–24
    complete hydatidiform mole, 20–21
    hydropic degeneration of the placenta, 22
    mole with coexisting fetus, 21–22
    partial mole, 21
Gestational viability, 11–12, 11t
    sonographic signs, 11–12
GGTP. *See* Gamma-glutamyl transpeptidase
GIFT. *See* Gamete intrafallopian transfer
GIP. *See* Glucose intolerance of pregnancy
Glioblastomas, 133, 134f
Glucose intolerance of pregnancy, 323
GnRH-a. *See* Gonadotropin-releasing hormone agonists
Gonadal dysgenesis, 426
Gonadal vein, 360
Gonadotropin-releasing hormone agonists (GnRH-a), 410, 413, 414, 416
Graafian follicle, 357f, 364, 366f
Grannum's placental grading system, 37, 37f, 40f
Granulosa cell tumors, 395–396
Grating lobe artifacts, 457, 457f
Great vessels (fetal)
    abnormalities, 172–191
    embryology, 156–157, 157f
    sonographic anatomy, 160–161, 161f
    transposition of, 164, 177–178, 182, 184, 186
Growth parameters, fetal, 67–83. *See also* Abdominal circumference; Biparietal diameter; Crown-rump length; Examinations; Femur length; Head circumference; Mean sac diameter
GTD. *See* Gestational trophoblastic disease
GTN (gestational trophoblastic neoplasia). *See* Gestational trophoblastic disease
Guided follicular aspiration, 419, 419f
Gynecology
    examinations, 463
    infertility, 409–419
    pediatric, 422–427
    pelvic anatomy and physiology, 345–366

Gynecology *(continued)*
    pelvic pathology, 371–401
    postmenopausal, 428–433
Gyri, 116

H

Hamartoma, renal fetal, 265
Hand (fetal), 199f
HC. *See* Head circumference
hCG. *See* Human chorionic gonadotropin, beta subunit
Head circumference (HC), 72t, 73–75, 74t, 75f, 468–469, 469t
Heart (fetal), 156–165, 172–191. *See also entries under* Cardiac; Cardiovascular system; Fetoplacental circulation
    abnormalities, 166t, 172–191
    apical five-chamber view, 164, 165f
    embryology, 6–8, 11f, 156–157
    fetal heart rate, 11, 11t, 83, 173, 189–191, 469f, 469t
    four-chamber view of fetal, 162–163, 162f
    LVOT view, 163, 163f
    rhythm abnormalities, 173, 189–191
    RVOT view, 164, 164f
    sonographic anatomy, 10–11, 159–165
Heart rate. *See* Fetal heart rate
Hemangiomas, 62–63, 188
    cardiac, 188
    umbilical cord, 62–63, 63f
Hematogenesis, 7
Hematoma. *See also* Hemorrhage
    in gestational sac, 16f
    postpartum, 334, 335f
    subchorionic, 41f
    umbilical cord, 58, 62, 64
Hematometrocolpos, 425, 425f
Hemolytic disease, 302
Hemorrhage. *See also* Hematoma
    intracranial hemorrhage in utero, 133–134
    marginal placental hemorrhage, 46
    postpartum, 332, 333f
    subchorionic, 17f, 46, 46f, 47f

Hemorrhagic ovarian cysts, 386–387, 387f
Hepatic calcifications, 238–239, 238f
Hepatic masses (fetal), 236–238
    cystic, 237, 237f
    solid, 236, 236f
Hepatic veins (fetal), 222, 222f
Hepatoblastoma, 237f
Hepatomegaly (fetal), 235, 235f, 303f
Hermaphroditism, 427. *See also* Pseudohermaphroditism
Herniation
    cloacal exstrophy, 230–231
    gastroschisis, 227–229
    limb–body wall complex, 229–230
    midgut (physiologic), 220–221, 226, 229
    omphalocele, 220–221, 226–227
Herpes simplex virus, 327–328
Heterotaxy syndrome, 185
Heterotopic pregnancy, 14, 18–19, 19f
Heterozygous achondroplasia, 204
High-risk pregnancies. *See* At-risk pregnancies
High short-axis view of fetal heart, 519f
Higher-order gestations, 313–314, 313f, 314f
Hindbrain, 112, 117–118, 118f
hMG. *See* Human menopausal gonadotropin
Holoprosencephaly, 126–128
    alobar, 126, 126f
    facial anomalies, 126, 127f
    lobar, 126–127, 126f
    semilobar, 126, 126f
Holoventricle, 126. *See also* Monoventricle
Homozygous dominant achondroplasia, 204
Hormone levels during menstrual cycle, 362f
Hormone replacement therapy (HRT), 429–430
HRT. *See* Hormone replacement therapy
HSV. *See* Herpes simplex virus
Human chorionic gonadotropin, beta subunit (beta-hCG), 4–5, 5t, 8, 10, 12, 15–16, 18, 20, 22, 273t, 274, 471, 471t
Human menopausal gonadotropin (hMG), 413–414
Humegon. *See* Human menopausal gonadotropin

Humerus, 199f
HyCoSy. *See* Hysterosalpingo contrast sonography
Hydatidiform mole
    with coexisting fetus, 21–22, 22f
    complete, 20–21, 20f, 21f
    partial, 21–22
Hydranencephaly, 124–125, 125f
Hydrocephalus, 122–123, 123f, 124f. *See also* Ventriculomegaly
Hydronephrosis, 258–259, 258f, 259f
Hydropic degeneration of the placenta, 22
Hydrops
    fetalis, 50, 167f, 302–304
    immune, 302
    nonimmune, 302, 303f, 304f
    placental, 35, 50
    risk factors, 302–303
Hydrosalpinx, 398f
Hyperechogenic bowel, 278–279
Hypertelorism, 96–98, 99f
Hypertensive disorders of pregnancy, 324–325
Hyperthermia, 440
Hypogastric arteries. *See* Iliac vessels
Hypomineralization of facial bones, 211f
Hypophosphatasia, 210
Hypoplastic left heart syndrome, 180–181, 181f
Hypoplastic right ventricle, 180–181, 182f
Hypoplastic thorax, 206f
Hypotelorism, 96, 98–99, 99f, 104
Hypothalamus, 114f, 410
    infertility and, 410
Hysterosalpingo contrast sonography (HyCoSy), 419, 472
Hysterosonography, 375f, 384f, 419

I

ICH. *See* Intracranial hemorrhage in utero
Identical twins. *See* Monochorionic/monoamniotic gestations
Idiopathic osteolyses, 209–210
    hypophosphatasia, 210
    osteogenesis imperfecta, 210

IHF. *See* Immune hydrops fetalis
Iliac bones, 347
Iliac vessels, 56f, 249f, 358, 358f, 360, 360f
Iliacus, 347
Ilium, 347f
Imaging artifacts. *See* Artifacts
Imaging modes, 442–444
Immature cystic teratoma, 393, 393f, 394f
Immune hydrops fetalis (IHF), 302
Imperforate anus, 233, 233f
Implantation bleeding, 4, 13
Implantation of conceptus, 5t, 6–8, 7f. *See also* Ectopic pregnancy
In vitro fertilization (IVF), 414–415, 472
Incompetent cervix, 321–322, 322f
Incomplete abortion, 15–16
Infantile polycystic kidney disease (IPKD), 253–255, 254f, 255f
Infarction. *See* Basal plate
Inferior vena cava, 157, 158f, 162, 167, 360
Infertility, 409–419
    causes, 410–413
    cervical factors, 411–412
    female, 410–413
    male, 410
    ovulation disorders, 410–411
    sonographic management, 415–419
    treatment, 413–415
    tubal factors, 411
    uterine factors, 412
Infundibulopelvic ligament, 348
Infundibulum, 356
Inhibin A (inhA), 272, 273, 273t, 471t
Iniencephaly, 140–141, 141f
Innominate artery. *See* Brachiocephalic artery
Instrumentation
    distance measurement accuracy, 474
    quality assurance, 473–474
    safety, 472–473
    sterility/cleanliness, 473–474

Instrumentation *(continued)*
    transducers, 448–457
    workstation image display, 474
Integration of data, 470
Interbrain, 116
Interligamentous fibroids, 377
Interocular distance. *See* Interorbital distance
Interorbital distance (IOD), 80, 80t, 81f, 92f, 96f, 99f
Intersex state. *See* Sexual ambiguity
Interthalamic adhesion, 116
Interventricular foramen, 156–157, 157f
Interventricular septum, 156–157, 162, 164, 173–174
Intervillous thrombosis, 41, 42f
Intracavitary approach, 465–466
    endovaginal, 465
    transesophageal, 465
    transrectal, 465
Intracostal approach, 464
Intracranial abnormalities
    cystic, 122–131
    solid, 132–137
Intracranial calcifications, 135, 309–310, 310f
Intracranial hemorrhage in utero, 133–134
Intracranial vasculature, 119
Intracranial vesicles and ventricles, 112–113
Intradecidual sign, 9
Intramural fibroids, 376
Intramural portion of fallopian tube, 356
Intraperitoneal fetal transfusion, 337
Intrauterine adhesions. *See* Asherman syndrome
Intrauterine contraceptive devices (IUDs/IUCDs), 412–413
    infertility and, 412–413, 413f
Intrauterine fetal transfusion, 337, 472
Intrauterine growth restriction (IUGR)
    asymmetric, 305–306
    Doppler evaluation, 304, 306–308
    etiology, 304–305
    symmetric, 305, 305f
    weight estimations, 308

Intrauterine pregnancy, 4–5, 6–10, 20
    sonographic signs, 8, 9f
Intravascular fetal transfusion, 337
Invasive mole, 23, 23f
Invasive procedures
    amniocentesis, 472
    amnioinfusion, 472
    amnioreduction, 472
    assisted reproductive techniques, 472
    chorionic villus sampling, 472
    contrast procedures, 472
    fetal blood sampling, 472
    intrauterine fetal transfusion, 472
    oocyte retrieval, 472
    sonographer's role, 471–472
    sonohysterography, 472
IOD. *See* Interorbital distance
IPKD. *See* Infantile polycystic kidney disease
Ischia, 346, 347f
Ischiopagus twinning, 320
Isthmic portion of fallopian tube, 356
Isthmus, uterine, 350
IUCDs. *See* Intrauterine contraceptive devices
IUDs. *See* Intrauterine contraceptive devices
IUGR. *See* Intrauterine growth restriction
IVF. *See* In vitro fertilization

J

Jeune thoracic dystrophy, 208–209
Jugular veins, 161

K

Karyotypes (human), 274–275, 282–286
    defined, 282
    normal, 275f
    with triploidy, 283f
    with trisomy 13, 285f
    with trisomy 18, 285f
    with trisomy 21, 284f

Kidneys (fetal), 248. *See also entries under* Renal
    abnormalities, 251–258
    embryology, 6–8, 248, 248f
    normal appearance, 249f
Knots (umbilical), 58, 59
    false, 59
    true, 59
Krukenberg tumors, 396–397, 397f

L

L/S ratio. *See* Lecithin/sphingomyelin (L/S) ratio
Labor
    preterm, 331
Laboratory values, 4. *See also* Maternal serum markers
    early pregnancy factor (EPF), 4
    human chorionic gonadotropin, beta subunit (beta-hCG), 4–5, 5t, 8, 10, 12, 15–16, 18, 20, 22, 273t, 274, 471, 471t
    progesterone, 4, 16
Lamina terminalis, 116
Laparoschisis. *See* Gastroschisis
Large for gestational age (LGA), 324
Last menstrual period (LMP), 4, 5, 68–69
Lateral cervical ligament, 348–349
Lateral ventricle, 469, 469t, 469f
Lecithin/sphingomyelin (L/S) ratio, 155
Left ventricular outflow tract view (fetal heart), 163, 518f
Leiomyomas, 376
    uterine, 328–329
Leiomyosarcoma, 377–378, 378f
Lemon sign, 142–143, 143f
Levator ani muscle group, 347, 347f
LGA. *See* Large for gestational age
LH. *See* Luteinizing hormone
Lie (fetal), 330–331, 331f
Ligaments, 348–349
    broad, 349
    cardinal, 348–349
    infundibulopelvic, 348
    lateral cervical, 349

    mesovarium, 348
    osseous pelvic, 348, 348f
    ovarian suspensory, 348, 348f
    pubic, 348
    pubovesicular, 349
    rectouterine, 349
    round, 349
    sacrococcygeal, 348
    sacroiliac, 348
    sacrosciatic, 348
    sacrospinous, 348
    uterine, 349, 349f
    utero-ovarian, 348
    uterosacral, 349
Limb–body wall complex, 229–230, 229f, 230f
Limb shortening, 201f, 202f
Linea terminalis, 347, 348f
Linear array transducers, 450, 450f
Lissencephaly, 135
Liver (fetal), 221–223, 222f
    abnormalities, 235–238
    anatomy, 221
    loss of parenchymal homogeneity, 235–236, 236f
    masses, 236f, 237f
LMP. *See* Last menstrual period
Lobar holoprosencephaly, 126–127, 126f, 128f
Long bones
    bowed, 211f
    lower extremity, 200f
    upper extremity, 199f
Long umbilical cord, 58, 59, 60
Longitudinal lie, 331
Looping, cardiac, 157
Low-lying placenta, 44f
Low-lying previa, 44–45
Low short-axis view of fetal heart, 519f
LUF syndrome. *See* Luteinized unruptured follicle syndrome
Lungs (fetal)
    abnormalities, 165–172
    amniotic fluid role, 153–156

Lungs (fetal) *(continued)*
    embryology, 151–152, 152f
    maturity studies, 155–156
    sonographic anatomy, 160
Luschka, foramina of, 116
Luteal phase of menstrual cycle, 366
Luteinization, 361
Luteinized unruptured follicle syndrome, 410
Luteinizing hormone (LH), 361
    during menstrual cycle, 362f
LVOT view. *See* Left ventricular outflow tract view

M

M-mode imaging, 444, 444f, 473
    atrial flutter, 190f
    atrioventricular block, 191f
    embryonic heart, 473f
    fetal heart rate, 11, 11f, 469f, 469t
    fetal tachycardia, 190f
    premature atrial contractions, 191f
    premature ventricular contractions, 190f
Macroglossia, 102f, 138f, 289f
Macrophthalmia, 138f
Macrosomia, 308, 323–324
Magendie, foramen of, 116
Male infertility. *See* Infertility
Malignant masses
    coexisting with pregnancy, 328, 330
    endometrial, 380–383, 382f
    gestational trophoblastic neoplasia, 22–23
    invasive mole, 23
    leiomyosarcoma, 377–378
    neuroblastoma, 264–265
    ovarian, 388–396, 390t, 391f, 395f
    pediatric, 423–424
    pregnancy-associated, 330
    scoring, 389, 389t
    tamoxifen-related, 430
    teratomas, 103
    Wilms tumor, 265
Malignant mixed germ cell tumors, 395
Malposition, uterine, 352–353
Mandibular prominences, 88, 88f
Marginal cord insertion, 61f
Marginal placental hemorrhage, 46, 46f
Marginal previa, 44, 44f
Marginal subchorionic hemorrhage, 46, 46f, 47f
Massa intermedia, 116
Masses. *See also* Cysts; Solid masses; *specific pathologies*
    cardiac, 187–188, 189f
    coexisting with pregnancy, 328–330
    cystic, 329–330
    fetal chest, 172f
    hepatic, 236f
    intracranial (fetal), 133
    malignant, 330
    measurement of, 468f
    ovarian, 329–330
    pediatric ovarian, 423–424
    pediatric uterine, 425–426
    pediatric vaginal, 426
    postmenopausal adnexal, 431
    postmenopausal ovarian, 430
    postmenopausal uterine, 430–431
    solid, 330
    uterine, 328–323, 376–379
Maternal complications, 302t, 321–330. *See also* Pelvic pathology
    coexisting masses, 328–329
    diabetes, 322–323
    hypertensive disorders of pregnancy, 324–325
    incompetent cervix, 321–322
    with multiple gestations, 311
    TORCH Infections, 325–328
    uterine rupture, 328
Maternal diabetes, 322–323
Maternal lakes, 41
Maternal serum alpha-fetoprotein (MSAFP), 273–274, 273t, 471t

Maternal serum markers, 272–274, 273t. *See also* Alpha-fetoprotein; Estriol; Human chorionic gonadotropin, beta subunit; Inhibin A; Laboratory values; Quad screen; Triple screen

Matrix array transducers, 451, 451f

Mature cystic teratomas, 392, 393f

Maxilla, 88, 89–91, 91f, 93

Maxillary prominences, 88, 88f

Maximum vertical pocket (MVP), 153, 155

MCA. *See* Middle cerebral arteries

MCKD. *See* Multicystic dysplastic kidney disease

MD gestation. *See* Monochorionic/diamniotic gestations

Mean sac diameter (MSD), 9, 10, 12, 14, 69–70

Measurement techniques, 466–469, 466t, 467f–469f, 469t

Mechanical bioeffects of ultrasound, 440–442

Mechanical index, 442

Meckel-Gruber syndrome, 291–292, 292f

Meconium peritonitis, 234, 234f

Median cleft facial syndrome, 93–94, 94f

Medulla (ovarian), 357, 357f

Medulla oblongata, 118, 118f, 120f

Medullary cone, 120

Megalencephaly, 136–137

Megaureter, congenital primary, 260–261

Membranes. *See* Embryonic membranes; Premature rupture of membranes; Preterm premature rupture of membranes

Menarche, 361

Menopause, 361, 428–433. *See also entries under* Postmenopausal

Menopur. *See* Human menopausal gonadotropin

Menstrual age, 4, 5, 5t, 6. *See also* Conceptual age; Gestational age

Menstrual cycle, 361–366
    hormone levels during, 362f
    ovarian response, 364–366
    uterine response, 361–364, 362f, 363f

Menstrual phase of menstrual cycle, 363

Menstruation, 361. *See also* Menstrual cycle

Mermaid syndrome, 290

Meromelia, 202, 202f

Mesencephalon. *See* Midbrain

Mesomelia, 201, 201f

Mesonephroi, 248, 248f

Mesovarium ligament, 348

Metanephroi, 248

Metastatic ovarian tumors, 396

Metatarsals, 200f

Metatropic dysplasia, 209. *See also* Gastroschisis

Metencephalon, 113f

MI. *See* Mechanical index

Microbubbles, 441, 441f

Microcephaly, 100, 135, 136f, 327f

Microencephaly, 135–136

Micrognathia, 101–102, 102f, 327f

Micromelia, 201, 201f, 204f, 207f

Microphthalmia, 96, 100–101, 101f

Micturition (fetal), 349

Midbrain, 112, 113f, 117, 117f

Middle cerebral arteries, 119, 119f
    Doppler studies, 307
    pulsatility index, 308f
    resistivity, 308f

Midgut herniation, 8, 12, 12f, 220–221, 221f
    vs. omphalocele, 220–221

Mid placental lesions, 40, 41, 41f
    maternal lakes, 41, 41f
    septal cysts, 41

Mirena. *See* Intrauterine contraceptive devices

Mirror-image artifacts, 456, 456f

Miscarriage. *See* Spontaneous abortion

MM gestation. *See* Monochorionic/monoamniotic gestations

Molar pregnancy, 20–22, 21f, 22f, 23f. *See also* Hydropic degeneration of the placenta; Persistent trophoblastic neoplasia
    complete, 20–21
    with coexisting fetus, 21–22
    partial, 21

MoM. *See* Multiples of the median

Momentum transfer, 441
Monochorionic/diamniotic gestations, 312, 313f, 314f
Monochorionic/monoamniotic gestations, 312, 312f, 314f
Monosomy, 282
Monoventricle, 126, 128f
Monozygotic twins, 312–313
Monro, foramina of, 115
Morgagni hernia, 168
Morula, 6, 6f
Motion mode. *See* M-mode imaging
MRD. *See* Multicystic renal dysplasia
MSAFP. *See* Maternal serum alpha-fetoprotein
MSD. *See* Mean sac diameter
Müllerian ducts, 247
    anomalies, 330f, 373–375, 373f
    arcuate uterus, 373
    bicornuate uterus, 373
    didelphic uterus, 373
    septate uterus, 373
    unicornuate uterus, 373
    uterine agenesis, 373
Multicystic dysplastic kidney disease (MCKD), 254t, 255–256
Multicystic renal dysplasia (MRD), 255–256, 255f, 256f
Multiple-gestation pregnancies, 311–321. *See also* Twin pregnancies
    clinical findings, 311–312
    dizygotic twins, 313
    evaluation protocols, 314–315
    fetal complications, 311
    higher-order, 313–314
    maternal complications, 311
    monozygotic twins, 312–313
    placentation/membranes, 312
Multiples of the median (MoM), 273
Musculature, pelvic, 347
Musculoskeletal system, 8, 201–214
MVP. *See* Maximum vertical pocket
Myomas, 376
Myxomas, cardiac, 187

N

Nabothian cysts, 372, 372f
Nasal bone length, 81–82
Neck (fetal), 87, 89–105
    abnormalities, 92, 92t, 101–105
    cysts, 103f
    embryology, 89–92
    teratomas, 104f
Negative frequency shift, 445
Neoplasms, genitourinary, 266f
Neoplastic markers, 471, 471t
Neoplastic ovarian masses, 388–397
    epithelial, 390–391
    germ cell, 392–395
    Krukenberg, 396–397
    metastatic, 396
    pediatric, 423–424
    scoring, 389–390, 389t
    sex cord stromal, 395–396
Neopores, 112
Nephroblastoma (Wilms tumor), 265
Neural plate, 7–8, 8f
Neural tube, 7–8, 8f, 112
Neural tube defects, 137–143, 137f
    anencephaly, 137–138
    cephalocele, 139–140
    encephalocele, 139–140
    exencephaly (acrania), 138–139
    iniencephaly, 140–141
    spina bifida, 141–143
Neuroblastomas, 264–266, 265f
Neurulation, 5, 7–8, 8f, 111–112, 112f
NIHF. *See* Nonimmune hydrops fetalis
Nomograms
    binocular distance, 96f
    fetal weight, 309f
    interocular distance, 96f
    middle cerebral artery pulsatility index, 308f
    umbilical artery pulsatility index, 307f

umbilical artery resistivity index, 306f
umbilical artery S/D ratios, 306f
Nonimmune hydrops fetalis (NIHF), 302
Non-neoplastic ovarian lesions, 384–388
Nonstress test (NST), 83, 83t
Nose (fetal), 91f, 92f
Notochord, 8f
NST. See Nonstress test
Nuchal cord, 59f
Nuchal thickening, 278, 278f
    measuring technique, 278
    vs. nuchal translucency, 278
    values, 278
Nuchal translucency, 12–13, 276–277
    abnormal, 13f
    measuring technique, 277, 277f, 494f
    values, 277
Nuchal umbilical cord, 59

O

Oblique lie, 331
Obstetric ultrasound practice guidelines, 491–498
Obstetrics
    at-risk pregnancies, 301–337
    exam protocols, 462–466
    fetal abdomen and pelvis, 219–245
    fetal biometry, 67–85
    fetal central nervous system, 111–149
    fetal chest, lungs, and heart, 151–195
    fetal face and neck, 87–109
    fetal genitourinary tract, 247–270
    fetal skeleton, 197–217
    first trimester, 3–29, 466
    multiple-gestation pregnancies, 301–342
    placenta, 31–52
    prenatal genetic workup, 271–300
    second/third trimesters, 466
    umbilical cord, 53–66
Obstructive cystic renal dysplasia (OCRD), 254t, 257–258, 257f
Obstructive uropathies, 258–264

Obturator artery, 358
Obturator internus, 347
Occipitofrontal diameter (OFD), 73, 75
OCRD. See Obstructive cystic renal dysplasia
OD. See Orbital diameter
OEIS complex, 230
OFD. See Occipitofrontal diameter
OHSS. See Ovarian hyperstimulation syndrome
Oligodendrogliomas, 133
Oligohydramnios, 154, 155, 155f, 166
    effect on head shape, 73
Omifin. See Clomiphene citrate
Omphalocele, 12, 220–221, 226–227, 226f, 227f
    vs. physiologic herniation, 220–221
Omphalomesenteric cyst, 63f
Omphalopagus twinning, 320
Oocyte during tubal transit, 6f
Oocyte retrieval, 415, 419, 472
Orbital diameter (OD), 80, 80t, 81f, 92f, 98t
Orbits, 88, 89, 92, 96, 98, 99–100
    abnormalities, 92, 96–101
    hypertelorism, 96–98
    hypotelorism, 96, 98–99, 104
    measurements, 80, 80t, 81f, 92f, 96f, 97t, 98t
Osseous pelvic ligaments, 348, 349f
Ossification centers, 198f
    vertebral, 119
Osteochondrodysplasias, 201–209, 201t, 201f, 202f
    achondrogenesis, 203–204
    achondroplasia, 204–205
    asphyxiating thoracic dystrophy, 208–209
    campomelic dysplasia, 207–208
    metatropic dysplasia, 209
    rhizomelic chondrodysplasia punctata, 209
    short rib–polydactyly syndrome, 206–207
    thanatophoric dysplasia, 205–206
Osteogenesis imperfecta, 210, 210f, 211f
Osteolyses (idiopathic), 209–210
    hypophosphatasia, 210
    osteogenesis imperfecta, 210

Outflow tracts (fetal heart), 157, 163, 164, 165, 175, 176–180, 183
    embryology, 157
    sonographic views, 163, 164
Ovarian/adnexal imaging, 466
Ovarian artery, 357f, 358
    resistivity indices, 360t
Ovarian cancer, 431–432
Ovarian choriocarcinoma, 395, 395f
Ovarian cortex, 356–357, 357f
Ovarian cysts. *See also* specific lesions
    coexisting with pregnancy, 329–330
    fetal, 240, 240f
    gynecologic, 346
    neoplastic, 388–397, 390t
    non-neoplastic (functional), 384–388, 424f
    pediatric, 346, 423–424
Ovarian hyperstimulation syndrome (OHSS), 414, 414f
Ovarian pathologies, 384–397. *See also* Neoplastic ovarian masses
    cancer, 431–432
    functional cysts, 384–388
    mass scoring system, 389t
    neoplastic masses, 388–397
    non-neoplastic lesions, 384–388
    ovarian torsion, 397
    pediatric pathologies, 423–427
Ovarian phases of menstrual cycle, 364–365, 365f
Ovarian suspensory ligaments, 348, 349f
Ovarian torsion, 397, 397f
Ovarian vein, 357f, 359f, 360
Ovarian venous plexus, 360, 360f
Ovarian venous thrombosis, 335f, 400–401, 401f
Ovaries, 346, 356–358
    adult, 356–358
    anatomy, 356–358
    histologic layers, 356–357
    measurement technique, 467f
    measurements, 346, 358, 423, 423t
    pediatric, 346, 423, 423t
    postmenopausal, 428, 429f
    vascular anatomy, 358–360
Oviducts. *See* Fallopian tubes
Ovulation, 4–6, 361, 366f
    failure, 410, 411f
Ovulatory phase of the menstrual cycle, 365

P

PACs. *See* Premature atrial contractions
Palate, 89f, 90f, 91–95, 91f, 95f, 104
    embryology, 88, 88f
    primary, 88, 92–93
    secondary, 88, 92–93
Palatine processes, 88
ParaGard. *See* Intrauterine contraceptive devices
Parameters, fetal growth. *See* Fetal growth parameters
Paraovarian cysts, 388, 388f
Partial mole, 21, 21f
Partial previa, 43, 43f
Parvovirus, 326, 326f
Patau syndrome. *See* Trisomy 13
Patient safety, 472–474
    ALARA principle, 473
    from bioeffects, 440, 472–473
    cleanliness, 474
    equipment, 474
Patients
    clinical information, 462
    communication, 462, 464
    history, 4, 462, 463
    identification, 462
    invasive procedures, 471–472
    pregnancy diagnosis, 4
    preparation, 462–463
    safety, 472–474
PBS. *See* Prune belly syndrome
PCOS. *See* Polycystic ovary syndrome
PDI. *See* Power Doppler imaging

Pediatric gynecologic pathologies
    germ cell tumors, 424
    gonadal dysgenesis, 426
    ovarian masses, 423–424
    ovarian torsion, 397, 397f, 424
    sexual ambiguity, 426–427
    uterine masses, 425
    vaginal masses, 423
Pediatric gynecologic sonography
    anatomy and physiology, 422–423
    indications, 423
    ovaries, 423, 423t
    pathologies, 423–427
    uterus, 422, 423t
Pediatric pelvic anatomy. *See* Pelvic anatomy
Pedunculated fibroids, 376
Pelvic anatomy
    adult anatomy, 346–360
        cervix, 350, 352–354
        endometrium, 350, 351–352
        fallopian tubes, 356
        musculature, 347, 347f
        osseous ligaments, 348
        ovarian suspensory ligaments, 348
        ovaries, 356–358
        pelvic cavities, 347–348
        pelvic recesses, 355
        skeletal structures, 346–347
        urinary bladder, 349
        uterine ligaments, 349
        uterine positional variants, 352
        uterus, 349–352
        vagina, 354–355
        vasculature, 358–361, 358f, 360f
    false pelvis, 347–348, 348f
    fetal anatomy, 225, 225f
    pediatric anatomy, 345–346, 422–423
        ovaries/adnexa, 346, 423, 423t
        uterus, 345–346, 422, 423t
    postmenopausal anatomy, 428–429
        ovaries, 428
        uterus, 428
    true pelvis, 347–348, 348f
Pelvic inflammatory disease (PID), 398, 398f
Pelvic pathology. *See also* Maternal complications; Pediatric gynecologic pathologies; Postmenopausal gynecologic pathologies
    adnexal, 398–401
    endometrial, 380–383
    ovarian, 384–397
    uterine, 372–379
    vaginal, 372
Pelvic physiology
    menstrual cycle, 361–366
    ovarian response, 364–366
    uterine response, 361–364
Pelvic recesses, 355, 355f
Pelvic ultrasound practice guidelines, 498–504
Pentalogy of Cantrell, 292–293, 292f
Pentasomy, 282–283, 287
Percutaneous umbilical blood sampling. *See* Cordocentesis
Pergonal. *See* Human menopausal gonadotropin
Pericardial effusion (fetal), 183, 186, 188–189, 189f, 303f
Persistent trophoblastic neoplasia, 22
Persistent truncus arteriosus, 173, 176, 178–179, 179f
Peurperium, 332
Phalanges. *See* Fingers
Pharyngeal arches, 89, 89f
Phased array transducers, 451, 451f
Philtrum, 88
Phosphatidylglycerol, 156
Physical examination, 4
    in pregnancy diagnosis, 4
Physical principles, 439–457
Physiologic herniation. *See* Midgut herniation
Physiologic ovarian cysts. *See* Functional ovarian cysts
Pia mater, 117
PID. *See* Pelvic inflammatory disease

Piezoelectric transducer elements, 448–451, 456
PIHD. *See* Pre-eclampsia
Piriformis, 347
Pituitary gland, 410
    infertility and, 410
Placenta, 31–49
    abnormalities, 35–50, 36t
        abruption, 35, 41, 42, 45–46, 47f
        of adherence, 47–49
        calcifications, 37, 40
        circummarginate, 38
        circumvallate, 38
        cystic lesions, 40–42
        hydrops, 35, 49, 50
        membranacea, 39
        molar, 20–23, 20f–23f
        of placental age, 37, 37f, 40f
        previa, 35, 42–45, 42f, 43f, 44f, 45f, 49
        of size/thickness, 36–37, 45
    chorionic villi, 33
    cord insertion, 56f
    cotyledons, 34, 40f, 41
    decidual layers, 32–33
    fetal portion, 34
    fetoplacental circulation, 157–159
    grading, 37
    maternal portion, 32, 34
    placentation, 32, 32f, 39
    sonographic appearance, 35, 38–50
    variants, 35–50
Placenta accreta, 47, 47f, 48f
Placenta increta, 47, 47f
Placenta membranacea, 39
Placenta percreta, 47, 47f, 49f
Placenta previa, 35, 42–45, 42f, 43f, 44f, 45f, 49
    complete, 42–43
    low-lying, 44–45
    marginal, 44
    partial, 43
    vasa previa, 40, 45

Placental abruption, 45–46
    concealed, 46
    external, 46
    fibroid-related, 377
Placental hydrops, 50f
Placental septa, 34, 40
Placental site trophoblastic tumor (PSTT), 23
Placental variants, 35–50, 36t
    accessory, 39–40
    extrachorial, 38–39
Pleural effusion, 152, 166–167, 167f, 172, 188
Polycystic ovary syndrome (PCOS), 388, 389f
    as cause of infertility, 411, 411f
Polydactyly, 202, 202f, 207f, 291f
Polyhydramnios, 154, 154f, 169, 171, 177, 231f
Polyps, endometrial, 383f, 384f
Pons, 118, 118f, 123f
Porencephaly, 134, 134f
Portal sinus, 158, 222, 222f
Posterior acoustic enhancement, 357f, 452, 453f
Posterior acoustic shadowing, 452, 452f
Posterior cerebral arteries, 119
Posterior cul-de-sac, 355, 355f
Posterior fossa, 112, 117–118
    Dandy-Walker malformation, 122, 129
Posterior urethral valves (PUV), 262–263, 263f
Postmenopausal gynecologic pathologies, 429–433
    cancer, 431–433
    with hormone replacement therapy, 429–430
    ovarian masses, 432f
    pelvic masses, 430–431
    postmenopausal vaginal bleeding, 429
    with tamoxifen, 430
Postmenopausal gynecologic sonography, 428–433
    anatomy and physiology, 428
    endometrium, 428f, 429t
    indications, 429
    ovaries, 428–429
    pathologies, 429–433
    uterus, 428, 428f

Postpartum conditions
    abscess, 334f
    hematoma, 335f
    hemorrhage (PPH), 332, 333f
    uterine anatomy, 332f

Postpartum risks. *See* Antepartum/postpartum risks

Potential spaces. *See* Pelvic recesses

Potter sequence, 253–258, 254t. *See also* Renal agenesis
    type I, 253–255, 254f, 255f
    type II, 255–256, 255f, 256f
    type III, 256, 256f
    type IV, 257–258, 257f

Pouch of Douglas, 355, 355f

Power Doppler imaging (PDI), 447–448, 447f, 448f

PPH. *See* Postpartum conditions

PPROM. *See* Preterm premature rupture of membranes

Practice guidelines (AIUM), 491–520
    fetal echocardiography practice guidelines, 515–520
    focused reproductive endocrinology and infertility scan practice guidelines, 512–515
    obstetric ultrasound practice guidelines, 491–498
    pelvic ultrasound practice guidelines, 498–504
    reproductive medicine ultrasound practice guidelines, 504–512
    sonohysterography practice guidelines, 501–504

Precocious puberty, 427
    pseudopuberty, 427
    true, 427

Pre-eclampsia, 324–325

Preexisting hypertension, 324–325

Pregnancy, 4–24
    diagnosis of, 4–5
    early time line, 5t, 6–8
    failed, 13–24
    normal, 4–13
    laboratory values, 4–5, 12
    sonographic signs, 8–12, 14–18, 20–23

Pregnancy-induced hypertensive disorder. *See* Pre-eclampsia

Premature atrial contractions, 190–191, 191f

Premature rupture of membranes (PROM), 331

Premature ventricular contractions, 190, 190f

Prenatal genetic testing. *See* Genetic testing

Preparation for an exam, 462–464
    patient preparation, 462–463
        gynecologic exam, 463
        obstetric exam, 463
    sonographer preparation, 462

Presacral teratomas (fetal), 240, 241f

Presentation (fetal), 330–331, 331f

Preterm labor, 331

Preterm premature rupture of membranes (PPROM), 331

Previa. *See* Placenta previa

Primary yolk sac, 6–7

Primitive streak, 7

Primordial gut, 220f

Probes. *See* Transducers

Proboscis, 127, 127f

Progesterone
    corpus luteum, 16, 329, 364, 366, 386
    and dysfunctional uterine bleeding, 380
    effect on endometrium, 350, 352
    and fibroids, 376
    in hormone replacement therapy, 429–430
    and infertility, 410, 412
    menstrual cycle levels, 361, 362f
    after menopause, 428
    in pregnancy diagnosis, 4

Prolapse
    of fibroids, 377
    of the umbilical cord, 58, 59–60

Proliferative phase of menstrual cycle, 361–363, 362f, 363f

PROM. *See* Premature rupture of membranes

Pronephroi, 248

Prosencephalon. *See* Forebrain

Protocols. *See* Examinations
Prune belly syndrome (PBS), 263–264, 264f
Pseudogestational sac, 9, 70
    of ectopic pregnancy, 19–20
Pseudoglandular phase of lung development, 152, 152f
Pseudohermaphroditism
    female, 427
    male, 427
Pseudomyxoma peritonei, 391, 391f
Pseudopuberty, 427
Psoas major, 347, 347f
PSTT. *See* Placental site trophoblastic tumor
PTA. *See* Persistent truncus arteriosus
Pubic bones, 347
Pubic ligament, 348
Pubic rami, 347, 348
Pubic symphysis, 347, 347f
Pubovesicular ligament, 349
PUBS. *See* Cordocentesis
Puerperal infection, 333
Pulmonary arteries (fetal), 157–159
Pulmonary development. *See* Lungs
Pulmonary hypoplasia, 160, 166, 166f, 167f, 169, 172, 176, 188
Pulmonary sequestration, 166, 167–168, 168f, 169, 170
Pulmonary surfactant, 152–153
Pulmonary veins, 157, 157f, 158f, 161, 167
Pulmonic maturity studies, 155–156
Pulsatility indices
    middle cerebral artery, 308f
    umbilical artery, 307, 307f
Pulsed-wave (PW) Doppler sonography, 473. *See also* Spectral Doppler sonography
    contraindications, 473
PUV. *See* Posterior urethral valves
PVCs. *See* Premature ventricular contractions
PW Doppler. *See* Spectral Doppler sonography
Pyelectasis, renal, 281, 281t, 281f
Pygopagus twinning, 320
Pyknosis, 441

Q

QA. *See* Quality assurance
Quad screen, 272
Quadruplets. *See* Higher-order gestations
Quality assurance, 473–474
    distance measurement accuracy, 474
    electrical/mechanical, 474
    sterility/cleanliness, 474
    transducer/system performance, 474
    workstation display, 474

R

Rachischisis, 142
Radial ray anomaly, 212, 212f, 293f
Radius (bone), 199f, 211f
Rarefaction, 440–441
Recesses, pelvic, 355, 355f
Rectouterine ligament, 349
Rectus abdominis, 347
Refraction artifacts, 454–455, 454f
Refractory shadows. *See* Refraction artifacts
Renal agenesis, 251–252. *See also* Potter sequence
    bilateral, 252, 253f
    Potter sequence, 253–258
    unilateral, 251–252, 252f
Renal arteries (fetal), 224
Renal capsule, 248
Renal cystic disease. *See also* Potter sequence
Renal duplications, 262, 262f
Renal ectopia, 252–253
    cross-fused, 253
Renal embryology, 248f
Renal hamartoma (fetal), 265
Renal pelvic measurements, 258, 258t
Renal pyelectasis, 281, 281t, 281f
Renal pyramids, 248
Reporting results, 470–471
Reproductive endocrinology and infertility scan practice guidelines, 512–515

Reproductive medicine ultrasound practice guidelines, 504–512
Repronex. See Human menopausal gonadotropin
Resistivity indices
    ovarian artery, 360t
    umbilical artery, 306, 306f
    uterine artery, 359t
Retained products of conception, 16f, 332, 333, 333f, 453f
Retroflexion, uterine, 352, 353f
Retroplacental space, 34f
Retroplacental vasculature, 34, 35, 43, 44
Retroversion, uterine, 352, 353f
Retroverted/retroflexed uterus, 352, 353f
Retzius, space of, 355, 355f
Reverberation artifacts, 452–454, 453f
Rh isoimmunization, 302
Rhabdomyoma, cardiac, 187, 189f
Rhabdomyosarcoma, vaginal, 426
Rhizomelia, 201, 201f
Rhizomelic chondrodysplasia punctata, 209
Rhombencephalon, 12–13, 113f, 115f. See also Hindbrain
    prominent, 12–13, 13f
Right ventricular outflow tract view (of fetal heart), 164, 518f
Ring of fire sign, 19, 19f
Rocker bottom foot, 214
Round ligaments, 349, 349f
Rubella, 326–327
RVOT view. See Right ventricular outflow tract view

S

Saccular phase. See Terminal sac phase of lung development
Sacral teratomas (fetal), 240
Sacrococcygeal ligaments, 348, 348f
Sacrococcygeal teratomas (fetal), 240, 241f
Sacroiliac ligaments, 348, 348f
Sacrosciatic ligaments, 348, 348f
Sacrospinous ligaments, 348
Sacrum, 347, 347f
Safety of patient
    ALARA principle, 473
    from bioeffects, 440, 472–473
Sagittal view of fetal heart, 519f
Salpinges. See Fallopian tubes
Sarcoma botryoides, 426, 426f
Sarcomas, intracranial, 133
Scalp edema, 140, 303f, 326f
Schizencephaly, 135, 135f
Scoring of ovarian masses, 389–390, 389t
SDMS. See Society of Diagnostic Medical Sonography
Second International Reference Preparation (2IS), 5, 5t, 8, 18
Second/third trimester examination protocols, 463, 464, 466
Secondary lobe artifacts
    grating lobes, 457, 457f
    side lobes, 456, 457f
Secondary yolk sac, 7, 7f, 10
Secretory phase of menstrual cycle, 352f, 362f, 364, 364f
Section-thickness artifacts, 455, 455f
Semilobar holoprosencephaly, 126, 126f, 128f
Septal cysts, 41
Septal defects
    atrial septal defect, 163, 173, 174–175, 176, 178, 181, 183
    atrioventricular septal defect, 173, 174, 175–176
    ventricular septal defect, 163, 173–174, 175, 176, 177, 178, 179, 180, 181, 182, 184
Septate uterus, 373, 373f, 375f
Septum pellucidum, 114
Septum primum, 156–157, 174
Sequences. See also Associations; Syndromes
    defined, 287
    Potter, 287
Sertoli-Leydig cell tumors, 396
Serum markers. See Maternal serum markers; *specific markers*

Sex cord stromal tumors, 395–396
　fibromas, 396
　granulosa cell tumors, 395–396
　Sertoli-Leydig cell tumors, 396
　thecomas, 396
Sexual ambiguity (intersex state), 426–427
Short-limb dysplasias. *See* Osteochondrodysplasias
Short rib–polydactyly syndrome (SRPS), 206–207, 207f
Short umbilical cord, 58–59
Shoulder presentation, 330
Side-lobe artifacts, 456, 457f
Single deepest pocket. *See* Maximum vertical pocket
Single-gene disease, 282
Single umbilical artery (SUA), 57, 57f, 58f, 61
Single ventricle anomalies, 180–182, 181f, 182f
　double-inlet left ventricle, 182, 184
　hypoplastic heart syndromes, 180–181, 184
　tricuspid atresia, 181–182
Sinus venosus, 156f, 174
Sirenomelia, 290, 290f
Situs abnormalities, 184–186
　situs ambiguous, 185
　situs inversus, 185
Skeletal dysplasias. *See* Osteochondrodysplasias
Skeleton (fetal), 197–214
　abnormalities, 201–214, 201t
　anatomy, 197–200
　embryology, 201–214
　facial anatomy, 198f
　lower extremity, 200
　pelvic anatomy, 346–347
　sonographic considerations, 202
　upper extremity, 199
Skull. *See* Calvaria
Slice-thickness artifacts. *See* Section-thickness artifacts
Small bowel obstruction, 232–233, 233f
Society of Diagnostic Medical Sonography, 462
Soft sonographic markers, 276

Solid masses. *See also* Cysts; Masses; *specific pathologies*
　chest, 172
　pelvic, 330
Somites, 7–8, 8f, 89
Sonographic approaches
　extracorporeal, 464–465
　intracavitary, 465–466
　transabdominal, 465f
　transperineal, 465f
　transvaginal, 465f
Sonographic signs. *See specific anatomy, conditions, and pathologies*
Sonohysterography, 472
　practice guidelines, 501–504
SP-A. *See* Surfactant-protein A
Space of Retzius, 355, 355f
Spalding's sign, 311, 311f
Spatial compounding, 442
Spatial frequency compounding, 443
Spectral Doppler sonography, 448, 448f
Spina bifida, 141–143, 143f
　aperta, 137f, 142, 142f
　occulta, 141–142, 141f
　rachischisis, 141f, 142
Spinal dysraphism. *See* Spina bifida
Spine, 118f, 119–120, 120f, 121f, 198f
Spiral arteries (placenta), 34
Spleen (fetal), 76f, 222f
　cysts, 239, 240f
　measurement, 82
　splenomegaly, 239
Splenomegaly (fetal), 239
Spontaneous abortion, 15–17, 22, 310. *See also* Fetal demise
　anembryonic pregnancy, 16
　blighted ovum, 16
　complete, 15
　elective, x
　etiologies, 15

incomplete, 15–16
risk factors, 15
subchorionic hemorrhage, 17
threatened, 16–17
SRPS. *See* Short rib–polydactyly syndrome
Stargazer posture, 140
Stein-Leventhal syndrome. *See* Polycystic ovary syndrome
Sterility/cleanliness, 474
Stomach (fetal), 224
Struma ovarii, 394, 394f
Stuck twin, 318–319, 319f
Sturge-Weber syndrome, 135
SUA. *See* Single umbilical artery
Subchorionic hemorrhage, 17, 17f, 45, 46
Subchorionic lesions, 40–41, 41f
Subclavian arteries, 161
Subcostal approach, 464
Submucosal fibroids, 376
Subserous fibroids, 377
Substernal approach, 464
Succenturiate lobe, 39, 39f, 40
Sulci, 116
Superior vena cava, 157, 158f, 160, 162, 174
Supertwins. *See* Higher-order gestations
Supine hypovolemic (hypotensive) syndrome, 465
Suprasternal approach, 464
Supraventricular tachycardia, 189–190, 190f
Surface rendering, 443
Surfactant-protein A (SP-A), 156
Suspensory ligament, 348
Sylvius, aqueduct of, 116, 117f
Symmetric intrauterine growth restriction, 305–306, 305f
Symphysis pubis, 347, 347f
Syncytiotrophoblast, 7, 7f, 32, 33, 34
Syndactyly, 202, 202f
Syndromes. *See also* Associations; Sequences
amniotic band, 287–288
Beckwith-Wiedemann, 288
caudal regression, 289
defined, 287
Ellis–van Creveld, 290–291
Meckel-Gruber, 291–292
pentalogy of Cantrell, 292–293
sirenomelia, 290
Synophthalmia. *See* Cyclopia

T

TA. *See* Truncus arteriosus
Tachycardia (fetal), 189–190, 190f
Talipes equinovarus (clubfoot), 208f, 212–213, 213f
Tamoxifen, 382, 430, 430f
Telencephalon, 113f
Tentorium cerebelli, 117, 117f
Teratomas
cardiac, 187
cerebral, 134f
epignathus, 102, 103, 104
immature cystic, 393, 393f, 394f
mature cystic, 392, 393f
neck, 103, 104f
ovarian, 392–394
presacral, 240, 241f
sacral, 240
sacrococcygeal, 241f
struma ovarii, 394
umbilical cord, 62, 63–64
Terminal sac phase of lung development, 152
TES. *See* Twin embolization syndrome
Testicular feminization syndrome, 427
Tetralogy of Fallot, 164, 173, 176–177, 176f, 184
Tetrasomy, 282–283, 287
Thalamus, 114f, 117f
Thanatophoric dysplasia, 167f, 205–206, 206f
Theca-lutein cysts, 21f, 329, 329f, 386, 387f
Thecomas, 396
Thermal bioeffects of ultrasound
hyperthermia, 440
thermal indices, 440

Thermal indices
- for bone (TIb), 440, 473
- for the cranium (TIc), 440
- for soft tissue (TIs), 440, 473

Third trimester examination protocols, 463, 464, 466
Thoracic cavity. *See* Chest
Thoracoabdominal syndrome. *See* Pentalogy of Cantrell
Thoracopagus twinning, 320
Thorax, bony, 159, 159f
Threatened abortion, 16–17
Three-dimensional (3D) ultrasound, 443, 443f
- anencephaly, 138f
- cleft lip, 95f
- clubfoot, 213f
- face, 89f, 91f
- hydropic facies, 304f
- macroglossia, 289f
- midgut herniation, 221f

Three-vessel trachea view of fetal heart, 518f
Thrombosis
- as a complication of pregnancy, 334–336
- intervillous, 42f
- ovarian venous, 335f, 401f
- umbilical vein, 58, 58f, 61

TI. *See* Thermal indices
Tibia, 200f, 210f
TOA. *See* Tubo-ovarian abscess
Toes, 200f
Tomographic slice ultrasound, 443–444
Tone. *See* Fetal tone
Tongue (fetal), 91f
Tooth buds, 91f
TORCH infections, 325–328
Torsion
- fibroids, 377
- ovarian, 397, 397f, 424
- umbilical cord, 58, 59

Toxoplasmosis, 325, 326f
Tracheal atresia, 166, 171, 171f, 172
Transabdominal approach, 464, 465f

Transcerebellar diameter, 81–82, 81f, 82t
Transducers, 448–451
- array configurations, 450–451
  - convex/curvilinear, 450–451, 450f
  - linear, 450, 450f
  - matrix, 451, 451f
  - phased, 451, 451f
- for continuous-wave Doppler, 446f
- endovaginal, 451, 451f
- frequency ranges, 449–450
- performance, 474

Transfusion
- intraperitoneal fetal, 337
- intravascular fetal, 337

Transitional cell tumors, 391
Translabial imaging. *See* Endovaginal and transperineal imaging
Transperineal imaging. *See* Endovaginal and transperineal imaging
Transposition of the great arteries. *See* Transposition of the great vessels
Transposition of the great vessels, 164, 176, 177–178, 177f, 178f, 182, 184, 186
Transvaginal imaging. *See* Endovaginal and transperineal imaging
Transvaginal oocyte retrieval, 419
Transvaginal sonography. *See* Endovaginal and transperineal imaging
Transverse lie, 331
Transvesicular approach, 464
TRAP. *See* Twin reversed arterial perfusion sequence
Tricuspid atresia, 173, 181–182, 181f, 182f
Tricuspid regurgitation, 183, 184, 187
Trident hand deformity, 206, 207f
Trilaminar embryonic disc, 7
Triple screen, 272
Triplets, 313f. *See also* Higher-order gestations
Triploidy, 282–283
- karyotype, 283f

Trisomy (defined), 282. *See also specific types*
Trisomy 13 (Patau syndrome), 285–286
- karyotype, 285f

Trisomy 18 (Edwards syndrome), 284–285
    karyotype, 285f
Trisomy 21 (Down syndrome), 283–284
    karyotype, 284f
    risk estimate, 277, 277t
Trophotropism, 60
True hermaphroditism, 427
True pelvis, 347–348, 348f
True precocious puberty, 427
Truncus arteriosus, 156–157, 157f, 162, 164, 173
    persistent, 176, 178–179, 179f
Tubal patency assessment, 419, 419f
Tubal transit of zygote, 6, 6f
Tubes. *See* Fallopian tubes
Tubo-ovarian abscess (TOA), 398–399, 453f
Tumors. *See* Cysts; Intracranial abnormalities; Masses
Tunic albuginea, 356
Turner syndrome, 286
Twin embolization syndrome, 318
Twin pregnancies, 311–321. *See also* Multiple-gestation pregnancies
    clinical findings, 311–312
    dizygotic twins, 313
    evaluation protocols, 314–315
    fetal complications, 311
    higher-order, 313–314
    maternal complications, 311
    molar, 22, 22f
    monozygotic twins, 312–313
    placentation/membranes, 312, 315f
Twin reversed arterial perfusion sequence, 317–318, 317f
Twin-twin transfusion syndrome, 316–317, 316f, 317f
Two-vessel cord. *See* Single umbilical artery

U

Ulna, 199f, 211f
Ultrasound
    bioeffects, 440–442
    Doppler, 444–448
    imaging artifacts, 451–457
    imaging modes, 442–444
    physical principles, 439–457
    system performance, 474
    transducers, 448–451
Umbilical arteries, 222–223
    Doppler evaluation, 306–307
    pulsatility index, 307, 307f
    resistivity index, 306, 306f, 307f
    S/D ratios, 306f
Umbilical cord, 53–64, 221
    abnormalities, 57–64, 57t
    anatomy and physiology, 54–56
    arteries, 53, 54, 55, 56f, 57, 63
    cord insertion, 55–62, 56f, 61f, 223, 223f
    cysts, 57, 62, 63f
    embryology, 53
    entanglement, 60f, 319–320, 320f
    in fetal circulation, 158
    knots, 58, 59
    long cord, 58, 59, 60
    masses, 57, 62–64
    nuchal cord, 59
    prolapse, 58, 59–60, 60f
    short cord, 58–59
    sonographic demonstration, 55, 57, 58, 59, 60, 61, 62, 63, 64
    stricture, 57, 58
    three-vessel, 55f
    veins, 53, 54, 55, 56f, 57, 63, 156f, 158, 221–222, 222f, 223f
    venous thrombosis, 58, 58f, 61
Unicornuate uterus, 373, 373f, 374f
Unilateral renal agenesis, 251–252, 252f
Uniparental disomy (UPD), 286–287
UPD. *See* Uniparental disomy
UPJ. *See* Ureteropelvic junction obstruction
Ureterocele, 260
    ectopic, 260f, 261f
Ureteropelvic junction obstruction (UPJ), 259–260, 260f
Ureters, 349, 357f
Urethra, 349

Urethral atresia, 263
Urethral sphincter, 349
Urinary bladder (adult), 349, 350f
    exam protocols, 463f
    gynecologic exam, 463
    obstetric exam, 463
    sonographic appearance, 453f
Urinary bladder (fetal), 248–249. See also Genitourinary system
    emptying and refilling, 249
    normal, 225, 225f
    sonographic appearance, 249
Urogenital system. See Genitourinary system
Uterine agenesis, 373
Uterine artery, 357f, 358, 358f, 359f
    resistivity indices, 359t
Uterine imaging, 466
Uterine ligaments, 349, 349f
Uterine pathologies, 372–375
    acquired, 375–379, 412
    Asherman syndrome, 375
    cancer, 432–433
    cervical, 372–373
    congenital, 372–375
    infertility-related, 412
    masses, 376–379, 425–426
    müllerian duct anomalies, 373–375
    pediatric, 425–426
    rupture, 328, 328f
Uterine phases of menstrual cycle, 361–364, 362f–364f
Uterine venous plexus, 359f, 360, 360f
Utero-ovarian ligament, 348
Uteroplacental circulation. See Fetoplacental circulation
Uterosacral ligament, 349, 349f
Uterovesical space, 355, 355f
Uterus. See also Uterine pathologies
    adult, 349–352
    anatomy, 349–352, 350f, 351f
    cervix, 350, 352–354
    corpus, 346, 350, 350f, 352, 352f, 353f
    fascial layers, 350
    fundus, 350, 350f
    isthmus, 350, 350f
    measurement technique, 467f
    measurements, 345–346, 346t, 423t
    neonatal, 422, 422f
    pediatric/premenarcheal, 345–346, 422, 422f, 423t
    positional variants, 352, 352f, 353f
    postmenarcheal, 422, 422f
    postmenopausal, 428, 428f
    response to menstrual cycle, 362–364, 362f–364f
    vessels, 358–361, 358f–361f
Uterus bicornis. See Bicornuate uterus
Uterus didelphys. See Didelphic uterus
Uterus subseptus. See Septate uterus
Uterus unicornis. See Unicornuate uterus

V

VACTERL association, 293, 293f
Vagina
    anatomy, 354–355, 354f–355f
    artery, 358
Vaginal pathologies
    agenesis, 372
    atresia, 372
    Gartner's duct cyst, 372
    hydrometrocolpos, 372
    imperforate hymen, 372
    masses (pediatric), 426
    persistent uterovaginal septum, 372
    postmenopausal bleeding, 429
Valves, cardiac (fetal), 156, 157–159, 158f, 162–165, 162f, 163f, 175–176, 178–184, 187
Vanishing twin, 315–316, 316f
Varices (umbilical), 62, 63, 63f
Vasa previa, 40, 45, 45f, 61

Vasculature, pelvic (adult), 358–360. *See also* Fetoplacental circulation; Heart
    arteries, 358–359
    veins, 360
Vasculogenesis, 7
Vein of Galen aneurysm/malformation, 130–131, 130f
Velamentous cord insertion, 57, 58, 60, 61–62, 62f
Venae cavae, 157
Venous thrombosis
    as complication of pregnancy, 334–336
    intervillous, 42f
    ovarian venous, 335f, 401f
    umbilical vein, 58, 58f, 61
Ventricles (brain), 112–113, 113f, 115–116, 115f, 116f, 117f
Ventricles (heart)
    anatomy and views, 162, 163, 164
    anomalies involving, 173–191
    measurement of, 169f
Ventricular septal defect (VSD), 163, 173–174, 173f, 174f, 175, 176, 176f, 177, 177f, 178, 179, 179f, 180, 181, 181f, 182, 182f, 184
Ventricular septal size, disproportionate, 182–184
    coarctation of the aorta, 173, 180, 182, 184
    Ebstein's anomaly, 163, 183, 190
Ventricular septations, 157, 163
Ventriculomegaly, 122, 124f, 326f, 327f. *See also* Hydrocephalus
Vermis. *See* Cerebellar vermis
Vertebrae (spinal), 119–120
Vertebral ossification centers, 119, 120f, 121f, 198f
Verumontanum, 263
Vesicular arteries, 358
VGA. *See* Vein of Galen aneurysm/malformation

Viability of pregnancy, 11–12, 11t
Villus. *See* Chorionic villi
Virchow's triad, 335
Volumetric ultrasound, 443–444, 443f
VSD. *See* Ventricular septal defect

W

Weight estimation (fetal), 308–309
Weight percentile chart, 309f
Wharton's jelly, 55, 55f, 58, 61
Willis, circle of, 118, 119f
Wilms tumor (nephroblastoma), 265
Wolffian ducts. *See* Müllerian ducts
Workstation display, 474

X

X chromosome, 247, 276
X-linked diseases, 282
XO syndrome. *See* Turner syndrome

Y

Y chromosome, 247, 276
Yolk sac, 6–8, 9, 10, 10f, 14, 18–20, 14f, 32f, 33, 33f
    primary, 6–7
    secondary, 7, 7f, 10
    tumors, 394–395

Z

ZIFT. *See* Zygote intrafallopian transfer
Zygote, 6
    tubal transit of, 6, 6f
Zygote intrafallopian transfer (ZIFT), 415, 472